AF731676

PULMONARY UPDATE

2023-2024

SECOND EDITION

Editor-in-Chief

MANU MADAN (MD, DM)

Consultant, Max Institute of Respiratory, Critical Care and Sleep Medicine
Max Super Speciality Hospital, Saket, New Delhi

Associate Editors

NIPUN MALHOTRA (MD, DM)

Assistant Professor
Department of Pulmonary Medicine
ESI Hospital, Basaidarapur, New Delhi, India

PANCHMI GUPTA (MS, DNB, FICO)

Senior Medical Officer
Department of Ophthalmology
Rajan Babu Institute of Pulmonary Medicine and Tuberculosis
New Delhi, India

Peepee Publishers and Distributors Private Limited®

PULMONARY UPDATE

Published by
Pawaninder P. Vij and Anupam Vij

Peepee Publishers and Distributors Private Limited
Head Office: 160, Shakti Vihar, Pitam Pura, Delhi-110 034 (India)

Correspondence Address:
7/31, First Floor, Ansari Road, Daryaganj
New Delhi-110 002 (India)
Ph: 41512412, 9811156083
e-mail: peepee160@yahoo.co.in
e-mail: peepee160@gmail.com
www.peepeepub.com
join us on facebook.com/pp.publishers

© 2025 Peepee Publishers and Distributors Private Limited

All rights reserved

No part of this publication may be reproduced or transmitted in any form or by any means, electronic, mechanical, photocopy, recording, translated, or any information storage and retrieval system, without permission in writing from the editor and the publisher.

This book has been published in good faith that the material provided by authors/contributors is original. Every effort is made to ensure accuracy of material, but publisher and printer will not be held responsible for any inadvertent errors. In case of any dispute, all legal matters to be settled under Delhi jurisdiction only.

First Edition: 2024

Second Edition: 2025

ISBN: 978-81-9833-669-9

DEDICATED TO

My parents and my family for guiding me and helping me achieve whatever I could do in my life, my wife for her continuous support, my teachers for all the guidance, and my patients for improving my skills to be a better doctor.

FOREWORD

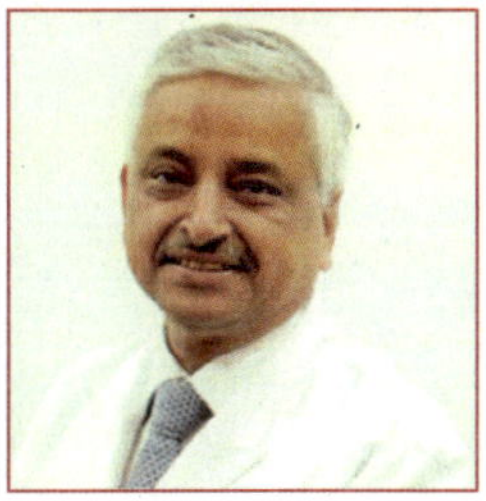

It is a great pleasure to once again write this foreword for the book **Pulmonary Update**, edited by Dr Manu Madan. This is the second update which is becoming an annual update of recent advances in Pulmonary Medicine. The book covers the recent advances in a very readable and comprehensive manner. Dr Manu Madan was a DM resident of Pulmonary, Critical Care and Sleep Medicine at AIIMS, New Delhi where I have seen him evolve from a student to a teacher. It is indeed a great effort by Dr. Madan to compile this academic update with writeups from bright and the best young brains in the field of Pulmonary Medicine.

The authors have made tremendous efforts and taken great pains in preparing this book. They have maintained simplicity and readability that would help students and experts alike. I find this book to be different from other books in Pulmonology as the approach and theme of this book are evidence-based. This book encapsulates the latest advances in the ever-evolving field of Pulmonary Medicine. It provides a guide to the cutting-edge advancements in landscape of Pulmonary Medicine.

This academic endeavour is going to be very useful for students of Pulmonary Medicine, Internal Medicine, and also practicing physicians to quickly brush up on the latest evidence related to a vast array of pulmonary medicine. I am confident that readers will find this book interesting and useful.

I congratulate Dr. Manu Madan and all the co-authors for the fine effort and am sure that this book will be very popular. Wishing the book a large readership and I am glad that this update has become an annual event.

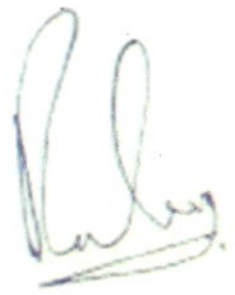

Prof. Dr. Randeep Guleria

M.D. (Medicine), D.M. (Pulmonary Medicine and Critical Care)
FAMS, DSc (Honoris Causa)

Former Director
All India Institute of Medical Sciences, New Delhi, India

Chairman
Institute of Internal Medicine and Respiratory and Sleep Medicine

Director
Medanta Medical School
Medanta–Gurugram, Haryana
Regn. No. DMC-81085

PREFACE

Pulmonary Update Book is an effort by renowned faculties from across India and Abroad, to keep pulmonary medicine students, physicians, and general medicine practitioners abreast with the latest in the field of pulmonary medicine. The book's target is to keep them updated, as well as encourage research in the field. It will also act as an interim guideline/ suggestion book for a topic that has no guidelines or has sporadic guidelines. It is not a textbook, but an update, which is aimed to be released regularly.

In this first edition, we had targeted articles published in indexed journals between January 2021 to August 2023. In this edition, we have included articles from August 2023 to August 2024. The initial part of the chapter includes relevant articles from this period in PICO format followed by a discussion, which will compare these new studies with existing literature and suggest a conclusion. Lastly, it will be followed by an algorithm with recommended changes. Studies have been classified as important and very important by highlighting them and giving them a light and a dark shade respectively.

All contributors (reviewers and authors) are esteemed faculties and need no introduction. I am highly thankful to all the authors, who have contributed to the book, giving their precious time in writing the chapter. Reviewers are important pillars of any book or article, and our book is no different. We request you all to let us know about any shortcomings and give your valuable feedback regarding the improvements needed to make this book more informative and practical in future editions.

Dr. Manu Madan

ACKNOWLEDGEMENTS

I thank the Almighty for giving me strength and guidance to complete this book. Writing a book is harder than I thought and more rewarding than I could have ever imagined. None of this would have been possible without the support of all the contributors. I thank all the authors, reviewers and the editors, who have put in their best efforts and helped me complete the task in due time. During the course of publishing the book, a number of revisions and updates were required, but this did not deter any author and editor from achieving our target.

I would like to express my gratitude to all my teachers, who have mentored me over the years right from my undergraduate days to my DM residency days. I am grateful to the almighty for blessing me with stalwarts of pulmonary medicine, Prof. (Dr.) Randeep Guleria, Prof. (Dr.) S. K. Chhabra, Prof. (Dr.) Ashok Shah, Prof. (Dr.) S. N. Gaur, Prof. (Dr.) Rajkumar, Prof. (Dr.) Anant Mohan, Dr. Karan Madan, Dr. Vijay Hadda, Dr. Pavan Tiwari, and Dr. Saurabh Mittal, as my teachers.

No words can describe the support rendered to me by my mother, Mrs. Asha Jain Madan, and my wife, Dr. Panchmi Gupta, in realizing this dream. I would like to thank all my friends for their words of encouragement, amongst them Dr. Nipun Malhotra, Dr. Vidushi Rathi, Dr. Pranav Ish, Dr. Nitesh Gupta, Dr. Kush Sharma, and Manish Sharma deserve a special mention.

Special thanks to all my seniors and colleagues at VMMC and Safdarjung Hospital who have helped me achieve this mammoth task. My heartfelt thanks to my head of department at Max Superspeciality Hospital, Saket, Dr. Vivek Nangia for his encouragement and support. I would also like to thank my students, who have inspired me to write this book. Gratitude is reserved for the publishers for being patient with a first-time author, right from the contract signing phase to the publishing phase, and helping me at each step to accomplish the task. Last but not least, I would like to acknowledge all our patients, who have been a constant source of improving my knowledge.

CONTRIBUTORS

Dr. Abhishek Chauhan (MD, DM)
Consultant, Yashoda Super Speciality Hospital, Kaushambi
Ghaziabad, Uttar Pradesh

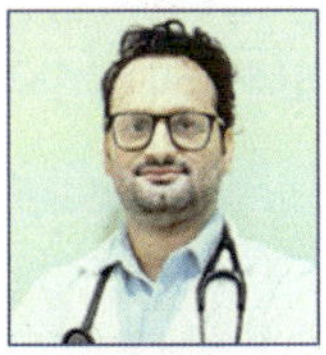

Dr. Aman Ahuja (DNB, DM)
Assistant Professor
Department of Pulmonary and Critical Care Medicine
Pt BDS PGIMS, Rohtak

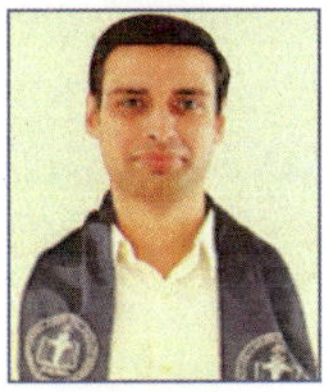

Dr. Amitesh Gupta (MD)
Assistant Professor, Department of Pulmonary Medicine, Maulana Azad Medical College and Associated Lok Nayak Hospital
New Delhi

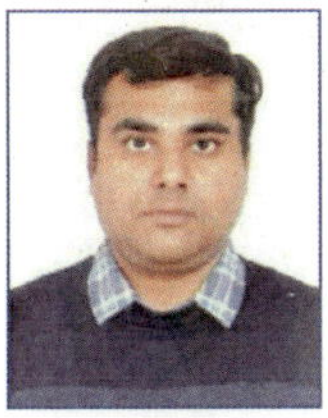

Professor (Dr.) Anant Mohan
(MD, PhD)
Head of Department
Department of Pulmonary
Critical Care and Sleep Medicine
AIIMS, New Delhi

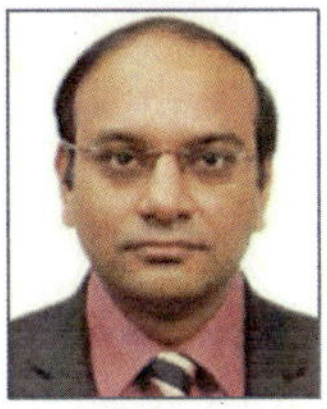

Dr. Arjun Khanna (MD, DM)
Senior Consultant and
Head of Department
Amrita Institute of Medical Sciences
Faridabad

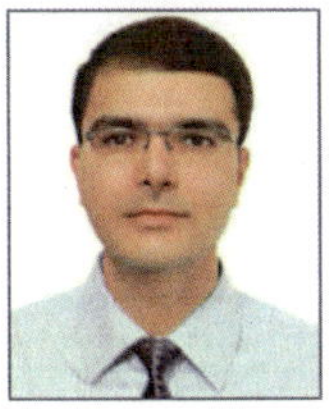

Dr. Arunachalam M
(DTCD, DNB, DM)
Senior Consultant and Head
Department of Pulmonology
Yatharth Superspeciality Hospital
Noida, UP

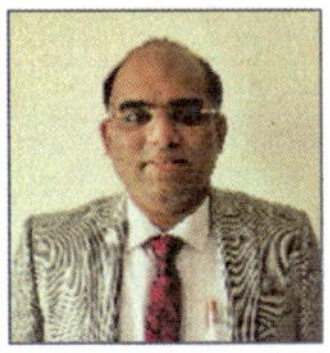

Dr. Ayush Goel (MD)
DM Resident
Department of Pulmonary
Critical Care and Sleep Medicine
AIIMS, New Delhi

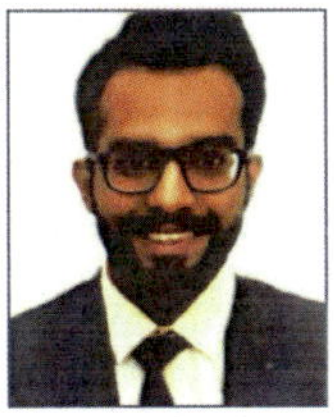

Dr. Bhushan Shah
(MD, DM Cardiology)
Assistant Professor
Department of Cardiology
AIIMS, Bhopal

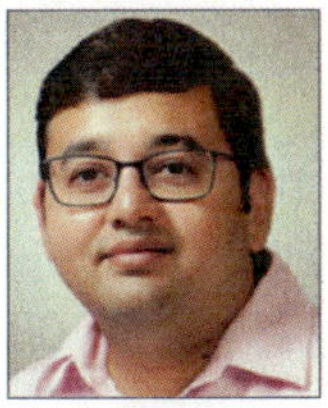

Dr. Ganesh Narwade (MD)
DM Resident
Department of Pulmonary Medicine
VMMC and SJH
New Delhi

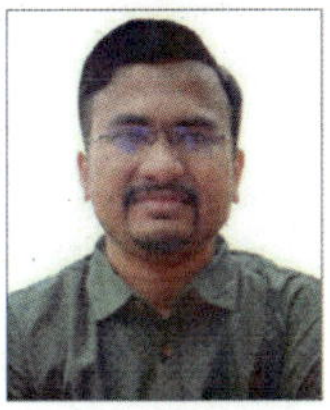

Dr. Gyanendra Agrawal (MD, DM)
Director, Respiratory and Critical Care Medicine
Max Super Speciality Hospital
Noida (Previously Jaypee Hospital)

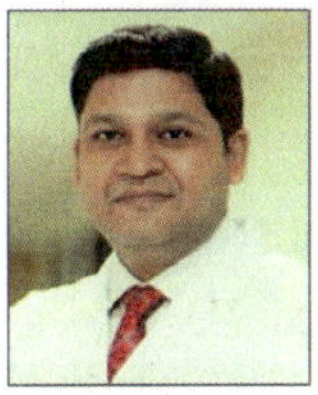

Dr. Hariharan Iyer (MD, DM)
Assistant Professor
Department of Pulmonary Medicine
AIIMS, Jodhpur

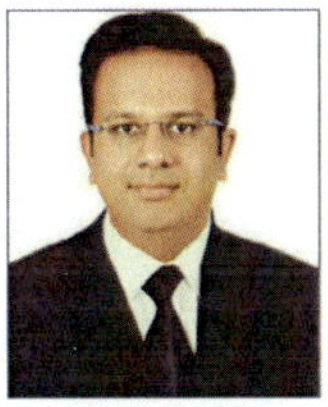

Dr. Irfan Shekh (MD, DM)
Associate consultant
Medanta, Gurugram, Haryana
Ex-Assistant Professor
Department of Pulmonary
Critical Care and Sleep Medicine
AIIMS, New Delhi

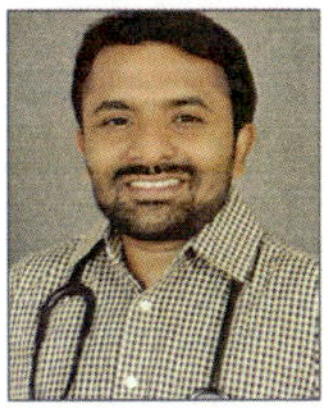

Dr. Jitendra Kumar Saini (MD)
Chest Specialist (SAG)
Head Department of Thoracic Oncology, National Institute of TB and Respiratory Diseases
New Delhi

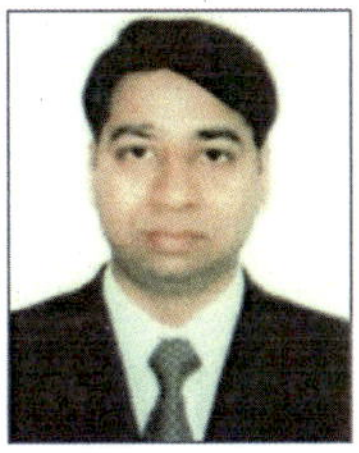

Dr. Karan Madan (MD, DM)
Additional Professor
Department of Pulmonary
Critical Care and Sleep Medicine
AIIMS, New Delhi

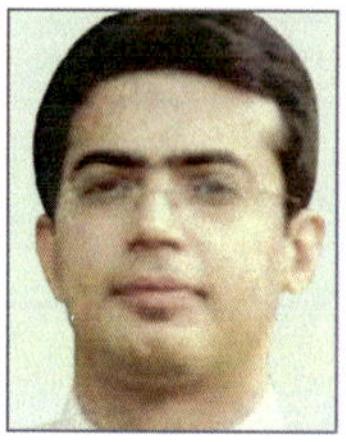

Dr. Mansi Gupta (MD, DM)
Associate Professor
Department of Pulmonary Medicine
SGPGI
Lucknow, UP

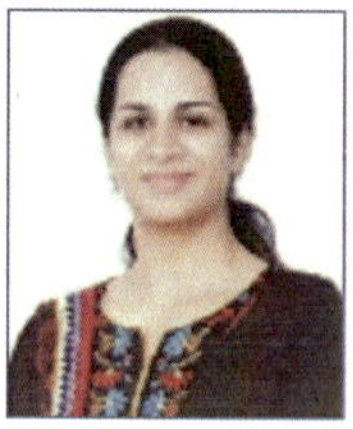

Dr. Naren Chandra (MD, DM)
Assistant Professor
Department of Pulmonary Medicine
VMMC and SJH
New Delhi

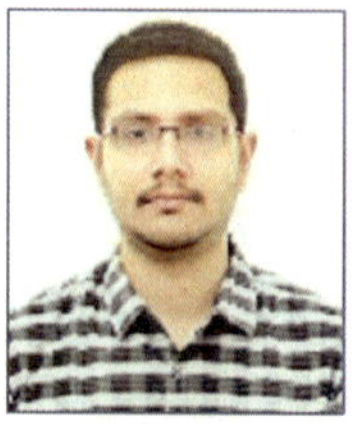

Dr. N. Murugan (MD)
Professor of Respiratory Medicine
Stanley Medical College
Chennai, Tamil Nadu

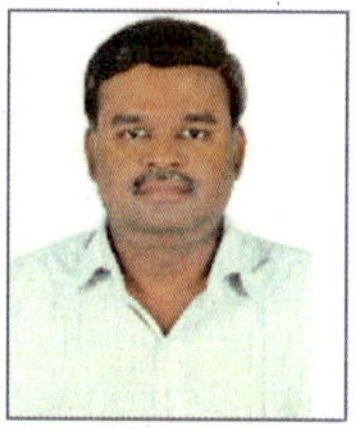

Dr. Nipun Malhotra (MD, DM)
Assistant Professor
Department of Respiratory Medicine
ESIC Basaidarapur
New Delhi

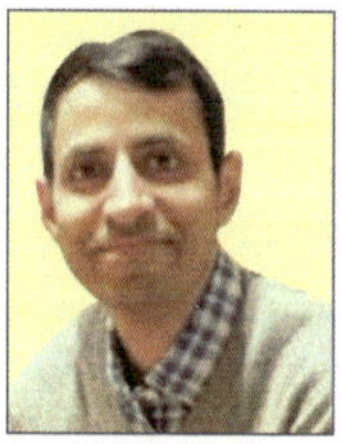

Dr. Nitesh Gupta (MD, DM)
Associate Professor
Department of Pulmonary Medicine
VMMC and SJH
New Delhi

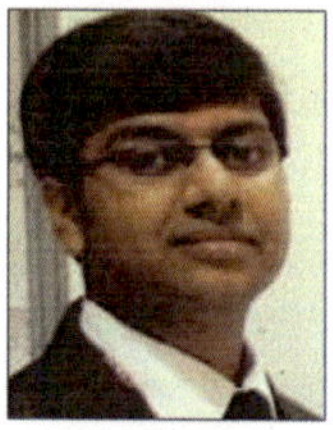

Dr. Parul Mrigpuri (MD)
Associate Professor
Department of Pulmonary Medicine
Vallabhbhai Patel Chest Institute
New Delhi

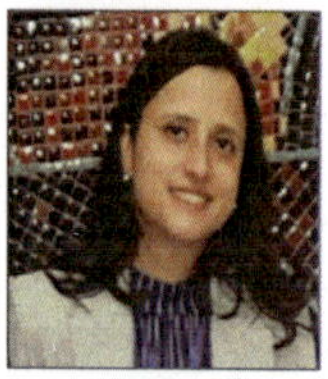

Dr. Pavan Tiwari (MD, DM)
Assistant Professor
Department of Pulmonary
Critical Care and Sleep Medicine
AIIMS, New Delhi

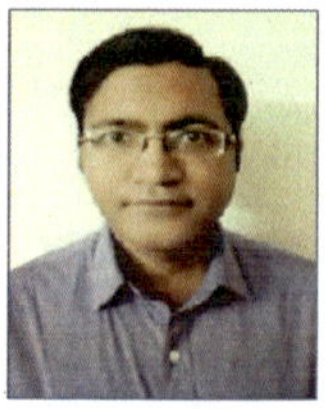

Dr. Pawan Singh (MD, DM)
Associate Professor
Department of Pulmonary and
Critical Care Medicine, Pt BDS
PGIMS, Rohtak

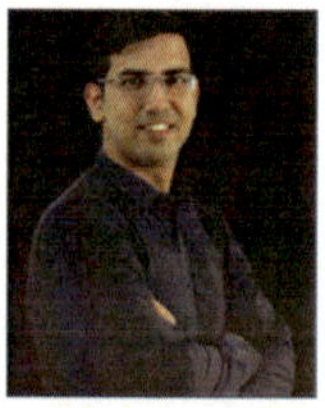

Dr. Pradeep Bajad (MD, DM)
Consultant and Assistant Professor
Amrita Hospital and School of
Medicine
Faridabad

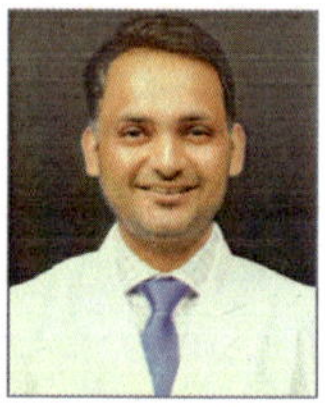

Dr. Rahul Roshan (MD, DM)
Principal Consultant
Department of Chest Diseases and
Allergic Disorders
BLK Max Hospital
New Delhi

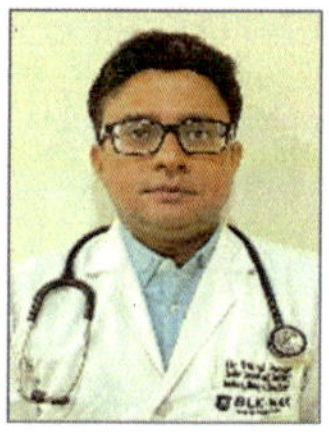

Dr. Rahul Tyagi (MD, DM)
Associate Professor
Army Institute of Cardio-Thoracic
Sciences
Pune

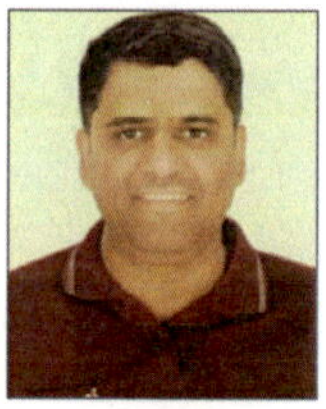

Dr. Rajnish Kaushik (MD, DM)
Assistant Professor
Department of Pulmonary Medicine
VMMC and SJH
New Delhi

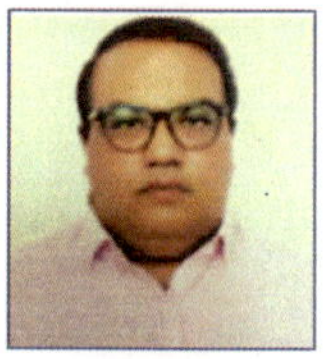

Dr. Rohit Kumar (MD, DM)
Associate Professor
Department of Pulmonary Medicine
VMMC and SJH
New Delhi

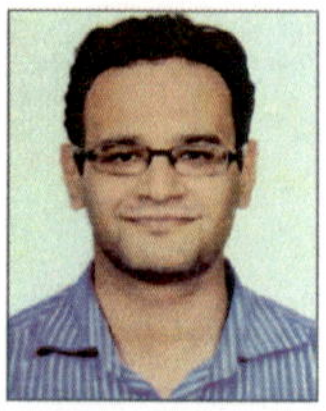

Dr. Rohit Vadala (MD, DM)
Consultant, Interventional
Pulmonologist
KIMS-Kingsway Hospital
Nagpur, Maharashtra

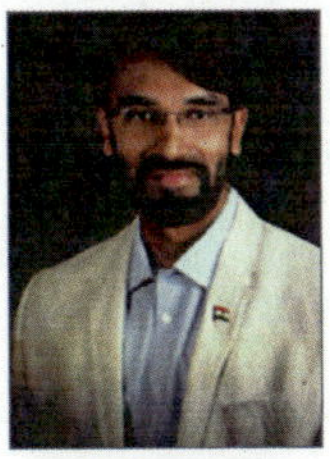

Dr. Ruchi Sharma (MD)
DM Cardiology resident
ESIC Medical College and Hospital
Faridabad, Haryana

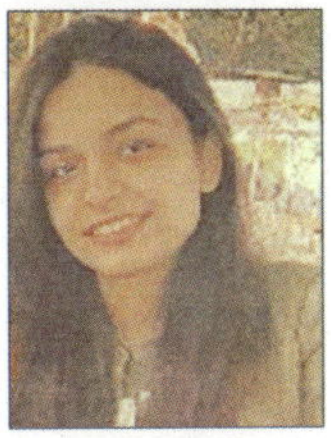

Dr. Rupak Singla (MD)
Head, Department of TB and
Respiratory Diseases
National Institute of TB and
Respiratory Diseases
New Delhi

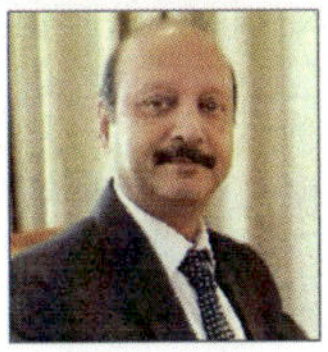

Dr. Saurabh Mittal (MD, DM)
Assistant Professor
Department of Pulmonary
Critical Care and Sleep Medicine
AIIMS, New Delhi

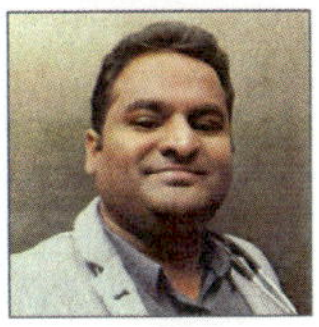

Dr. Sharada V. Kutty (MD, DM)
Associate Professor
Department of General Medicine
AIIMS, Mangalagiri
Andhra Pradesh

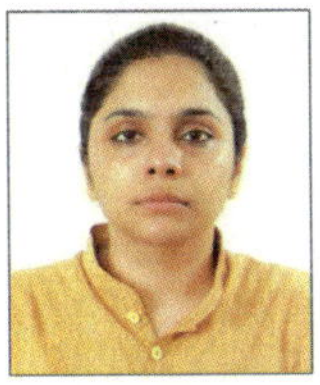

Dr. Shekhar Kunal
(MD, DM Cardiology)
Assistant Professor
Department of Cardiology
ESI Hospital
Faridabad

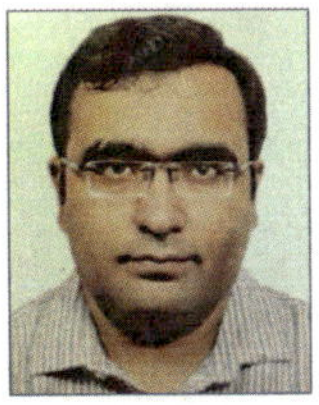

Dr. Shrinath V. (MD)
Senior Resident
Army Institute of Cardio-Thoracic
Sciences
Pune

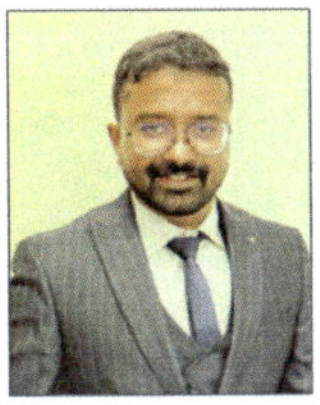

Dr. Shweta Bansal (MD, DM)
Senior Consultant and Unit Head
Artemis Hospital
Gurugram, Haryana

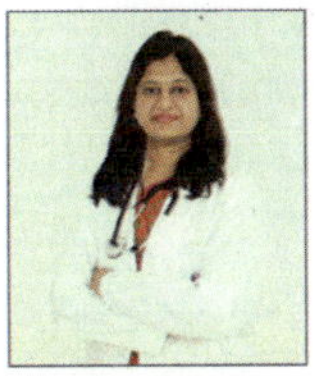

Dr. Sourabh Pahuja (MD, DM)
Senior Consultant and Assistant
Professor
Amrita Hospital and School of
Medicine
Faridabad

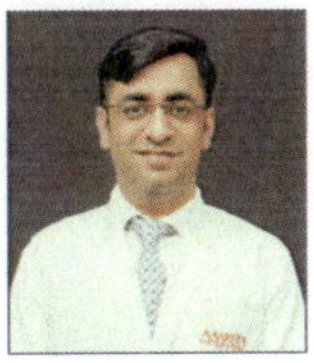

Dr. Sreyas Sharma (MD)
DM resident, Department of Pulmonary
Medicine, VMMC and SJH
New Delhi

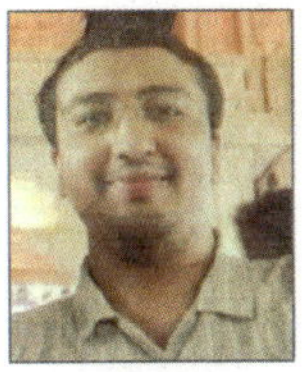

Dr. Srinivas Rajagopala (MD, DM)
Senior Consultant and Director
Transplant Pulmonology
Heart-Lung Transplant Unit
Kauvery Hospitals
Chennai

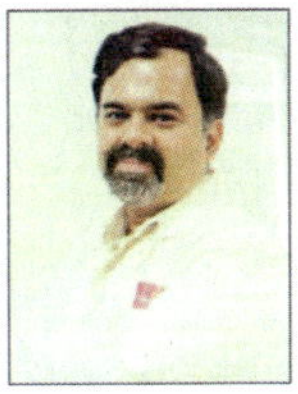

Dr. Sujay Halkur Shankar (MD)
DM Resident
Department of Pulmonary
Critical Care and Sleep Medicine
AIIMS, New Delhi

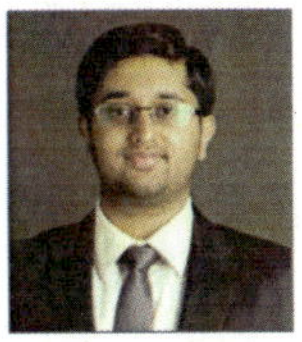

Dr. Sumita Agrawal (MD, DM)
Consultant and Head of Pulmonary
Critical Care and Sleep Medicine
Medical Superintendent
Medipulse Hospital
Jodhpur

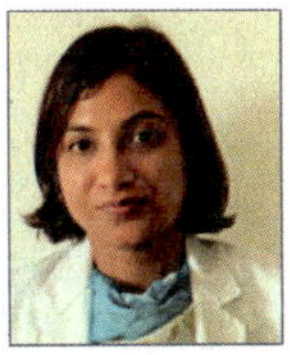

Dr. Tejas M. Suri (MD, DM)
Assistant Professor
Department of Pulmonary
Critical Care and Sleep Medicine
AIIMS, New Delhi

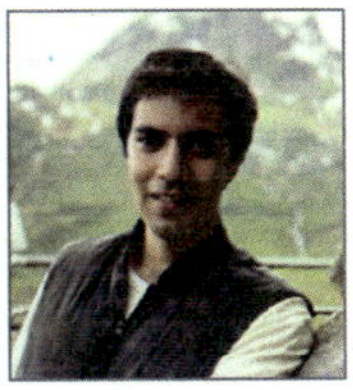

Dr. Vidushi Rathi (MD, DM)
Assistant Professor
Department of Pulmonary Medicine
Vallabhbhai Patel Chest Institute
New Delhi

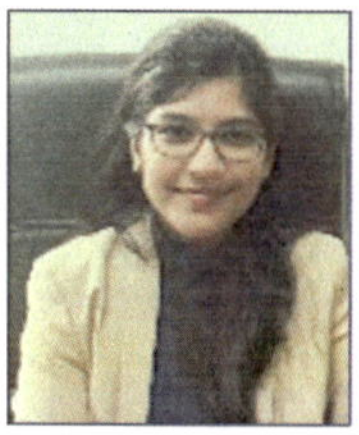

Dr. Vijay Hadda (MD)
Additional Professor
Department of Pulmonary
Critical Care and Sleep Medicine
AIIMS, New Delhi

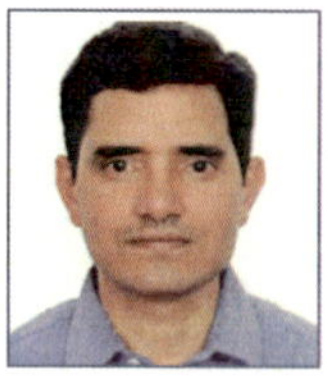

Dr. Yash Kedia (MD)
DM Resident
Department of Pulmonary Medicine
VMMC and SJH
New Delhi

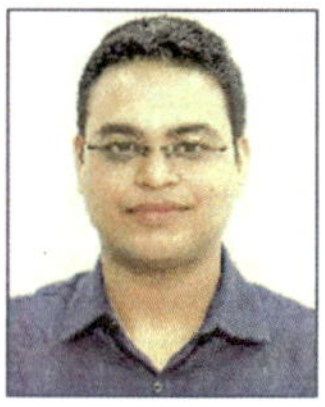

Dr. Zubair Ahmad Thoker
(MD, DM)
Consultant Pulmonology
Paras Hospital, Srinagar
Jammu and Kashmir

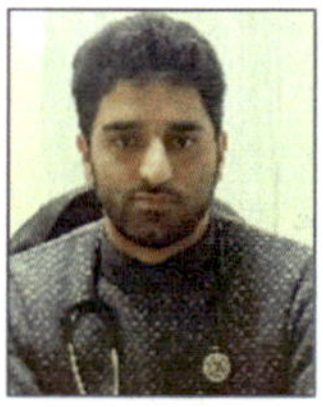

INTERNATIONAL CONTRIBUTORS

Dr. Archana Sasi
(MD, DM Medical Oncology)
Advanced Clinical Fellow Division of Leukemia, Dana Farber Cancer Institute, Boston
USA

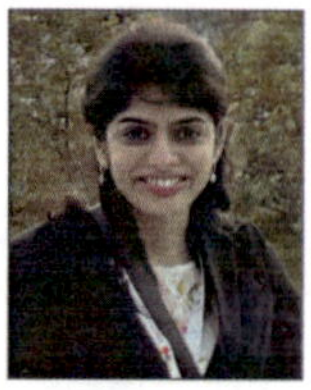

Dr. Mahendran Arul Janakiammal
(MD, DM)
Clinical Fellow in Transplant Medicine, Royal Brompton and Harefield Hospital, Guys and St. Thomas's Trust, London, UK

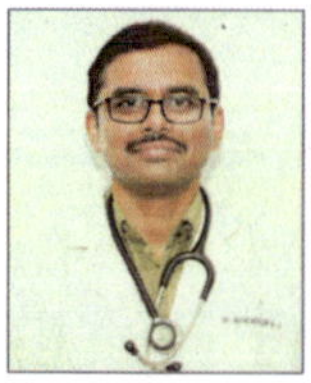

Dr. Caleb Bonds (MD)
Fellow, Critical Care Medicine
University of California
Riverside, USA

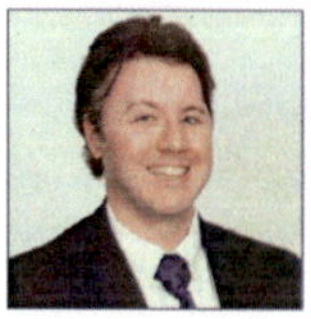

Dr. Deny Sung (MD)
Fellow, Critical Care Medicine
University of California
Riverside, USA

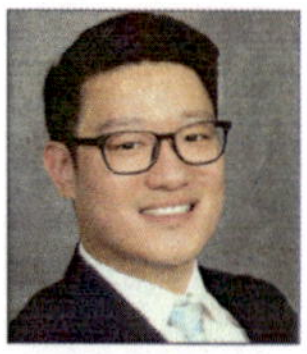

Dr. Jasmin Chovatiya (MD)
Fellow, Critical Care Medicine
University of California
Riverside, USA

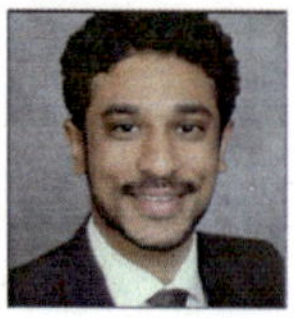

Dr. Jonathan Scheel (DO)
Chief Fellow, Critical Care Medicine
University of California
Riverside, USA

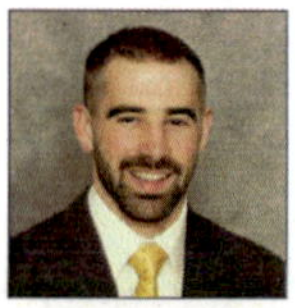

Dr. Kshitij Chatterjee (MD)
Health Sciences Assistant Clinical Professor, Associate Program Director
Critical Care Medicine Fellowship
University of California
Riverside, USA

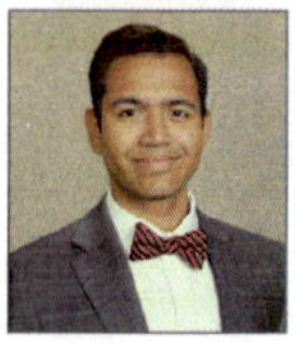

Dr. Prasad Nadendla (MD)
Fellow, Critical Care Medicine
University of California
Riverside, USA

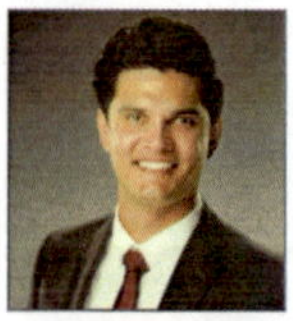

Dr. Roshan Roy (MD)
Fellow, Critical Care Medicine
University of California
Riverside, USA

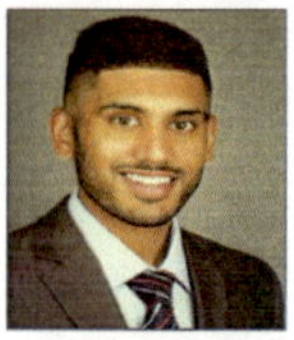

Dr. Sudeshna Ghosh (MD)
Fellow, Critical Care Medicine
University of California
Riverside, USA

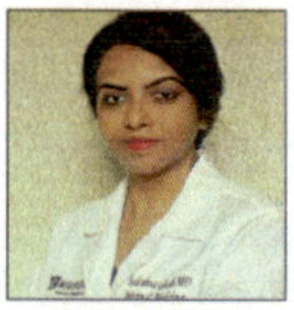

Dr. Sukhdev Singh (MD)
Fellow, Critical Care Medicine
University of California
Riverside, USA

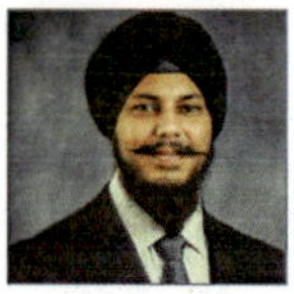

CONTENTS

CHAPTER 1

Bronchial Asthma

Authors: Dr. Rahul Tyagi, Dr. Shrinath V

Reviewer: Dr. Pavan Tiwari

INTRODUCTION

Bronchial asthma treatment has, for a long time, been largely dominated by metered dose inhalers and nebulizer therapy. Inhaled corticosteroids still form the backbone of asthma treatment. The recognition of asthma as a heterogeneous disease paved the way for identifying various phenotypes and endotypes. Although these phenotypes and endotypes have a common characteristic of chronic inflammation and reversible airway obstruction, they differ in other characteristics like the underlying mechanism of inflammation, clinical presentation, and response to treatment. As we enter the era of precision medicine, future asthma treatment will likely be dominated by biological therapies focused on the underlying inflammatory mechanism and guided by accurate biomarkers. A recent meta-analysis of 48 studies found that the use of licensed biological agents was associated with a 44% reduction in asthma exacerbation, a 60% reduction in hospitalization, and an improvement in lung function.[1] In this chapter, we will discuss the recent updates in the field of biomarkers and biologics in bronchial asthma.

Methodology

A PubMed search was carried out with keywords {"Asthma" AND ("Omalizumab" OR "Benralizumab" OR "Dupilumab" OR "Reslizumab" OR "Tezepelumab")}. Articles between the timespan of 1st August 2023 to August 2024 were reviewed.

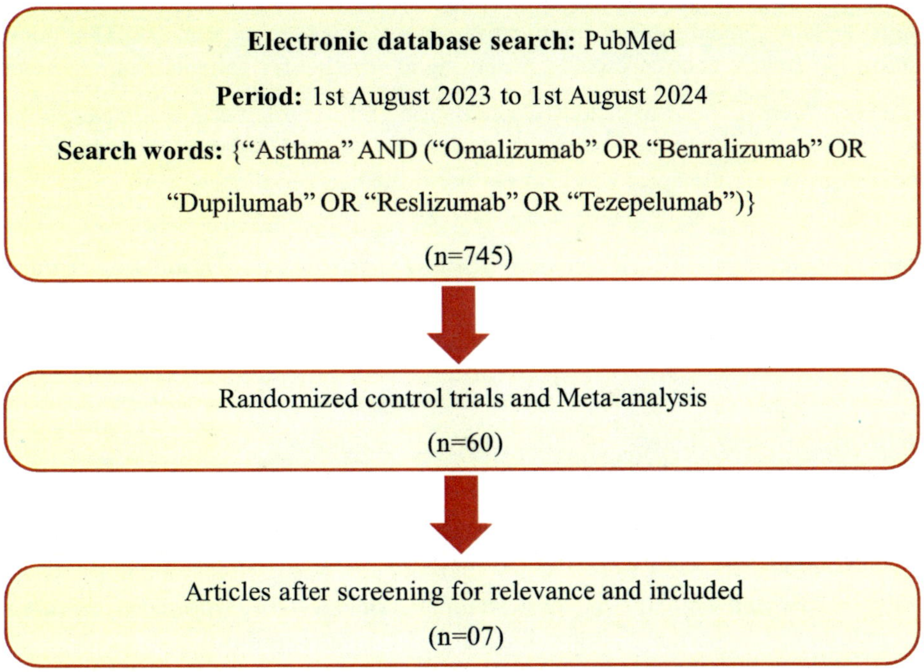

Analysis of Literature

- ***Efficacy of Tezepelumab in Severe, Uncontrolled Asthma: Pooled Analysis of the PATHWAY and NAVIGATOR Clinical Trials. (Am J Respir Crit Care Med, 2023)*[2]**
  - *Population:* Inadequately controlled severe asthma patients were randomized. (n=1334)
  - *Intervention:* Tezepelumab- 210 mg every 4 weeks. (n=665)
  - *Control:* Placebo. (n=669)
  - *Outcome:* Annual exacerbation rate was decreased by 60% in Tezepelumab arm. (rate ratio=0.40, [95% CI, 0.34-0.48]) irrespective of T2 high or T2 low phenotypes. Exacerbation-related hospitalization or emergency visits also decreased in the Tezepelumab arm (by 79%, RR=0.21, 95% CI; 0.13-0.35) without an increase in adverse events. Improvement in asthma control was also observed.
  - *Conclusion:* Monthly Tezepelumab can decrease exacerbations and also the need for hospitalization or ER visit due to severe uncontrolled asthma.

- ***Comparing bronchial thermoplasty with biologicals for severe asthma: Systematic review and network meta-analysis. (Respiratory Medicine. 2023)*[3]**
  - *Population:* Patients with severe asthma. (29 RCTs, n=15,547)
  - *Intervention:* RCTs on either bronchial thermoplasty or biological treatments (e.g., omalizumab, mepolizumab, benralizumab, reslizumab, dupilumab).
  - *Control:* Placebo or standard of care.
  - *Outcome:* Asthma Control Questionnaire (ACQ), Asthma Quality of Life Questionnaire (AQLQ), the number of patients experiencing $\geq$1 asthma exacerbation, annualized exacerbation rate ratio (AERR), oral corticosteroid dose reduction (OCDR), and morning peak expiratory flow rate (amPEF).
  - *Conclusion:* Despite the lack of head-to-head comparative trials, this NMA suggests that BT is non-inferior to biologicals in terms of quality-of-life scores, and represents a promising alternative for patients with severe asthma.
  - *Critical appraisal:* There were no head-to-head RCTs comparing BT to biologicals in severe asthma. Drawing any strong conclusions from this meta-analysis alone, should therefore be avoided. Further, a comparison of adverse events or patient preference for one of the therapies was also not performed.

- ***Biologic agents licensed for severe asthma: A systematic review and meta-analysis of randomised controlled trials. (European Respiratory Review. 2024)*[1]**
  - *Population:* Adults and adolescents diagnosed with severe asthma.
  - *Intervention:* Biologic agents such as omalizumab, mepolizumab, reslizumab, benralizumab, and dupilumab.
  - *Control:* Placebo or standard therapy (e.g., high-dose corticosteroids).
  - *Outcome:* Reduction in asthma exacerbations, improvement in lung function, improvement in asthma control measures, reduction in systemic corticosteroid use, adverse events associated with biologic therapy.
  - *Conclusion:* **Licensed asthma biologics reduce exacerbations and hospitalisations, improve lung function, asthma control and quality of life, and limit the use of systemic corticosteroids, with a favourable safety profile. These effects are more prominent in patients with evidence of T2 inflammation.**

- ***Reduction of daily maintenance inhaled corticosteroids in patients with severe eosinophilic asthma treated with Benralizumab (SHAMAL): A randomised, multicentre, open label, phase 4 study. (Lancet. 2024)[4]***
  - o *Population:* Patients with severe eosinophilic asthma under 18 years with a 5-point ACQ score of less than 1.5 and who have received at least 3 consecutive doses of Benralizumab. (n=168)
  - o *Intervention:* Tapering high dose ICS to medium dose ICS, low dose ICS and later as-needed ICS over 32 weeks. (n=125)
  - o *Control:* Continued high dose ICS + Formoterol and Benralizumab 8 weekly injection. (n=43)
  - o *Outcome:* Proportion of patients who reduced their ICS dose at the end of 32 weeks. In total 92% participants were able to reduce ICS-formoterol dose. Out of these, 61% reduced to as-needed only, 17% to low dose, and 15% to medium dose. Rate of adverse events was similar between dose reduction and continued high dose groups.
  - o *Conclusion:* Patients controlled on Benralizumab can have meaningful reductions in ICS therapy while maintaining asthma control.
  - o *Critical appraisal:* This is a phase IV post-marketing trial and therefore provides an insight on the safety and effectiveness in the public use setting. However, the sample size is small. Trials with bigger sample sizes are needed to draw concrete conclusions.

- ***Combination of omalizumab with allergen immunotherapy versus immunotherapy alone for allergic diseases: A meta-analysis of randomized controlled trials. (Int Forum Allergy Rhinol. 2024)[5]***
  - o *Population:* Patients with atopy predominant uncontrolled bronchial asthma with documental sensitivity to perennial aeroallergens. (11 RCTs, n=901)
  - o *Intervention:* Omalizumab in combination with allergen immunotherapy (AIT).
  - o *Control:* Patients only on AIT.
  - o *Outcome:* Patients receiving combination therapy had significantly fewer asthma exacerbations (odds ratio=0.32, 95% CI; 0.18-0.59, p=0.0003) compared to AIT alone. Combination therapy also caused a sustained unresponsiveness to allergens (odds ratio=6.77, 95% CI; 2.10-21.80, p=0.001, I^2=36%). There were improvements in severity score and daily rescue medication use in the combination group compared to AIT alone.
  - o *Conclusion:* Combination of Omalizumab with AIT significantly improved the efficacy and safety of AIT.
  - o *Critical appraisal:* Omalizumab and AIT have complementary actions and were also found to be complementary in reducing asthma exacerbations. **However, whether combination therapy achieves a meaningful reduction in ICS-LABA consumption or a meaningful improvement in asthma control was not evaluated.** Further, the total duration for which Omalizumab and AIT are required for sustained benefits was not evaluated. Patient acceptance is also an issue with using two different modalities that are injectables, and was also not evaluated.

☞

- ***Efficacy and safety of biologics for oral corticosteroid-dependent asthma: A systematic review and network meta-analysis. (The Journal of Allergy and Clinical Immunology: In Practice. 2023)***[6]
    - *Population:* Oral corticosteroid (OCS) dependent patients with asthma.
    - *Intervention:* Benralizumab, Dupilumab, Mepolizumab, Tralokinumab, Tezepelumab, and Reslizumab.
    - *Control:* ICS + LABA and oral corticosteroids.
    - *Outcome:* Compared with placebo, benralizumab, dupilumab, and mepolizumab were efficacious in achieving a reduction in the OCS dose whereas tralokinumab, tezepelumab, and subcutaneous reslizumab were ineffective. An indirect comparison found no significant differences among benralizumab, dupilumab, and mepolizumab.
    - *Conclusion:* In OCS-dependent patients with asthma, benralizumab, dupilumab, and mepolizumab were superior to placebo in reducing the OCS dose.

☞

- ***Titration of anti-IL-5 biologics in severe asthma: An open-label randomised controlled trial. (the OPTIMAL study) (European Respiratory Journal. 2024)***[7]
    - *Population:* Severe asthma patients aged >18yrs who have received anti-IL5 biological treatment for at least 12 months. (n=73)
    - *Intervention:* Down-titration of biologics over 52 weeks following "OPTIMAL algorithm". (n=37)
    - *Control:* Continued normal dosing of biologics. (n=36)
    - *Outcome:* 78% of patients randomized to the intervention arm tolerated down-titration of treatment. Compared to the control arm the intervention arm tended to have more exacerbations during the study (32% vs 17%) but it was not statistically significant. Lung function and symptom scores remained stable and comparable in both study arms.
    - *Conclusion:* The study offers proof for the concept of down-titration of anti-IL5 biologics. "OPTIMAL algorithm" provides a potential framework for the down-titration of biologics in patients well controlled on anti-IL5 therapy.
    - *Critical appraisal:* The effectiveness and safety of biologics, new and old, continues to be evaluated in RCTs. These agents are costly and have a parenteral route of administration. Whether these agents require life-long continuation for sustained benefits or can be stopped at some point of time remains unclear. The current trial is therefore an important piece of evidence. It showed that down-titration after one year of therapy may lead to an increase in exacerbations. This supports the view that biologic therapy and its duration need to be individualized under precision medicine.

DISCUSSION

Biomarkers

The cornerstone of personalized medicine is precision in diagnosis, endotyping of disease, and tailored therapy to target underlying inflammation. Based on the underlying pathology of inflammation, there are two broad endotypes: "T2 high" and "T2 low" asthma.[8] T2 high asthma consists of an atopic-eosinophilic endotype and non-atopic eosinophilic endotype while T2 low asthma consists of neutrophilic and pauci-granulocytic endotype. T2 high is the most common endotype, constituting 55% of asthma patients, the atopic-eosinophilic phenotype being the commonest. Neutrophilic endotypes constitute 20% of cases, paucigranulocytic endotypes constitute 18% and the rest 7% have mixed pathobiology.[8] Recognizing these endotypes is vital for selecting appropriate biological therapeutic agents. Phenotypes and biomarkers point to the underlying endotype. Phenotypes are clinically observable patient characteristics while biomarkers are indicators that can be objectively measured. As patients can have overlapping phenotypes, better biomarkers are the future in guiding precision medicine in asthma.

Biomarkers in T2 inflammation

T2 airway inflammation is characteristically eosinophil driven. T helper 2 (Th2) and innate lymphoid cells (ILC2) are primarily responsible for this eosinophilic inflammation. Markers of T2 inflammation that have been studied and commonly used in clinical practice are as follows:

Blood eosinophils

Eosinophils, along with their mediators, play a dominant role in various inflammation. **Eosinophil development and differentiation in bone marrow is driven by IL 5 in response to infective, inflammatory, or allergic stimuli**. These eosinophils released into the blood are recruited into tissues driven by chemokines mainly of the eotaxin family. Blood eosinophilia is one of the simplest and easily available markers of eosinophilic airway inflammation. **Large cohort studies have shown a moderate to good correlation between blood eosinophilia and sputum eosinophilia.**[9] The cut-off of blood eosinophil level to predict eosinophilic airway inflammation is a topic of debate with many clinical trials having used blood eosinophil levels ranging from 150 to 400 for biological therapy.[10] **In real-life studies it was demonstrated that a blood eosinophil level > 300 cells/µL correlated with a risk of asthma exacerbation, decline in respiratory function, mortality, and increased systemic corticosteroid dependence.**[11] **If the blood eosinophil count is < 150 cells/µL, sputum eosinophilia is unlikely especially when FeNO is < 25 ppb.**[12] The use of blood eosinophil count as a biomarker of airway eosinophilic inflammation is limited by other conditions that can elevate blood eosinophils, especially parasitic infections. Even with this limitation, blood eosinophil level remains a useful biomarker. It has been found to be better than serum IgE, FeNO, and serum periostin levels in predicting airway eosinophilia, exacerbation, and response to treatment.[10] Therefore, blood eosinophil count is a good biomarker for bronchial asthma, but its accuracy can be increased when combined with other markers of T2 inflammation.

Sputum eosinophil

Differential sputum count is performed after cytospin centrifugation and staining of sputum. Studies evaluating the normal eosinophil percentage in induced sputum of non-smoking healthy candidates have reported a mean value ranging from 0.3 to 0.6%.[9] **Any sputum differential eosinophil count > 2% was reproducible and cut-off > 3% has the highest power to distinguish between eosinophilic and non-eosinophilic airway inflammation.**[13] **Patients with elevated sputum eosinophil levels have been found to have better response to steroid therapy and those with > 5% sputum eosinophil count have been shown to have a shorter time to exacerbation.**[9] Though it is a potent biomarker of underlying T2 airway inflammation, an elevated sputum eosinophil level can be seen even in mild asthma and does not serve to differentiate between mild and severe asthma.

Cytokines

IL5 is an essential contributor to eosinophil proliferation, differentiation, and maturation. Increased IL 5 production leads to increased eosinophil production and decreased apoptosis. **IL4, IL5, and IL13 in sputum and bronchoalveolar lavage, along with TSLP, IL 33, and IL 25 in epithelium, are markers of T2 airway inflammation**. Though these cytokines are the gold standard for clinical research, they may not be feasible for routine clinical practice due to poor availability and high cost.

FeNO (Fraction of exhaled nitric oxide)

Nitric oxide is produced by airway epithelium due to the upregulation of nitric oxide synthase by IL 13 and is therefore a specific marker for T2 high airway inflammation.[12] The measurement is non-invasive and simple, though it requires an exhalation flow of 50 ml/s. FeNO is also a predictor of airway hyperresponsiveness and can be used to monitor treatment compliance with inhaled corticosteroid therapy. Healthy individuals have a FeNO level between 10 – 20 ppb. **A FeNO level < 25 ppb indicates that eosinophilic airway inflammation is less likely and corresponds to a sputum eosinophil count of < 3%. For a patient aged between 12 to 80 years, a FeNO level of > 50 ppb is highly associated with eosinophilic airway inflammation**. The negative predictive value of FeNO for eosinophilic inflammation is more than its positive predictive value.[10] Though a good biomarker, it is affected by various confounding factors, such as smoking, diet, nasal polyps, age, height, weight, and atopy.

Immunoglobulin E (IgE)

IgE is an immunoglobulin that induces type 1 inflammatory reaction and anaphylaxis. IgE is also a component of T2 inflammation and serves both as a marker of T2 inflammation and specific sensitization to seasonal and perennial allergens. Thus, both total and specific IgE levels are important as a biomarker for asthma. Though it is a marker of atopy, serum IgE levels does not consistently distinguish between atopic and non-atopic asthma.[9] The importance of this biomarker lies in the identification of T2 airway inflammation, the identification of subtypes that will better respond to anti-IgE therapy, and the determination of the optimal dose of Omalizumab. **The International Severe Asthma Registry (ISAR) takes a cut-off of 75 kU/L as significantly raised IgE level in severe asthma.**[9]

Serum periostin

Periostin is an extracellular matrix protein produced by airway epithelial cells and epithelial fibroblasts. It is induced by IL 4 and IL 13. It has been shown to enhance eosinophilic tissue infiltration and is a biomarker for T2-high asthma. **What makes serum periostin stand out from the rest of the T2 biomarkers is that it is implicated in airway remodelling and, therefore, it is associated with chronic rather than acute T2 airway inflammation.**[14-15] **Elevated periostin levels correlate with airway eosinophilia, decline in FEV1 and predict response to ICS. One of the most critical roles of serum periostin is the identification of smokers with asthma who can have T2 inflammation.** Asthmatics who smoke are difficult to manage as the smoke induces a non-T2 airway inflammation, and smoking intervenes with other biomarkers of airway inflammation like FeNO. In a study by Thomson NC et al, it was demonstrated that though smokers with asthma had a low serum periostin level, 40% of them had a serum periostin level above the group median. This subgroup of patients may benefit from anti-T2 interventions.[16] Sputum periostin can be a more organ-specific biomarker for eosinophilic inflammation than serum periostin.[10] **The use of serum periostin is limited by a lack of standardized measurement techniques and reference values.**

Biomarkers in non-T2 inflammation

Sputum neutrophils

Unlike the eosinophilic airway inflammation of T2 high asthma, the mechanism of neutrophilic inflammation of the airway seen in T2 low asthma is unclear. The cut-off for sputum neutrophils is also not well defined as even in healthy individual's neutrophils are the predominant cells in sputum.[17] **Sputum neutrophils greater than 61-76% may indicate an underlying neutrophil-predominant airway inflammation.**[10]

Interleukins 17 and 8

Neutrophil airway inflammation is driven by the Th17 immune response. Interleukin 17, released as a response to airway infection, irritants, and pollution, leads to neutrophil recruitment through IL 8. Studies have demonstrated elevated IL17 levels in induced sputum, BAL and bronchial biopsy of patients with severe asthma.[12] Though they are potential biomarkers and IL 17-targeted therapies are under development, technical challenges and cost limit their use in routine practice. **More validated trials linking sputum IL 17 and IL 8 levels to sputum neutrophil levels are required to identify a cut-off value for non-T2 airway inflammation.**

Other potential biomarkers

TNF-α and IFN-γ are other potent markers of T2-low asthma but more studies are required to evaluate whether they are validated for clinical use.[12,18]

Biomarkers indicative of airway remodeling

Bronchoscopy

Airway remodelling is seen in chronic airway inflammation due to asthma and is characterized by smooth muscle thickening, epithelial metaplasia, mucus hypersecretion, and basement membrane fibrosis. **Bronchial biopsy and histopathological evaluation of bronchial basement membrane thickness are the gold standard for detecting airway remodelling, but they are invasive procedures.**

Galectin-3 (Gal 3)

Galectin 3 regulates epithelial proliferation, remodelling, and eosinophilic inflammation. Detected in bronchial epithelial biopsy samples by immunostaining, it can be a valuable biomarker for airway remodelling. In a study by Ricco et al., it was demonstrated that **the presence of galectin 3 in bronchial biopsy specimens is a marker of response to Omalizumab therapy in reducing the respiratory membrane thickness.**[19]

YKL – 40

YKL 40 is a chitinase-like protein associated with airway remodelling. Serum levels of YKL 40 show a significant correlation with bronchial wall thickness measured by high-resolution computerized tomography.[20] **Higher levels of YKL-40 are associated with increased exacerbation, therapy resistance, poor symptom control and lung function.** The highest level of YKL 40 is seen in neutrophilic and obesity-related asthma phenotypes. Its clinical utility is limited by its poor specificity, as higher levels are also seen in COPD, lung malignancies, infections and autoimmune disorders.[21]

Upcoming biomarkers

Genomic biomarkers

Chromosome 17q21 is the focus of interest of all genomic studies on asthma as it contains many genes directly involved in asthma pathology. Several genes like CLC, EMR4P, IL-5RA, FRRS1, HRH4, SLC29A1, SIGLEC8 and IL1RL1 have been identified which are related to asthma pathophysiology causing airway inflammation through IL5/JAK/STAT and IL33/ST2/

IRAK/TRAF pathway.[15,22] The future of precision medicine lies in the identification of IL33R, CCR3, and TSLP receptor expression to identify eosinophilic asthma and IFN and TNF gene expression to identify neutrophilic asthma.

Proteomic and metabolomic biomarkers

Exhaled breath pH and volatile organic compounds (VOCs) have been studied in asthma. A lower exhaled breath pH has been associated with refractory asthma, obesity-associated asthma, high BAL neutrophils, impaired lung function and associated GERD.[23] Numerous volatile organic compounds have been evaluated for their usefulness in diagnosing asthma, assessing disease control and endotyping. Though results to date are promising, validation in independent prospective cohorts is needed as breathomics might be the future of asthma precision medicine.[24]

Microbiota and respiratory infection biomarkers

Recent studies have investigated lung and gut microbiota and its potential influence on disease pathology. In adult asthmatics increased histamine-secreting bacteria in the gut has been associated with increased asthma severity.[25] **Predominance of Proteobacteria in lung microbiota may be associated with severe asthma and poor asthma control.**[26] Metabolites of lung microbes may be a potential biomarker in asthma.

Updates in the management of bronchial asthma

Triple inhalation therapy in asthma

Once daily triple agent dry powder inhaler therapy containing fluticasone furoate, umeclidinium and vilanterol (FF/UMEC/VI) has been approved by FDA for use in moderate to severe asthma. A large, randomized control trial **(CAPTAIN trial)** of 2439 patients investigating triple therapy (fluticasone furoate, umeclidinium and vilanterol) and dual therapy fluticasone furoate and vilanterol) in 6 different dose combinations demonstrated a statistically significant improvement in lung function with triple therapy compared to dual therapy with no significant improvement in exacerbation rate.[27] Other triple therapies under investigation include beclomethasone-glycopyrronium-formoterol and mometasone-glycopyrrolate-indacaterol. **Two parallel 52-week randomized trials (TRIMARAN and TRIGGER) demonstrated a modest improvement in lung function with beclomethasone-glycopyrronium-formoterol triple therapy compared to beclomethasone-formoterol dual therapy with inconsistent effect on improvement in the rate of exacerbation.**[28] **Mometasone-glycopyrrolate-indacaterol triple therapy has also been shown to improve lung function when compared to mometasone-indacaterol dual therapy.**[29] **For patients with severe asthma poorly controlled on dual inhaler therapy use of a triple combination of ICS+LABA+LAMA is a reasonable treatment choice before considering costlier treatment options.**

Biologics in Bronchial Asthma

Anti-IgE monoclonal antibody (Omalizumab)

Omalizumab was the first biologic approved by FDA for use in severe asthma.

Mechanism of action: Omalizumab binds to Fc segment of free IgE in serum thereby preventing it from binding to receptors on mast cells and basophils.[18]

Approved use:

a. **It is approved for subcutaneous administration in persons 6 years of age or older who have moderate-to-severe allergic asthma**. Predictive markers for response to Omalizumab in moderate-to-severe asthma include history of atopy, a positive skin-prick test or allergen-specific IgE to a perennial aeroallergen, total serum IgE levels and weight within dosing range. The dosing range of serum total IgE is 30 – 700 IU/ml in United States and 30 – 1500 IU/ml in Europe.

b. Symptomatic chronic spontaneous urticaria.

c. Nasal polyps with inadequate response to nasal corticosteroids.

Dose in asthma: The dose of Omalizumab varies from 75mg to 375mg every 2 to 4 weeks and depends on the patient's body weight and pre-treatment total IgE levels. Dose can be calculated using serum total IgE and body weight table or as **0.016 mg/kg per IU/ml of IgE per month.**[18] Total IgE levels may be elevated post-treatment and therefore cannot be used as a marker of response to therapy. Omalizumab dose should not be adjusted based on total IgE levels evaluated during treatment or < 1yr following interruption of therapy. If Omalizumab therapy has been interrupted for more than a year, total IgE levels can be re-evaluated for dosage determination. No dose adjustments are required for renal and hepatic impairment. Omalizumab is given for atleast 3 – 6 months before evaluation for response.

Method of administration: Omalizumab is subcutaneously administered into clean skin of the upper arm, abdomen or thigh. **Doses more than 150 mg should be divided over > 1 injection site with each site separated by at least 1 inch**. It should not be injected into moles, scars, bruises, tender areas or broken skin. Patients should be observed for 2 hours after the initial 3 injections as the risk of anaphylaxis is maximum during this period. For subsequent injections, patients may be observed for only 30 minutes.

Adverse effect: Omalizumab is well tolerated, with the most common adverse event being injection site reaction; occasional cases of headache and rare cases of thromboembolism (<3%) and anaphylaxis have been reported. **It is generally well tolerated with anaphylaxis reported in 0.1 to 0.2% of patients, especially with the first three doses**. Due to the potential risk of anaphylaxis, it is recommended that the drug be administered in a health care setup.

Evidence: In a study including 1070 moderate-to-severe allergic asthma patients randomised to receive Omalizumab or placebo; a composite endpoint for Omalizumab response (no exacerbation and one of the following: reduced symptom score, reduced usage of rescue medication, improved lung function, improved quality of life) was met at 16 weeks by 64% patients. **The Extra trial had 850 patients with severe asthma randomised to Omalizumab or placebo; a 48 week follow-up showed a 25% reduction in asthma exacerbation in the Omalizumab group with improvement in symptom control and reduced mean daily albuterol dose.**[30] In the post hoc analysis of the Extra trial, Omalizumab was seen to reduce exacerbation in patients with high, but not low, bronchodilator reversibility regardless of the presence of fixed airway obstruction.[31] **In a meta-analysis, evaluating real-world data of Omalizumab; in moderate-to-severe allergic asthma, Omalizumab therapy improved lung function (mean improvement in FEV1 was 160, 220 and 250ml at 16 weeks, 6 months and 12 months), improvement in asthma symptom control, a significant reduction in the rate of exacerbation, oral corticosteroid use and unscheduled physician visit.**[32] **In a recent meta-analysis of 14 studies on the use of Omalizumab for ABPA, the use of Omalizumab causes reduction in annualized exacerbation rate, reduction in use of oral corticosteroids, improvement in FEV1 and has better asthma symptom control**. Greater improvement was seen with treatment > 12 months.[33] A meta analysis of 11 RCTs concluded that Omalizumab when compared with allergen immunotherapy (AIT) enhanced the safety and efficacy of AIT.[5]

Anti-IL5 therapy

Interleukin 5 is the cytokine responsible for eosinophil hematopoiesis, development, recruitment and survival. Mepolizumab and Reslizumab are anti-IL5 monoclonal antibodies while Benralizumab is an anti-IL5 receptor alpha antibody.

Mepolizumab

Mechanism of action: Mepolizumab reduces the production and survival of eosinophil by inhibiting IL5 signaling.

Approved use:

a. **Patients more than 6 years of age with severe eosinophilic asthma**. The blood eosinophilic cut off for use of Mepolizumab is taken as 150/µL. A higher baseline blood eosinophil level and late age of asthma onset predicts better response to Mepolizumab therapy while male sex and BMI ≥30 kg/m^2 predict poor response.[34] As per **DREAM and MENSA study, inclusion criteria for Mepolizumab therapy should include severe asthma with blood eosinophil levels >150/µL or a documented level >300/µL anytime in the previous one year along with two or more exacerbations in previous 12 months.**[35]

b. Eosinophilic granulomatosis with polyangiitis (EGPA): can be used as an adjunct to corticosteroid therapy to induce remission.

c. Hyper eosinophilic syndrome

d. Rhinosinusitis with nasal polyps

Dose in asthma: 100mg once every 4 weeks. A minimum of 3 to 6 months of treatment is suggested to determine efficacy. No dosing modification required for hepatic or renal impairment.

Method of administration: Mepolizumab is subcutaneously administered into clean skin of upper arm, abdomen on thigh. It should not be injected into moles, scars, bruises, tender areas or broken skin.

Adverse effects: Generally well tolerated, with local site reaction being the most common adverse effect. Post-injection headache and herpes zoster infection have also been reported.

Evidence: In a double-blind, placebo-controlled randomised trial (SIRUS trial) to assess the steroid-sparing effect of Mepolizumab in severe eosinophilic asthma, it was demonstrated that Mepolizumab had 2.39 times greater likelihood of reducing oral corticosteroid use. The median percentage reduction from baseline in the glucocorticoid dose was 50% in the Mepolizumab group than in the placebo group. The Mepolizumab group also had a relative reduction of 32% in the annualized rate of exacerbation and also had better symptom control on objective assessment.[36] In another placebo-controlled randomised trial in severe refractory eosinophilic asthma, Mepolizumab was associated with significantly fewer exacerbations, improved quality of life, significantly lower blood and sputum eosinophil levels.[37] In a large randomised, double-blind placebo-controlled trial (MENSA trial) by Ortega et al., 576 patients with severe eosinophilic asthma (severe asthma with peripheral eosinophil count > 150/ µL or a count of > 300/µL anytime in previous 1 year) were randomised to receive subcutaneous Mepolizumab, intravenous Mepolizumab and placebo. **There was a 47% decrease in exacerbation rate among patients receiving intravenous Mepolizumab and 53% among those receiving subcutaneous Mepolizumab. The Mepolizumab group showed an increase in FEV1 at the end of 32 weeks of therapy with a mean increase of 100 ml in intravenous Mepolizumab and 98ml in patients with subcutaneous Mepolizumab.**[35] In patients with chronic rhinosinusitis with nasal polyps Mepolizumab has been shown to improve the sense of smell.[38]

Reslizumab

Mechanism of action: By inhibiting IL5 signaling, Reslizumab reduces the production and survival of eosinophil, thereby decreasing eosinophilic airway inflammation.

Approved use:

Approved as an add on therapy in patients **aged ≥ 18 years with severe eosinophilic asthma inadequately controlled on standard therapy. Expert opinion is to reserve the use of Reslizumab for patients with peripheral blood eosinophilia ≥400 cells/µL.**

Dose in asthma: 3mg/kg once every 4 weeks. A minimum of 4 months of treatment is suggested to determine efficacy. No dosing adjustment needed for renal or hepatic impairment.

Method of administration: Reslizumab is given as an intravenous infusion. Infusion must be given over 20 to 50 min with flushing of the line with normal saline post completion of infusion. Avoid intravenous bolus or push. Do not infuse concomitantly with other drugs in the same line. Patient should be observed post infusion for anaphylaxis.

Adverse effect: Has an FDA black box warning for anaphylaxis (0.3% cases). Increased blood creatine phosphokinase levels and oropharyngeal pain have been observed.

Evidence: Reslizumab has been demonstrated to improve asthma control, lung function and attain a reduction in sputum eosinophil count in randomised control trial on severe eosinophilic asthma.[39] **In a systematic review of 5 RCTs, Reslizumab has been shown to reduce asthma exacerbation and improve asthma control without much steroid-sparing effect.**[40] Similar results in reduction of exacerbation have been shown by two multicentre, parallel, double-blind, randomised, placebo controlled phase 3 trials. Reslizumab at a dose of 3mg/kg in severe eosinophilic asthma has been proven to improve health related quality of life (HRQoL) and to improve lung function (mean improvement in FEV1 by 160 ml) after 16 weeks of therapy.[41] In a phase 3 study in patients with poorly controlled asthma, Reslizumab failed to show significant improvement in lung function among patients with a peripheral blood eosinophil count less than 400 cells/μL while a significant improvement was noted in those with eosinophil counts above this threshold.[42]

Benralizumab

Mechanism of action: Benralizumab binds to the alpha subunit of IL 5 receptor and inhibits its signaling resulting in reduced production and survival of eosinophils and basophils. It causes apoptosis of eosinophils and basophils via antibody-mediated cytolysis.

Approved use: Approved as an add-on therapy in **patients aged >12 years with severe eosinophilic asthma inadequately controlled on standard therapies**. A peripheral blood eosinophil level of **>150/μL is generally taken as a cut-off** for Benralizumab therapy.

Dose in asthma: 30 mg every 4 weeks for the first 3 doses then once every 8 weeks. A minimum of 4 months of treatment is suggested to determine efficacy. No dosing adjustment for hepatic or renal dysfunction.

Method of administration: Benralizumab is subcutaneously administered into clean skin of upper arm, abdomen on thigh. It should not be injected into moles, scars, bruises, tender areas or broken skin.

Adverse effect: Mostly well tolerated with headache and pharyngitis being the most commonly reported side effects.

Evidence: Phase 3 double-blinded placebo control trial (SIROCCO trial) results demonstrated that Benralizumab was effective in 4 weekly and 8 weekly doses to reduce the rate of exacerbation, improve symptom control and improve lung function when compared with placebo in patients with severe asthma with peripheral eosinophil level more than 300/μL over 48 weeks.[43] These results were replicated in a similar trial **(CALIMA trial)** wherein both 4 weekly and 8 weekly dosing reduced the rate of exacerbation in severe eosinophilic asthma with peripheral eosinophil levels more than 300/μL when assessed over 60 weeks.[44] In the multicentre **ANDHI trial**, assessing 656 adults with severe eosinophilic asthma (peripheral blood eosinophil counts ≥150/μL and 2 or more exacerbations in the previous year), patients were randomized to Benralizumab or placebo group for 24 weeks; Benralizumab was shown to decrease annual asthma exacerbations when compared with placebo.[45] In the **ZONDA trial**, Benralizumab at 28 weeks of therapy in severe eosinophilic asthma patients was able to decrease oral corticosteroid dose by 75% from baseline compared with 25% in the placebo group.[46] Oral steroids were successfully tapered off in 62% of 598 participants of the **PONENTE study** with Benralizumab therapy.[47] The 2024 phase 4 RCT **(SHAMAL trial)** demonstrated that in severe eosinophilic asthma controlled with Benralizumab therapy reduction of ICS dose can be carried out while maintaining the asthma control.[4] However, larger sample sized trials are required to draw concrete conclusions.

Anti-IL4 receptor therapy

Dupilumab

Mechanism of action: Dupilumab binds to IL-4R alpha receptor and inhibits IL-4 and IL-13 signaling and inflammatory response.

Approved use:

a. Patients **aged ≥6 years with moderate to severe eosinophilic or oral glucocorticoid dependent asthma uncontrolled on standard therapy with peripheral blood eosinophil count ≥150/µL.**

b. Asthma with comorbid moderate to severe atopic dermatitis.

c. Atopic dermatitis.

d. Eosinophilic esophagitis.

e. Prurigo nodularis.

f. Rhinosinusitis with nasal polyposis.

Dose in asthma: There are two dosing regimens:

a. 400 mg once (given as 200 mg injections) followed by 200 mg every 2 weeks.

b. **600 mg once (given as 300 mg injections) followed by 300 mg every 2 weeks. (Preferred for oral steroid-dependent asthma and in those complicated with severe atopic dermatitis).**

No dosing adjustment for hepatic or renal dysfunction. Response to treatment is assessed after 4 months of therapy.

Method of administration: Given subcutaneously into the upper arm, thigh, or lower abdomen. It should not be injected into moles, scars, bruises, tender areas, or broken skin. Thigh injection resulted in slightly higher exposure than upper arm injection, and abdomen injection resulted in exposure like or slightly lower than thigh injection; however, these differences were found to be not clinically significant.[48]

Adverse effect: Local site reaction and upper respiratory tract infection are the most reported adverse effect of Dupilumab. As IL-4/IL-13 acts as a restrain on Th17-mediated inflammation, inhibition of these cytokines can precipitate Th17 inflammatory diseases like seronegative arthritis, psoriasis and iridocyclitis.[49]

Evidence: In a multicentre trial, 1902 patients aged 12 years or older with poorly controlled asthma were randomly assigned to one of the two dosing regimens of dupilumab and to placebo, administered every two weeks for 52 weeks. The Dupilumab group had reduction in annualised exacerbation rate by 50% when compared to placebo. There was a statistically significant increase in FEV1 with both doses of Dupilumab. In a post hoc analysis of the study, Dupilumab improved exacerbation in patients with peripheral blood eosinophil levels ≥150/µL regardless of the IgE levels. A clinically meaningful improvement in asthma control was seen in patients with peripheral blood eosinophil levels greater than 500/µL.[50] Dupilumab also has a glucocorticoid-sparing effect with a 70% reduction in the dose of oral steroids at the end of 24 weeks of therapy with 300 mg every 2 weekly doses.[51]

Anti thymic stromal lymphopoietin (anti-TSLP)

TSLP is an epithelial cell-derived cytokine released in response to a range of epithelial insults (allergens, viruses, bacteria, pollutants, smoke) that is responsible for the initiation and persistence of inflammation in asthma.[52] Inhibition of TSLP is a novel approach to treating the diverse phenotypes and endotypes of asthma.

Tezepelumab

Mechanism of action: Binding of Tezepelumab to TSLP prevents TSLP from interacting with the heterodimeric TSLP receptor thereby reducing inflammation mediated by eosinophils, IgE, IL-5 and IL-13.

Approved use: Approved as an **add-on therapy in patients ≥12 years of age with severe asthma not controlled with standard medication**. A minimum baseline level of blood eosinophil or FeNO is not required.

Dose in asthma: 210 mg every 4 weeks. No dosing adjustment for hepatic or renal dysfunction. Response to treatment is assessed after 4 months of therapy.

Method of administration: Given subcutaneous into upper arm, thigh or lower abdomen. It should not be injected into moles, scars, bruises, tender areas or broken skin.

Adverse effect: Injection site reaction, arthralgias, back pain and pharyngitis has been reported.

Evidence: In the **PATHWAY trial**, 550 patients with moderate to severe asthma with at least two asthma exacerbations or one that required hospitalisation in the previous year despite standard therapy were assigned to placebo or one of the three different doses of Tezepelumab (70mg, 210mg or 280 mg 4 weekly). After 52 weeks the Tezepelumab group had a similar decrease in exacerbation rate when compared with placebo. **The treatment arm also showed a small improvement in symptom control, quality of life and a significant reduction in emergency department visits**. Improvements were similar regardless of baseline blood eosinophil count, FeNO or presence of perennial allergy.[53,54] A post hoc analysis of data of the PATHWAY trial to assess the efficacy of Tezepelumab in participants with perennial allergy and meeting the criteria for Omalizumab demonstrated that Tezepelumab decreased annualised asthma exacerbation rate by 66% to 78% in patients with perennial allergy and 67% to 71% in patients without perennial allergy. **Tezepelumab improved prebronchodilator FEV1, and reduced blood eosinophil and FeNO irrespective of perennial allergy status.**[55] **In the NAVIGATOR trial, 1059 patients (618 with eosinophil count ≥300/µL, 441 with eosinophil count less than 300/µL) were randomised to 210 mg every 4-weekly dose of Tezepelumab or placebo. At the end of 52 weeks, the Tezepelumab group had a 56% relative reduction in exacerbation rate**. Patients with peripheral blood eosinophil count < 300/µL had a clinically significant but smaller reduction in exacerbation than compared with patients with higher eosinophil levels. Tezepelumab was associated with fewer exacerbations requiring hospitalisation. There was small, clinically non-significant improvement in asthma control and quality of life along with a modest improvement in prebronchodilator FEV1.[53]

In the SOURCE trial, 210 mg every 4-weekly dose of Tezepelumab had no overall significant effect on oral glucocorticoid reduction. However, there was evidence of improved glucocorticoid requirement in subgroups of patients with blood eosinophil count ≥150/µL.[56] A systematic review demonstrated better performance of Tezepelumab over placebo in decreasing asthma exacerbation, asthma control, reducing blood eosinophil count, IgE levels and FeNO.[57]

Other upcoming biologics in asthma

- **Anti-IL13 antibodies (Lebrikizumab and Tralokinumab):** IL-13 promotes IgE production by B cells, generation of eosinophil chemo-attractants and contractility of airway smooth muscle. In a randomized trial of 2148 patients with uncontrolled asthma, lebrikizumab (37.5mg or 125 mg) or placebo was administered every 4 weekly for 52 weeks. **The trial demonstrated inconsistent results in terms of a clinically significant reduction in exacerbation.**[58] Randomized trials have shown inconsistent results in terms of lung function improvement with the use of Lebrikizumab.[59,60] **Trials of Tralokinumab have also shown inconsistent effects.**[61,62]
- **Anti-IL23 antibody (Risankisumab):** IL-23 causes the release of cytokines from Th2 lymphocytes and promotes proliferation of Th17 lymphocytes. Risankisumab is an anti-IL-23p19 monoclonal antibody; though it's used in psoriasis, its use in asthma remains doubtful with randomized trials failing to demonstrate benefit.[63]

- **Anti-IL33 (Itepekimab) and IL33/ST2 (Astegolimab) antibodies:** IL33 is released with airway epithelial cells, endothelial cells and mast cells in response to cell damage caused by irritants. IL-33 in-turns activate both the innate and adaptive immune system leading to airway inflammation. A phase 2 randomised study comparing 4 subcutaneous regimens (Itepekimab, Dupilumab, Itepekimab + Dupilumab, placebo) demonstrated an improvement in lung function due to monotherapy with Itepekimab and Dupilumab when compared to placebo. Combination therapy did not cause an improvement in lung function.[64] A phase 2 multicenter randomized trial (ZENYATTA) on Astegolimab demonstrated a reduction in exacerbation when compared to placebo.[65]
- **Prostaglandin D2 receptor antagonist (Fevipiprant):** Prostaglandin D2 is the predominant prostaglandin produced by mast cells which can cause bronchoconstriction and chemokinetic action. Randomized trials have demonstrated a clinically significant reduction in the rate of exacerbation with Fevipiprant at a dose of 450 mg daily along with small improvement in lung function.[66,67] Fevipiprant is being evaluated in severe asthma.[67] It was previously evaluated for non-severe asthma and was found to have a role akin to montelukast. However, **neither is fevipiprant a part of routine practice nor has the GINA guidelines recognised it as a drug for management of asthma.**

How to choose a biologic for severe asthma?

- **In India, currently omalizumab, mepolizumab, and benralizumab are approved for use in asthma. Presently, Dupilumab is not approved in India for asthma (currently approved for atopic dermatitis in India).**
- **We recommend pheno-endotyping of all severe asthma patients prior to choosing an add-on biologic agent.**
- For severe asthma, **patients not dependent on oral corticosteroids** and having poor symptom control, blood eosinophil and FeNO can be used to decide add on therapy.
- **Blood eosinophils are < 150 cells/µL and FeNO < 25 ppb**:
  - o **History of perennial allergy or atopy present: Omalizumab** therapy is recommended (provided IgE level is within dosing range).
  - o There is **no history of perennial allergy or atopy: Consider Tezepelumab** therapy (Not yet available in India).
- **Blood eosinophils are < 150 cells/µL and FeNO > 25 ppb**:
  - o **History of perennial allergy or atopy present: Omalizumab therapy** (provided IgE level is within dosing range) **or Dupilumab therapy** is recommended.
  - o **No history of perennial allergy or atopy: Dupilumab or Tezepelumab therapy** is recommended.
- **Blood eosinophils are > 1500 cells/µL:**
  - o **Mepolizumab, Reslizumab or Benralizumab** therapy is recommended after **ruling out other hyper-eosinophilic conditions**.
- **Blood eosinophils levels between 50 - 1500 cells/µL:**
  - o The therapy depends on the **dominant biomarker** and underlying co-morbidities.
- **Steroid-dependent severe asthma patients:**
  - o **Mepolizumab, Reslizumab or Benralizumab therapy is recommended if there is current or recent history of increased serum eosinophil levels.**
  - o **Dupilumab therapy is recommended if there is no current or recent history of increased serum eosinophil levels.**
- Adequate safety and efficacy data is available for Omalizumab, Benralizumab, Mepolizumab, Reslizumab and Tezepelumab. **All these agents are USA FDA-approved as add-on treatments** for severe asthma. A choice of biologic can be made

based on the pheno-endotype of the patient, local availability and cost. **As per a recent network meta-analysis, for patients of eosinophilic asthma, there is very little to differentiate between mepolizumab, benralizumab and dupilumab in terms of safety and efficacy. In India presently Omalizumab, Benralizumab and Mepolizumab are only the ones available for use.**

- **In case of insignificant response to prescribed biologic over 4-6 months, switchover to other eligible biologics may be done.**

Clinical response and clinical remission in severe asthma patients treated with biologics

- **Clinical response:** Severe asthma patients following 12 months of treatment with biologics has ≥50% reduction in exacerbation and/or a ≥50% reduction in maintenance oral corticosteroid dose.[68] **As per data of Danish Severe Asthma Register following 12 months of biologic therapy 79% of patients showed clinical response.**

- **Clinical remission: Severe asthma patients following 12 months of treatment with biologics have Asthma Control Questionnaire (ACQ)-5 <1.5, need no oral corticosteroids for disease control and FEV1 above the lower limit of normal or no more than 100ml less than baseline.** As per a retrospective, observational analysis of severe asthma patients registered in UK Severe Asthma Registry, 18% of severe patients attained clinical remission following 12 months of biologics therapy.[69]

When to stop biologic therapy in severe asthma?

Although the patient selection, initiation and dosing of biological therapy is well established by guidelines and numerous randomised control trials it is largely unknown as to how long the therapy is to be continued. Sudden cessation of therapy has been shown to increase the risk of exacerbations in severe eosinophilic asthma patients who were well controlled on Mepolizumab.[70]

Taking cues from down titration of biologics in rheumatic diseases once disease control has been attained, trials have tested down-titration of biologics once clinical remission is attained. **The OMADORE study and OPTIMAL study have explored protocol based down-titration of Omalizumab and anti-IL5 therapy respectively.**[7,71] Further studies on long term prognosis of titration and potential adjustments to these titration algorithms are required to enable clinical implementation guidelines. **Presently, GINA guidelines note that whether benefits are sustained after cessation of biologics and the duration of treatment required to have sustained benefits are unclear. Biologics are part of precision medicine and therefore the duration needs to be individualized to each patient. When a biologic is used, an initial duration of 4 months of therapy should be given before assessing for response. If there is no response, switching to another biologic is advised. If there is response after 4 months of use, the biologic should be continued for 6-12 months. Following this a reassessment of response should be done. If there is a good response, re-evaluate the patient every 3-6 months and consider the following steps in order:**

1. First consider tapering down OCS.
2. If asthma is well controlled at 3-6 months, consider tapering down ICS-LABA from high-dose to as low a dose as possible. Do not stop ICS-LABA maintenance.
3. If asthma is well controlled at 3-6 months, consider the need for ongoing biologic therapy and whether it can be tapered down to a full withdrawal or not. The risk of losing asthma control is a possibility that should be discussed during this step.

There are no RCTs that have evaluated these steps in order. However, **GINA guidelines recommend the order based on 'observed benefit, potential side-effects, cost, and patient preference'. It is equally important to individualize the withdrawal of therapy in severe asthma as it is to initiate. Patients should actively participate in the decision making process.**

Management of Severe Asthma

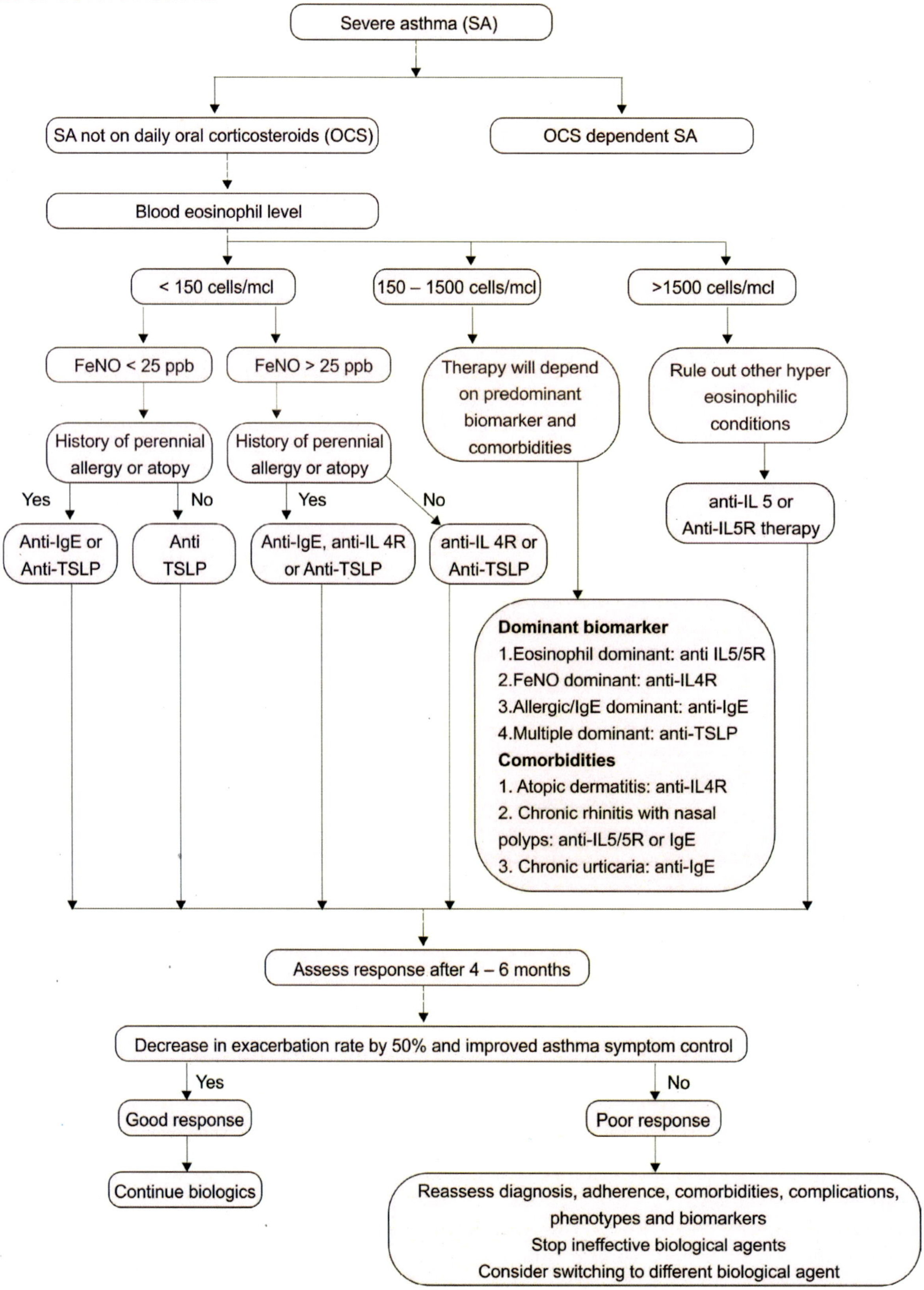

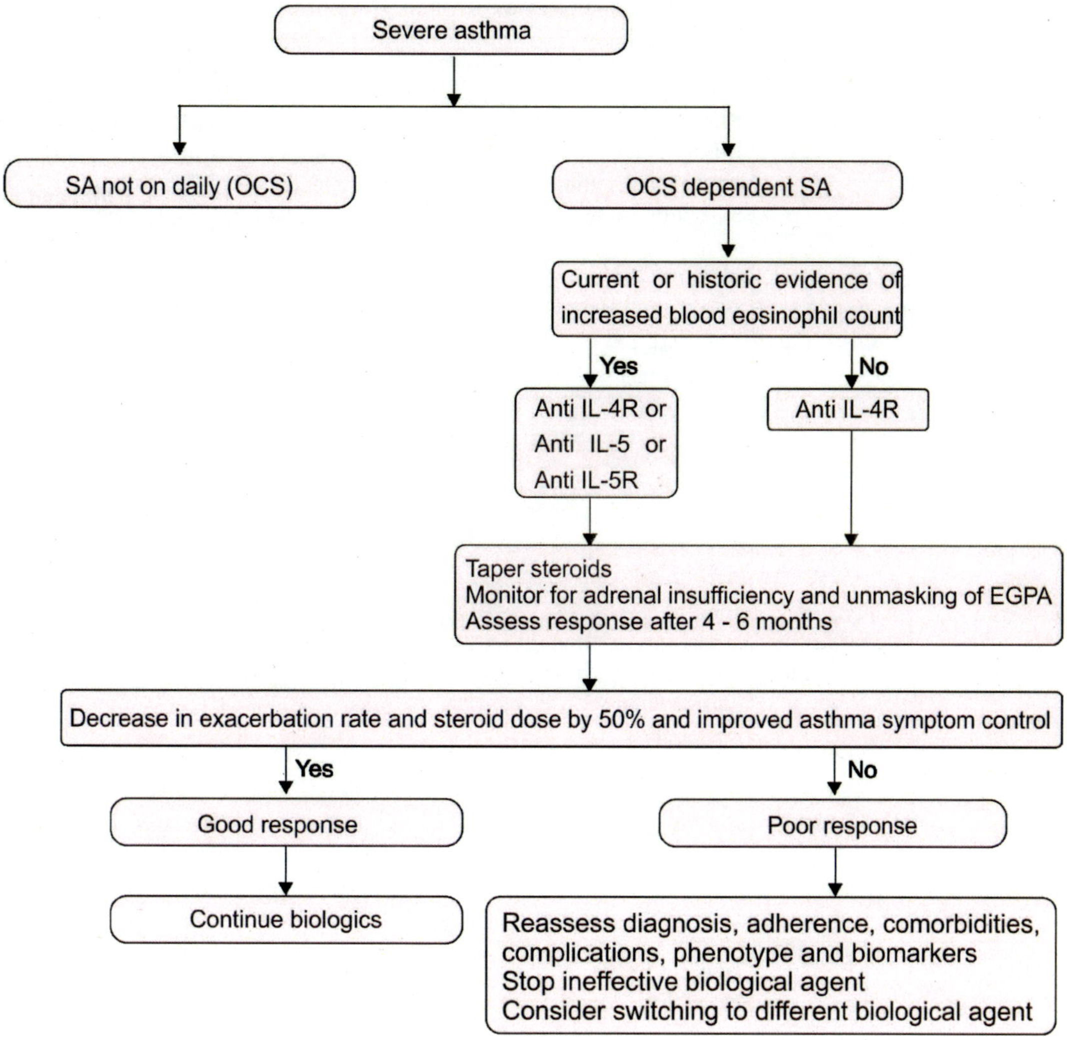
Severe asthma
SA not on daily (OCS)
OCS dependent SA
Current or historic evidence of increased blood eosinophil count
Yes
No
Anti IL-4R or Anti IL-5 or Anti IL-5R
Anti IL-4R
Taper steroids
Monitor for adrenal insufficiency and unmasking of EGPA
Assess response after 4 - 6 months
Decrease in exacerbation rate and steroid dose by 50% and improved asthma symptom control
Yes
No
Good response
Poor response
Continue biologics
Reassess diagnosis, adherence, comorbidities, complications, phenotype and biomarkers
Stop ineffective biological agent
Consider switching to different biological agent

Summary of Biologics in Severe Bronchial Asthma

S. no.	Name	Target	Biological effect	Dosing	Indication
1	Omalizumab*	IgE	Prevents binding of IgE to its receptors on mast cells and basophils	Varies from 75 mg to 375 mg every 2 to 4 weeks and depends on patient's weight and total IgE levels Or 0.016 mg/kg per IU/ml of IgE per month	Moderate to severe allergic asthma IgE ≥ 30 IU/ml and within dosing range Sensitisation on skin prick test
2	Mepolizumab*	IL 5	Inhibits IL5 signalling	100 mg SC every 4 weeks	Severe eosinophilic asthma with blood eosinophil level ≥ 300/microL at anytime in last 1 year
3	Reslizumab	IL 5	Inhibits IL5 signalling	3 mg/kg IV very 4 weeks	Severe eosinophilic asthma with blood eosinophil level ≥ 400/microL
4	Benralizumab*	Alpha subunit of IL 5 receptor	Inhibits IL 5 signalling resulting in reduced production and survival of eosinophils and basophils	30 mg SC every 4 weeks for the first 3 doses then once every 8 weeks	Severe eosinophilic asthma with blood eosinophil level ≥ 300/microL at any time in last 1 year
5	Dupilumab	IL 4R alpha receptor	Inhibits IL 4 and IL 13 signalling and inflammatory response.	400 mg SC once (given as 200 mg injections) followed by 200 mg every 2 weeks	Severe eosinophilic asthma with blood eosinophil level ≥ 150/microL or FeNO ≥ 25 ppb
6	Tezepelumab	TSLP	Inhibits TSLP signalling	210 mg SC every 4 weeks	Severe asthma with high or low eosinophil levels, oral corticosteroid dependent asthma

* Currently available in India

REFERENCES

1. Kyriakopoulos C, Gogali A, Markozannes G, Kostikas K. Biologic agents licensed for severe asthma: a systematic review and meta-analysis of randomised controlled trials. Eur Respir Rev. 2024 Apr 30;33(172):230238.

2. Corren J, Menzies-Gow A, Chupp G, Israel E, Korn S, Cook B, et al. Efficacy of Tezepelumab in Severe, Uncontrolled Asthma: Pooled Analysis of the PATHWAY and NAVIGATOR Clinical Trials. Am J Respir Crit Care Med. 2023 Jul 1;208(1):13–24.

3. Fong KY, Zhao JJ, Syn NL, Nair P, Chan YH, Lee P. Comparing bronchial thermoplasty with biologicals for severe asthma: Systematic review and network meta-analysis. Respir Med. 2023 Sep;216:107302.

4. Jackson DJ, Heaney LG, Humbert M, Kent BD, Shavit A, Hiljemark L, et al. Reduction of daily maintenance inhaled corticosteroids in patients with severe eosinophilic asthma treated with benralizumab (SHAMAL): a randomised, multicentre, open-label, phase 4 study. The Lancet. 2024 Jan;403(10423):271–81.

5. Zhang Y, Zhang M, Zhang J, Li Q, Lu M, Cheng L. Combination of omalizumab with allergen immunotherapy versus immunotherapy alone for allergic diseases: A meta-analysis of randomized controlled trials. Int Forum Allergy Rhinol. 2024 Apr;14(4):794–806.

6. Phinyo P, Krikeerati T, Vichara-Anont I, Thongngarm T. Efficacy and Safety of Biologics for Oral Corticosteroid–Dependent Asthma: A Systematic Review and Network Meta-Analysis. J Allergy Clin Immunol Pract. 2024 Feb;12(2):409–20.

7. Soendergaard MB, Bjerrum AS, Rasmussen LM, Lock-Johansson S, Hilberg O, Hansen S, et al. Titration of anti-IL-5 biologics in severe asthma: an open-label randomised controlled trial (the OPTIMAL study). Eur Respir J. 2024 Aug;64(2):2400404.

8. Levy BD, Noel PJ, Freemer MM, Cloutier MM, Georas SN, Jarjour NN, et al. Future Research Directions in Asthma. An NHLBI Working Group Report. Am J Respir Crit Care Med. 2015 Dec 1;192 (11):1366–72.

9. Guida G, Bagnasco D, Carriero V, Bertolini F, Ricciardolo FLM, Nicola S, et al. Critical evaluation of asthma biomarkers in clinical practice. Front Med. 2022 Oct 10;9:969243.

10. Gvalani A, Athavale A, Gupta D. Biomarkers in severe asthma: Identifying the treatable trait. Lung India. 2023;40(1):59.

11. Israel, E, Canonica, GW, Brusselle, G, Yang, S, Howarth, PH, Martin, AL, et al. Real-life effectiveness of mepolizumab in severe asthma: a systematic literature review. J Asthma. 2022 Nov 2;59(11):2201–17.

12. Habib N, Pasha MA, Tang DD. Current Understanding of Asthma Pathogenesis and Biomarkers. Cells. 2022 Sep 5;11(17):2764.

13. Simpson JL, McElduff P, Gibson PG. Assessment and Reproducibility of Non-Eosinophilic Asthma Using Induced Sputum. Respiration. 2010;79(2):147–51.

14. Takayama G, Arima K, Kanaji T, Toda S, Tanaka H, Shoji S, et al. Periostin: A novel component of subepithelial fibrosis of bronchial asthma downstream of IL-4 and IL-13 signals. J Allergy Clin Immunol. 2006 Jul;118(1):98–104.

15. Fouka E, Domvri K, Gkakou F, Alevizaki M, Steiropoulos P, Papakosta D, et al. Recent insights in the role of biomarkers in severe asthma management. Front Med. 2022 Sep 26;9:992565.

16. Thomson NC, Chaudhuri R, Spears M, Haughney J, McSharry C. Serum periostin in smokers and never smokers with asthma. Respir Med. 2015 Jun;109(6):708–15.

17. Simpson JL, Scott R, Boyle MJ, Gibson PG. Inflammatory subtypes in asthma: Assessment and identification using induced sputum. Respirology. 2006 Jan;11(1):54–61.

18. Brusselle GG, Koppelman GH. Biologic Therapies for Severe Asthma. Taichman DB, editor. N Engl J Med. 2022 Jan 13;386(2):157–71.

19. Riccio AM, Mauri P, De Ferrari L, Rossi R, Di Silvestre D, Benazzi L, et al. Galectin-3: an early predictive biomarker of modulation of airway remodeling in patients with severe asthma treated with omalizumab for 36 months. Clin Transl Allergy. 2017 Dec;7(1):6.

20. Konradsen JR, James A, Nordlund B, Reinius LE, Söderhäll C, Melén E, et al. The chitinase-like protein YKL-40: A possible biomarker of inflammation and airway remodeling in severe pediatric asthma. J Allergy Clin Immunol. 2013 Aug;132(2):328-335.e5.

21. Specjalski K, Romantowski J, Niedoszytko M. YKL-40 as a possible marker of neutrophilic asthma. Front Med. 2023 Feb 8;10:1115938.

22. Lemonnier N, Melén E, Jiang Y, Joly S, Ménard C, Aguilar D, et al. A novel whole blood gene expression signature for asthma, dermatitis, and rhinitis multimorbidity in children and adolescents. Allergy. 2020 Dec;75(12):3248–60.

23. Liu L, Teague WG, Erzurum S, Fitzpatrick A, Mantri S, Dweik RA, et al. Determinants of Exhaled Breath Condensate pH in a Large Population With Asthma. Chest. 2011 Feb;139(2):328–36.

24. Peel AM, Wilkinson M, Sinha A, Loke YK, Fowler SJ, Wilson AM. Volatile organic compounds associated with diagnosis and disease characteristics in asthma – A systematic review. Respir Med. 2020 Aug;169:105984.

25. Barcik W, Boutin RCT, Sokolowska M, Finlay BB. The Role of Lung and Gut Microbiota in the Pathology of Asthma. Immunity. 2020 Feb;52(2):241–55.

26. Huang YJ, Nariya S, Harris JM, Lynch SV, Choy DF, Arron JR, et al. The airway microbiome in patients with severe asthma: Associations with disease features and severity. J Allergy Clin Immunol. 2015 Oct;136(4):874–84.

27. Lee LA, Bailes Z, Barnes N, Boulet LP, Edwards D, Fowler A, et al. Efficacy and safety of once-daily single-inhaler triple therapy (FF/UMEC/VI) versus FF/VI in patients with inadequately controlled

asthma (CAPTAIN): a double-blind, randomised, phase 3A trial. Lancet Respir Med. 2021 Jan;9(1):69–84.

28. Virchow JC, Kuna P, Paggiaro P, Papi A, Singh D, Corre S, et al. Single inhaler extrafine triple therapy in uncontrolled asthma (TRIMARAN and TRIGGER): two double-blind, parallel-group, randomised, controlled phase 3 trials. The Lancet. 2019 Nov;394(10210):1737–49.

29. Kerstjens HAM, Maspero J, Chapman KR, Van Zyl-Smit RN, Hosoe M, Tanase AM, et al. Once-daily, single-inhaler mometasone–indacaterol–glycopyrronium versus mometasone–indacaterol or twice-daily fluticasone–salmeterol in patients with inadequately controlled asthma (IRIDIUM): a randomised, double-blind, controlled phase 3 study. Lancet Respir Med. 2020 Oct;8(10):1000–12.

30. Hanania NA, Alpan O, Hamilos DL, Condemi JJ, Reyes-Rivera I, Zhu J, et al. Omalizumab in Severe Allergic Asthma Inadequately Controlled With Standard Therapy: A Randomized Trial. Ann Intern Med. 2011 May 3;154(9):573.

31. Hanania NA, Fortis S, Haselkorn T, Gupta S, Mumneh N, Yoo B, et al. Omalizumab in Asthma with Fixed Airway Obstruction: Post Hoc Analysis of EXTRA. J Allergy Clin Immunol Pract. 2022 Jan;10(1):222–8.

32. Bousquet J, Humbert M, Gibson PG, Kostikas K, Jaumont X, Pfister P, et al. Real-World Effectiveness of Omalizumab in Severe Allergic Asthma: A Meta-Analysis of Observational Studies. J Allergy Clin Immunol Pract. 2021 Jul;9(7):2702–14.

33. Jin M, Douglass JA, Elborn JS, Agarwal R, Calhoun WJ, Lazarewicz S, et al. Omalizumab in Allergic Bronchopulmonary Aspergillosis: A Systematic Review and Meta-Analysis. J Allergy Clin Immunol Pract. 2023 Mar;11(3):896–905.

34. Harvey ES, Langton D, Katelaris C, Stevens S, Farah CS, Gillman A, et al. Mepolizumab effectiveness and identification of super-responders in severe asthma. Eur Respir J. 2020 May;55(5):1902420.

35. Ortega HG, Liu MC, Pavord ID, Brusselle GG, FitzGerald JM, Chetta A, et al. Mepolizumab treatment in patients with severe eosinophilic asthma. N Engl J Med. 2014 Sep 25;371(13):1198–207.

36. Bel EH, Wenzel SE, Thompson PJ, Prazma CM, Keene ON, Yancey SW, et al. Oral glucocorticoid-sparing effect of mepolizumab in eosinophilic asthma. N Engl J Med. 2014 Sep 25;371(13):1189–97.

37. Haldar P, Brightling CE, Hargadon B, Gupta S, Monteiro W, Sousa A, et al. Mepolizumab and exacerbations of refractory eosinophilic asthma. N Engl J Med. 2009 Mar 5;360(10):973–84.

38. Mullol J, Lund VJ, Wagenmann M, Han JK, Sousa AN, Smith SG, et al. Mepolizumab improves sense of smell in severe chronic rhinosinusitis with nasal polyps: SYNAPSE. Rhinol J. 2023 Jan 1;0(0):0–0.

39. Castro M, Mathur S, Hargreave F, Boulet LP, Xie F, Young J, et al. Reslizumab for poorly controlled, eosinophilic asthma: a randomized, placebo-controlled study. Am J Respir Crit Care Med. 2011 Nov 15;184(10):1125–32.

40. Agache I, Beltran J, Akdis C, Akdis M, Canelo-Aybar C, Canonica GW, et al. Efficacy and safety of treatment with biologicals (benralizumab, dupilumab, mepolizumab, omalizumab and reslizumab) for severe eosinophilic asthma. A systematic review for the EAACI Guidelines - recommendations on the use of biologicals in severe asthma. Allergy. 2020 May;75(5):1023–42.

41. Bjermer L, Lemiere C, Maspero J, Weiss S, Zangrilli J, Germinaro M. Reslizumab for Inadequately Controlled Asthma With Elevated Blood Eosinophil Levels: A Randomized Phase 3 Study. Chest. 2016 Oct;150(4):789–98.

42. Corren J, Weinstein S, Janka L, Zangrilli J, Garin M. Phase 3 Study of Reslizumab in Patients With Poorly Controlled Asthma: Effects Across a Broad Range of Eosinophil Counts. Chest. 2016 Oct;150(4):799–810.

43. Bleecker ER, FitzGerald JM, Chanez P, Papi A, Weinstein SF, Barker P, et al. Efficacy and safety of benralizumab for patients with severe asthma uncontrolled with high-dosage inhaled corticosteroids and long-acting β2-agonists (SIROCCO): a randomised, multicentre, placebo-controlled phase 3 trial. Lancet Lond Engl. 2016 Oct 29;388(10056):2115–27.

44. FitzGerald JM, Bleecker ER, Nair P, Korn S, Ohta K, Lommatzsch M, et al. Benralizumab, an anti-interleukin-5 receptor α monoclonal antibody, as add-on treatment for patients with severe, uncontrolled, eosinophilic asthma (CALIMA): a randomised, double-blind, placebo-controlled phase 3 trial. Lancet Lond Engl. 2016 Oct 29;388(10056):2128–41.

45. Harrison TW, Chanez P, Menzella F, Canonica GW, Louis R, Cosio BG, et al. Onset of effect and impact on health-related quality of life, exacerbation rate, lung function, and nasal polyposis symptoms for patients with severe eosinophilic asthma treated with benralizumab (ANDHI): a randomised, controlled, phase 3b trial. Lancet Respir Med. 2021 Mar;9(3):260–74.

46. Nair P, Wenzel S, Rabe KF, Bourdin A, Lugogo NL, Kuna P, et al. Oral Glucocorticoid-Sparing Effect of Benralizumab in Severe Asthma. N Engl J Med. 2017 Jun 22;376(25):2448–58.

47. Menzies-Gow A, Gurnell M, Heaney LG, Corren J, Bel EH, Maspero J, et al. Oral corticosteroid elimination via a personalised reduction algorithm in adults with severe, eosinophilic asthma treated with benralizumab (PONENTE): a multicentre, open-label, single-arm study. Lancet Respir Med. 2022 Jan;10(1):47–58.

48. Zheng Y, Abuqayyas L, Megally A, Fuhr R, Salapa K, Downie J, et al. Tezepelumab Pharmacokinetics, Safety, and Tolerability After Administration via Vial-and-syringe, Accessorized Prefilled Syringe, or Autoinjector: A Randomized Trial in Healthy Volunteers. Clin Ther. 2021 Jan;43(1):142-155.e5.

49. Bridgewood C, Wittmann M, Macleod T, Watad A, Newton D, Bhan K, et al. T Helper 2 IL-4/IL-13 Dual Blockade with Dupilumab Is Linked to Some Emergent T Helper 17 Type Diseases, Including Seronegative Arthritis and Enthesitis/Enthesopathy, but Not to Humoral Autoimmune Diseases. J Invest Dermatol. 2022 Oct;142(10):2660–7.

50. Rabe KF, Pavord ID, Castro M, Wechsler ME, Daizadeh N, Kapoor U, et al. Dupilumab efficacy and safety in patients with asthma and blood eosinophils ≥500 cells·µL-1. Eur Respir J. 2022 Jun; 59(6):2102577.

51. Rabe KF, Nair P, Brusselle G, Maspero JF, Castro M, Sher L, et al. Efficacy and Safety of Dupilumab in Glucocorticoid-Dependent Severe Asthma. N Engl J Med. 2018 Jun 28;378(26):2475–85.

52. Parnes J, Molfino NA, Colice G, Martin U, Corren J, Menzies-Gow A. Targeting TSLP in Asthma. J Asthma Allergy. 2022 Jun;Volume 15:749–65.

53. Menzies-Gow A, Corren J, Bourdin A, Chupp G, Israel E, Wechsler ME, et al. Tezepelumab in Adults and Adolescents with Severe, Uncontrolled Asthma. N Engl J Med. 2021 May 13;384(19):1800–9.

54. Corren J, Garcia Gil E, Griffiths JM, Parnes JR, van der Merwe R, Salapa K, et al. Tezepelumab improves patient-reported outcomes in patients with severe, uncontrolled asthma in PATHWAY. Ann Allergy Asthma Immunol. 2021 Feb;126(2):187–93.

55. Corren J, Ambrose CS, Salapa K, Roseti SL, Griffiths JM, Parnes JR, et al. Efficacy of Tezepelumab in Patients with Severe, Uncontrolled Asthma and Perennial Allergy. J Allergy Clin Immunol Pract. 2021 Dec;9(12):4334-4342.e6.

56. Wechsler ME, Menzies-Gow A, Brightling CE, Kuna P, Korn S, Welte T, et al. Evaluation of the oral corticosteroid-sparing effect of tezepelumab in adults with oral corticosteroid-dependent asthma (SOURCE): a randomised, placebo-controlled, phase 3 study. Lancet Respir Med. 2022 Jul;10(7):650–60.

57. Shaban Abdelgalil M, Ahmed Elrashedy A, Awad AK, Reda Gad E, Ali MM, Abdelmoez Farahat R, et al. Safety and efficacy of tezepelumab vs. placebo in adult patients with severe uncontrolled asthma: a systematic review and meta-analysis. Sci Rep. 2022 Dec 3;12(1):20905.

58. Hanania NA, Korenblat P, Chapman KR, Bateman ED, Kopecky P, Paggiaro P, et al. Efficacy and safety of lebrikizumab in patients with uncontrolled asthma (LAVOLTA I and LAVOLTA II): replicate, phase 3, randomised, double-blind, placebo-controlled trials. Lancet Respir Med. 2016 Oct;4(10):781–96.

59. Corren J, Lemanske RF, Hanania NA, Korenblat PE, Parsey MV, Arron JR, et al. Lebrikizumab Treatment in Adults with Asthma. N Engl J Med. 2011 Sep 22;365(12):1088–98.

60. Noonan M, Korenblat P, Mosesova S, Scheerens H, Arron JR, Zheng Y, et al. Dose-ranging study of lebrikizumab in asthmatic patients not receiving inhaled steroids. J Allergy Clin Immunol. 2013 Sep;132(3):567-574.e12.

61. Panettieri RA, Sjöbring U, Péterffy A, Wessman P, Bowen K, Piper E, et al. Tralokinumab for severe, uncontrolled asthma (STRATOS 1 and STRATOS 2): two randomised, double-blind, placebo-controlled, phase 3 clinical trials. Lancet Respir Med. 2018 Jul;6(7):511–25.

62. Piper E, Brightling C, Niven R, Oh C, Faggioni R, Poon K, et al. A phase II placebo-controlled study of tralokinumab in moderate-to-severe asthma. Eur Respir J. 2013 Feb;41(2):330–8.

63. Brightling CE, Nair P, Cousins DJ, Louis R, Singh D. Risankizumab in Severe Asthma — A Phase 2a, Placebo-Controlled Trial. N Engl J Med. 2021 Oct 28;385(18):1669–79.

64. Wechsler ME, Ruddy MK, Pavord ID, Israel E, Rabe KF, Ford LB, et al. Efficacy and Safety of Itepekimab in Patients with Moderate-to-Severe Asthma. N Engl J Med. 2021 Oct 28;385(18):1656–68.

65. Kelsen SG, Agache IO, Soong W, Israel E, Chupp GL, Cheung DS, et al. Astegolimab (anti-ST2) efficacy and safety in adults with severe asthma: A randomized clinical trial. J Allergy Clin Immunol. 2021 Sep;148(3):790–8.

66. Maspero J, Agache IO, Kamei T, Yoshida M, Boone B, Felser JM, et al. Long-term safety and exploratory efficacy of fevipiprant in patients with inadequately controlled asthma: the SPIRIT randomised clinical trial. Respir Res. 2021 Dec;22(1):311.

67. Brightling CE, Gaga M, Inoue H, Li J, Maspero J, Wenzel S, et al. Effectiveness of fevipiprant in reducing exacerbations in patients with severe asthma (LUSTER-1 and LUSTER-2): two phase 3 randomised controlled trials. Lancet Respir Med. 2021 Jan;9(1):43–56.

68. Hansen S, Baastrup Søndergaard M, Von Bülow A, Bjerrum AS, Schmid J, Rasmussen LM, et al. Clinical Response and Remission in Patients With Severe Asthma Treated With Biologic Therapies. CHEST. 2024 Feb;165(2):253–66.

69. McDowell PJ, McDowell R, Busby J, Eastwood MC, Patel PH, Jackson DJ, et al. Clinical remission in severe asthma with biologic therapy: an analysis from the UK Severe Asthma Registry. Eur Respir J. 2023 Dec;62(6):2300819.

70. Moore WC, Kornmann O, Humbert M, Poirier C, Bel EH, Kaneko N, et al. Stopping *versus* continuing long-term mepolizumab treatment in severe eosinophilic asthma (COMET study). Eur Respir J. 2022 Jan;59(1):2100396.

71. Domingo C, Pomares X, Navarro A, Amengual MJ, Montón C, Sogo A, et al. A step down protocol for omalizumab treatment in oral corticosteroid dependent allergic asthma patients. Br J Clin Pharmacol. 2018 Feb;84(2):339–48.

CHAPTER 2

Chronic Obstructive Pulmonary Disease

Author: Dr. Hariharan Iyer

Reviewer: Dr. Mansi Gupta

INTRODUCTION

COPD is a chronic disease of the airways caused by multifactorial etiologies. It is responsible for significant mortality and morbidity. Understanding this disease, including its treatment, is ever-changing, with newer concepts emerging every year. This review will focus on the latest updates in the diagnosis and management of COPD.

Methodology

A PubMed search was done using the search terms "COPD", or "Chronic Obstructive Pulmonary Disease", or "chronic obstructive pulmonary disease". The search term was limited to Randomised Control Trials between 1st August 2023 and 1st August 2024. A total of 238 articles were screened. Of these, 27 articles that were irrelevant to the discussion were removed. The remaining articles were analysed and included for discussion. Additional helpful articles were also added to facilitate the flow of the article for driving through the relevant points.

Electronic database search: PubMed

Period: 1st August 2023 to 1st August 2024

Search term used: "COPD" or "Chronic Obstructive Pulmonary Disease" or "chronic obstructive pulmonary diseases"

(n=238)

↓

Articles analysed: 25

Flowchart 1: Search term used and selection of eligible and excluded articles

Analysis of Literature

1. Diagnosis of COPD

- ***Early detection of chronic obstructive pulmonary disease in primary care: A randomised controlled trial. (DISCO Trial) (Br J Gen Pract. 2023)***[1]

  - *Population:* Patients of age group 40–80 years without prior asthma or COPD. (n=3,162)

    General physicians were randomly allocated to one of four groups: control (standard of care), GOLD questions (adapted from symptoms and risk factors identified by GOLD), COPD coordination, and GOLD questions with COPD coordination. New cases of COPD were confirmed by spirometry: post-bronchodilator forced expiratory volume in 1 second over forced vital capacity of <0.7. A dedicated COPD coordinator ensured COPD coordination, reminding patients of specialised COPD appointments (including spirometry) and verifying whether spirometries were performed.

  - *Intervention:*

    Group 1: Control group. (n=802, 25%)

    Group 2: GOLD questions. (n=820, 26%)

    Group 3: COPD coordination. (n=802, 25%)

    Group 4: GOLD questions with COPD coordination. (n=738, 23%)

  - *Outcome:* In the control group, COPD was not evoked, and no spirometry was prescribed. All new cases of COPD diagnosed (n = 24, 0.8%) were in the intervention groups, representing 6.8% of patients who performed spirometry. Statistically, significantly more new cases of COPD were detected with COPD coordination (P = 0.01).

  - *Conclusion:* Easy-to-implement interventions, such as the GOLD questions and COPD coordination, can identify new cases of COPD. Studies are needed to identify the most appropriate case-finding strategies for GPs to detect COPD in primary care in each country.

- ***Early Diagnosis and Treatment of COPD and Asthma - A Randomized, Controlled Trial. UCAP Trial. (NEJM. 2024)***[2]

  - *Population:* Symptomatic patients with undiagnosed asthma or COPD, detected on spirometry. (n=508)

  - *Intervention:* Guideline-based care initiated by a pulmonologist and asthma-COPD educator. (n=253)

  - *Control:* Usual care by primary care practitioner. (n=255)

  - *Outcome:* Annualized rate of a primary-outcome event was lower in the intervention group than in the usual-care (0.53 vs. 1.12 events per person-year; incidence rate ratio, 0.48; 95% CI, 0.36 to 0.63; P<0.001). At 12 months, the SGRQ score was lower than the baseline score by 10.2 points in the intervention group and by 6.8 points in the usual-care group (difference, –3.5 points; 95% CI, –6.0 to –0.9), and the CAT score was lower than the baseline score by 3.8 points and 2.6 points, respectively (difference, –1.3 points; 95% CI, –2.4 to –0.1). The FEV_1 increased by 119 ml in the intervention group and by 22 ml in the usual-care group (difference, 94 ml; 95% CI, 50 to 138). Incidence of adverse events similar.

  - *Conclusion:* Patients who received pulmonologist-supervised treatment had less subsequent health care utilisation for respiratory illness than those who received usual care.

  - *Critical appraisal:* The trial was not powered to detect differences in secondary outcomes. The trial's population was Canadian health care, so generalisation of results may not be appropriate. The intervention group is an ideal situation that may not be available in resource-limited settings. Adherence to guidelines in the intervention group was not monitored.

2. Management of Stable COPD

- ***Ensifentrine, a Novel Phosphodiesterase 3 and 4 Inhibitor for the Treatment of Chronic Obstructive Pulmonary Disease: Randomized, Double-Blind, Placebo-controlled, Multicenter Phase III Trials (summary of the ENHANCE 1 and 2 Trials). (ENHANCE Trials; Am J Respir Crit Care Med. 2023)*** [3]
  - *Population:* Moderate to severe COPD patients aged 40-80 years. (n=1549)

    Totals of 760 (ENHANCE-1) and 789 (ENHANCE-2) patients were randomised and treated.
  - *Intervention:* Twice daily Ensifentrine 3 mg. (n=479)
  - *Comparator:* Placebo. (n=284)
  - *Outcome:* Ensifentrine treatment improved average FEV_1 area under the curve at 0–12 hours versus placebo (ENHANCE-1, 87 ml [95% CI 55 to 119]; ENHANCE-2, 94ml [65 - 124]; (P <0.001). Significantly improved symptoms and quality of life (SGRQ) in the treatment group compared to placebo at Week 24 in ENHANCE-1 but not in ENHANCE-2. The rate of moderate or severe exacerbations was lesser than placebo over 24 weeks along with increased time to first exacerbation. Adverse event rates were similar in both groups.
  - *Conclusion:* Ensifentrine significantly improved lung function in both trials and reduced the rate of exacerbation in COPD patients.
  - *Critical appraisal:* Patients receiving concurrent dual LAMA/LABA, or triple therapy were excluded.

- ***A Double-Blind, Randomized, Placebo-controlled Trial of Long-Term Doxycycline Therapy on Exacerbation Rate in Patients with Stable Chronic Obstructive Pulmonary Disease. (Am J Respir Crit Care Med. 2023)*** [4]
  - *Population:* Moderate to very severe COPD with a history of exacerbation. (n=222)
  - *Intervention:* 12 months of doxycycline 100 mg once daily. (n=110)
  - *Comparator:* Placebo. (n=112)
  - *Outcome:* No difference in COPD exacerbation rates between the two groups (rate ratio [RR], 0.86; 95% CI, 0.67–1.10; *P* = 0.23). In preplanned subgroup analysis, doxycycline significantly reduced the exacerbation rate in those with severe COPD (*P* = 0.019) and in those with an eosinophil count <300 cells/µl (*P* = 0.01). Health status measured by SGRQ was 5.2 points worse in the doxycycline group at 12 months (*P* <0.007).
  - *Conclusion:* Doxycycline did not significantly reduce the exacerbation rate over 12 months, but those with more severe COPD or blood eosinophil counts <300 cells/µl may have benefitted from doxycycline therapy.
  - *Critical appraisal:* Antibiotic resistance was not evaluated, which may have influenced the outcome.

- ***Chronic Obstructive Pulmonary Disease Self-Management in Three Low- and Middle-Income Countries: A Pilot Randomized Trial. (Am J Respir Crit Care Med. 2023)*** [5]
  - *Population:* Patients with COPD Group B-D. (n=239)
  - *Intervention:* Multicomponent, Community Health Worker supported intervention. (n=120)
  - *Comparator:* Standard of care and COPD education. (n=119)

- *Outcome:* At the end of one year, there was no difference in mean total SGRQ score between the two groups (34.7 vs. 34.0 points; p = 0.71). The intervention arm had a higher proportion of hospitalisations than the control arm (10% vs. 5.2%; adjusted odds ratio, 2.2; 95% confidence interval, 0.8, 7.5; $P = 0.15$) at 12 months.
- *Conclusion:* No difference in SGRQ score in those receiving community health worker-based intervention for COPD.
- *Critical appraisal:* The study was not powered to detect differences in clinical outcomes at each study site. The higher percentage of participants with group D COPD in the intervention arm could have led to a bias. Data on the availability of primary care and pulmonary physicians are not available. The intervention did not include inhaler education but focused on training and support to identify COPD exacerbations and make informed decisions on when to seek care. A large proportion of participants died or were lost to follow-up in the control arm.

- ***Dupilumab for COPD with Blood Eosinophil Evidence of Type 2 Inflammation. (NOTUS Trial) (NEJM. 2024)***[(6)]
  - *Population:* COPD patients with a blood eosinophil count of 300 cells/microliter, on background triple inhaler therapy or LAMA–LABA alone (if ICS contraindicated) for at least three months and at a stable dose for at least one month. They must have had at least two moderate or one severe exacerbation in the past year, at least one moderate exacerbation requiring treatment with systemic steroids, and at least one exacerbation while receiving background triple inhaler therapy. (n=935)
  - *Intervention:* Subcutaneous Dupilumab 300 mg. (n=470)
  - *Comparator:* Placebo. (n=465)
  - *Outcome:* Annual rate of moderate or severe exacerbations: 0.86 (95% C.I. 0.70 to 1.06) with dupilumab and 1.30 (95% CI, 1.05 to 1.60) with placebo; the rate ratio compared with placebo was 0.66 (95% CI, 0.54 to 0.82; P<0.001). Prebronchodilator FEV_1 increased from baseline to week 12 with dupilumab (least-squares mean change, 139 ml [95% CI, 105 to 173]) compared with placebo (least-squares mean change, 57 ml [95% CI, 23 to 91]), with a significant least-squares mean difference at week 12 of 82 ml (P<0.001) and at week 52 of 62 ml (P = 0.02). There was no significant change in SGRQ scores from baseline to 52 weeks and adverse events between the two groups.
  - *Conclusion:* In patients with COPD and type 2 inflammation, as indicated by elevated blood eosinophil counts, dupilumab was associated with fewer exacerbations and better lung function than placebo.
  - *Critical appraisal:* Pharma company-sponsored trial. The sample size for the week-52 endpoints was reduced owing to the early primary analysis, which reduced the statistical power for some week-52 endpoints. Enrollment of predominantly the White population. The trial was conducted during the global COVID-19 pandemic, which led to disruptions in health care and changes in behaviours that, at times, decreased exposure to viral respiratory infections.

- ***Icenticaftor, a CFTR Potentiator, in COPD: A Multicenter, Parallel-Group, Double-Blind Clinical Trial. (Am J Respir Crit Care Med. 2023)***[7]
  - *Population:* COPD on triple therapy for at least three months. (n=599)
  - *Intervention:*

    Group 1: Icenticaftor 450 mg B.I.D. (n= 99)

    Group 2: Icenticaftor 300 mg B.I.D. (n=250)

    Group 3: Icenticaftor 150 mg B.I.D. (n=124)

Group 4: Icenticaftor 75 mg B.I.D. (n=126)

Group 5: Icenticaftor 25 mg B.I.D. (n=124)

Group 6: Placebo B.I.D. for 24 weeks (n=251)

- o *Outcome:* After 12 weeks, there was no dose-response relationship for change from baseline through FEV_1 with treatment; however, it was observed for E-RS cough and sputum score. A dose-response relationship was observed after 24 weeks through FEV_1, E-RS cough and sputum and total scores, rescue medication use, and fibrinogen. A dose of 300 mg b.i.d. was consistently the most effective. All treatments are well tolerated.
- o *Conclusion:* The primary endpoint was negative, as Icenticaftor did not improve trough FEV_1 over 12 weeks. However, it improved trough FEV1, reduced cough, sputum, and rescue medication use, and lowered fibrinogen concentrations at 24 weeks.

☞

- ***Effectiveness of clinical pharmacist intervention on medication adherence in patients with chronic obstructive pulmonary disease - A randomised controlled study. (Patient Educ Couns. 2024)***[8]
  - o *Population:* COPD outpatients. (n=180)
  - o *Intervention:* Pharmacist-delivered education emphasised medication adherence, disease, and medication knowledge. (n=91)
  - o *Comparator:* Control group. (n=89)
  - o *Outcome:* The two groups significantly improved medication adherence rate (90.1% vs. 66.3%, $p < 0.001$). Patient behaviour was the most common barrier to non-adherence but was effectively reduced at the endpoint. The Modified Medical Research Council (mMRC) dyspnea scale and inhalation technique improved significantly in intervention patients.
  - o *Conclusion:* Pharmacist intervention can considerably improve medication adherence and knowledge of COPD patients.
  - o *Critical appraisal:* This was a single-centre study. Adherence was self-reported, so there was a chance of recall bias. The study was short. Objective outcome measures such as spirometry were not included in the analysis.

☞

- ***Atomization efficacy of a novel micro-dose mesh nebulizer (CVS-100) versus the traditional mesh nebulizer (M102) in adults with chronic obstructive pulmonary disease: A randomized non-inferiority clinical trial. (Respir Med. 2023)***[9]
  - o *Population:* Stable COPD patients. (n=64)
  - o *Intervention:* Nebulised Combivent (Compound Ipratropium Bromide Solution) with CVS-100 (microdose mesh Nebuliser)
  - o *Comparator:* Nebulised Combivent (Compound Ipratropium Bromide Solution) with M-102 (traditional mesh nebuliser)
  - o *Outcome:* No significant differences between the two groups were found in FEF50%, FEF75%, FEF 25-75%, and MVV before and after nebulisation.
  - o *Conclusion:* A novel micro-dose mesh nebuliser (CVS-100) was found to be non-inferior to the traditional mesh nebuliser (M102) regarding the change in FEV1% pred from baseline after nebulisation.
  - o *Critical appraisal:* Small sample size.

- ***Bronchodilator Efficacy of High-Flow Nasal Cannula in COPD: Vibrating Mesh Nebulizer Versus Jet Nebulizer. (Respir Care. 2024)***[10]
  - *Population:* Stable COPD patients. (n=17)
  - *Intervention:*

    Group 1: Salbutamol via high-flow nasal cannula with vibrating mesh nebuliser (HFNC-VMN).

    Group 2: Salbutamol via jet nebuliser (after a 4-hour washout before cross-over).
  - *Outcome:* The difference between respiratory resistance at 5 Hz and 20 Hz significantly decreased after HFNC-VMN compared to baseline (P = .02), while no significant change was observed after the jet nebuliser (P = .056). Area of reactance and resonant frequency of reactance both significantly decreased (P = .035 and P = .03, respectively), and respiratory reactance at 5 Hz significantly increased (P = .02) in the HFNC-VMN group compared to baseline, with no significant changes with the jet nebuliser. HFNC-VMN had a shorter nebulisation time (6 [5-9] min vs 20 [16-22] min, respectively, P < .001).
  - *Conclusion:* Bronchodilator therapy via HFNC-VMN was not inferior to a jet nebuliser for subjects with stable COPD and can significantly improve airway oscillometry mechanics and decrease nebulisation time compared to the jet nebuliser.
  - *Critical appraisal:* Small sample size.

- ***Efficacy and safety of aclidinium/formoterol versus monotherapies and aclidinium versus placebo in Chinese and other Asian patients with moderate-to-severe COPD: The AVANT Phase 3 study. (Respir Med. 2023)***[11]
  - *Population:* Moderate to severe stable COPD patients.

    A 24-week, randomised, parallel-group, double-blind, double-dummy, placebo-controlled study to assess the efficacy and safety of aclidinium/formoterol 400 µg/12 µg combination vs monotherapies and aclidinium vs placebo (1:1:1:1) in Asian patients (< ~70% of whom were Chinese) with moderate-to-severe stable COPD.
  - *Intervention:*

    Group 1: Aclidinium bromide/Formoterol Fumarate (AB/FF). (n=265)

    Group 2: Aclidinium bromide (AB). (n=267)

    Group 3: Formoterol fumarate (FF). (n=265)

    Group 4: Placebo. (n=269)
  - *Outcome:* At 24 weeks, AB/FF demonstrated improvements from baseline in 1-h morning post-dose FEV_1 vs AB (least squares [LS] mean 92 mL; 95% confidence interval [CI] 60, 124 mL; p < 0.001), and in trough FEV_1 vs FF (LS mean 85 mL; 95% CI 53, 117 mL; p < 0.001). AB improved trough FEV_1 vs placebo (LS mean 134 mL; 95% CI 103, 166 mL; p < 0.001). Improvement in transition dyspnea index focal score at Week 24 for AB/FF vs placebo (LS mean 0.8; 95% CI 0.2, 1.3; p = 0.005) but not for AB vs placebo (LS mean 0.4; 95% CI –0.1, 1.0; p = 0.132). SGRQ total scores improved for AB/FF vs placebo (LS mean –4.0; 95% CI –6.7, –1.4; p = 0.003) and AB vs placebo (LS mean –2.9; 95% CI –5.5, –0.3; p = 0.031). Adverse events (AE), serious AEs and AEs leading to medication discontinuation were similar in the two groups.
  - *Conclusion:* In patients with moderate-to-severe, stable COPD, aclidinium provided clinically meaningful bronchodilation vs placebo, while AB/FF provided higher bronchodilation than monotherapies. In addition, while symptoms and quality of life were observed with aclidinium, those improvements were clinically meaningful for aclidinium/formoterol compared with placebo. Moreover, aclidinium/formoterol was well tolerated, with comparable rates of treatment-emergent AEs across treatment groups.

- *Critical appraisal:* The study was conducted during COVID-19, mainly on Chinese patients, hence fewer patient visits. This might have led to under-reporting of mild symptoms. The study was not powered to report exacerbation rates.

3. Management of AECOPD

- ***Extracorporeal Carbon Dioxide Removal to Avoid Invasive Ventilation During Exacerbations of Chronic Obstructive Pulmonary Disease: VENT-AVOID Trial - A Randomized Clinical Trial. (Am J Respir Crit Care Med. 2024)***[12]
  - *Population*: AECOPD patients. (n=65)
  - *Intervention:* Standard care with veno-venous. $ECCO_2R$ (NIV stratum: $n = 26$; IMV stratum: $n = 32$).
  - *Comparator:* Standard care alone (NIV stratum: $n = 22$; IMV stratum: $n = 33$).
  - *Outcome:* Median ventilator-free days within the first five days post-randomization (VFD-5) between the arms controlled by strata ($P = 0.36$) did not differ in the two groups. In the NIV stratum, the median VFD-5 for both arms was five days (median shift = 0.0; 95% confidence interval [CI]: 0.0-0.0). In the IMV stratum, the median VFD-5 in the standard care and $ECCO_2R$ arms were 0.25 and 2 days, respectively; median shift = 0.00 (95% confidence interval: 0.00-1.25). In the NIV stratum, all-cause in-hospital mortality was significantly higher in the $ECCO_2R$ arm (22% vs. 0%, $P = 0.02$), with no difference in the IMV stratum (17% vs. 15%, $P = 0.73$).
  - *Conclusion:* $ECCO_2R$, compared with standard care, did not improve VFD-5 in AECOPD.
  - *Critical appraisal:* The trial stopped early due to the slow enrollment rate.

- ***Blood eosinophil-guided oral prednisolone for COPD exacerbations in primary care in the UK (STARR2): A non-inferiority, multicentre, double-blind, placebo-controlled, randomised controlled trial self-management intervention for patients following hospitalisation for acute exacerbation of chronic obstructive pulmonary disease (AECOPD). (Lancet Respir Med. 2024)***[13]
  - *Population:* COPD patients with a history of at least one exacerbation in the previous 12 months requiring systemic corticosteroids with or without antibiotics.
  - *Intervention:* Blood eosinophil-directed treatment (BET; to receive oral prednisolone 30 mg once daily if eosinophil count was high [≥2%] or placebo if eosinophil count was low [<2%]). (n=73)
  - *Comparator:* Standard care treatment (ST; to receive prednisolone 30 mg once daily irrespective of the point-of-care eosinophil result). (n=71)
  - *Outcome:* 14 (19%) treatment failures at 30 days post-exacerbation in the BET group and 23 (32%) in the ST group. As per non-inferiority analysis, BET was non-inferior to ST. Frequency of adverse events were similar between the study groups.
  - *Conclusion:* Blood eosinophil-directed prednisolone therapy at the time of an acute exacerbation of COPD is non-inferior to standard care and can be used to safely reduce systemic glucocorticoid use in clinical practice.
  - *Critical appraisal:* Error in randomisation code detected after 60 randomisations and hence statistical compromise noted. Low number of exacerbations associated with a low eosinophil count which is not consistent with secondary care and hospital datasets. Steroid course recommended in this study is 14 days, which is not consistent with international guidelines.

☞

- ***High flow nasal cannula oxygen therapy versus non-invasive ventilation for acute exacerbations of chronic obstructive pulmonary disease with acute- moderate hypercapnic respiratory failure: a randomized controlled non- inferiority trial. (Crit Care. 2024)***[14]
  - o *Population:* AECOPD patients with baseline arterial blood gas pH between 7.25 to 7.35 and $PaCO_2 \geq 50$ mmHg admitted to intensive care units (ICUs) (n=225)
  - o *Intervention:*

    Group 1: HFNC. (n=113)

    Group 2: NIV. (n=112)
  - o *Outcome:* Failure rate: HFNC group 25.7%, NIV group: 14.3%; difference between groups 11.38% (95% CI 0.25-21.20, P = 0.033). This was higher than the non-inferiority cut-off of 9%. Treatment failure occurred in 28/110 (25.5%) in the HFNC group and 15/109 (13.8%) patients in the NIV group (risk difference, 11.69%; 95% CI 0.48-22.60). Intubation rate in the HFNC group vs NIV group (14.2% vs 5.4%, P = 0.026). The treatment switch rate, ICU/ hospital length of stay or 28-day mortality was similar in both groups. (all P > 0.05).
  - o *Conclusion:* HFNC was not non-inferior to NIV and resulted in a higher rate of treatment failure than NIV when used as the initial respiratory support for AECOPD patients with acute-moderate hypercapnic respiratory failure.
  - o *Critical appraisal:* This was a single-centre study with no blinding. The initial gas flow rate of HFNC in this study was 40 L/min. It is worth exploring whether other flow rates would have a better effect on carbon dioxide removal. Switching from HFNC to NIV was subjective.

4. Miscellaneous concepts in COPD

☞

- ***Clinical course of COPD patients with exercise-induced elevation of pulmonary artery pressure or less severe pulmonary hypertension presenting with respiratory symptoms and the impact of bosentan intervention-prospective, single-centre, randomized, parallel-group study. (BMC Pulm Med. 2024)***[15]
  - o *Population:* COPD patients diagnosed as having WHO functional class II, III or IV) with eePAP (exercise-induced elevation of Pulmonary Artery Pressure) or less severe PH whose respiratory symptoms were stable but remained and gradually progressed even after COPD therapy. (n=29)
  - o *Intervention:* Bosentan treated group. (n=14)
  - o *Comparator:* Untreated group. (n=15)
  - o *Outcome:* No death occurred in the drug-treated group; 5 patients died in the untreated group. Significant differences were noted in hospital-free survival (686.00 ± 55.87 days vs. 499.94 ± 53.27 days; hazard ratio [HR], 0.18; P = 0.026) and overall survival (727 days vs. 516.36 ± 55.38 days; HR, 0.095; P = 0.030) in all causes of death analysis, but not in overall survival in respiratory-related death analysis. Bosentan was not associated with increased adverse events, including requiring O_2 inhalation.
  - o *Conclusion:* The prognosis for COPD patients with eePAP or less severe PH presenting with respiratory symptoms was very poor, and bosentan tended to improve their prognosis and suppress ADL (Activities of Daily Living) deterioration without worsening respiratory failure.
  - o *Critical appraisal:* The study was underpowered due to the small sample size for clinically meaningful conclusions.

- ***Inhaled treprostinil in pulmonary hypertension associated with COPD: PERFECT study results. (Eur Respir J. 2024)***[16]
    - o *Population:* Patients with PH-COPD (mean pulmonary arterial pressure ≥30 mmHg and pulmonary vascular resistance ≥4 WU). (n=124)
    - o *Intervention:* iTRE up to 12 breaths (72 µg) 4 times daily. (n=66)
    - o *Comparator:*Placebo. (n=58)
    - o *Outcome:* The study was terminated early as iTRE increased the risk of serious adverse events and suggested an increased mortality risk. The change in 6MWD was numerically worse with iTRE exposure than with placebo exposure.
    - o *Conclusion:* The risk-benefit observations associated with iTRE in patients with PH-COPD did not support the continuation of the PERFECT study. The results of this study do not support iTRE as a viable treatment option in patients with PH-COPD.

- ***Lifestyle Intervention and Excess Weight in Chronic Obstructive Pulmonary Disease (COPD): INSIGHT COPD Randomized Clinical Trial. (Ann Am Thorac Soc. 2023)***[17]
    - o *Population:* Overweight Patients with COPD. (N=684)
    - o *Intervention:* Lifestyle intervention. The intervention was a self-directed video program delivering the Diabetes Prevention Program's Group Lifestyle Balance curriculum.
    - o *Comparator:* Usual care.
    - o *Outcome:* Participants were obese (body mass index, 33.0 ± 4.6 kg/m^2) with moderate COPD. At 12 months, participants randomised to the intervention arm walked farther (P = 0.02), had less dyspnea at the 6-minute-walk test (adjusted difference, -0.36 [95% CI, -0.63 to -0.09]; P = 0.008), and had more significant weight loss (adjusted difference, -1.34 kg [95% CI, -2.33 to -0.34 kg]; P = 0.008). The intervention did not improve the odds of clinically meaningful thresholds of walk distance (98.4 ft) or dyspnea (1 unit) but did achieve meaningful thresholds of weight loss (3% and 5%).
    - o *Conclusion:* Among participants with COPD who were overweight or obese, a self-guided low-intensity video-based lifestyle intervention led to modest weight loss but did not lead to clinically significant improvements in physical functional status and dyspnea.

- ***Nutritional Support in Malnourished Outpatients with Chronic Obstructive Pulmonary Disease (COPD): A Randomized Controlled Pilot Study. (Nutrients. 2024)***[18]
    - o *Population:* Malnourished Outpatients with COPD. (n=33)
    - o *Intervention:* Routine care plus counselling + recommended to purchase powdered Oral Nutritional Supplements. (n=21)
    - o *Comparator:* Routine care plus free provision of powdered Oral Nutritional Supplements. (n=12)
    - o *Outcome:* There were no differences between the groups in weight, quality of life, and nutritional intake at baseline or week 12. However, overall protein intake and quality of life improved in the whole cohort. Adherence to supplements was associated with weight gain.

- *Conclusion:* Improvements in nutritional intake in malnourished patients of COPD are associated with adherence to the supplements.
- *Critical appraisal:* Small sample size.

• ***Combined Effect of Early Nutrition Therapy and Rehabilitation for Patients with Chronic Obstructive Pulmonary Disease Exacerbation: A Prospective Randomized Controlled Trial. (Nutrients. 2024)***[19]

- *Population:* Patients hospitalized for COPD exacerbation. (n=42)
- *Intervention:* Pulmonary Rehabilitation (PR) with regular diet. (n=21)
- *Comparator:* PR with nutritional intake. (n=21)
- *Outcome:* The intervention group showed a greater change in quadriceps strength. Lean body mass and skeletal muscle indices markedly decreased in the control group but were maintained in the intervention group. Logistic regression analysis identified nutritional therapy as a significant factor associated with increased muscle strength. There were no serious adverse events in either group.
- *Conclusion:* Nutritional therapy combined with PR is safe and effective for improving exercise function while maintaining body composition in patients with COPD exacerbation.
- *Critical appraisal:* Small sample.

• ***Tailored psychological intervention for anxiety or depression in COPD (TANDEM): A randomised controlled trial. (Eur Respir J. 2023)***[20]

- *Population:* People with COPD and moderate to very severe airway obstruction and Hospital Anxiety and Depression Scale subscale scores indicating mild to moderate anxiety (HADS-A) and/or depression (HADS-D). (n=423)
- *Intervention:* Tailored psychological intervention on a cognitive behavioural approach. (n=242)
- *Comparator:* Usual care. (n=181)
- *Outcome:* No improvement in anxiety or depression at six months in the intervention group.
- *Conclusion:* No improvement in anxiety or depression at six months with tailored cognitive behavioural therapy.

• ***Valaciclovir for Epstein-Barr Virus Suppression in Moderate-to-Severe COPD: A Randomized Double-Blind Placebo-Controlled Trial. (Chest. 2023)***[21]

- *Population:* Stable moderate-to-severe COPD and sputum EBV (measured using quantitative polymerase chain reaction). (n=84)
- *Intervention:* Valaciclovir (1 g tid). (n=43)
- *Comparator:* Placebo for 8 weeks. (n=41)
- *Outcome:* A more significant number of participants in the valaciclovir group achieved EBV suppression (n = 36 [87.8%] vs n = 17 [42.5%]; $P < .001$) along with a significant reduction in sputum EBV titer compared with placebo ($P = .002$). Although a 24-mL numerical FEV_1 increase was present in the valaciclovir group, this was not statistically significant. Reduction in sputum white cell count was noted in the valaciclovir group compared to placebo ($P = .003$).
- *Conclusion:* Valaciclovir is safe and effective for EBV suppression in COPD, however it is not associated with improvements in FEV1.
- *Critical appraisal:* Study did not have adequate power to detect changes in lung function. Missing data in some patients due to COVID restriction.

- ***Efficacy of different respiratory supports to prevent hypoxia during flexible bronchoscopy in patients of COPD: A triple-arm, randomised controlled trial. (BMJ Open Respir Res. 2023)***[22]

  - *Population:* Patients with COPD undergoing bronchoscopy. (n=90)
  - *Intervention:*

    Group 1: Conventional oxygen therapy (COT). (n=30)

    Group 2: Non-Invasive Ventilation (NIV). (n=30)

    Group 3: High flow oxygen therapy (HFOT). (n=30)
  - *Outcome:* SpO_2 during bronchoscopy (FB) lowest in the COT group (COT: 87.03±5.7% vs HFOT: 95.57±5.0% vs NIV: 97.40±1.6%, p<0.001). Secondary objectives were similar except for respiratory rate (breaths-per-minute), which was highest in the COT group (COT: 20.23±3.1 vs HFOT: 18.57±4.1 vs NIV: 16.80±1.9, p<0.001). Post FB partial pressure of oxygen in arterial blood was highest in the NIV group (p<0.001), and partial pressure of carbon dioxide in arterial blood was similar in the three arms. Operator's ease-of-performing-procedure least in the NIV group based on the Visual Analogue Scale (p<0.01). Nasal pain was higher in the NIV group compared to the other two groups (p<0.01).
  - *Conclusion:* NIV and HFOT are superior to COT in preventing hypoxia during bronchoscopy, but NIV is associated with poor patient tolerance and less operator ease of performing the procedure.
  - *Critical appraisal:* This was a single-centre study. The estimated sample size could not be reached. An in-house modified NIV mask was used, which was not externally validated.

5. Pulmonary Rehabilitation in COPD

- ***Laryngeal widening and adequate ventilation by expiratory pressure load training improve aerobic capacity in COPD: A randomised controlled trial. (Thorax. 2023)***[23]

  - *Population:* Stable COPD patients in condition to tolerate CPET. (n=40)
  - *Intervention:* Expiratory pressure load training (EPT). (n=20)
  - *Comparator:* Control. (n=20)
  - *Outcome:* EPT increased: (1) endurance time, p=0.0008 (GOLD I-II); p=0.0006 (GOLD III-IV); (2) peak oxygen uptake (p=0.0086 in GOLD I-II; p=0.0004 in GOLD III-IV); (3) glottic dilatation ratio at maximum collapse on laryngoscopy in the submaximal exercise (p=0.0062 in GOLD I-II; p=0.0001 in GOLD III-IV); and (4) the inflexion point of expiratory tidal volume relative to minute ventilation during the incremental exercise (p=0.0015 in GOLD I-II; p=0.0075 in GOLD III-IV) compared with controls. Across GOLD grades, the responses of the glottic dilatation ratio at maximum collapse and the expiratory tidal volume at the inflexion point were selected as more influential variables correlating with the improvement in peak oxygen uptake and endurance time, respectively.
  - *Conclusion:* EPT improved aerobic capacity and endurance time with larger laryngeal widening and adequate ventilation despite advanced COPD.
  - *Critical appraisal:* Small sample size of 47 patients. Patients can still exercise without dyspnoea even if they are hypoxemic after EPT because ventilatory limitation rather than hypoxaemia is often the cause of exercise limitation in COPD.

- **Determination of the minimal important difference for inspiratory muscle strength in people with severe and very severe COPD. *(Clin Rehabil. 2023)***[24]

  - *Population:* People with severe to very severe COPD undergoing a pulmonary rehabilitation program (Post hoc analysis of a randomised controlled trial (EMI2 study). (n=73)

- *Intervention:* Patients followed a standardised pulmonary rehabilitation program five days a week for four weeks. The program included aerobic training, ground-based outdoor walking training, and lower and upper limb muscle strengthening.
- *Outcome:* At the end of the PR program, MIP improved by 14.8 ± 14.9 cmH_2O ($p < 0.05$). The receiver operating characteristic curve analysis reported a minimally significant difference of 13.5 cmH_2O (sensibility: 75% specificity: 67.5%). Using distribution-based methods, the estimate of minimal important difference was 7.9 cmH_2O (standard error of measurement method) and 10.9 cmH_2O (size effect method).
- *Conclusion:* Measuring the minimally important difference is a simple tool for assessing changes in inspiratory muscle strength during a pulmonary rehabilitation program. We propose a minimally important difference of 13.5 cmH_2O for improving MIP.
- *Critical appraisal:* The EMI2 study was underpowered for this post-hoc analysis.

- ***Effect of respiratory muscle training in patients with stable chronic obstructive pulmonary disease: A systematic review and meta-analysis. (Heliyon. 2024)***[25]
  - *Population:* Individuals with stable COPD. Included 12 RCTs with a total of 453 individuals.
  - *Intervention:* Respiratory muscle training (RMT) including: 'inspiratory muscle training (IMT), respiratory muscle endurance training (RMET), expiratory muscle training, pranayama breathing training'. A few studies also included IMT with pulmonary rehabilitation or with cycle ergometer training.
  - *Comparator:* 'Sham training or health education'.
  - *Outcome and Conclusion:* 1. Significant improvement was noted in maximal inspiratory pressure (PImax) with RMT alone. 2. A non-significant improvement was noted in FEV_1/FVC and FEV_1 when RMT was added to other interventions compared to these interventions alone. 3. No significant difference was noted in dyspnea during exercise, dyspnea during daily life, six minute walk distance, or maximal expiratory pressure (PEmax). 4. A significant worsening of FEV_1/FVC was noted when RMT was used alone.
  - *Critical appraisal:* The analysis included a limited number of trials. For obvious technical and practical reasons, blinding was not possible in any of these RCTs. The analysis did not evaluate adverse events of RMT.

DISCUSSION

COPD is a heterogeneous lung condition characterised by chronic respiratory symptoms (dyspnea, cough, sputum production and/or exacerbations) due to abnormalities of the airways (bronchitis, bronchiolitis) and/or alveoli (emphysema) that cause persistent, often progressive, airflow obstruction. This review will discuss the newer concepts in COPD in the last year.

Diagnosis of COPD

The diagnosis of COPD is usually made with a combination of exposure to various risk factors such as smoking, indoor biomass fuel and spirometry. However, a sizeable population with COPD remains underdiagnosed. Recently, some studies have been done to identify patients with risk factors or symptoms of COPD, thereby enabling early diagnosis and effective treatment. A French study used specific questions about COPD and the involvement of a dedicated coordinator in patients aged 40-80 years and found that active COPD screening led to the identification of newer cases of COPD than standard care.[1] Another study was done on patients in the community with respiratory symptoms without diagnosed lung disease involving a pulmonologist and an asthma-COPD educator. This study also found that identifying undiagnosed COPD and asthma patients led to lower healthcare utilisation for respiratory illness and SGRQ and CAT scores.[2] ***We do not routinely recommend early diagnosis of COPD in community settings, but it may be done in a research setting as it can lead to reduced healthcare utilisation.***

Management of Stable COPD

Bronchodilators are the cornerstone of COPD management. However, certain newer therapies have been investigated as supportive or add-on therapies in the last year.

Role of PDE3-PDE4 inhibitors

Ensifentrine is a dual PDE3 and PDE4 inhibitor with anti-inflammatory and bronchodilator properties. This drug was investigated in two trials, ENHANCE 1 and ENHANCE 2. Ensifentrine improved lung function, reduced the rate of exacerbation, and increased the time to first exacerbation in patients with COPD.[3] ***In patients of chronic bronchitis with severe COPD and a history of exacerbations, PDE4 inhibitors such as Roflumilast can improve lung function and reduce exacerbations as per GOLD guidelines.*** On the other hand, Ensifentrine is a novel, inhaled PDE3 and PDE4 having both bronchodilator effect and anti-inflammatory effect, may help in alleviating dyspnea and decreasing exacerbations.

Role of Doxycycline in reducing exacerbations

Exacerbations in COPD increase morbidity and mortality and are associated with a decline in lung functions. A trial was conducted in the UK in patients with moderate to severe COPD with a history of exacerbations to investigate the role of long-term doxycycline at a dose of 100 mg for 12 months. Although the study did not find a difference in exacerbation rate, doxycycline reduced exacerbation in patients of severe COPD and eosinophil count less than 300/microlitre.[4] ***We do not recommend routine use of doxycycline on a long-term basis for reducing exacerbations in COPD.***

Role of Dupilumab in COPD

A significant population of patients with COPD continue to have exacerbations despite maximal therapy. A proportion of the above patients have Th-2-mediated inflammation. Dupilumab is a monoclonal antibody targeting IL-4 and IL-13, mediators of Th-2 inflammation. To investigate the safety and efficacy of dupilumab, the NOTUS trial was conducted in patients with COPD with a blood eosinophil count of more than 300 per microlitre.[6] The patients received subcutaneous dupilumab 300 micrograms every two weeks for a duration of 52 weeks. The study showed the favourable response of dupilumab in reducing the annualised rate of moderate to severe exacerbations and improving lung function at week 12 compared to the placebo. ***We recommend that***

dupilumab be used on a case-to-case basis for patients of COPD with eosinophil counts of more than 300 and repeated exacerbations despite maximal inhaled therapy.

Role of Icenticaftor, a CFTR potentiator in COPD

Reduction of cough and sputum production in chronic bronchitis patients is seldom addressed. CFTR dysfunction is associated with altered movement of electrolytes across the cell, disrupting the mucociliary clearance in such patients. Icenticaftor is a drug that potentiates ions' movement across the channels, thereby improving mucociliary clearance. This drug was investigated for treatment in COPD patients with chronic bronchitis phenotype at variable doses. The study found that at a dose of 300mg for six months, Icenticaftor reduced cough and sputum production but did not improve the FEV1 levels.[7] ***We do not recommend the routine use of Icenticaftor in chronic bronchitis due to the lack of large-scale studies supporting its use in the current scenario.***

Management of COPD in low-resource settings is challenging. A community health worker (CHW) supported the self-management of COPD, which was investigated in three resource-limited countries. However, the study did not find any difference in the SGRQ score, rate of exacerbations, hospitalisations and quality of life with this approach.[5]

Adherence to inhalers and their correct use is a cornerstone in the management of COPD. A study was done in Vietnam to evaluate the role of pharmacists in improving adherence to medications in COPD patients. This study found that medication adherence, mMRC dyspnea score, and correct inhaler technique were significantly enhanced in the pharmacist-delivered education group.[8] ***We recommend education and training on inhaled bronchodilator therapy and ensuring regular compliance with it to enhance the benefit of therapy in COPD.***

Role of Nebulisers

Effective nebulisation is critical to drug delivery and optimal outcomes in patients with COPD. A novel micro dose mesh nebuliser was compared with the traditional mesh nebuliser device. The device was found to be non-inferior to the conventional mesh nebuliser device in terms of change in FEV1 % from baseline.[9] Another study found that in patients with COPD, a vibrating mesh nebuliser along with HFNC is non-inferior to the conventional jet nebuliser in terms of airway oscillatory mechanics.[10]

Role of LABA/LAMA in COPD

LABA/LAMA combination is a well-documented therapy in patients with COPD that provides bronchodilation and symptom control. AVANT was a study conducted to investigate the efficiency of this combination in the Asian population. The study found that the aclidinium bromide/ formoterol combination was more effective in providing bronchodilation than placebo and monotherapies with an acceptable safety profile.[11] ***We concur with the GOLD guidelines for managing stable COPD. The cornerstone of this management is bronchodilators, i.e. LABA + LAMA in Group B, LABA + LAMA in Group E and the addition of ICS in the cases where blood eosinophil is more than or equal to 300 per microlitre.***

Management of AECOPD

Exacerbation of COPD is a change in the symptoms of COPD beyond day-to-day variation that mandates a shift in baseline therapy. The severity of exacerbation is variable. However, exacerbations are associated with significant morbidity and mortality in COPD.

Role of Extracorporeal CO_2 removal:

Hypercapnic respiratory failure is commonly encountered in clinical settings in COPD patients. The management of such patients is usually NIV or Invasive mechanical ventilation in severe cases. The VENT-AVOID was a randomised control trial in AECOPD patients either on NIV or IMV. The trial randomly assigned patients either to veno-venous extracorporeal CO_2 removal or standard care. However, the trial showed no significant difference in the ventilator-free days five days after randomisation.[12] **We do not recommend** ***extracorporeal CO_2 removal for hypercapnic respiratory failure.***

Eosinophil-guided steroid treatment in AECOPD

Systemic steroids are used for short-term management in AECOPD. However, in certain patients, treatment failure and hyperglycaemia can occur even with this short course of treatment. Blood eosinophil count-guided treatment can help direct the treatment with systemic steroids judiciously. In the STARR2 trial, patients with AECOPD were randomised to receive blood eosinophil-guided therapy with steroids (30 mg) if their eosinophil count was more than or equal to 2% and to placebo if the same was less than 2%. The other group was a standard treatment group, which received 30 mg of prednisolone in all patients. This study found that eosinophil-guided treatment is non-inferior to standard practice in reducing treatment failure rates at the end of 30 days.[13] ***We concur with the GOLD guidelines in the use of oral steroids for five days in AECOPD. However, eosinophil-guided use of oral steroids may be tried on a case-to-case basis for minimising inadvertent use of steroids and their side effects.***

Role of HFNC in AECOPD

NIV is the standard of care for the management of acute hypercapnic respiratory failure in patients with AECOPD. However, there are some problems concerning discomfort due to mask and air leaks in some patients, which can compromise adequate ventilation. HFNC is also used in some studies in patients with AECOPD with hypercapnic respiratory failure due to its effects of reducing the intrinsic PEEP by its high flow and prevention of bronchoconstriction due to its warmed, humidified air. A non-inferiority trial in patients with AECOPD with pH 7.25-7.35 and pCO_2 more than 50 mmHg was conducted in the Chinese population. This study has shown that HFNC is not non-inferior to NIV in preventing intubation or reducing treatment failure rates in patients of AECOPD with moderate-severe hypercapnic respiratory failure. NIV also reduced the $PaCO_2$ at 48 hours after initiation compared to HFNC.[14] This study cautions against the use of HFNC in all patients of AECOPD with hypercapnic respiratory failure. An earlier meta-analysis found lesser intubation rates and better respiratory rate with the use of HFNC compared to NIV in hypercapnic AECOPD.[31] The current role of HFNC in hypercapnic COPD is controversial based on the contradictory results. ***We do not recommend the routine use of HFNC for hypercapnic AECOPD. However, it may be tried on a case-to-case basis and in research settings.***

Miscellaneous concepts in COPD

Management of Pulmonary Hypertension in COPD

Pulmonary hypertension is a common complication of COPD. It is associated with increased mortality, decreased exercise capacity and reduced quality of life. In some patients with mild COPD, with significant symptom burden, there may exist pulmonary artery hypertension. A study investigated the efficacy of bosentan in COPD patients with exercise-induced elevated pulmonary artery pressure or mild PAH. In this small group of patients, bosentan improved hospital-free and overall survival.[15] The results of this study are encouraging and may be used to investigate the efficacy of anti-PH therapies in a more extensive group of patients. Another study with inhaled treprostinil (iTRE) showed that iTRE increased the risk of serious adverse events and suggested an increased risk of mortality.[16] ***We do not recommend using bosentan or inhaled treprostinil for pulmonary hypertension in patients with COPD.***

Lifestyle measures in COPD

INSIGHT was a randomised trial aimed at investigating whether lifestyle intervention aimed at weight loss measures would lead to improvement in physical status in obese patients with COPD. However, this intervention did not lead to clinically meaningful improvements in physical status or dyspnea.[17] Malnourishment is an essential factor in COPD, which is primarily due to inflammatory mediators, and they can lead to an adverse outcome. Hence, nutritional supplementation to maintain adequate body mass index is emphasised in these patients. A small study found that nutritional support significantly improves nutrition status and quality of life in patients with COPD who are malnourished.[18] This effect of enhanced nutritional support was also replicated in another study where nutritional support was combined with pulmonary rehabilitation. The study found enhanced quadriceps strength and maintained muscle mass in patients supplemented with protein-rich food.[19] ***We recommend nutritional therapy to maintain the body mass index in patients with COPD.***

Intervention for anxiety and depression in COPD

Anxiety and depression are some of the main comorbidities in COPD, which are often under-recognized. They impact the overall prognosis of the disease. The TANDEM trial investigated the role of a tailored psychological intervention based on a cognitive behavioural approach for COPD patients suffering from anxiety and depression. However, this was a negative trial which did not find the role of cognitive behavioural therapy to help reduce the symptoms of anxiety and depression nor improve the disease-related quality of life.[20] ***We do not recommend the routine use of cognitive behavioural therapy for anxiety and depression in patients with COPD.***

Valaciclovir for EBV suppression in COPD

In a trial, patients with elevated EBV counts in sputum were given valaciclovir for eight weeks.[21] However, the drug did not improve FEV1. ***We do not recommend the routine use of valaciclovir for EBV suppression in COPD.***

Efficacy of respiratory support patients during flexible bronchoscopy in COPD

COPD patients undergoing bronchoscopy frequently experience hypoxia during the procedure. Three modalities, i.e. conventional oxygen therapy, high flow oxygen therapy (HFOT), and non-invasive ventilatory support, were investigated to prevent intra-procedure hypoxia. Both NIV and HFOT were better than conventional oxygen therapy in reducing hypoxia. However, NIV was associated with reduced operator ease and patient comfort, thereby providing HFOT as a good alternative in COPD patients to prevent hypoxia during bronchoscopy.[22] ***We recommend the use of NIV or HFNC in high-risk patients of COPD undergoing bronchoscopy to prevent hypoxia.***

Pulmonary Rehabilitation in COPD

COPD patients have exercise intolerance due to limitations in their aerobic capacity. Pulmonary rehabilitation is an essential aspect of the comprehensive management of COPD patients. Reports have indicated narrowing of the glottis during expiration during exertion, leading to exercise intolerance. A randomised trial investigated the utility of expiratory pressure load training for three months in COPD patients to widen the glottis and improve aerobic capacity. The results favoured this modality in improving aerobic capacity and endurance time with larger laryngeal widening in COPD patients.[23] ***We do not recommend using laryngeal widening as a routine for COPD patients.***

Recent studies have shown the beneficial effects of inspiratory muscle training, chest wall mobilisation, endurance, and resistance training in COPD patients.[24-28] A meta-analysis found a significant improvement in maximal inspiratory pressure (PImax) with respiratory muscle training (RMT).[25] It also found a non-significant improvement in FEV_1/FVC and FEV_1. Inspiratory muscle training. Components of RMT include inspiratory or expiratory muscle training, respiratory muscle endurance training, or 'pranayama'. It is likely that the benefit of respiratory muscle training is achieved when used as part of pulmonary rehabilitation (PR) programs. The ATS guidelines on (2023) also strongly recommend PR in stable COPD to improve exercise capacity, dyspnea, and health related quality of life.[29] They also noted no significant adverse events with PR in this setting. They strongly recommended PR after a severe exacerbation of COPD within three weeks of hospitalization. In this setting, PR significantly reduces the risk of rehospitalization in addition to other above mentioned benefits.[29] Comparing telerehabilitation with in-center PR, the ATS panel found similar improvements with either setting. They have, therefore, recommended giving the choice to the individual. ***We recommend pulmonary rehabilitation as an integral part of COPD management.*** The benefits of PR diminish within 12 months of completing the program. Based on the previously published evidence, the benefit of maintenance PR on exercise capacity or health related quality of life is inconsistent. Further, maintenance PR is unable to reduce hospitalizations.

However, there are no significant adverse events of maintenance PR. Looking at the inconsistent evidence but absence of adverse events, the ATS suggest using 'either supervised maintenance PR or usual care' after the initial PR program.

Vaccinations in stable COPD

The GOLD guidelines (2023) recommended routine vaccination stable COPD individuals: influenza (killed or live inactivated), pneumococcal (one dose of PCV20 alone or one dose of PCV15 followed by one dose of PPSV23), SARS-CoV-2, TdaP (for individuals who were not vaccinated in adolescence), and herpes zoster (if age >50 years). The GOLD 2024 guidelines additionally recommended RSV vaccination.

CONCLUSIONS

There have been many new changes in the understanding of COPD concerning diagnosis and management. The above review helps to focus on these updates and keep the physician abreast of recent developments in this disease in the last year.

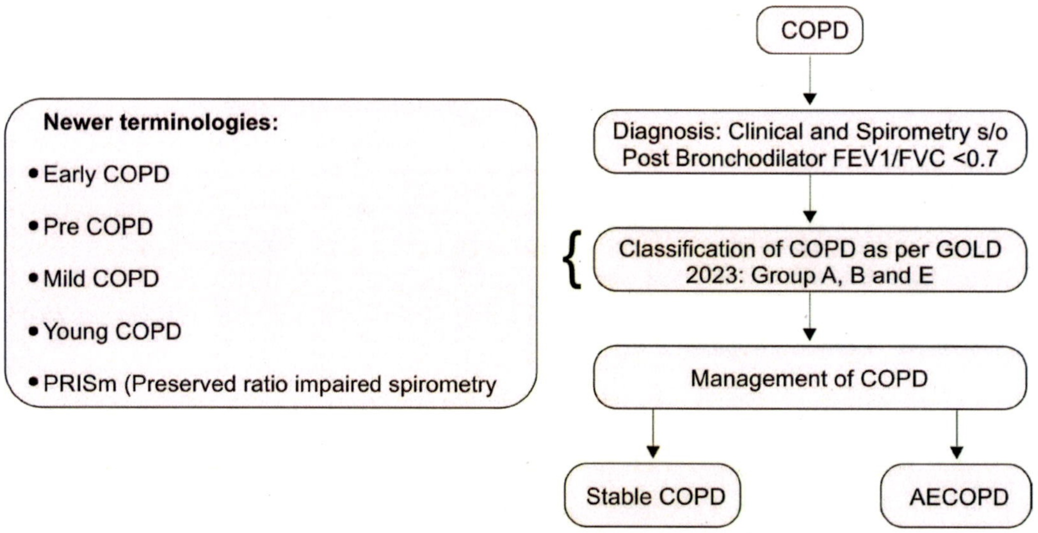

Flowchart 2: Diagnosis and Management of Stable COPD
Adapted from reference (30)

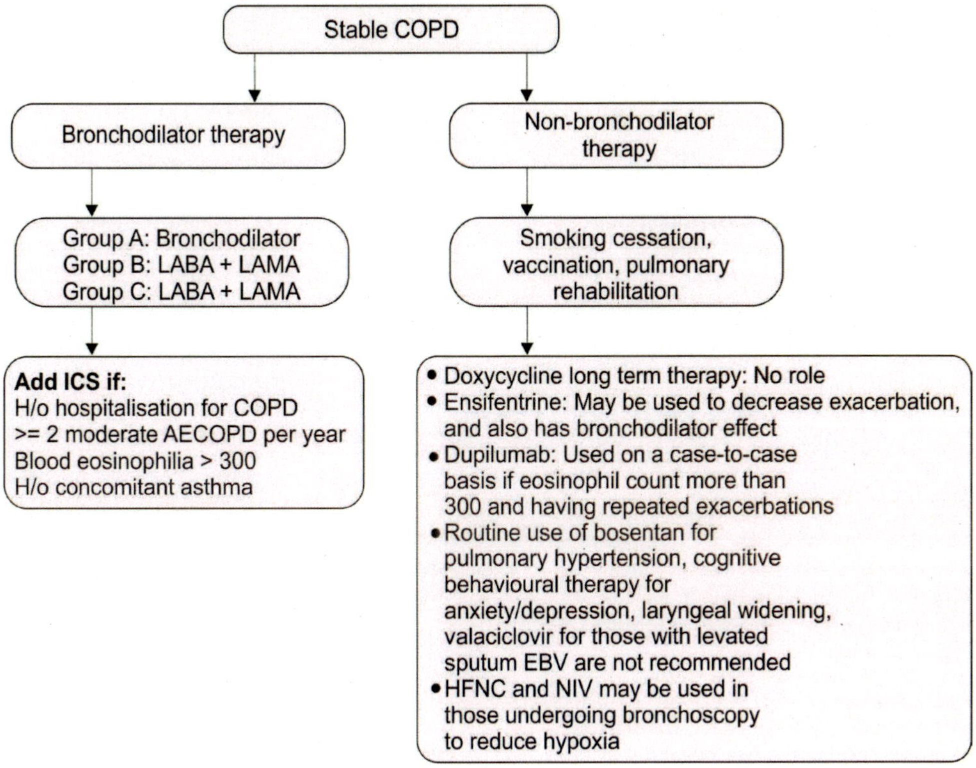

Management of Stable COPD

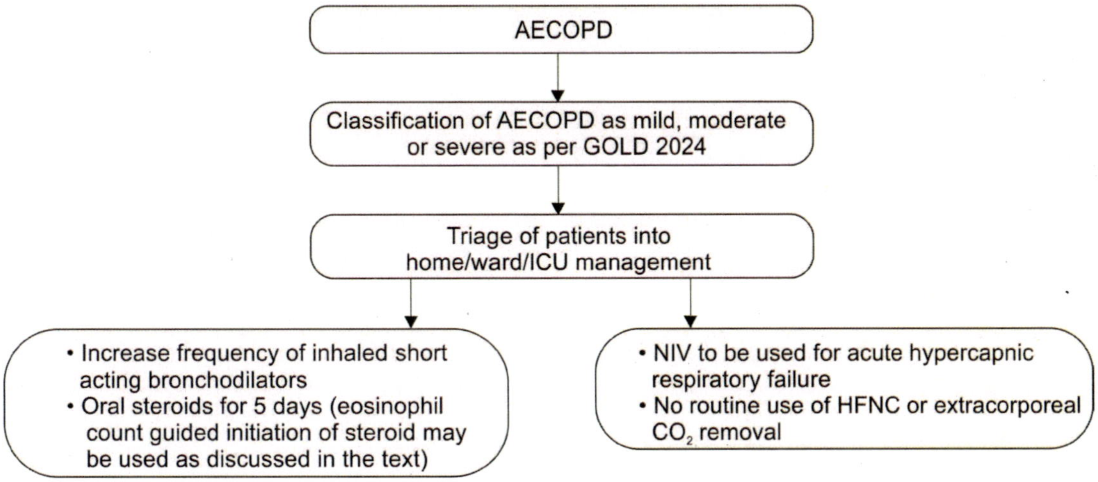

Management of Acute Exacerbation of COPD

REFERENCES

1. Chapron A, Andres E, Fiquet L, Pelé F, Allory E, Le Pabic E, et al. Early detection of chronic obstructive pulmonary disease in primary care: a randomised controlled trial. Br J Gen Pract J R Coll Gen Pract. 2023 Dec;73(737):e876–84.

2. Aaron SD, Vandemheen KL, Whitmore GA, Bergeron C, Boulet LP, Côté A, et al. Early Diagnosis and Treatment of COPD and Asthma - A Randomized, Controlled Trial. N Engl J Med. 2024 Jun 13;390(22):2061–73.

3. Anzueto A, Barjaktarevic IZ, Siler TM, Rheault T, Bengtsson T, Rickard K, et al. Ensifentrine, a Novel Phosphodiesterase 3 and 4 Inhibitor for the Treatment of Chronic Obstructive Pulmonary Disease: Randomized, Double-Blind, Placebo-controlled, Multicenter Phase III Trials (the ENHANCE Trials). Am J Respir Crit Care Med. 2023 Aug 15;208(4):406–16.

4. Allinson JP, Vlies BH, Brill SE, Law M, Burnside G, Finney LJ, et al. A Double-Blind, Randomized, Placebo-controlled Trial of Long-Term Doxycycline Therapy on Exacerbation Rate in Patients with Stable Chronic Obstructive Pulmonary Disease. Am J Respir Crit Care Med. 2023 Sep 1;208(5):549–58.

5. Pollard SL, Siddharthan T, Hossen S, Rykiel NA, Flores-Flores O, Alupo P, et al. Chronic Obstructive Pulmonary Disease Self-Management in Three Low- and Middle-Income Countries: A Pilot Randomized Trial. Am J Respir Crit Care Med. 2023 Nov 15;208(10):1052–62.

6. Bhatt SP, Rabe KF, Hanania NA, Vogelmeier CF, Bafadhel M, Christenson SA, et al. Dupilumab for COPD with Blood Eosinophil Evidence of Type 2 Inflammation. N Engl J Med. 2024 Jun 27;390(24):2274–83.

7. Martinez FJ, Criner GJ, Gessner C, Jandl M, Scherbovsky F, Shinkai M, et al. Icenticaftor, a CFTR Potentiator, in COPD: A Multicenter, Parallel-Group, Double-Blind Clinical Trial. Am J Respir Crit Care Med. 2023 Aug 15;208(4):417–27.

8. Nguyen T, Truong MTX, Lam DN, Nguyen HTT, Huynh AM, Duong VK, et al. Effectiveness of clinical pharmacist intervention on medication adherence in patients with chronic obstructive pulmonary disease - A randomized controlled study. Patient Educ Couns. 2024 Jan;118:108037.

9. Qu Y, Gong Y, Li L, Song Y, Song Y, Hou D, et al. Atomization efficacy of a novel micro-dose mesh nebulizer (CVS-100) versus the traditional mesh nebulizer (M102) in adults with chronic obstructive pulmonary disease: A randomized non-inferiority clinical trial. Respir Med. 2023 Dec;219:107434.

10. Arunsurat I, Rittayamai N, Chuaychoo B, Tangchityongsiva S, Promsarn S, Yuenyong S, et al. Bronchodilator Efficacy of High-Flow Nasal Cannula in COPD: Vibrating Mesh Nebulizer Versus Jet Nebulizer. Respir Care. 2024 Jan 24;69(2):157–65.

11. Sun Y, Molins E, Daoud SZ, Trivedi R, Stewart C, Lamarca R, et al. Efficacy and safety of aclidinium/formoterol versus monotherapies and aclidinium versus placebo in Chinese and other Asian patients with moderate-to-severe COPD: The AVANT Phase 3 study. Respir Med. 2023 Nov;218:107393.

12. Duggal A, Conrad SA, Barrett NA, Saad M, Cheema T, Pannu S, et al. Extracorporeal Carbon Dioxide Removal to Avoid Invasive Ventilation During Chronic Obstructive Pulmonary Disease Exacerbations: VENT-AVOID Trial - A Randomized Clinical Trial. Am J Respir Crit Care Med. 2024 Mar 1;209(5):529–42.

13. Ramakrishnan S, Jeffers H, Langford-Wiley B, Davies J, Thulborn SJ, Mahdi M, et al. Blood eosinophil-guided oral prednisolone for COPD exacerbations in primary care in the UK (STARR2): a non-inferiority, multicentre, double-blind, placebo-controlled, randomised controlled trial. Lancet Respir Med. 2024 Jan;12(1):67–77.

14. Tan D, Wang B, Cao P, Wang Y, Sun J, Geng P, et al. High flow nasal cannula oxygen therapy versus non-invasive ventilation for acute exacerbations of chronic obstructive pulmonary disease with acute-moderate hypercapnic respiratory failure: a randomized controlled non-inferiority trial. Crit Care Lond Engl. 2024 Jul 18;28(1):250.

15. Kashiwada T, Tanaka Y, Tanaka T, Okano T, Saito Y, Seike M, et al. Clinical course of COPD patients with exercise-induced elevation of pulmonary artery pressure or less severe pulmonary hypertension presenting with respiratory symptoms and the impact of bosentan intervention-prospective, single-centre, randomized, parallel-group study. BMC Pulm Med. 2024 Feb 17;24(1):90.

16. Nathan SD, Argula R, Trivieri MG, Aziz S, Gay E, Medarov B, et al. Inhaled treprostinil in pulmonary hypertension associated with COPD: PERFECT study results. Eur Respir J. 2024 Jun 6;63(6):2400172.

17. Au DH, Gleason E, Hunter-Merrill R, Barón AE, Collins M, Ronneberg C, et al. Lifestyle Intervention and Excess Weight in Chronic Obstructive Pulmonary Disease (COPD): INSIGHT COPD Randomized Clinical Trial. Ann Am Thorac Soc. 2023 Dec;20(12): 1743–51.

18. Conway V, Hukins C, Sharp S, Collins PF. Nutritional Support in Malnourished Outpatients with Chronic Obstructive Pulmonary Disease (COPD): A Randomized Controlled Pilot Study. Nutrients. 2024 May 30;16(11).

19. Oyama Y, Tatsumi H, Takikawa H, Taniguchi N, Masuda Y. Combined Effect of Early Nutrition Therapy and Rehabilitation for Patients with Chronic Obstructive Pulmonary Disease Exacerbation: A Prospective Randomized Controlled Trial. Nutrients. 2024 Mar 5;16(5).

20. Taylor SJC, Sohanpal R, Steed L, Marshall K, Chan C, Yaziji N, et al. Tailored psychological intervention for anxiety or depression in COPD (TANDEM): a randomised controlled trial. Eur Respir J. 2023 Nov;62(5).

21. Linden DA, Guo-Parke H, McKelvey MC, Einarsson GG, Lee AJ, Fairley DJ, et al. Valaciclovir for Epstein-Barr Virus Suppression in Moderate-to-Severe COPD: A Randomized Double-Blind Placebo-Controlled Trial. Chest. 2023 Sep;164(3):625–36.

22. Sharma VK, Singh PK, Govindagoudar MB, Thulasi A, Chaudhry D, Shriram CP, et al. Efficacy of different respiratory supports to prevent hypoxia during flexible bronchoscopy in patients of COPD: a triple-arm, randomised controlled trial. BMJ Open Respir Res. 2023 Nov;10(1).

23. Miki K, Tsujino K, Fukui M, Miki M, Kitajima T, Sumitani H, et al. Laryngeal widening and adequate ventilation by expiratory pressure load training improve aerobic capacity in COPD: a randomised controlled trial. Thorax. 2023 Dec 15;79(1):23–34.

24. Beaumont M, Couasnon C, Péran L, Berriet AC, Ber CL, Pichon R. Determination of the minimal important difference for inspiratory muscle strength in people with severe and very severe COPD. Clin Rehabil. 2023 Nov;37(11):1521-1532.

25. Huang Z, Li Z, Yan M, Zheng J, Huang W, Hong L, et al. Effect of respiratory muscle training in patients with stable chronic obstructive pulmonary disease: A systematic review and meta-analysis. Heliyon. 2024 Mar 27;10(7):e28733.

26. Tsui AYY, Chau RMW, Cheing GLY, Mok TYW, Ling SO, Kwan CHY, et al. Effect of chest wall mobilization on respiratory muscle function in patients with severe chronic obstructive pulmonary disease (COPD): A randomized controlled trial. Respir Med. 2023 Dec;220:107436.

27. Pancera S, Lopomo NF, Porta R, Sanniti A, Buraschi R, Bianchi LNC. Effects of Combined Endurance and Resistance Eccentric Training on Muscle Function and Functional Performance in Patients With Chronic Obstructive Pulmonary Disease: Randomized Controlled Trial. Arch Phys Med Rehabil. 2024 Mar;105(3):470–9.

28. Cui S, Ji H, Li L, Zhu H, Li X, Gong Y, et al. Effects and long-term outcomes of endurance versus resistance training as an adjunct to standard medication in patients with stable COPD: a multicenter randomized trial. BMC Pulm Med. 2024 Apr 22;24(1):196.

29. Rochester CL, Alison JA, Carlin B, Jenkins AR, Cox NS, Bauldoff G, et al. Pulmonary Rehabilitation for Adults with Chronic Respiratory Disease: An Official American Thoracic Society Clinical Practice Guideline. Am J Respir Crit Care Med. 2023 Aug 15;208(4):e7-e26.

30. Agustí A, Celli BR, Criner GJ, Halpin D, Anzueto A, Barnes P, et al. Global Initiative for Chronic Obstructive Lung Disease 2023 Report: GOLD Executive Summary. Eur Respir J. 2023 Apr 1;61(4):2300239.

31. Du Y, Zhang H, Ma Z, Liu J, Wang Z, Lin M, et al. High-Flow Nasal Oxygen versus Noninvasive Ventilation in Acute Exacerbation of Chronic Obstructive Pulmonary Disease Patients: A Meta-Analysis of Randomized Controlled Trials. Can Respir J. 2023 Jun 30;2023:7707010.

CHAPTER

3

Bronchiectasis

Authors: Dr. Pawan Singh, Dr. Aman Ahuja

Reviewer: Dr. Rohit Kumar

INTRODUCTION

Bronchiectasis is defined as abnormal permanent dilation of the bronchi. It is characterized by excessive mucus production and recurrent chest infections. Multiple aetiologies can cause bronchiectasis, which can be seen in all age groups but is frequently seen in the elderly, except in Asia, where relatively younger people are affected.[1,2]

Methodology

A PubMed and Cochrane dataset search was done with Boolean search keywords ('Bronchiectasis' OR 'ABPA' OR 'Cystic Fibrosis'). Articles between the period of 1st August 2023 to 1st Aug 2024 were reviewed. Publications were limited to human studies in the English language. We enrolled a total of 3 RCTs with 1 long-term follow-up, 1 real-life study & 2 systematic reviews in the list of studies related to bronchiectasis updates which were found eligible for practice-changing updates and likely to have some impact on upcoming treatment strategy.

Electronic database search: Pubmed and Cochrane

Period: 1st August 2023 to 1st August 2024

Search words: 'Bronchiectasis' OR 'Cystic Fibrosis' OR 'ABPA'

(n=79)

↓

Articles after screening for relevance and included in the review

(n=7)

Analysis of Literature

- ***Safety and Efficacy of the Epithelial Sodium Channel Blocker Idrevloride in People with Primary Ciliary Dyskinesia (CLEAN-PCD): A Multinational, Phase 2, Randomised, Double-Blind, Placebo-Controlled Crossover Trial. (Lancet Resp. Med. 2023)***[3]
    - *Population:* Primary ciliary dyskinesia (PCD) patients aged 12 years and older with a confirmed diagnosis with percentage predicted FEV1 (ppFEV1) ranging from 40% to <90%, recruited across 32 hospitals in North America and Europe. (n=123).

- *Intervention:* Administration of nebulized idrevloride, an epithelial sodium channel (ENaC) blocker, at a dose of 85 µg, either alone or in combination with hypertonic saline (4.2% NaCl). The treatment was given twice daily for 28 days, followed by a 28-day washout period, with an optional extension for an additional 28 days with the co-administration of oral ivacaftor.
- *Comparator:* Placebo.
- *Implementation arms:*

  Sequence 1: Idrevloride in hypertonic saline during Treatment Period 1, followed by hypertonic saline alone during Treatment Period 2.

  Sequence 2: Hypertonic saline alone during Treatment Period 1, followed by idrevloride in hypertonic saline during Treatment Period 2.

  Sequence 3: Idrevloride alone during Treatment Period 1, followed by placebo during Treatment Period 2.

  Sequence 4: Placebo during Treatment Period 1, followed by idrevloride alone during Treatment Period 2.
- *Outcome:* The primary outcome was the absolute change in ppFEV1 from baseline after 28 days of treatment. ppFEV1 significantly improved with idrevloride in hypertonic saline compared to hypertonic saline alone. However, no significant differences were observed when comparing idrevloride alone to placebo, or in the parallel comparisons of idrevloride in hypertonic saline versus idrevloride alone or placebo.
- *Conclusion:* Idrevloride in hypertonic saline was safe and associated with improved lung function over a 28-day period in people compared with hypertonic saline alone.

☞

- ***Intravenous N-acetylcysteine in Respiratory Disease with Abnormal Mucus Secretion. (European Review for Medical and Pharmacological Sciences. 2023)[4]***
  - o *Population:* Hospitalized adult patients with abnormal mucus secretion across 28 centers in China. (n=333)
  - o *Intervention:* 600 mg of intravenous (IV) N-acetylcysteine (NAC) twice daily for 7 days.
  - o *Comparator:*

    a) 30 mg of IV ambroxol hydrochloride twice daily.

    b) Placebo for 7 days.
  - o *Outcome:* The primary goal was to determine whether NAC was superior to placebo and non-inferior to ambroxol in terms of reducing sputum viscosity and facilitating mucus expectoration. NAC demonstrated a statistically significant improvement over placebo in both sputum viscosity (mean difference of 0.24 ± 0.763, $p < 0.001$) and expectoration difficulty (mean difference of 0.29 ± 0.783, $p = 0.002$). Additionally, NAC was shown to be non-inferior to ambroxol, with mean changes in sputum viscosity (–1.2 vs. –1.2) and expectoration difficulty scores (–1.4 vs. –1.3) falling within the pre-specified non-inferiority margin.
  - o *Conclusion:* IV NAC might be useful in patients with abnormal mucus secretion.

- ***Improvement in Lung Clearance Index and Chest Computed Tomography Scores with Elexacaftor/Tezacaftor/Ivacaftor Treatment in People with Cystic Fibrosis Aged 12 Years and Older - The RECOVER Trial. (AJRCCM. 2023)[5]***
  - o *Population:* Cystic fibrosis patients aged ≥12 years (n=117) who carried heterozygous or homozygous mutations for F508 deletion. This study was a prospective, observational study.

- *Intervention:* Elexacaftor/Tezacaftor/Ivacaftor (ETI) combination therapy was initiated and participants were followed up for 12 months.
- *Outcomes:* Improvement in lung clearance index, spirometry, and quality of life. ETI is associated with significant improvements in lung function and quality of life in cystic fibrosis patients.
- *Conclusion:* ETI is associated with improvements in $LCI_{2.5}$, spirometry, PRAGMA-CF CT scores, improved nutrition and quality of life.

• ***Long-term Safety and Efficacy of Elexacaftor/Tezacaftor/Ivacaftor in People with Cystic Fibrosis and at Least One F508del Allele: 144-Week Interim Results from a 192-Week Open-Label Extension Study. (ERJ. 2023)***[6]

- *Population:* Cystic fibrosis (CF) patients, aged ≥12 years, who have at least one F508del allele. The participants were enrolled in a 192-week open-label extension study after completing either a 24-week or 4-week parent study. The study was conducted across 110 sites in North America, Europe, and Australia. (n=506)
- *Intervention:* Participants received a daily regimen of elexacaftor (ELX) 200 mg once daily, tezacaftor (TEZ) 100 mg once daily, and ivacaftor (IVA) 150 mg every 12 hours. The primary focus was to assess the long-term safety and efficacy of this triple combination therapy over a 144-week interim period.
- *Comparator:* Outcomes were compared with the placebo and active treatment arms from the previous parent studies.
- *Outcome:* The study found that the combination therapy of ELX/TEZ/IVA led to sustained and statistically significant improvements in key outcomes. The mean absolute increase in FEV1 percentage predicted from baseline was 14.8 percentage points (95% CI 13.3–16.3) for those who had previously received placebo, and 14.1 percentage points (95% CI 12.6–15.6) for those who had received ELX/TEZ/IVA in the parent study. Sweat chloride concentrations significantly decreased by 50.5 mmol/L (95% CI –53.4 to –47.7) in the placebo crossover group and by 47.2 mmol/L (95% CI –49.9 to –44.4) in the continuous treatment group. Moreover, the annualized pulmonary exacerbation rate was reduced to 0.20 events per 48 weeks (95% CI 0.16–0.24), showcasing the therapy's ability to maintain long-term clinical benefits ($p < 0.001$ for all key measures).
- *Conclusion:* Patients receiving the intervention had sustained improvements in lung function, respiratory symptoms, CF transmembrane conductance regulator function, pulmonary exacerbation rates and nutritional status.

• ***Nebulized amphotericin B for preventing exacerbations in allergic bronchopulmonary aspergillosis: A systematic review and meta-analysis. (Pulm Pharmacol Ther. 2023)***[7]

- *Population:* Allergic bronchopulmonary aspergillosis patients from 5 studies. (n=188)
- *Intervention:* Nebulized amphotericin B (NAB) therapy.
- *Outcomes:* Frequency of subjects remaining exacerbation-free one year after initiating NAB, time to first exacerbation and the safety of NAB therapy. There was no difference in pooled risk difference of exacerbation between NAB and placebo. 76% (62–88) subjects remained exacerbation free with NAB at one year. NAB increased time to first exacerbation. There were no serious adverse events reported with NAB.
- *Conclusion:* NAB does not enhance exacerbation-free status at one year. However, there is weak evidence indicating it may delay ABPA exacerbations.

☞

- ***Dipeptidyl peptidase-1 inhibition with brensocatib reduces the activity of all major neutrophil serine proteases in patients with bronchiectasis: results from the WILLOW trial. (Respir Res. 2023)***[8]
  - *Population:* Patients with non-CF bronchiectasis and chronic sputum production in a Phase 2 RCT. (n=255)
  - *Intervention:* Brensocatib (oral DPP-1 inhibitor) once daily for 24 weeks. (n=170)
  - *Comparator:* Placebo. (n=85)
  - *Outcome:* Reduction in neutrophil serine protease activity. Brensocatib reduces neutrophil serine protease activity and leads to clinical improvements in non-CF bronchiectasis patients.
  - *Conclusion:* The anti-inflammatory effect of Brensocatib may be beneficial in patients of non-CF bronchiectasis.

☞

- ***The Efficacy and Safety of Inhaled Antibiotics for the Treatment of Bronchiectasis in Adults: Updated Systematic Review and Meta-Analysis. (Chest. 2024)***[9]
  - *Population:* Bronchiectasis patients diagnosed by CT imaging from 20 studies. (n=3,468)
  - *Intervention:* Inhaled antibiotics (included - DPI or inhaled liposomal ciprofloxacin, tobramycin DPI, or nebulized gentamicin, tobramycin, liposomal amikacin, ceftazidime, colistimethate sodium, and aztreonam).
  - *Comparator:* Placebo or standard care without inhaled antibiotics.
  - *Outcome:* Primary-Exacerbation frequency. Secondary: Severe exacerbations, bacterial load, symptoms, quality of life, and FEV1. Inhaled antibiotics reduced number of patients with exacerbations (risk ratio, 0.85; 95% CI, 0.75-0.96). A slight reduction in exacerbation frequency (rate ratio [RR], 0.78; 95% CI, 0.68-0.91). Probable reduction in severe exacerbations (RR, 0.48; 95% CI, 0.31–0.74). Likely slight increase in time to the first exacerbation (hazard ratio, 0.80; 95% CI, 0.68-0.94). Slight increase in the Quality-of-Life Questionnaire-Bronchiectasis respiratory symptom score (mean difference, 2.51; 95% CI, 0.44–4.31). Reduction in St. George Respiratory Questionnaire scores (mean difference, –3.13; 95% CI, –5.93 to –0.32). Nebulized antibiotics lead to a consistent reduction in bacterial load with no change in FEV1. Adverse effects were comparable to placebo.
  - *Conclusion:* Inhaled antibiotics resulted in a slight reduction in exacerbations and a probable reduction in severe exacerbations.

DISCUSSION

The pathogenesis of bronchiectasis is described by Cole's vicious vortex hypothesis. It states that environmental insults with the background of genetic susceptibility and impaired mucociliary clearance led to the colonization of microbes in the airway. This causes self-perpetuating airway inflammation and damage.

Bronchiectasis diagnosis is confirmed on high-resolution CT scan (HRCT) of the chest. **The direct sign of bronchiectasis includes increased broncho-arterial ratio (Signet-ring sign), contour abnormalities, visibility of the airways in the lung periphery (with in 1 cm of costal pleura) and lack of normal bronchial tapering, while indirect signs include bronchial wall thickening, bronchial mucus impaction, mosaic attenuation, and bronchial artery hypertrophy.**

The most common cause of bronchiectasis in the US registry is Non-tuberculous Mycobacterium (NTM) infection.[10] **In contrast <5% of cases have NTM as a cause in Korean, Australian, Indian, and European registries.**[1,2,11,12] **In these registries, idiopathic and post-infective were the most common cause except in Indian registry where tuberculosis was the leading cause of bronchiectasis.** The most common organism isolated in bacterial cultures of patients with bronchiectasis is Pseudomonas aeruginosa. Other frequent isolates include Haemophilus influenzae, Enterobacteriaceae, and Staphylococcus aureus. The isolation of pseudomonas is associated with recurrent exacerbations, decline in lung function and worse prognosis.

Even after the decrease in the incidence of serious childhood infection and improvement in vaccination, the prevalence of bronchiectasis has increased. Increased prevalence can be attributed to better diagnostic modalities and the use of CT scan. It continues to be a neglected disease among physicians. Till date, we don't have any licensed therapy for bronchiectasis. The management is further hampered by the widespread use of inhaled corticosteroids and inadequate bronchial toileting.

Due to distinct pathology and management, bronchiectasis is classified as cystic fibrosis and non-cystic fibrosis bronchiectasis (NCFB). Cystic fibrosis is due to a genetic defect in gene coding for cystic fibrosis transmembrane conductance regulator. This alteration causes increased sodium absorption and decreased chloride ions in secretions leading to bronchiectasis. In NCFB, the dilatation of the airways hampers mucociliary clearance and mucus stasis favours the colonisation of microorganisms. Effective management requires a multidisciplinary approach aimed at controlling infections, reducing inflammation, and maintaining lung function. The management of CF bronchiectasis involves a comprehensive approach that includes antibiotic therapy, airway clearance techniques, anti-inflammatory treatments, bronchodilators, muco-active agents, nutritional support, and, in some cases, surgical interventions. Regular monitoring and a multidisciplinary team are crucial to optimizing patient outcomes and improving quality of life.

Elexacaftor/Tezacaftor/Ivacaftor is a groundbreaking triple combination therapy for cystic fibrosis (CF) approved by US FDA in 2019. This therapy targets the defective CFTR protein caused by specific genetic mutations, particularly the F508del mutation, which is the most common CF mutation. Elexacaftor/Tezacaftor/Ivacaftor has been approved for use in younger patients, including those aged 6 to 11 years. The interim analysis of long-term follow-up published recently adds to the evidence of long-term efficacy and safety of triple drug combination in cystic fibrosis with CFTR mutation.[6] **A new triple-combination therapy (vanzacaftor, tezacaftor, and deutivacaftor) is expected to set a higher standard for CF treatment and has been approved by the FDA in December 2024.**

Exacerbations of bronchiectasis are acute episodes characterized by a significant worsening of respiratory symptoms, especially sputum production, and shortness of breath. Exacerbations are often triggered by infections, leading to heightened inflammation and further lung damage, rarely underlying disease worsening can cause bronchiectasis exacerbations like in ABPA. Management typically involves antimicrobial therapy based on respiratory culture data, along with measures to improve airway clearance and reduce inflammation. Preventive strategies, such as vaccination and regular physiotherapy, are crucial in reducing the frequency and severity of exacerbations. Effective management of exacerbations is essential to improve the quality of life and decelerate disease progression in patients with bronchiectasis.

Allergic Bronchopulmonary Aspergillosis

The International Society for Human and Animal Mycology (ISHAM) has recently updated its guidelines for the management of Allergic Bronchopulmonary Aspergillosis (ABPA).[13] These updates reflect advancements in diagnostics and therapeutics, aiming to improve patient outcomes. Here are the key changes:

1. Screening and Diagnosis

- **Screening: The updated guidelines recommend screening for *Aspergillus fumigatus* sensitization using fungus-specific IgE in all newly diagnosed asthmatic adults at tertiary care centers.** For children, screening is recommended only for those with difficult-to-treat asthma.
- **Diagnosis:** ABPA diagnosis now requires a combination of clinical, radiological, and immunological criteria. Specifically, patients must have a predisposing condition or compatible clinical presentation, along with fungal sensitization and serum total IgE $\geq$500 IU/mL. Additionally, two of the following are required: fungal-specific IgG, peripheral blood eosinophilia, or suggestive imaging. (Figure 1)

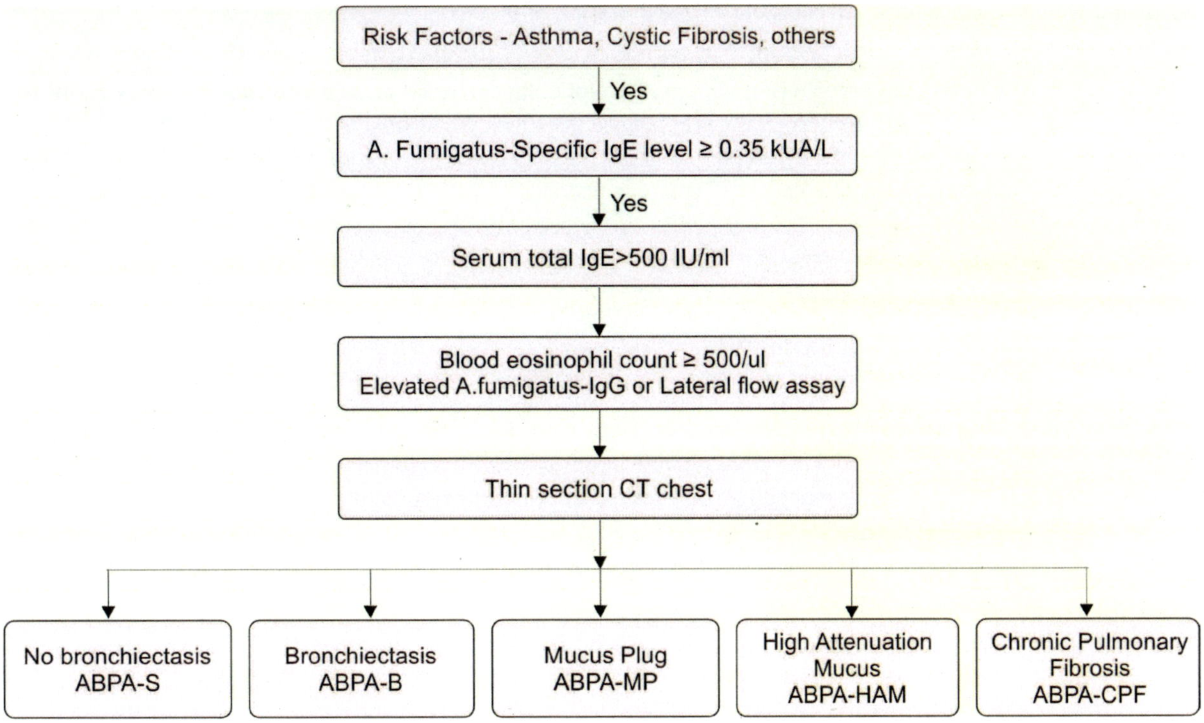

Figure 1: Diagnostic Algorithm for Allergic Bronchopulmonary Aspergillosis (ABPA)

2. Classification

- **ABPA vs. ABPM:** The guidelines distinguish between ABPA (caused by *Aspergillus spp.*) and Allergic Bronchopulmonary Mycosis (ABPM, caused by fungi other than *Aspergillus spp.*). ABPM diagnosis requires repeated growth of the causative fungus from sputum.

3. Treatment Recommendations

- **Asymptomatic Patients:** Routine treatment is not recommended for asymptomatic ABPA patients. (Table 1)
- **Acute ABPA:** For newly diagnosed or exacerbated ABPA, oral prednisolone or itraconazole monotherapy is recommended.
- **Recurrent Exacerbations:** For recurrent ABPA exacerbations, a combination of prednisolone and itraconazole is recommended.

4. Assessment of Treatment Response

- **Multidimensional Criteria:** An objective multidimensional criterion has been devised to assess treatment response. This includes clinical, radiological, and immunological parameters to provide a comprehensive evaluation of patient progress.

While nebulised LAmB has shown some positive secondary outcomes, ISHAM does not currently recommend it as a routine maintenance therapy for ABPA due to the lack of significant reduction in severe clinical exacerbations. Further research is needed to establish its role in the long-term management of ABPA.

Table 1: Management of ABPA

Stage	**Management**
Stage 0	Management of underlying bronchial asthma (universal) and observation ABPA therapy may not be required
Stage 1 (acute)	Prednisolone for 4 months. Alternatively, itraconazole or voriconazole for 4–6 months
Stage 2 (response)	Monitoring with total IgE, spirometry, quality-of-life questionnaires, and chest radiograph
Stage 3 (exacerbation)	Prednisolone, itraconazole, or **combination** of prednisolone and itraconazole
Stage 4 (remission)	Monitoring with total IgE, spirometry, quality-of-life questionnaires, and chest radiograph
Stage 5	**Control of exacerbation** with prednisolone, itraconazole, or their combination followed by any of the following: itraconazole, low-dose glucocorticoids, omalizumab, monthly pulses of methylprednisolone or nebulized amphotericin B
Stage 6	Pharmacological control of asthma, glucocorticoids or azoles or their combination, depending on the disease activity. Pulmonary rehabilitation, long-term oxygen therapy, domiciliary non-invasive ventilation, and lung transplantation, as indicated

Primary Ciliary Dyskinesia

The management of primary ciliary dyskinesia has seen significant advancements with improved diagnostic techniques, enhanced mucociliary clearance strategies, and novel therapeutic approaches. Sodium channel blockers like idrevloride represent a novel therapeutic approach for improving mucociliary clearance in patients with primary ciliary dyskinesia.[3] Idrevloride has shown promise in clinical trials, but it is not yet widely available for routine clinical use. Ongoing research and further clinical trials are needed to confirm its long-term efficacy and safety. If future studies continue to show positive results, idrevloride and other ENaC blockers could become an integral part of the therapeutic arsenal for managing PCD.

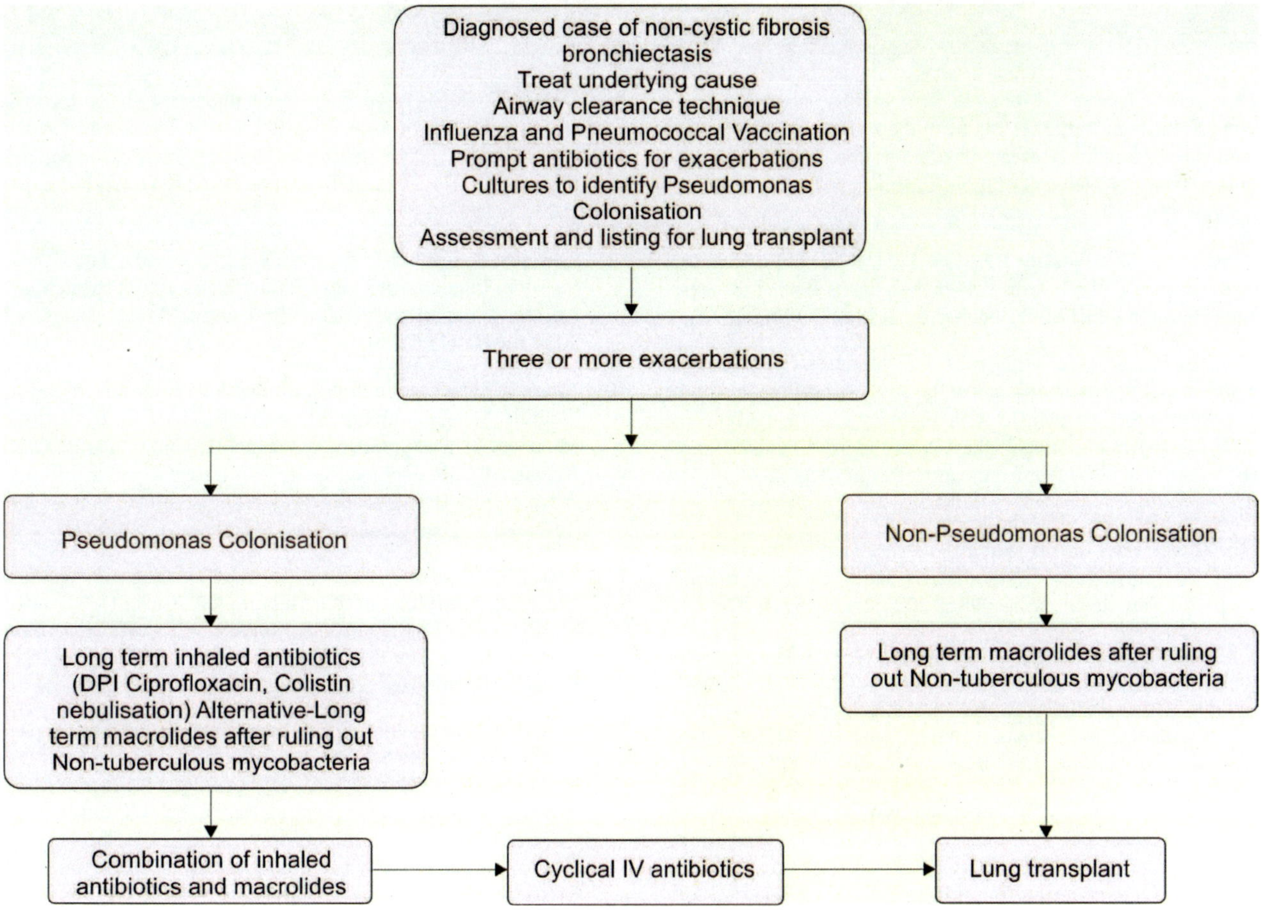

Flowchart: Management Algorithm of Non-cystic Fibrosis Bronchiectasis

REFERENCES

1. Dhar R, Singh S, Talwar D, Mohan M, Tripathi SK, Swarnakar R, et al. Bronchiectasis in India: results from the European Multicentre Bronchiectasis Audit and Research Collaboration (EMBARC) and Respiratory Research Network of India Registry. Lancet Glob Health. 2019;7(9):e1269-e79.

2. Choi H, Lee H, Ra SW, Kim HK, Lee JS, Um SJ, et al. Clinical Characteristics of Patients with Post-Tuberculosis Bronchiectasis: Findings from the KMBARC Registry. J Clin Med. 2021;10(19).

3. Ringshausen FC, Shapiro AJ, Nielsen KG, Mazurek H, Pifferi M, Donn KH, et al. Safety and efficacy of the epithelial sodium channel blocker idrevloride in people with primary ciliary dyskinesia (CLEAN-PCD): a multinational, phase 2, randomised, double-blind, placebo-controlled crossover trial. Lancet Respir Med. 2024;12(1): 21-33.

4. Tang W, Zhu D, Wu F, Xu JF, Yang JP, Deng ZP, et al. Intravenous N-acetylcysteine in respiratory disease with abnormal mucus secretion. Eur Rev Med Pharmacol Sci. 2023;27(11):5119-27.

5. McNally P, Lester K, Stone G, Elnazir B, Williamson M, Cox D, et al. Improvement in Lung Clearance Index and Chest Computed Tomography Scores with Elexacaftor/Tezacaftor/Ivacaftor Treatment in People with Cystic Fibrosis Aged 12 Years and Older - The RECOVER Trial. Am J Respir Crit Care Med. 2023;208(9):917-29.

6. Daines CL, Tullis E, Costa S, Linnemann RW, Mall MA, McKone EF, et al. Long-term safety and efficacy of elexacaftor/tezacaftor/ivacaftor in people with cystic fibrosis and at least one F508del allele: 144-week interim results from a 192-week open-label extension study. Eur Respir J. 2023;62(6).

7. Muthu V, Dhooria S, Sehgal IS, Prasad KT, Rudramurthy SM, Aggarwal AN, et al. Nebulized amphotericin B for preventing exacerbations in allergic bronchopulmonary aspergillosis: A systematic review and meta-analysis. Pulm Pharmacol Ther. 2023;81:102226.

8. Cipolla D, Zhang J, Korkmaz B, Chalmers JD, Basso J, Lasala D, et al. Dipeptidyl peptidase-1 inhibition with brensocatib reduces the activity of all major neutrophil serine proteases in patients with bronchiectasis: results from the WILLOW trial. Respir Res. 2023;24(1):133.

9. Cordeiro R, Choi H, Haworth CS, Chalmers JD. The Efficacy and Safety of Inhaled Antibiotics for the Treatment of Bronchiectasis in Adults: Updated Systematic Review and Meta-Analysis. Chest. 2024 Jul;166(1):61-80.

10. Aksamit TR, O'Donnell AE, Barker A, Olivier KN, Winthrop KL, Daniels MLA, Johnson M, Eden E, Griffith D, Knowles M, Metersky M, Salathe M, Thomashow B, Tino G, Turino G, Carretta B, Daley CL; Bronchiectasis Research Registry Consortium. Adult Patients With Bronchiectasis: A First Look at the US Bronchiectasis Research Registry. Chest. 2017 May;151(5):982-992.

11. Visser SK, Bye PTP, Fox GJ, Burr LD, Chang AB, Holmes-Liew CL, King P, Middleton PG, Maguire GP, Smith D, Thomson RM, Stroil-Salama E, Britton WJ, Morgan LC. Australian adults with bronchiectasis: The first report from the Australian Bronchiectasis Registry. Respir Med. 2019 Aug;155:97-103.

12. Chalmers JD, Polverino E, Crichton ML, Ringshausen FC, De Soyza A, Vendrell M, Burgel PR, Haworth CS, Loebinger MR, Dimakou K, Murris M, Wilson R, Hill AT, Menendez R, Torres A, Welte T, Blasi F, Altenburg J, Shteinberg M, Boersma W, Elborn JS, Goeminne PC, Aliberti S; EMBARC Registry Investigators. Bronchiectasis in Europe: data on disease characteristics from the European Bronchiectasis registry (EMBARC). Lancet Respir Med. 2023 Jul;11(7):637-649.

13. Agarwal R, Sehgal IS, Muthu V, Denning DW, Chakrabarti A, Soundappan K, et al. Revised ISHAM-ABPA working group clinical practice guidelines for diagnosing, classifying and treating allergic bronchopulmonary aspergillosis/mycoses. European Respiratory Journal. 2024;63(4):2400061.

CHAPTER 4

Interstitial Lung Disease

Authors: Dr. Ayush Goel, Dr. Sujay Halkur Shankar, Dr. Irfan Shekh

Reviewer: Dr. Pavan Tiwari

INTRODUCTION

Interstitial lung diseases are a heterogeneous group of diffuse parenchymal lung disorders characterized by inflammation and fibrosis. ILDs may be related to underlying systemic disease, environmental exposure, and smoking or can occur without any known etiological context thus posing a diagnostic and therapeutic challenge for clinicians. In this chapter, we will be discussing the recent advances in the diagnosis and management of interstitial lung disease.

Methodology

A PubMed search was carried out using the following search terms. Articles published in English between 1st August 2023 to 1st August 2024 were reviewed. 236 articles were identified and were screened for relevance. Finally, 23 articles have been selected for this review.

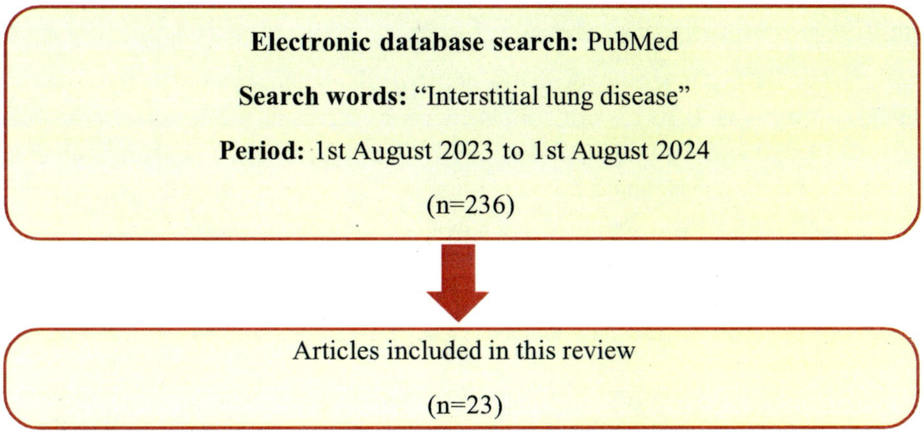

Analysis of Literature

Diagnostics

☞

- ***Transbronchial cryobiopsy followed by as-needed surgical lung biopsy versus immediate surgical lung biopsy for diagnosing interstitial lung disease (the COLD study): A randomised controlled trial. (Lancet Respir Med. 2024)[1]***
  - o *Population:* ILD patients requiring histopathological evidence for final MDT diagnosis. (n=55)
  - o *Intervention:* Step-up strategy (Transbronchial cryobiopsy followed by surgical lung biopsy if inconclusive) (n=28).
  - o *Control:* Immediate surgical lung biopsy. (n=27)
  - o *Outcome:* Primary outcome was unexpected chest tube drainage (any chest tube requirement after transbronchial cryobiopsy or need for chest tube > 24 hours after surgical lung biopsy). Unexpected chest tube drainage occurred in 11% (4 - 27%) in the intervention arm and in 46% (2 - 65%) in the control arm with an absolute risk reduction of 35% (11-56%; p = 0·0058). In the step-up strategy, the multidisciplinary team diagnostic yield after transbronchial cryobiopsy alone was 82% (64 – 92%), which increased to 89% (73 – 96%) when subsequent SLB was performed after inconclusive transbronchial cryobiopsy. In the immediate surgical lung biopsy strategy, the multidisciplinary team diagnostic yield was 88% (69 – 97%). Total in-hospital stay was 1 day (IQR 1 – 1) in the step-up group versus 5 days (IQR 4 – 6) in the SLB group. 01 (4%) serious adverse event occurred in step-up strategy versus 12 (50%) in the immediate SLB strategy.
  - o *Conclusion:* A diagnostic strategy starting with transbronchial cryobiopsy, followed by SLB when transbronchial cryobiopsy is inconclusive, appears to result in a significant reduction of patient burden and in-hospital stay with a similar diagnostic yield versus immediate SLB.
  - o *Critical appraisal:* The RCT provides evidence to optimize the balance between the risk from lung biopsy and getting a histological diagnosis. For a majority of patients and clinicians, the approach of utilizing TBLC to reduce the need for surgical lung biopsy is pragmatic and improves net diagnostic rate. However, some patients may not want two procedures for diagnosis and may prefer undergoing surgical lung biopsy directly. This may also be suitable for centers with high volume and experience with surgical lung biopsy.

Idiopathic pulmonary fibrosis

- ***Bexotegrast in Patients with Idiopathic Pulmonary Fibrosis: The INTEGRIS-IPF Clinical Trial. (Am J Respir Crit Care Med. 2024)[2]***
  - o *Population*: Subjects diagnosed with IPF with FVC $\geq$45% and DLCO $\geq$30% with or without background antifibrotics. (n=119, Phase 2a, multicenter trial)
  - o *Intervention*: 40mg, 80mg, 160mg, or 320mg Bexotegrast once daily for 12 weeks.
  - o *Control*: Matching placebo for 12 weeks. (3:1 randomization).

- *Outcome:* Primary outcome was treatment emergent adverse events (TEAE). 81.8% subjects were on background antifibrotics. TEAE were comparable between treatment (69.7%) and placebo (67.7%) with grade 3 or higher adverse events seen in 6.7% and 6.5% in the intervention and placebo arms respectively. The most common adverse event was diarrhea (16.9%). The pooled change in FVC over the study period was -3.6mL in the Bexotegrast group compared with -110.5mL in the placebo group.
- *Conclusion:* Bexotegrast showed acceptable safety and tolerability in subjects with IPF with secondary outcomes showing evidence of antifibrotic action.
- *Critical appraisal:* This was a phase 2a trial and should not be used to conclude efficacy of the drug in IPF. However, Bexotegrast appears to be a promising therapeutic option for IPF, if proven in Phase 3 trials.

- ***Pamrevlumab for Idiopathic Pulmonary Fibrosis: The ZEPHYRUS-1 Randomized Clinical Trial. (JAMA. 2024)***[3]
  - *Population:* Subjects diagnosed with IPF not on background antifibrotics at enrolment (n = 356, Phase 3 trial).
  - *Intervention:* Intravenous Pamrevlumab (30 mg/kg) administered 3 weekly for 48 weeks.
  - *Control:* Intravenous placebo for 48 weeks (1:1 randomization).
  - *Outcome:* The primary outcome was absolute change in FVC from baseline to week 48. There was no significant between-group difference for absolute change in FVC from baseline to week 48 in the pamrevlumab group vs the placebo group; mean between-group difference, 70 mL [95% CI, -60 to 190 mL], P = .29). There was no significant difference between the two groups in treatment-related adverse events.
  - *Conclusion:* Pamrevlumab did not benefit patients with IPF over placebo in change in FVC.

- ***Zinpentraxin Alfa for Idiopathic Pulmonary Fibrosis: The Randomized Phase III STARSCAPE Trial. (Am J Respir Crit Care Med. 2024)***[4]
  - *Population:* Subjects diagnosed with IPF.
  - *Intervention:* Intravenous zinpentraxin alpha 10mg/kg every 4 weeks. (n=331)
  - *Control:* Intravenous placebo. (n=333)
  - *Outcome:* Primary outcome was absolute change from baseline to week 52 in the FVC. The trial was terminated early after a prespecified futility analysis showed no benefit over placebo. In the final analysis, absolute change from baseline to Week 52 in FVC was similar between placebo and zinpentraxin alfa (– 214.89 mL vs –235.72 mL; p = 0.5420); there were no apparent treatment effect on secondary endpoints of change in baseline to week 52 in the percent predicted FVC and 6-minute walk distance. The adverse effects were similar between the placebo group and the zinpentraxin alpha group (72.3% vs 74.6%).
  - *Conclusion:* Zinpentraxin alfa did not benefit patients with IPF over placebo.

- ***Nalbuphine Tablets for Cough in Patients with Idiopathic Pulmonary Fibrosis. (NEJM Evid. 2023)***[5]
  - *Population:* Cross-over trial including subjects diagnosed with IPF (n=41) with 22-day treatment periods separated by a 2-week washout period.
  - *Intervention:* Nalbuphine extended release tablets (NAL ER) 27 mg once a day titrated to 162 mg twice at day 16 followed by placebo.
  - *Control:* Placebo followed by NAL ER 27 mg once a day titrated to 162 mg twice a day.

- *Outcome:* The primary outcome was percent change from baseline in hourly daytime objective cough frequency as measured by an electronic cough monitor. There was a 75.1% reduction in daytime objective cough frequency during the NAL ER treatment period versus the placebo treatment period of 22.6% (52.5% placebo-compared reduction; $p < 0.001$) at day 21. There was a 76.1% (83.1 - 69.1) decrease in the 24-hour objective cough frequency with NAL ER, versus a 25.3% (43.9 - 6.7) decrease with placebo (50.8% placebo-compared reduction). Nausea, fatigue, constipation, and dizziness were more common with NAL ER than with placebo.
- *Conclusion:* In this short-term crossover trial, NAL ER reduced cough in individuals with IPF.

- ***Morphine for treatment of cough in idiopathic pulmonary fibrosis (PACIFY COUGH): A prospective, multicentre, randomised, double-blind, placebo-controlled, two-way crossover trial. (Lancet Respir Med. 2024)***[6]
  - *Population:* Subjects diagnosed with IPF within 5 years with self-reported cough > 8 weeks with cough VAS > 30mm (n=44, Phase 2 RCT).
  - *Intervention:* Morphine (controlled-release tablets) 5mg twice a day for 14 days followed by placebo.
  - *Control:* Placebo for 14 days followed by Morphine (controlled-release tablets) 5mg twice a day. Cross-over was done after a 7-day washout period.
  - *Outcome:* The primary outcome was percentage change in objective awake cough frequency from baseline at day 14 as measured by a cough monitor. In the intention-to-treat analysis, morphine reduced objective awake cough frequency by 39.4% (– 54.4 to –19.4; $p = 0.0005$) compared with placebo. Mean daytime cough frequency reduced from 21.6 (SE 1.2) coughs per hour at baseline to 12.8 (SE 1.2) coughs per hour with morphine, whereas cough rates did not change with placebo (21.5 [SE 1.2] coughs per hour to 20.6 [1.2] coughs per hour).
  - *Conclusion:* In patients with cough related to idiopathic pulmonary fibrosis, low dose controlled-release morphine significantly reduced objective cough counts over 14 days compared with placebo. Morphine shows promise as an effective treatment to palliate cough in patients with IPF.
  - *Critical appraisal:* This was a Phase 2 trial and should not be used as evidence for efficacy of the drug in this setting. However, there is a gross scarcity of effective treatment modalities for persistent cough in IPF. Previously, opioids were used in this setting based on evidence from refractory cough not necessarily in IPF. This RCT also carries significance in palliation of symptoms in advanced IPF.

- ***Comparison of Pirfenidone and Nintedanib: Post Hoc Analysis of the CleanUP-IPF Study. (Chest. 2024)***[7]
  - *Population:* IPF patients on nintedanib or perfenidone.
  - *Method:* A post-hoc analysis was performed using the Clinical Efficacy of Antimicrobial Therapy Strategy Using Pragmatic Design in IPF (CleanUP-IPF) trial (No. NCT02759120). Participants who reported using pirfenidone or nintedanib on enrolment into the trial were included in the primary analysis.
  - *Outcomes:* 407 subjects reported using pirfenidone (n=264, 65%) or nintedanib (n = 143, 35%). The pirfenidone group had more participants with a history of coronary artery disease than the nintedanib group (34.1% vs 20.3%).

Patients treated with nintedanib had a higher 12-month FVC than those treated with pirfenidone (mean difference, 106 mL; 95% CI, 34 - 178). There were no significant differences in overall survival and non-elective respiratory hospitalization between the pirfenidone and nintedanib groups.

- *Conclusion:* Subjects with IPF who used nintedanib had a slower 12-month FVC decline than pirfenidone in a post hoc analysis of a clinical trial.
- *Critical appraisal:* This was a post-hoc analysis and not a head-to-head efficacy and safety finding RCT between the two drugs.

- ***Efficacy and Safety of Pirfenidone in Advanced Versus Non-Advanced Idiopathic Pulmonary Fibrosis: Post-Hoc Analysis of Six Clinical Studies. (Adv Ther. 2023)***[8]
  - *Population:* IPF patients (n=1247). Data were included from the ASCEND, CAPACITY (004 and 006), RECAP (advanced IPF defined as percent predicted forced vital capacity [%FVC] < 50% and/or percent predicted carbon monoxide diffusing capacity [%DLco] < 35% at baseline); PASSPORT (advanced IPF defined as baseline %FVC < 50%); and SP-IPF (advanced IPF defined as %DLco ≤ 40% at screening and at risk of group 3 pulmonary hypertension).
  - *Outcomes:* In the pooled ASCEND/CAPACITY studies, the annual mean rate of FVC decline from baseline to week 52 was significantly lower for pirfenidone versus placebo in advanced ($p = 0.0035$) and non-advanced IPF ($p = 0.0001$). Rate of all-cause mortality over 52 weeks was numerically lower for pirfenidone versus placebo in advanced and non-advanced IPF. In RECAP, the mean annual rate of FVC decline from baseline to week 180 of pirfenidone treatment was similar in patients with advanced (-141.5 mL) and non-advanced IPF (-153.5 mL).
  - *Conclusion:* These results highlight the benefit of pirfenidone treatment in patients with advanced and non-advanced IPF.

- ***Inhaled pirfenidone solution (AP01) for IPF: A randomised, open-label, dose-response trial. (Thorax, 2023)***[9]
  - *Population:* Subjects diagnosed with IPF within 5 years with FVC between 40 – 90% who are ineligible, unwilling or intolerant for oral anti-fibrotics. (Phase 1b, dose-response trial)
  - *Intervention 1:* Inhaled pirfenidone AP01 50mg once a day. (n=46)

    2: Inhaled pirfenidone AP01 100mg twice a day. (n=45)
  - *Outcome:* The most common treatment-related adverse events were all mild or moderate and included cough (15.4%), rash (12.1%), nausea (8.8%), throat irritation (5.5%), fatigue (4.4%) and taste disorder, dizziness and dyspnoea (3.3%). Changes in FVC percentage predicted over 24 and 48 weeks, respectively, were -2.5 (-5.3 to 0.4, -88 mL) and -4.9 (-7.5 to -2.3,-188 mL) in the 50 mg once per day, and 0.6 (-2.2 to 3.4, 10 mL) and -0.4 (-3.2 to 2.3, -34 mL) in the 100 mg two times per day group.
  - *Conclusion:* **Side effects commonly associated with oral pirfenidone in other clinical trials were less frequent with AP01. Mean FVC% predicted remained stable in the 100 mg two times per day group.**

CTD associated ILD

- ***2023 American College of Rheumatology (ACR)/American College of Chest Physicians (CHEST) Guideline for the Treatment of Interstitial Lung Disease in People with Systemic Autoimmune Rheumatic Diseases. (Arthritis Rheumatol. 2024)***[10]

- ***2023 American College of Rheumatology (ACR)/American College of Chest Physicians (CHEST) Guideline for the Screening and Monitoring of Interstitial Lung Disease in People with Systemic Autoimmune Rheumatic Diseases. (Arthritis Rheumatol. 2024)***[11]

☞

- ***Tocilizumab in Patients with Systemic Sclerosis-associated Interstitial Lung Disease: A Systematic Review and Meta-Analysis. (Ann Am Thorac Soc. 2024)[12]***
  - o *Population:* SSc-ILD patients treated with tocilizumab from 5 studies.
  - o *Outcomes:* The absolute decrease from baseline in FVC for the tocilizumab arm was 118 mL, 241 mL, and 129 mL less than the placebo arm at 24, 48, and 96 weeks, respectively, favoring tocilizumab. The mean decrease in FVC% predicted at 48 weeks was 6.50% less and the risk of decrease > 10% was 66% less in the tocilizumab arm. Patients were 1.97 times more likely to have any increase in FVC% predicted if they received tocilizumab in place of placebo. When the placebo arm was given tocilizumab from 48 to 96 weeks, the mean change in absolute FVC was 54.90 mL less and the mean change in FVC% predicted was 1.30% less. For DLco percentage predicted, at 48 weeks there was 1.50% less change and from 48 to 96 weeks there was 5.40% less change in the tocilizumab arm.
  - o *Conclusion:* Tocilizumab use in patients with SSc-ILD is associated with less disease progression and a better toxicity profile than placebo.

- ***Nintedanib Therapy Alone and Combined with Mycophenolate in Patients with Systemic Sclerosis-associated Interstitial Lung Disease: Systematic Reviews and Meta-analysis. (Ann Am Thorac Soc. 2024)[13]***
  - o *Population* Patients with SSc-ILD should be treated with nintedanib alone or with a combination of nintedanib plus mycophenolate.
  - o *Outcome:* For nintedanib therapy alone, the systematic review included 3 studies and revealed that disease progression was less in the nintedanib arm (the annual rate of decline in FVC was 44.5 mL less, the absolute change from baseline was 46.4 mL less, and FVC % predicted was 1.2% less) compared with placebo. Gastrointestinal side effects and treatment discontinuation were twice as common in the nintedanib group compared to placebo.
  - o *Conclusion:* The use of nintedanib alone and in combination with mycophenolate in patients with SSc-ILD is associated with a significant reduction in disease progression compared with placebo but at the cost of increased gastrointestinal side effects and treatment discontinuation.

☞

- ***Rituximab in Patients with Systemic Sclerosis-associated Interstitial Lung Disease: A Systematic Review and Meta-Analysis. (Ann Am Thorac Soc. 2024)[14]***
  - o *Population:* Studies using rituximab to treat patients with SSc-ILD. The comparator group was selected to be placebo or mycophenolate. The final analysis included 3 studies.
  - o *Outcomes:* Rituximab significantly improved the FVC % predicted (mean difference, 3.13% [0.37 - 5.90]) and the modified Rodnan Skin Score (mean difference, -7.01 [11.46 to -2.56]) at 24 - 48 weeks.
  - o *Conclusion:* Rituximab use in patients with SSc-ILD is associated with stabilization of lung function.

- ***Cyclophosphamide in Patients with Systemic Sclerosis-associated Interstitial Lung Disease: A Systematic Review and Meta-Analysis. (Ann Am Thorac Soc. 2024)[15]***
  - o *Population:* Studies using cyclophosphamide to treat patients with SSc-ILD. The comparator group included placebo and mycophenolate. A total of 5 studies were included in the final analysis.

- *Outcomes:* Compared with placebo, there was a 2.83% (0.8 – 4.87) reduction in the decline at 12 months for FVC % predicted using cyclophosphamide. There were improvements in breathlessness (Transition Dyspnea Index mean difference, 2.90 [1.94-3.86]) and disability (Health Assessment Questionnaire-Disability Index MD, -0.16 [-0.28 to -0.04]). There were increased risks of leukopenia and constitutional symptoms using cyclophosphamide, but no difference in mortality.
- *Conclusion:* Cyclophosphamide is effective in SSc-ILD compared with placebo, with an increased risk of side effects.

☞

- ***The prevalence and risk factors of rheumatoid arthritis-associated interstitial lung disease: A systematic review and meta-analysis. (Ann Med. 2024)***[16]
  - *Population:* Studies reporting the prevalence and risk factors of Rheumatoid arthritis from 56 studies (n = 11851 patients)
  - *Outcomes:* The pooled prevalence of RA-ILD was 18.7% (15.8 - 21.6) with significant heterogeneity (I^2 = 96.4%). The risk factors for RA-ILD included male sex (OR = 1.92 [1.70 - 2.16]), older age (WMDs = 6.89, [3.10 - 10.67]), smoking history (OR = 1.91 [1.48 - 2.47]), pulmonary comorbidities predicted (HR = 2.08 [1.89 - 2.30]), longer RA duration (OR = 1.03 [1.01 - 1.05]), older age of RA onset (WMDs = 4.46 [0.63 - 8.29]), positive RF (HR = 1.15 [0.75 - 1.77]; ORs = 2.11 [1.65 - 2.68]), positive ACPA (OR = 2.11 [1.65 - 2.68]), higher ESR (OR = 1.008 [1.002 - 1.014]), moderate and high DAS28 (≥ 3.2) (OR = 1.87 [1.36 - 2.58]), rheumatoid nodules (OR = 1.87 [1.18 - 2.98]), leflunomide use (OR = 1.42 [1.08 - 1.87]), and steroid use (HR = 1.70 [1.13 - 2.55]). The use of biological agents was a protective factor (HR = 0.77 [0.69 - 0.87]).
  - *Conclusion:* The pooled prevalence of RA-ILD was approximately 18.7%. **13 risk factors for RA-ILD were identified, including male sex, older age, having a smoking history, pulmonary comorbidities, older age of RA onset, longer RA duration, positive RF, positive ACPA, higher ESR, moderate and high DAS28 (≥ 3.2), rheumatoid nodules, leflunomide use and steroid use. Additionally, biological agents use was a protective factor.**

☞

- ***Rituximab in the treatment of progressive interstitial lung disease associated with the anti-synthetase syndrome. (Arthritis Res Ther. 2024)***[17]
  - *Population:* Multicentre retrospective observational study including patients with Anti-synthetase syndrome associated ILD (ASS-ILD) that started treatment with RTX (Injection RTX -1gm on day 0 and 15 and then every 6 months) due to recurrent or ongoing progressive ILD despite therapy with glucocorticoids and immunosuppressants (n=28).
  - *Outcome:* After 6 months of treatment, RTX reversed the decline in PFT parameters: Δ%pFVC +6.29% (-10.07 to 2.51; p = 0.002) and Δ%pDLCO +6.15% (-10.86 to -1.43; p = 0.013). 24 patients completed 1 year of therapy and 22 2 years, maintaining the response in PFT: Δ%pFVC: +9.93% (-15.61 to -4.25; p = 0.002) and Δ%pDLCO: +7.66% (-11.67 to -3.65; p < 0.001). Prednisolone could be discontinued in 18% of cases. In 33% of patients who required oxygen therapy at the start of treatment, it could be discontinued. The frequency of adverse events reached 28.5% of cases.
  - *Conclusion:* RTX appears to be effective as rescue therapy in most patients with recurrent or progressive ASS-ILD unresponsive to conventional treatment. The use of RTX was well tolerated in the majority of patients.

Hypersensitivity pneumonitis

- ***Pirfenidone in fibrotic hypersensitivity pneumonitis: A double-blind, randomised clinical trial of efficacy and safety. (Thorax. 2023)***[18]
    - o *Population:* Patients with fibrotic HP and evidence of progression (n = 40 with 2:1 randomization).
    - o *Intervention:* Oral Pirfenidone (2403mg/day) over 52 weeks.
    - o *Control:* Placebo.
    - o *Outcome:* Primary outcome was the mean absolute change in the percent predicted of FVC. There was no significant between-group difference in FVC% at week 52 (mean difference -0.76% [-6.34 to 4.82]). Pirfenidone resulted in a lower rate of decline in the adjusted FVC% at week 26 and improved PFS (HR 0.26 [0.12 to 0.60]).
    - o *Conclusion:* The trial was underpowered to detect a difference in the primary end point. Pirfenidone was found to be safe and improved PFS in patients with FHP.

Sarcoidosis

- ***Diagnostic Yield and Safety of the 19-Gauge versus 22-Gauge Endobronchial Ultrasound-Guided Transbronchial Needle Aspiration Needle in Subjects with Sarcoidosis (GUESS). (Respiration. 2024)***[19]
    - o *Population:* Patients with suspected sarcoidosis with mediastinal lymphadenopathy taken up for EBUS-TBNA. (n = 150, sarcoidosis diagnosed in 116 patients).
    - o *Intervention:* Use of 19-G needle. (n=60)
    - o *Control:* Use of 22-G needle. (n=56)
    - o *Outcome:* Primary outcome was diagnostic sensitivity (granulomas in patients finally diagnosed with sarcoidosis). The diagnostic sensitivity of the 19-G needle (45/60, 75.0%) was not higher (p = 0.52) than the 22-G needle (39/56, 69.6%). We obtained adequate aspirates in 90.0% and 85.7% of subjects in the respective groups (p = 0.48). The operators had greater difficulty puncturing lymph nodes with the 19-G needle (p = 0.03), while the operator-assessed cough intensity was similar in the groups (p = 0.41).
    - o *Conclusion:* 19-G needle was not superior to the 22-G in diagnostic sensitivity, specimen adequacy, or safety of EBUS-TBNA in sarcoidosis. Puncturing the lymph nodes was more difficult with the 19-G needle.

- **High-dose (40 mg) versus low-dose (20 mg) prednisolone for treating sarcoidosis: A randomised trial. (SARCORT trial). (Eur Respir J. 2023)**[20]
    - o *Population:* Patients of pulmonary sarcoidosis (1:1 randomization). This RCT was conducted in India (PGIMER, Chandigarh). Patients with indications for high-dose corticosteroids (like vision-threatening sarcoidosis, cardiac sarcoidosis) were excluded.
    - o *Intervention:* High dose prednisolone (40mg/day tapered over 6 months). (n=43)
    - o *Control:* Low dose prednisolone (20mg/day tapered over 6 months). (n=43)

- *Outcome:* Primary outcome was treatment failure or relapse at 18 months after randomization. 20 (46.5%) subjects had relapse or treatment failure in the high-dose group and 19 (44.2%) in the low-dose group (p = 0.75). The mean time to relapse/treatment failure was similar between the groups (high-dose 307 days *versus* low-dose 269 days, p = 0.27). The overall response, the changes in FVC at 6 and 18 months and the incidence of adverse effects were similar. Changes in HRQoL scores did not differ between the study groups. Frequency of treatment related adverse events were similar between the groups.
- *Conclusion:* High-dose prednisolone was not superior to a lower dose in improving outcomes or the HRQoL in sarcoidosis and was associated with similar adverse effects.
- *Critical appraisal:* This was a well conducted RCT and may prove to be a practice altering study. However, the single center and the non-blinded design are chief weaknesses. It also did not include patient related outcomes as an evaluation target. The study did not need to include a placebo arm since the efficacy of steroids in sarcoidosis has already been established. The trial was conducted in India, and therefore the evidence is more applicable to the Indian population.

Non-IPF fibrosing ILD

☞

- ***Impact of antifibrotic therapy on disease progression, all-cause mortality, and risk of acute exacerbation in non-IPF fibrosing interstitial lung diseases: evidence from a meta-analysis of randomized controlled trials and prospective controlled studies. (Ther Adv Respir Dis. 2024)***[21]
  - *Population:* Non-IPF fibrosing ILDs from 9 studies. (n=1990)
  - *Outcome:* Antifibrotic therapy reduced the rate of patients with disease progression (5 trials with 1741 subjects; RR = 0.56 [0.42 - 0.75]; $p < 0.0001$; $I^2 = 0$; high-certainty evidence). Antifibrotic therapy did not significantly decrease all-cause mortality (9 trials with 1990 subjects; RR = 0.76 [0.55 - 1.03]; p = 0.08; $I^2 = 0$; low-certainty evidence). However, in patients with progressive fibrosing ILDs (PF-ILD), antifibrotic therapy decreased all-cause mortality (4 trials with 1100 subjects; RR = 0.69 [0.48 - 0.98]; p = 0.04; $I^2 = 0$; low-certainty evidence).
  - *Conclusion:* Study supports the use of antifibrotic agents in patients with PF-ILDs, which could slow disease progression and decrease all-cause mortality.

Granulomatous lymphocytic ILD

- ***The efficacy and safety of systemic corticosteroids as first line treatment for granulomatous lymphocytic interstitial lung disease. (J Allergy Clin Immunol. 2023)***[22]
  - *Population:* Granulomatous lymphocytic interstitial lung disease patients (GL-ILD). (n=79)
  - *Intervention:* Steroids (>0.3mg/kg prednisolone equivalent) without other immunosuppression. (n=56)
  - *Comparator:* Patients with GL-ILD who had not received any immunosuppression. (n=23)
  - *Outcome:* Treatment with high-dose corticosteroids significantly improved HRCT scores and forced vital capacity. DLco significantly improved in both groups. Of 18 patients, for whom extended follow-up data was available, 13 achieved a long-term, maintenance therapy independent remission. All patients with relapse were retreated with corticosteroids, but only one-fifth of them responded. Two opportunistic infections were found in the corticosteroid treatment group, while overall infection rate was similar between cohorts.

- *Conclusion:* Induction therapy with high-dose corticosteroids improved HRCT scans and PFT results of patients with GL-ILD and achieved long-term remission in 42% of patients. It was not associated with major side effects. Low-dose maintenance therapy provided no benefit and efficacy was poor in relapsing disease.

Miscellaneous

- ***Prognosis of Lung Transplantation in Patients with Acute Exacerbations of Interstitial Lung Disease: A Meta-Analysis Based on Cohort Studies. (Ann Thorac Cardiovasc Surg. 2024)***[23]
  - *Population:* Patients with acute exacerbation of interstitial lung disease (AE-ILD) treated with lung transplantation compared to those with stable interstitial lung disease (ILD) from 5 cohort studies.
  - *Outcome:* The results showed that regarding perioperative outcomes, the AE-ILD group did not differ from the stable-ILD group in the incidence of ACR (RR = 0.34, p = 0.44) and the incidence of PGD III (RR = 0.53, p = 0.43), but had a longer LOS (mean difference = 9.15, p = 0.02). Regarding prognosis, the two also did not differ in 90-day OS (RR = 0.97, p = 0.59), 1-year OS (RR = 1.05, p = 0.66), and 3-year OS (RR = 0.91, p = 0.76).
  - *Conclusion:* Study concluded that the efficacy of lung transplantation in patients with AE-ILD is not inferior to that of patients with stable ILD. Lung transplantation is one of the potential treatments for patients with AE-ILD.

- ***The outcome of 12-week corticosteroid therapy in COVID-19-related diffuse interstitial lung abnormalities. (Med J Malaysia. 2024)***[24]
  - *Population:* Moderate to severe COVID -19 patients with diffuse interstitial lung abnormalities on CT. (n=330)
  - *Intervention:* 12 weeks of oral prednisolone.
  - *Outcome:* On follow-up at 12 weeks, the CT patterns showed improvement in ground-glass opacities, perilobular density and consolidation. There was an improvement in the mean (SD) CT score before and after prednisolone therapy, with values of 17.3 (5.3) and 8.6 (5.5), respectively ($p < 0.001$). The median mMRC was 1 (IQR 0 - 1), and 98.8% had a radiological response. The common side effects of prednisolone therapy were weight gain (13.9%), hyperglycaemia (1.8%) and cushingoid habitus (0.6%).
  - *Conclusion:* A 12-week treatment with prednisolone showed significant improvement in CT scores with minimal residual dyspnoea and was relatively safe. Longer duration of steroids may be beneficial in moderate to severe COVID-19- related DILA.

- ***Oxygen therapy for exercise capacity in fibrotic interstitial lung disease: A systematic review and meta-analysis of randomised controlled trials. (Respir Med. 2024)***[25]
  - *Population:* Fibrosing ILD patients from 14 studies.
  - *Outcomes:* Oxygen therapy improved SpO_2 during exercise (mean difference, MD = 6.26 %), exercise duration (MD = 122.15 s), fatigue (standard mean difference, SMD = -0.30), and dyspnoea (MD = -0.75 Borg score units). High-flow oxygen systems tended to be more effective than low-flow systems in improving exercising SpO_2, duration, fatigue, dyspnoea, and heart rate.
  - *Conclusion:* Short-term use of oxygen supplementation can improve SpO_2, exercise capacity, fatigue, and dyspnoea among patients with fILD. Further analyses demonstrates that HFNCs yield more favourable outcomes, yet not reaching statistical significance except for improving SpO_2 and fatigue.

DISCUSSION

Interstitial lung abnormalities

Interstitial lung abnormalities (ILAs) are defined as incidental findings on chest CT scans, typically identified in patients who are not suspected of having ILD at the time of imaging. These abnormalities are characterized by nondependent changes affecting more than 5% of any lung zone and are often found in older individuals and smokers. ILAs represent a spectrum of early interstitial changes that may progress to more significant fibrosing interstitial lung diseases, such as pulmonary fibrosis.[26]

The classification of ILAs includes subtypes such as non-subpleural, subpleural non-fibrotic, and subpleural fibrotic patterns, which are used to assess the potential for progression to clinically significant ILD. The presence of ILAs has been associated with worsened clinical outcomes, increased mortality, and a higher incidence of complications, such as sepsis-related acute respiratory distress syndrome (ARDS) and treatment-related complications in lung cancer patients. The traction bronchiectasis/bronchiolectasis index is emerging as a promising imaging biomarker for prognostic risk stratification.[26–28]

The treatment of ILAs following COVID-19 involves a multifaceted approach, as these conditions can vary in severity and progression. Research indicates that a significant proportion of patients hospitalized with COVID-19 develop ILAs, with some progressing to irreversible fibrotic changes. Approximately 30% of these patients exhibit ILAs post-hospitalization, and up to one-third may develop irreversible fibrosis. Some treatment strategies that have been studied include Nintedanib, Tacrolimus, and Interferon alpha. **A recent retrospective study looked at the role of steroids in the management of COVID-associated ILA which showed improvement in CT scores with 98.8% subjects having radiologic response.[24,29–31] However due to paucity of evidence, at this point of time suggesting any treatment for COVID related fibrosis is not possible.**

CTD associated ILD

Connective tissue diseases (CTD) are a variety of systemic autoimmune disorders leading to immune-mediated destruction of organs mediated by circulating autoantibodies. ILD frequently complicates the course of patients with auto-immune myopathy, systemic sclerosis, Sjogren's syndrome, rheumatoid arthritis, and systemic lupus erythematosus (SLE) with estimated prevalence of 40%, 30-40%, 40%, 10%, and 8-12% respectively.[32] **The diagnosis of CTD associated ILD is made when a patient satisfies the classification criteria of the suspected CTD plus a high resolution computed tomographic (HRCT) scan of the thorax showing evidence of interstitial lung disease.** Most guidelines suggest testing for autoantibodies even in the absence of overt clinical features of CTD to differentiate CTD associated ILD from IIPs. ANA, anti-ccp, rheumatoid factor, and myositis panel are recommended in all patients.[33,34]

The optimal treatment strategy for individual CTD associated ILD is currently unknown. The key guidelines from the American College of Rheumatology (ACR) for treating ILD in patients with systemic autoimmune rheumatic diseases (SARDs) emphasize evidence-based recommendations tailored to specific conditions and disease progressions. **A significant aspect of these guidelines is the strong recommendation against using glucocorticoids as a first-line therapy for systemic sclerosis-associated ILD (SSc-ILD) and after ILD progression in these patients.** This recommendation is based on the potential adverse effects and limited efficacy of glucocorticoids in this context. **However, glucocorticoids are conditionally recommended for first-line ILD treatment in other SARDs, reflecting their potential utility in different autoimmune contexts. For SSc-ILD specifically, the guidelines recommend the use of mycophenolate as a primary treatment option.** Other suggested treatments include cyclophosphamide, rituximab, tocilizumab, nintedanib, and the combination of nintedanib with mycophenolate, highlighting a range of therapeutic options based on current evidence and expert consensus.[10,35]

The 2023 ACR guidelines, developed in collaboration with the American College of Chest Physicians, provide evidence-based recommendations for screening and monitoring ILD in patients with SARDs such as rheumatoid arthritis, systemic sclerosis, idiopathic inflammatory myopathies, mixed connective tissue disease, and Sjögren's syndrome. **The guidelines conditionally recommend the use of pulmonary function tests (PFTs) and high-resolution computed tomography (HRCT) for screening, while strongly advising against surgical lung biopsy for this purpose. For monitoring, PFTs, HRCT, and ambulatory desaturation testing are conditionally recommended, with a focus on identifying ILD risk factors and determining appropriate testing frequency.**[11]

Sarcoidosis

Sarcoidosis is a complex systemic disease characterized by the formation of non-caseating granulomas in various organs and tissues. The disease is of unknown etiology although it is thought to involve an abnormal immune response potentially triggered by environmental factors, infections, or genetic predispositions. **The hallmark of sarcoidosis is the presence of non-caseating epithelioid cell granulomas, which distinguishes it from other granulomatous diseases like tuberculosis, where caseation is present.** These granulomas can affect any organ, but the lungs and thoracic lymph nodes are most commonly involved, occurring in over 90% of cases. Other frequently affected organs include the skin, eyes, and extra-thoracic lymph nodes, with less common involvement of the liver, heart, nervous system, and kidneys.[36,37]

Diagnosis typically involves clinical evaluation, histological confirmation of non-necrotizing granulomatous inflammation, and exclusion of other causes of granulomatous disease. Endobronchial ultrasound-guided transbronchial needle aspiration (EBUS-TBNA) plays a significant role in the diagnosis of pulmonary sarcoidosis, offering a minimally invasive approach with a high diagnostic yield. Sarcoidosis often requires tissue sampling for definitive diagnosis. Traditional bronchoscopic techniques like bronchoalveolar lavage and transbronchial lung biopsy have been used historically but are less sensitive compared to EBUS-TBNA. Recent studies have compared EBUS-TBNA with other endosonographic techniques. **For instance, a randomized clinical trial found that the granuloma detection rate for EBUS-TBNA was 70%, comparable to 68% for endoscopic ultrasound-guided fine-needle aspiration (EUS-B-FNA), indicating that both methods are effective for diagnosing sarcoidosis.** Advancements in EBUS-guided procedures, such as EBUS-guided transbronchial mediastinal cryobiopsy (EBUS-TMC), have shown even higher diagnostic yields. **EBUS-TMC achieved a 92.8% diagnostic yield for sarcoidosis, surpassing the 78.5% yield of EBUS-TBNA, suggesting that newer techniques may further enhance diagnostic accuracy.**[38–40] One recent study investigated the diagnostic yield and safety of 19-gauge (G) versus 22-G needles in endobronchial ultrasound-guided transbronchial needle aspiration (EBUS-TBNA) for sarcoidosis. A total of 150 subjects with suspected sarcoidosis and enlarged thoracic lymph nodes were randomized to receive either needle type. The primary outcome, diagnostic sensitivity, showed no significant difference between the 19-G (75.0%) and 22-G (69.6%) needles. Sample adequacy was also similar, with 90.0% for the 19-G and 85.7% for the 22-G. However, operators reported greater difficulty in puncturing lymph nodes with the 19-G needle, while cough intensity was comparable between groups ($p=0.41$). The only complication noted was transient hypoxemia in two subjects from each group.[19]

The primary goals of treatment are to prevent or minimize organ damage, relieve symptoms, and improve the patient's quality of life. **Glucocorticoids (GC) are a cornerstone in the management of pulmonary sarcoidosis, primarily due to their effectiveness in reducing inflammation and improving symptoms. According to the European Respiratory Society (ERS) clinical practice guidelines, glucocorticoids are recommended as the first-line treatment for symptomatic sarcoidosis, including pulmonary manifestations**. One major gap is the absence of consensus on monitoring disease activity and treatment efficacy. Additionally, the long-term use of glucocorticoids is associated with significant adverse effects, which necessitates the exploration of alternative therapies and steroid-sparing strategies. The evidence also highlights the need for a more structured approach to treatment initiation and duration.[40,41] **The SARCORT trial investigated the effectiveness of high-dose (40 mg/day) versus low-dose (20 mg/day) prednisolone in treating pulmonary sarcoidosis.** Conducted as a single-centre, open-label, parallel-group, randomised controlled trial ($n = 86$). The primary outcome measured was the frequency of relapse or treatment failure at 18 months. **Results showed that 46.5% of subjects in the high-dose group experienced relapse or treatment failure compared to 44.2% in the low-dose group, with no significant difference. The mean time**

to relapse was also similar between groups, and other outcomes, including changes in FVC and HRQoL scores, did not differ significantly.[20]

Granulomatous lymphocytic ILD

Granulomatous lymphocytic interstitial lung disease (GL-ILD) is a rare and severe form of interstitial lung disease primarily associated with common variable immunodeficiency (CVID). It is characterized by the presence of lymphocytic aggregates and granulomas in the lung tissue, leading to significant respiratory complications and increased mortality rates among affected patients. GL-ILD can occur in 10-30% of individuals with CVID and is often linked to other immunological abnormalities, such as autoimmune cytopenias and splenomegaly. The pathogenesis of GL-ILD remains poorly understood, but it is thought to involve B-cell dysregulation and aberrant immune responses.[42,43]

The most prevalent CT features include bronchiectasis, non-perilymphatic nodules, consolidations, ground-glass opacities (GGO), and reticulations, with a notable predominance in the lower lung fields. Specifically, traction bronchiectasis and interlobular septal thickening are significant indicators of disease progression. The presence of multiple small nodules, consolidations, and reticulations is particularly suggestive of GL-ILD, differentiating it from other conditions like sarcoidosis.[44,45] Diagnostic criteria typically include the presence of lymphatic infiltrates and non-caseating granulomas in lung biopsies, alongside radiological findings such as ground-glass opacities, reticular patterns, and nodules on high-resolution CT scans. The Baumann and Hartmann scoring systems for CT scans have shown high reproducibility in diagnosing GLILD, with the Baumann method being particularly predictive. Additionally, integrating clinical parameters, laboratory results, and imaging findings can enhance diagnostic accuracy, potentially reducing the need for invasive procedures like lung biopsies.[46,47]

Granulomatous lymphocytic interstitial lung disease (GLILD) is primarily treated with systemic corticosteroids, which are considered the first-line therapy. High-dose corticosteroids have shown significant improvements in pulmonary function tests (PFTs) and HRCT scores, with about 42% of patients achieving long-term remission without major side effects. However, responses can be inconsistent, and relapses are common upon tapering. Rituximab has emerged as a promising steroid-sparing option, demonstrating substantial improvements in symptoms and PFTs in some cases. Additionally, mycophenolate mofetil (MMF) has been associated with long-term effectiveness, allowing for corticosteroid weaning while maintaining lung function.[22,48,49]

Idiopathic pulmonary fibrosis

IPF is a chronic interstitial lung disease characterized by inflammation, fibrosis, and destruction of lung architecture. **The mean age of onset is around 65 years with 70% of the patients being male and having a history of cigarrete smoking.** Histopathology shows focal areas of fibroblastic foci with hyperplastic alveolar epithelial cells alternating with nearly normal lung tissue. HRCT findings include predominant subpleural involvement, apico-basal gradient, interstitial thickening, architectural distortion, traction bronchiectasis and honey combing.[50] **Genomic classifiers have been recently introduced for clinical use. Lung tissue obtained by transbronchial forceps biopsy undergoes whole-transcriptome RNA sequencing followed by gene expression analysis.** The pattern of gene expression is subjected to machine learning, and then a diagnostic feature is categorized as present or absent. **The Envisia classifier distinguishes usual interstitial pneumonia (UIP) from non-UIP histopathology, helping clinicians and multidisciplinary teams make a diagnosis of idiopathic pulmonary fibrosis (IPF) in patients without a definite UIP pattern at chest imaging. This obviates the need for more invasive surgical lung biopsy.**

The treatment of IPF has undergone major changes over the years. Before the results of the PANTHER-IPF trial, treatment was primary focussed on the use of immunosuppressive treatment aimed at reducing inflammation and fibrosis. **The PANTHER-IPF which compared a combination of prednisone, Azathioprine and N-acetylcysteine to placebo showed an increased risk of hospitalization, adverse effect, and death.**[51] The focus was then shifted to anti-oxidant and anti-fibrotic drugs which reduce collagen production by suppressing TGF-B, VEGF, FGF and PDGF signalling pathways. In the CAPACITY trial, mean FVC change at week 72 was -8% in the pirfenidone arm compared to -12.4% in the placebo arm (difference 4.4% CI 0.7-9.1).[52]

In the INPULSIS 2 trial, the adjusted annual rate of change in FVC was -113.6ml with Nintedanib versus -207.3ml with placebo.[53] Despite these effective anti-fibrotic agents, time to exacerbation, hospitalisation rates, and long-term survival of IPF has not improved. The five-year survival without lung transplantation ranges from 20-40%.[54]

Alteration of the lung micro-biome has been associated with the pathogenesis of IPF. Previous small-scaled studies have looked at antibiotics to improve outcomes with varying results. The CleanUP-IPF trial looked at Trimethoprim-Sulfamethoxazole or Doxycycline but failed to show reduction in time to first non-elective respiratory hospitalisation (HR: 1.04, 20.4events vs 18.5 events per 100 patient years).[55] Another small sized RCT showed worse outcomes with the addition of nebulised N-acetylcysteine to Pirfenidone.[56] The search for newer investigational treatments for IPF continue. Early studies using preferential phosphodiesterase 4B inhibitor (BI 101550) have shown promise albeit with higher drug discontinuation rates.[57]

The recommended dose of Pirfenidone is 2403mg/day which can be associated with high rates of nausea (36%), dyspepsia (19%) and vomiting (14%).[52] In routine practice a lot of patients aren't able to increase the dose beyond 1800mg due to adverse effects putting a doubt over its efficacy. A retrospective cohort study however showed that the mean annual FVC decline wasn't significantly different in patients who received <1800mg/day of pirfenidone compared to standard arm.[58] One study explored the impact of dietary fat types on gastrointestinal (GI) adverse events (AEs) in patients with idiopathic pulmonary fibrosis (IPF) treated with pirfenidone. Conducted as a multicenter, non-randomized trial across several European countries including 86 subjects monitored over 16 weeks, **the research found that a diet high in saturated fatty acids (SFA) was associated with worse tolerability and a higher incidence of GI AEs compared to a diet rich in monounsaturated fatty acids (MUFA). The findings suggest that dietary modifications could serve as a crucial strategy to mitigate pirfenidone-related GI AEs.**[59]

Acute exacerbation of IPF is defined as acute worsening of symptoms (typically <30days) with CT evidence of new onset ground glass opacities/consolidation not fully explained by heart failure or pulmonary embolism. Risk factors include immunosuppression, infections, and aspiration. It is associated with worse outcomes with median survival being three to four months. **The evidence for treatment options is mostly anecdotal or from observational studies. The most frequently used agent is a trial of glucocorticoids.**[60] Even high dose glucocorticoids have been used. Further immunosuppression using intravenous CYC has shown to increase all cause mortality at 3 months (45% vs 31%).[61]

Up to 80% of patients with IPF may have chronic cough. It is mostly non-productive and tends to occur more during daytime. Chronic cough is a very disabling symptom and can lead to difficulty sleeping, musculo-skeletal pain, urinary incontinence, decreased social interaction and reduced exercise tolerance. **Pathophysiology of cough in IPF is multi-factorial: increased cough reflex hypersensitivity due to fibrosis and alteration of nerve endings, gastro-esophageal reflux, micro-aspiration and concomitant OSA to name a few. Treatment is mainly focussed on treating co-morbidities contributing to cough and use of anti-fibrotic agents.**[62] Randomised trials using azithromycin or inhaled compounds like Cromolyn sodium have failed to show any significant change in cough related QoL or 24 hour cough count.[63]

Progressive pulmonary fibrosis

Interstitial lung diseases other than IPF can also show evidence of worsening pulmonary fibrosis despite appropriate treatment. Ever since the advent of anti-fibrotic drugs and their use in IPF, trials have been conducted to look at their efficacy in reducing fibrosis in non-IPF ILD. These trials have been heterogenous in the way they defined patients as having progressive fibrosing ILD.

ATS 2022 update coined the term progressive pulmonary fibrosis to group together patients having non-IPF ILD who might benefit from anti-fibrotic treatment. In a patient with ILD of known or unknown etiology other than IPF who has radiological evidence of pulmonary fibrosis, **PPF is defined as at least two of the following three criteria occulting within the past year with no alternative explanation: worsening respiratory symptoms, absolute decline in FVC >5% predicted or in DLCO >10% predicted within 1year of follow-up, or radiological evidence of disease progression (new reticulation, honey combing or traction bronchiectasis).**[64]

The INBUILD trial showed that the use of Nintedanib in PF-ILD who have progressed after appropriate immunosuppressive treatment reduced the rate of FVC decline at 52weeks from -187ml/yr to -80.8ml/yr ($p<0.001$). Proportion of patients with further progression (>10% absolute decline) was significantly less in the Nintedanib arm (40.4% vs 54.7%).[65] **In the SENCIS trial patients with SSc-ILD with >10% fibrosis on CT were given Nintedanib. Around 50% of the patients were still receiving MMF. Nintedanib reduced the annual rate of FVC decline from -93.3ml/yr to -52.4ml/yr.**[66]

The **RELIEF trial** looked at use of Pirfenidone in patients with PF-ILD other than IPF. There was a significant reduction in rate of annual FVC decline as well in the proportion of patients with >10% FVC decline per year (20% vs 40%).[67] **The TRAIL1 study evaluated the efficacy of pirfenidone among RA-ILD patients with at least 10% fibrosis on HRCT.** Although the trial reach not significance for its primary composite outcome of death and %FVC reduction >10% over 52weeks, **decline in %FVC was significantly lower in patients with UIP pattern ILD who received Pirfenidone (3.6%, $p<0.001$).**[68]

Although these trials have paved the way for the use of Nintedanib and pirfenidone in patients with non-IPF fibrosing ILD, a few important questions loom at large regarding the timing of initiation.

FLOWCHARTS

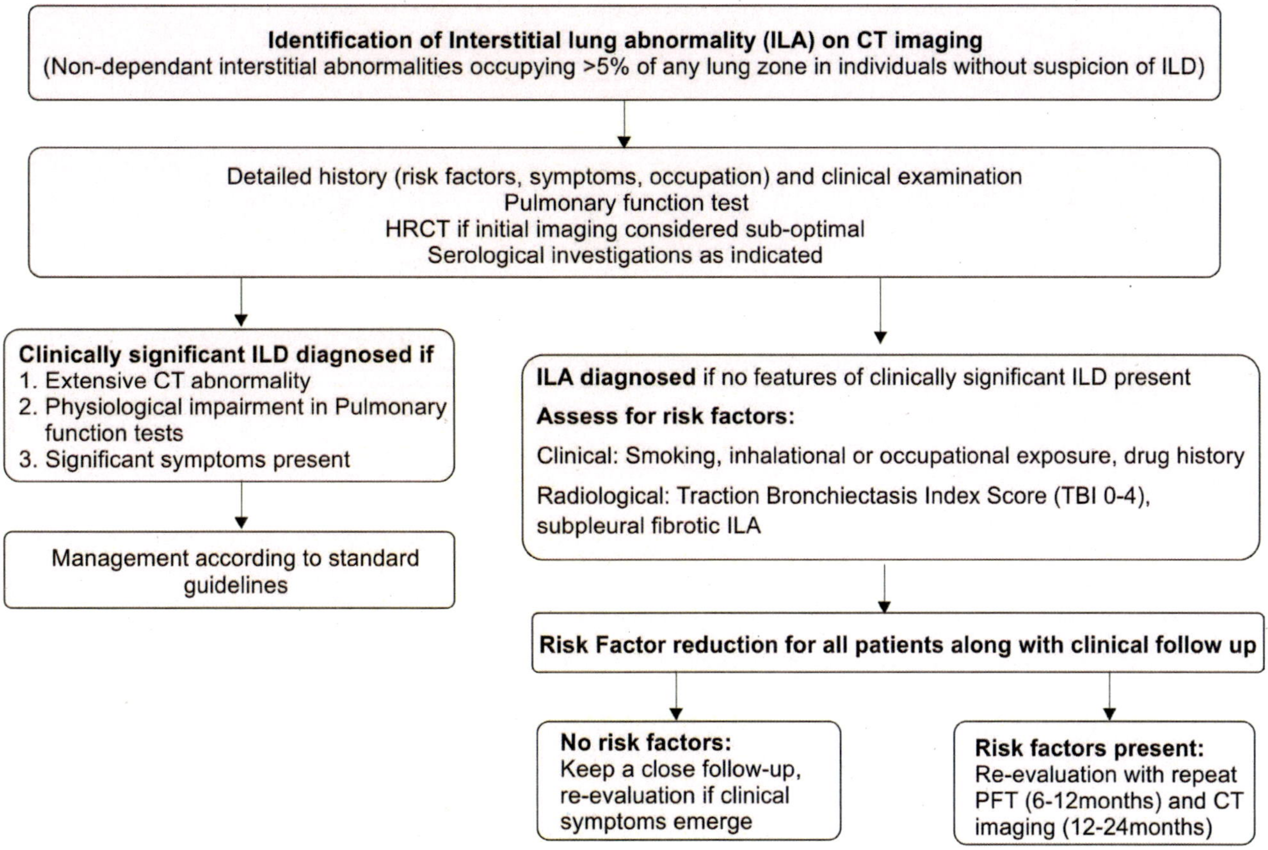

A. Management of ILA

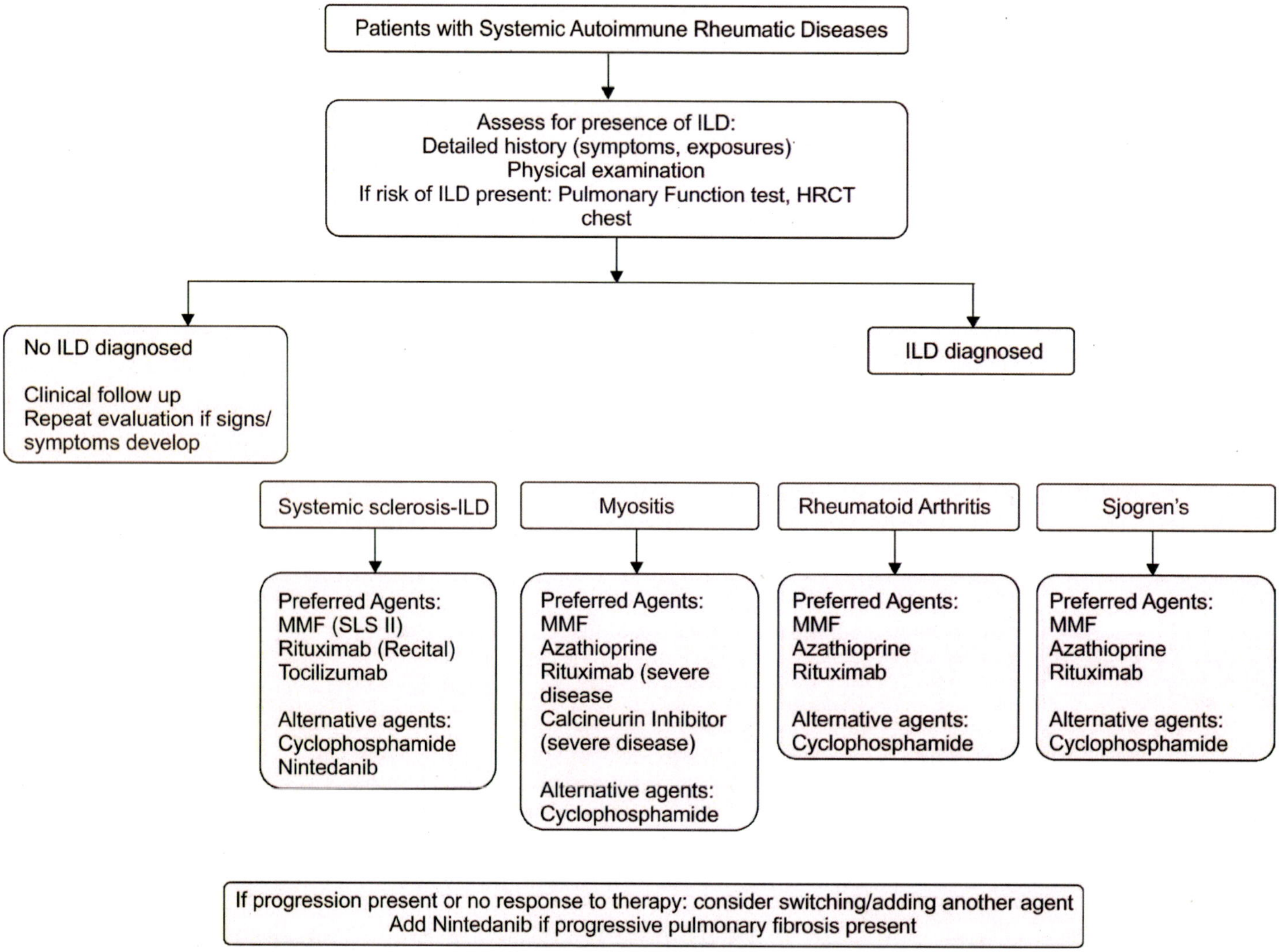

B. Management of CTD-ILD

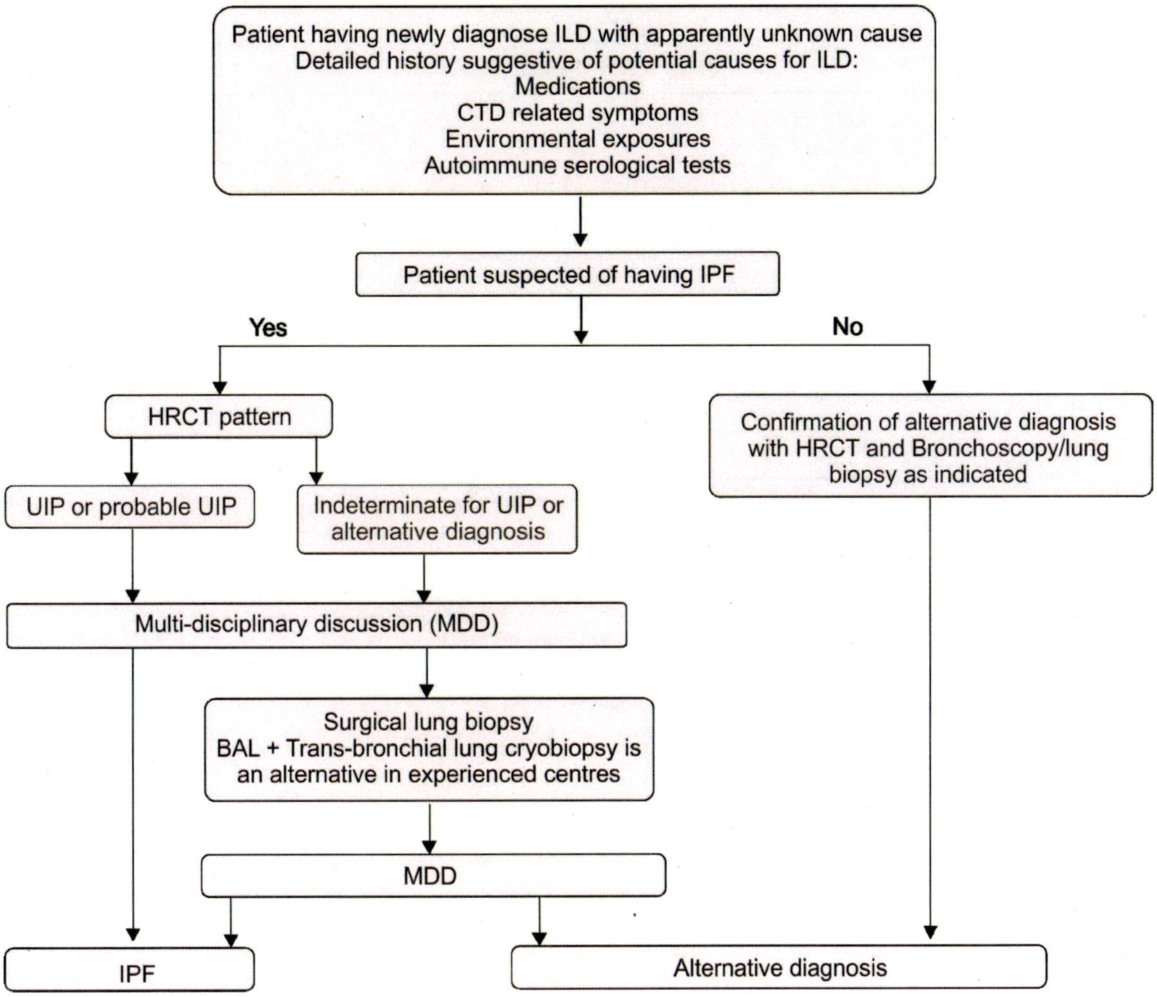

C. Diagnosis of IPF

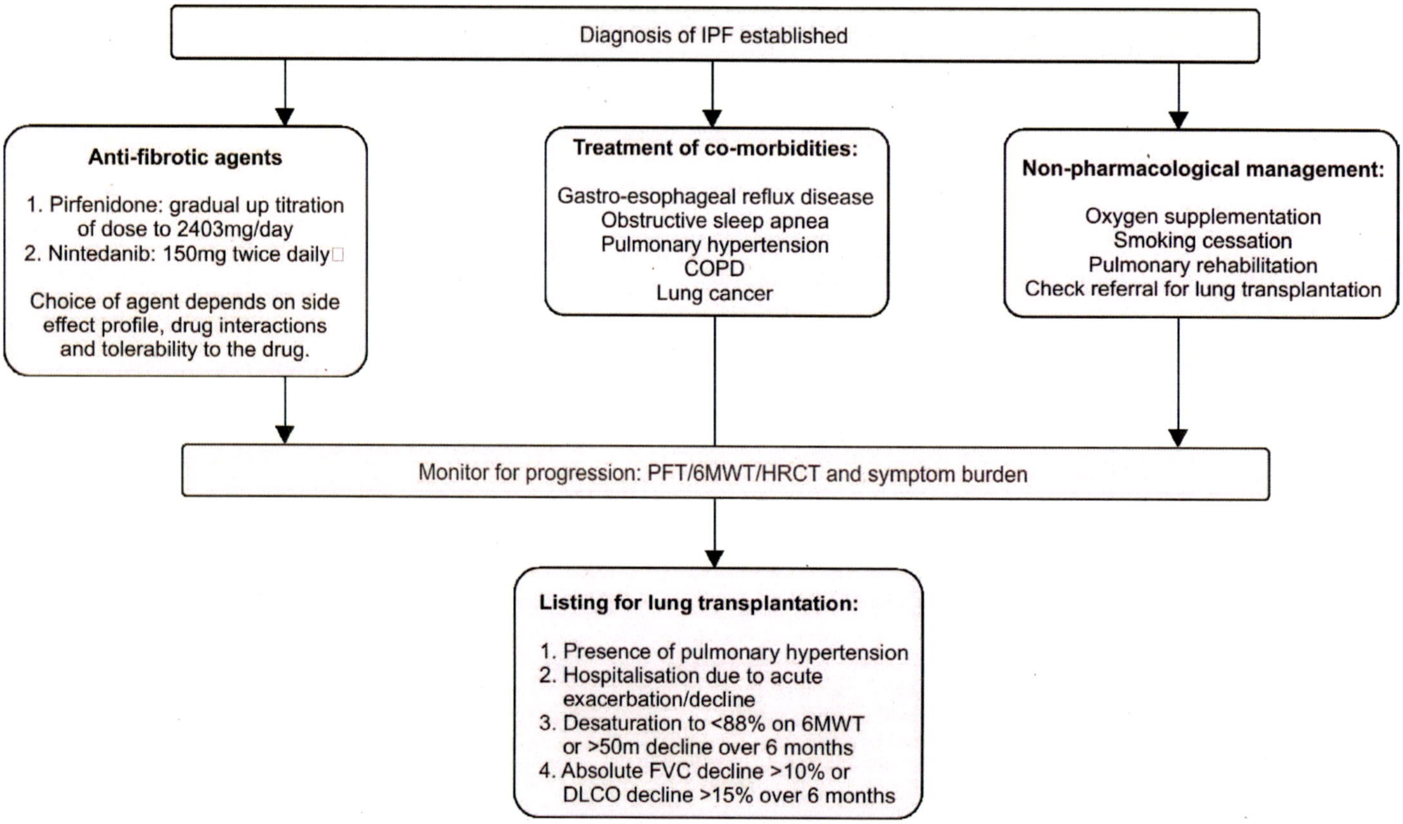

D. Treatment of IPF

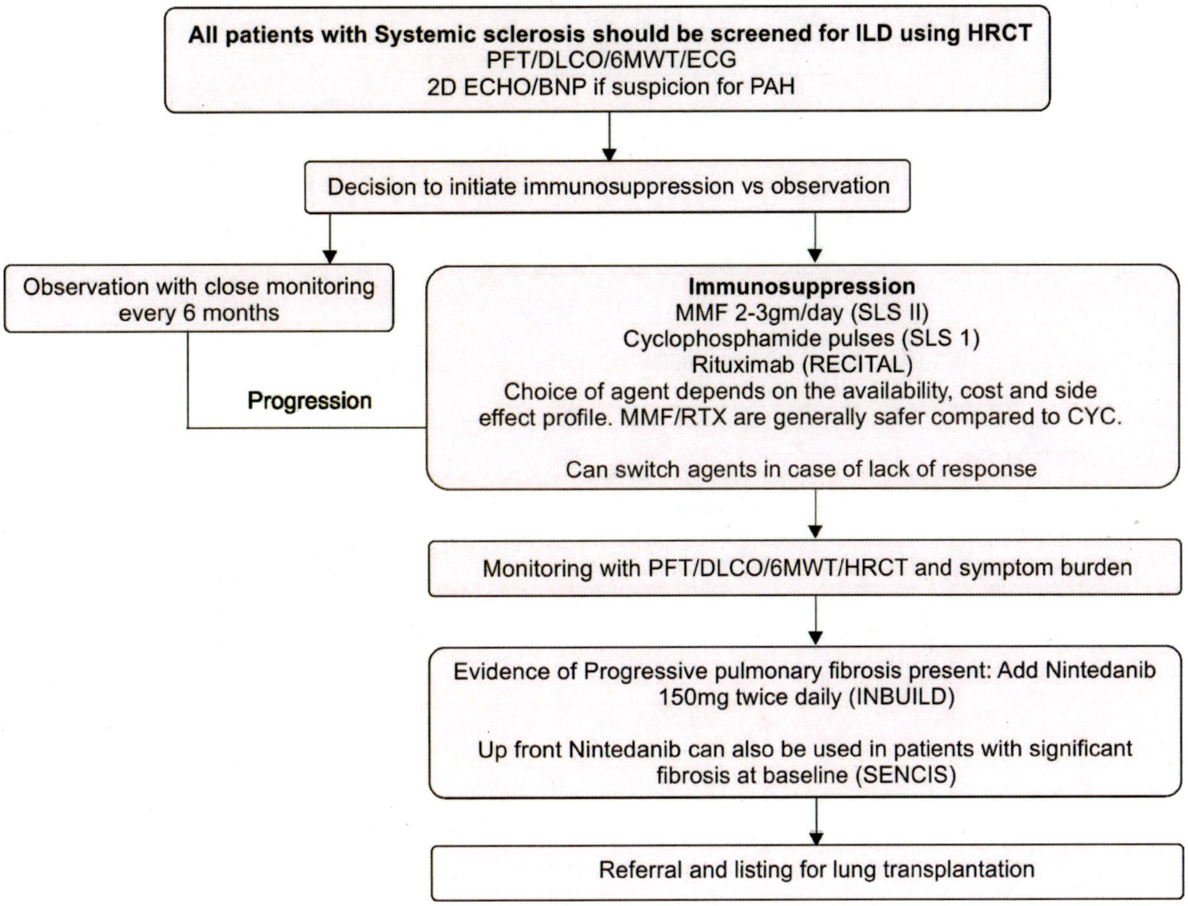

E. Diagnosis and Management of SSc-ILD

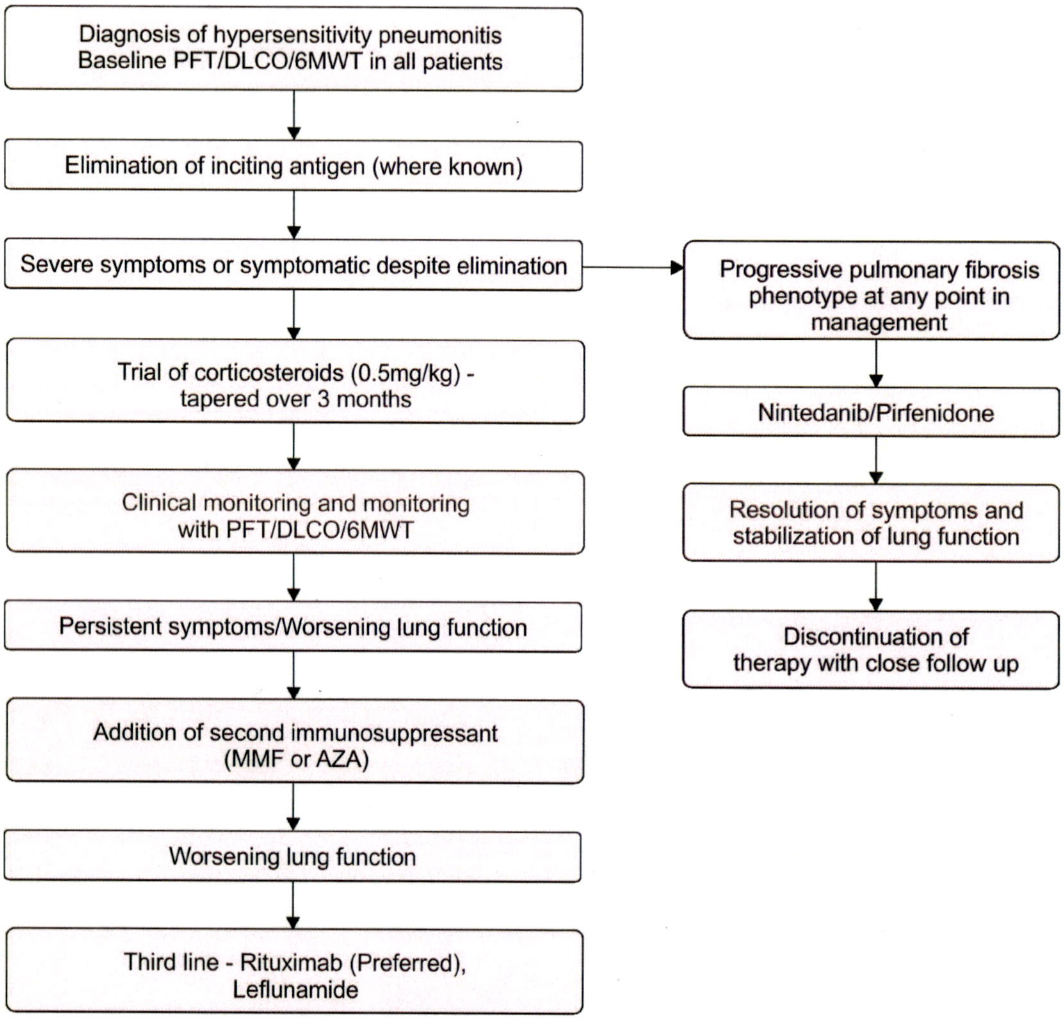

F. Treatment of hypersensitivity pneumonitis

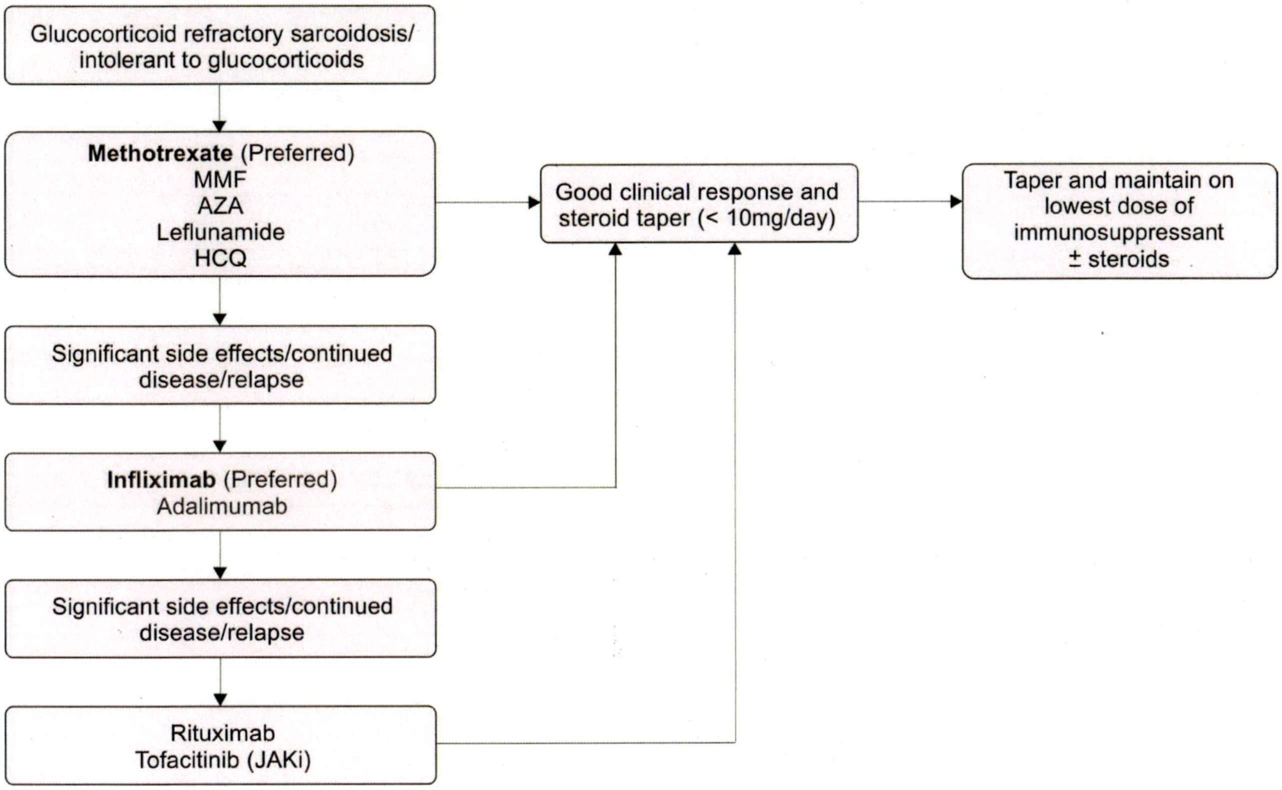

G. Treatment of refractory sarcoidosis

REFERENCES

1. Kalverda KA, Ninaber MK, Wijmans L, Thüsen J von der, Jonkers RE, Daniels JM, et al. Transbronchial cryobiopsy followed by as-needed surgical lung biopsy versus immediate surgical lung biopsy for diagnosing interstitial lung disease (the COLD study): a randomised controlled trial. The Lancet Respiratory Medicine. 2024 Jul 1;12(7):513–22.
2. Lancaster L, Cottin V, Ramaswamy M, Wuyts WA, Jenkins RG, Scholand MB, et al. Bexotegrast in Patients with Idiopathic Pulmonary Fibrosis: The INTEGRIS-IPF Clinical Trial. Am J Respir Crit Care Med. 2024 Aug 15;210(4):424–34.
3. Raghu G, Richeldi L, Fernández Pérez ER, De Salvo MC, Silva RS, Song JW, et al. Pamrevlumab for Idiopathic Pulmonary Fibrosis: The ZEPHYRUS-1 Randomized Clinical Trial. JAMA. 2024 Aug 6;332(5):380–9.
4. Richeldi L, Schiffman C, Behr J, Inoue Y, Corte TJ, Cottin V, et al. Zinpentraxin Alfa for Idiopathic Pulmonary Fibrosis: The Randomized Phase III STARSCAPE Trial. Am J Respir Crit Care Med. 2024 May 1;209(9):1132–40.
5. Maher TM, Avram C, Bortey E, Hart SP, Hirani N, Molyneux PL, et al. Nalbuphine Tablets for Cough in Patients with Idiopathic Pulmonary Fibrosis. NEJM Evid. 2023 Aug;2(8):EVIDoa2300083.
6. Wu Z, Spencer LG, Banya W, Westoby J, Tudor VA, Rivera-Ortega P, et al. Morphine for treatment of cough in idiopathic pulmonary fibrosis (PACIFY COUGH): a prospective, multicentre, randomised, double-blind, placebo-controlled, two-way crossover trial. Lancet Respir Med. 2024 Apr;12(4):273–80.
7. Kim JS, Murray S, Yow E, Anstrom KJ, Kim HJ, Flaherty KR, et al. Comparison of Pirfenidone and Nintedanib: Post Hoc Analysis of the CleanUP-IPF Study. Chest. 2024 May;165(5):1163–73.
8. Behr J, Nathan SD, Costabel U, Albera C, Wuyts WA, Glassberg MK, et al. Efficacy and Safety of Pirfenidone in Advanced Versus Non-Advanced Idiopathic Pulmonary Fibrosis: Post-Hoc Analysis of Six Clinical Studies. Adv Ther. 2023 Sep;40(9):3937–55.
9. West A, Chaudhuri N, Barczyk A, Wilsher ML, Hopkins P, Glaspole I, et al. Inhaled pirfenidone solution (AP01) for IPF: a randomised, open-label, dose-response trial. Thorax. 2023 Sep;78(9):882–9.
10. Johnson SR, Bernstein EJ, Bolster MB, Chung JH, Danoff SK, George MD, et al. 2023 American College of Rheumatology (ACR)/ American College of Chest Physicians (CHEST) Guideline for the Treatment of Interstitial Lung Disease in People with Systemic Autoimmune Rheumatic Diseases. Arthritis Rheumatol. 2024 Aug;76(8):1182–200.
11. Johnson SR, Bernstein EJ, Bolster MB, Chung JH, Danoff SK, George MD, et al. 2023 American College of Rheumatology (ACR)/ American College of Chest Physicians (CHEST) Guideline for the Screening and Monitoring of Interstitial Lung Disease in People with Systemic Autoimmune Rheumatic Diseases. Arthritis Rheumatol. 2024 Aug;76(8):1201–13.
12. Ghazipura M, Macrea M, Herman D, Barnes H, Knight SL, Silver RM, et al. Tocilizumab in Patients with Systemic Sclerosis-associated Interstitial Lung Disease: A Systematic Review and Meta-Analysis. Ann Am Thorac Soc. 2024 Feb;21(2):328–37.
13. Herman D, Ghazipura M, Barnes H, Macrea M, Knight SL, Silver RM, et al. Nintedanib Therapy Alone and Combined with Mycophenolate in Patients with Systemic Sclerosis-associated Interstitial Lung Disease: Systematic Reviews and Meta-analysis. Ann Am Thorac Soc. 2024 Mar;21(3):474–85.
14. Macrea M, Ghazipura M, Herman D, Barnes H, Knight SL, Silver RM, et al. Rituximab in Patients with Systemic Sclerosis-associated Interstitial Lung Disease: A Systematic Review and Meta-Analysis. Ann Am Thorac Soc. 2024 Feb;21(2):317–27.
15. Barnes H, Ghazipura M, Herman D, Macrea M, Knight SL, Silver RM, et al. Cyclophosphamide in Patients with Systemic Sclerosis-associated Interstitial Lung Disease: A Systematic Review and Meta-Analysis. Ann Am Thorac Soc. 2024 Jan;21(1):122–35.
16. Wang HF, Wang YY, Li ZY, He PJ, Liu S, Li QS. The prevalence and risk factors of rheumatoid arthritis-associated interstitial lung disease: a systematic review and meta-analysis. Ann Med. 2024 Dec;56(1): 2332406.
17. Narváez J, Cañadillas E, Castellví I, Alegre JJ, Vicens-Zygmunt V, Bermudo G, et al. Rituximab in the treatment of progressive interstitial lung disease associated with the antisynthetase syndrome. Arthritis Res Ther. 2024 Jun 18;26(1):122.
18. Fernández Pérez ER, Crooks JL, Lynch DA, Humphries SM, Koelsch TL, Swigris JJ, et al. Pirfenidone in fibrotic hypersensitivity pneumonitis: a double-blind, randomised clinical trial of efficacy and safety. Thorax. 2023 Nov;78(11):1097–104.
19. Dhooria S, Sehgal IS, Prasad KT, Muthu V, Dogra P, Saini M, et al. Diagnostic Yield and Safety of the 19-Gauge versus 22-Gauge Endobronchial Ultrasound-Guided Transbronchial Needle Aspiration Needle in Subjects with Sarcoidosis (GUESS). Respiration. 2024;103(6):336–43.
20. Dhooria S, Sehgal IS, Agarwal R, Muthu V, Prasad KT, Dogra P, et al. High-dose (40 mg) versus low-dose (20 mg) prednisolone for treating sarcoidosis: a randomised trial (SARCORT trial). Eur Respir J. 2023 Sep;62(3):2300198.
21. Li DY, Liu X, Huang JY, Hang WL, Yu GR, Xu Y. Impact of antifibrotic therapy on disease progression, all-cause mortality, and risk of acute exacerbation in non-IPF fibrosing interstitial lung diseases: evidence from a meta-analysis of randomized controlled trials and prospective controlled studies. Ther Adv Respir Dis. 2024;18:17534666241232561.
22. Smits B, Goldacker S, Seneviratne S, Malphettes M, Longhurst H, Mohamed OE, et al. The efficacy and safety of systemic corticosteroids as first line treatment for granulomatous lymphocytic interstitial lung disease. J Allergy Clin Immunol. 2023 Aug;152(2):528–37.

23. Yang L, Xiang Z, Dai M, Zhang Q, Zhou Y. Prognosis of Lung Transplantation in Patients with Acute Exacerbations of Interstitial Lung Disease: A Meta-Analysis Based on Cohort Studies. Ann Thorac Cardiovasc Surg. 2024;30(1):24–00086.

24. Ng BH, Azmi MI, Abeed NNN, Low HJ, Soo CI, Jailaini MFM, et al. The outcome of 12-week corticosteroid therapy in COVID-19-related diffuse interstitial lung abnormalities. Med J Malaysia. 2024 May;79(3):296–305.

25. Lin LY, Wu YC, Wu JS, Tai HY, Huang TW, Cheng WH. Oxygen therapy for exercise capacity in fibrotic interstitial lung disease: A systematic review and meta-analysis of randomised controlled trials. Respir Med. 2024 Jun;227:107657.

26. Wada N, Hunninghake GM, Hatabu H. Interstitial Lung Abnormalities: Current Understanding. Clin Chest Med. 2024 Jun;45(2):433–44.

27. Koh KH, Tan MO, Chuah TY. Do not dismiss interstitial lung abnormalities. Proceedings of Singapore Healthcare. 2023 Dec 1;32:20101058231215174.

28. Jin GY. Interstitial Lung Abnormality in Asian Population. Tuberc Respir Dis (Seoul). 2024 Apr;87(2):134–44.

29. Robertshaw M, Kershaw CD. Post COVID Interstitial Lung Abnormalities-Incidence and Management. Curr Pulmonol Rep. 2023;12(2):64–9.

30. Ohgushi M, Ogo N, Yanagihara T, Harada Y, Sumida K, Egashira A, et al. Tacrolimus Treatment for Post-COVID-19 Interstitial Lung Disease. Intern Med. 2022 Feb 15;61(4):585–9.

31. Zhou Q, MacArthur MR, He X, Wei X, Zarin P, Hanna BS, et al. Interferon-α2b Treatment for COVID-19 Is Associated with Improvements in Lung Abnormalities. Viruses. 2020 Dec 30;13(1):44.

32. Fischer A, Strek ME, Cottin V, Dellaripa PF, Bernstein EJ, Brown KK, et al. Proceedings of the American College of Rheumatology/Association of Physicians of Great Britain and Ireland Connective Tissue Disease-Associated Interstitial Lung Disease Summit: A Multidisciplinary Approach to Address Challenges and Opportunities. Arthritis Rheumatol. 2019 Feb;71(2):182–95.

33. Singh S, Sharma BB, Bairwa M, Gothi D, Desai U, Joshi JM, et al. Management of interstitial lung diseases: A consensus statement of the Indian Chest Society (ICS) and National College of Chest Physicians (NCCP). Lung India. 2020;37(4):359–78.

34. Raghu G, Remy-Jardin M, Myers JL, Richeldi L, Ryerson CJ, Lederer DJ, et al. Diagnosis of Idiopathic Pulmonary Fibrosis. An Official ATS/ERS/JRS/ALAT Clinical Practice Guideline. Am J Respir Crit Care Med. 2018 Sep 1;198(5):e44–68.

35. Raghu G, Montesi SB, Silver RM, Hossain T, Macrea M, Herman D, et al. Treatment of Systemic Sclerosis-associated Interstitial Lung Disease: Evidence-based Recommendations. An Official American Thoracic Society Clinical Practice Guideline. Am J Respir Crit Care Med. 2024 Jan 15;209(2):137–52.

36. Sève P, Pacheco Y, Durupt F, Jamilloux Y, Gerfaud-Valentin M, Isaac S, et al. Sarcoidosis: A Clinical Overview from Symptoms to Diagnosis. Cells. 2021 Mar 31;10(4):766.

37. Rossides M, Darlington P, Kullberg S, Arkema EV. Sarcoidosis: Epidemiology and clinical insights. J Intern Med. 2023 Jun;293(6):668–80.

38. Benzaquen S, Matta A, Sultan S, Sarvottam K. Role of Bronchoscopy in Diagnosis of Sarcoidosis. Clin Chest Med. 2024 Mar;45(1):25–32.

39. Crombag LMM, Mooij-Kalverda K, Szlubowski A, Gnass M, Tournoy KG, Sun J, et al. EBUS versus EUS-B for diagnosing sarcoidosis: The International Sarcoidosis Assessment (ISA) randomized clinical trial. Respirology. 2022 Feb;27(2):152–60.

40. Poletti V, Petrarulo S, Piciucchi S, Dubini A, De Grauw AJ, Sultani F, et al. EBUS-guided cryobiopsy in the diagnosis of thoracic disorders. Pulmonology. 2024 Jan 4;S2531-0437(23)00223-4.

41. Sellarés J, Francesqui J, Llabres M, Hernandez-Gonzalez F, Baughman RP. Current treatment of sarcoidosis. Curr Opin Pulm Med. 2020 Sep;26(5):591–7.

42. Cinetto F, Scarpa R, Carrabba M, Firinu D, Lougaris V, Buso H, et al. Granulomatous Lymphocytic Interstitial Lung Disease (GLILD) in Common Variable Immunodeficiency (CVID): A Multicenter Retrospective Study of Patients From Italian PID Referral Centers. Front Immunol. 2021;12:627423.

43. Beaton TJ, Gillis D, Morwood K, Bint M. Granulomatous lymphocytic interstitial lung disease: limiting immunosuppressive therapy-a single-centre experience. Respirol Case Rep. 2020 Jul;8(5):e00565.

44. Scarpa R, Cinetto F, Milito C, Gianese S, Soccodato V, Buso H, et al. Common and Uncommon CT Findings in CVID-Related GL-ILD: Correlations with Clinical Parameters, Therapeutic Decisions and Potential Implications in the Differential Diagnosis. J Clin Immunol. 2023 Nov;43(8):1903–15.

45. Fraz MSA, Moe N, Revheim ME, Stavrinou ML, Durheim MT, Nordøy I, et al. Granulomatous-Lymphocytic Interstitial Lung Disease in Common Variable Immunodeficiency-Features of CT and 18F-FDG Positron Emission Tomography/CT in Clinically Progressive Disease. Front Immunol. 2020;11:617985.

46. Meerburg JJ, Hartmann IJC, Goldacker S, Baumann U, Uhlmann A, Andrinopoulou ER, et al. Analysis of Granulomatous Lymphocytic Interstitial Lung Disease Using Two Scoring Systems for Computed Tomography Scans-A Retrospective Cohort Study. Front Immunol. 2020;11:589148.

47. Cabanero-Navalon MD, Garcia-Bustos V, Forero-Naranjo LF, Baettig-Arriagada EJ, Núñez-Beltrán M, Cañada-Martínez AJ, et al. Integrating Clinics, Laboratory, and Imaging for the Diagnosis of Common Variable Immunodeficiency-Related Granulomatous-Lymphocytic Interstitial Lung Disease. Front Immunol. 2022;13:813491.

48. Tessarin G, Baronio M, Gazzurelli L, Rossi S, Chiarini M, Moratto D, et al. Rituximab Monotherapy Is Effective as First-Line Treatment for Granulomatous Lymphocytic Interstitial Lung Disease (GLILD) in CVID Patients. J Clin Immunol. 2023 Nov;43(8):2091–103.

49. Bintalib HM, Lowe DM, Mancuso G, Gkrepi G, Seneviratne SL, Burns SO, et al. Corticosteroid-induced remission and mycophenolate maintenance therapy in granulomatous lymphocytic

interstitial lung disease: long-term, longitudinal change in lung function in a single-centre cohort. ERJ Open Res. 2022 Oct;8(4):00024–2022.

50. Glass DS, Grossfeld D, Renna HA, Agarwala P, Spiegler P, DeLeon J, et al. Idiopathic pulmonary fibrosis: Current and future treatment. The Clinical Respiratory Journal. 2022;16(2):84–96.

51. Prednisone, Azathioprine, and N-Acetylcysteine for Pulmonary Fibrosis | NEJM [Internet]. [cited 2023 May 10]. Available from: https://www.nejm.org/doi/full/10.1056/nejmoa1113354

52. Noble PW, Albera C, Bradford WZ, Costabel U, Glassberg MK, Kardatzke D, et al. Pirfenidone in patients with idiopathic pulmonary fibrosis (CAPACITY): two randomised trials. The Lancet. 2011 May 21;377(9779):1760–9.

53. Efficacy and Safety of Nintedanib in Idiopathic Pulmonary Fibrosis | NEJM [Internet]. [cited 2023 May 10]. Available from: https://www.nejm.org/doi/full/10.1056/nejmoa1402584

54. Martinez FJ, Collard HR, Pardo A, Raghu G, Richeldi L, Selman M, et al. Idiopathic pulmonary fibrosis. Nat Rev Dis Primers. 2017 Oct 20;3(1):1–19.

55. Martinez FJ, Yow E, Flaherty KR, Snyder LD, Durheim MT, Wisniewski SR, et al. Effect of Antimicrobial Therapy on Respiratory Hospitalization or Death in Adults With Idiopathic Pulmonary Fibrosis: The CleanUP-IPF Randomized Clinical Trial. JAMA. 2021 May 11;325(18):1841–51.

56. Sakamoto S, Kataoka K, Kondoh Y, Kato M, Okamoto M, Mukae H, et al. Pirfenidone plus inhaled N-acetylcysteine for idiopathic pulmonary fibrosis: a randomised trial. Eur Respir J. 2021 Jan;57(1):2000348.

57. Richeldi L, Azuma A, Cottin V, Hesslinger C, Stowasser S, Valenzuela C, et al. Trial of a Preferential Phosphodiesterase 4B Inhibitor for Idiopathic Pulmonary Fibrosis. N Engl J Med. 2022 Jun 9;386(23):2178–87.

58. Hwang H, Lee JK, Choi SM, Lee YJ, Cho YJ, Yoon HI, et al. Efficacy of lower dose pirfenidone for idiopathic pulmonary fibrosis in real practice: a retrospective cohort study. Korean J Intern Med. 2022 Mar;37(2):366–76.

59. Molina-Molina M, Shull JG, Vicens-Zygmunt V, Rivera-Ortega P, Antoniou K, Bonella F, et al. Gastrointestinal pirfenidone adverse events in idiopathic pulmonary fibrosis depending on diet: the MADIET clinical trial. Eur Respir J. 2023 Oct;62(4):2300262.

60. Juarez MM, Chan AL, Norris AG, Morrissey BM, Albertson TE. Acute exacerbation of idiopathic pulmonary fibrosis—a review of current and novel pharmacotherapies. J Thorac Dis. 2015 Mar;7(3):499–519.

61. Naccache JM, Jouneau S, Didier M, Borie R, Cachanado M, Bourdin A, et al. Cyclophosphamide added to glucocorticoids in acute exacerbation of idiopathic pulmonary fibrosis (EXAFIP): a randomised, double-blind, placebo-controlled, phase 3 trial. Lancet Respir Med. 2022 Jan;10(1):26–34.

62. Manen MJG van, Birring SS, Vancheri C, Cottin V, Renzoni EA, Russell AM, et al. Cough in idiopathic pulmonary fibrosis. European Respiratory Review. 2016 Sep 1;25(141):278–86.

63. Azithromycin for the Treatment of Chronic Cough in Idiopathic Pulmonary Fibrosis: A Randomized Controlled Crossover Trial - PubMed [Internet]. [cited 2023 May 10]. Available from: https://pubmed.ncbi.nlm.nih.gov/34015241/

64. Raghu G, Remy-Jardin M, Richeldi L, Thomson CC, Inoue Y, Johkoh T, et al. Idiopathic Pulmonary Fibrosis (an Update) and Progressive Pulmonary Fibrosis in Adults: An Official ATS/ERS/JRS/ALAT Clinical Practice Guideline. Am J Respir Crit Care Med. 2022 May;205(9):e18–47.

65. Nintedanib in Progressive Fibrosing Interstitial Lung Diseases | NEJM [Internet]. [cited 2023 May 10]. Available from: https://www.nejm.org/doi/full/10.1056/NEJMoa1908681

66. Distler O, Highland KB, Gahlemann M, Azuma A, Fischer A, Mayes MD, et al. Nintedanib for Systemic Sclerosis-Associated Interstitial Lung Disease. N Engl J Med. 2019 Jun 27;380(26):2518–28.

67. Behr J, Prasse A, Kreuter M, Johow J, Rabe KF, Bonella F, et al. Pirfenidone in patients with progressive fibrotic interstitial lung diseases other than idiopathic pulmonary fibrosis (RELIEF): a double-blind, randomised, placebo-controlled, phase 2b trial. Lancet Respir Med. 2021 May;9(5):476–86.

68. Solomon JJ, Danoff SK, Woodhead FA, Hurwitz S, Maurer R, Glaspole I, et al. Safety, tolerability, and efficacy of pirfenidone in patients with rheumatoid arthritis-associated interstitial lung disease: a randomised, double-blind, placebo-controlled, phase 2 study. Lancet Respir Med. 2023 Jan;11(1):87–96.

CHAPTER

5 ANCA Associated Vasculitis

Author: Dr. Zubair Ahmad Thoker

Reviewer: Dr. Vijay Hadda

INTRODUCTION

Anti-neutrophil cytoplasmic antibody-associated vasculitis (AAV) is a systemic autoimmune disease characterized by inflammation of the small blood vessels, which consists of granulomatosis with polyangiitis (GPA), microscopic polyangiitis (MPA) and eosinophilic granulomatosis with polyangiitis (EGPA). The persistent systemic inflammation induced by AAV may result in multiple organs damage, including the kidneys and lungs. AAV can present as a mild disease in a routine outdoor clinic of a pulmonary physician or as a severe form of disease requiring admission to the intensive care unit. Hence, all pulmonary and critical care physicians should have a good understanding of this challenging but potentially treatable disease. Successful treatment of AAV focuses on suppressing disease activity while minimizing treatment-related toxicity. An update on newer treatment modalities and newer guidelines on diagnosis and treatment is pivotal in making crucial decisions during the management of AAV. In this chapter, we have provided a brief overview of current treatment and management and recent studies conducted on AAV.

Methodology

A PubMed search was carried out with the search term "(ANCA Associated Vasculitis)". Randomized control trials and meta-analyses published between August 2023 to August 2024 were reviewed. Our search resulted in 17 articles that were screened for relevance; and finally, 7 studies were selected to be included in this update.

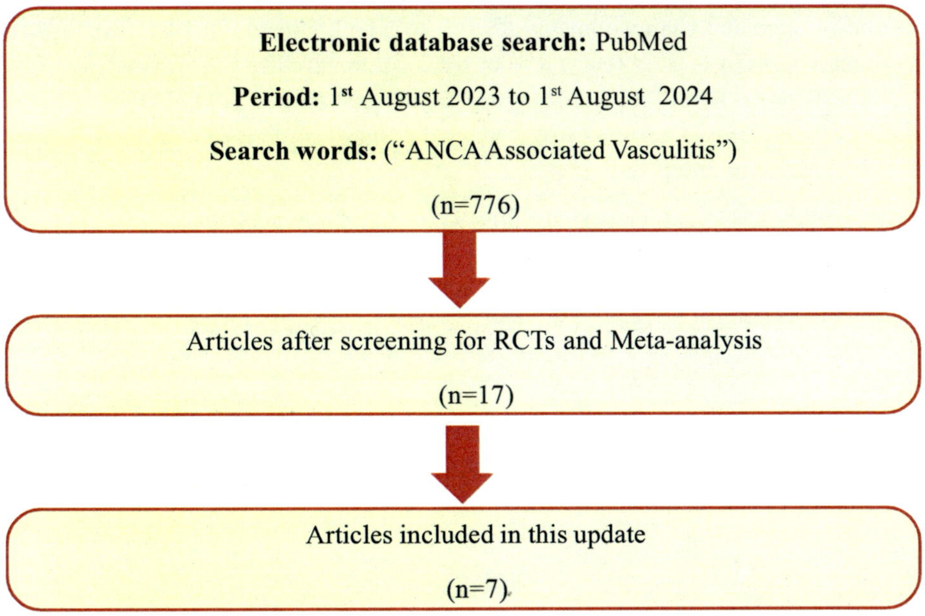

Analysis of Literature

- ***Cardiovascular and cerebrovascular outcomes in anti-neutrophil cytoplasmic antibody-associated vasculitis: A systematic review with meta-analysis. (Autoimmunity Reviews. 2024)***[1]
  - o *Population:* AAV patients from 14 studies (N= 20,096. 5757 events over 46,495 person-years)
  - o *Outcome: Cardiovascular and cerebrovascular events were assessed.* AAV patients showed an 83% increased risk (RR - 1.83, 95% CI 1.37–2.45) of incident type-specific cardiovascular and cerebrovascular diseases (CCVD), 48% for coronary artery disease (RR - 1.48, 95% CI 1.26–1.75), and 56% for cerebrovascular accident (RR - 1.56, 95% CI 1.22–1.99). For type-specific CCVD, the risks of myocardial infarction, stroke, and heart failure increased by 67%, 97%, and 72% respectively.
  - o *Conclusion and comments:* AAV is associated with increased risks of overall and type-specific CCVD, especially within the initial two years after AAV diagnosis. However, the included studies showed significant heterogeneity.

☞

- ***The impact of treatment with avacopan on health-related quality of life in antineutrophil cytoplasmic antibody-associated vasculitis: A post-hoc analysis of data from the ADVOCATE trial. (Lancet Rheumat. 2023)***[2]
  - o *Population:* Patients with ANCA-associated vasculitis. (n=331)

    All the patients received either cyclophosphamide (followed by azathioprine) or rituximab
  - o *Intervention:* Oral Avacopan (C5a receptor antagonist) at a dose of 30 mg twice daily. (n=166)
  - o *Comparator:* Oral Prednisone 30 mg followed by a tapering dose. (n=165)
  - o *Outcome:* Health related quality of life assessed by least squares mean change from baseline in SF- 36 version 2, EQ-5D-5L visual analogue scale, EQ-5D health utility scores, and SF-6D health utility scores at weeks 26 and 52 between two groups. The LS mean change from baseline in the SF-36 Physical Component Summary (PCS) score was greater in the avacopan group at week 26, with a between-group difference of 2.8 (95% CI 0.4 to 5.2). The LS mean change from baseline was greater in the avacopan group than in the prednisone taper group across all of the SF-36 domains measured except social functioning at week 26, with larger relative between-group difference for the role physical, bodily pain and vitality domains at week 26. The LS mean (95% CI) difference between groups for change from baseline was 4.7 (95% CI 0.0 to 9.3) at week 52 for the EQ-5D- 5L VAS and 0.04 (95% CI 0.00 to 0.09) for the EQ-5D-5L index. Least squares means a change from baseline in EQ-5D-5L visual analogue scale, EQ-5D health utility scores, and SF-6D health utility scores were significantly greater at week 52 in the avacopan group compared with the prednisone group.
  - o *Conclusion:* Patients with ANCA associated vasculitis who received Avacopan reported statistically significant and clinically meaningful improvements in health-related quality of life at 26 and 52 weeks and in health utility EQ-5D and SF-6D scores at 52 weeks.

- ***Efficacy and safety of Avacopan in patients with ANCA associated vasculitis receiving rituximab in a randomised trial. (Ann Rheum Dis. 2024)[3]***
  - *Population:* Patients with AAV (GPA or MPA) receiving background rituximab induction therapy. (n=214)
  - *Intervention:* Avacopan 30 mg twice daily for 52 weeks plus prednisone-matching placebo. (n=107)
  - *Comparator:* Tapered prednisone over 20 weeks plus Avacopan-matching placebo for 52 weeks. (n=107)
  - *Outcome:* Remission at week 26, sustained remission (defined as remission at week 26 and at week 52 with no receipt of GCs for AAV 4 weeks before week 52 and no relapse between weeks 26 and 52), Glucocorticoid Toxicity Index (GTI), estimated glomerular filtration rate, urinary albumin to creatinine ratio and safety, were assessed. Remission at week 26 was observed in 77.6% (83/107) patients in the avacopan group and 75.7% (81/107) patients in the prednisone taper group (difference 3.0 % points; 95% CI –8.3 to 14.2). Sustained remission at week 52 was observed in 71% (76/107) patients in the avacopan group and 56.1% (60/107) patients in the prednisone taper group (difference, 16.5% points; 95% CI 4.3 to 28.6). The relapse rate after remission at any time was 8.7% (9/104 patients) in the avacopan group compared with 20.2% (21/104 patients) in the prednisone taper group. The recovery of renal function and speed of reduction in albuminuria favoured the avacopan group. GC-induced toxicity, as assessed by GTI, was greater in the prednisone taper group than in the avacopan group. Serious adverse events occurred in 34.6% and 39.3% of patients in the avacopan and prednisone taper groups, respectively.
  - *Conclusion:* The efficacy of treatment with Avacopan compared with a prednisone taper was similar at week 26 and greater at week 52, with a favourable safety profile. In addition, Avacopan was associated with improved renal outcomes and lower glucocorticoid toxicity. This demonstrates the efficacy and safety of Avacopan and its potential role as a standard therapy along with rituximab for the treatment of AAV to induce and sustain remission. Longer follow-up is important to better understand the benefits and risks of the adjunctive use of avacopan therapy for AAV.

- ***Association Between Plasma Rituximab Concentration and the Risk of Major Relapse in Antineutrophil Cytoplasmic Antibody-Associated Vasculitides During Rituximab Maintenance Therapy in a RCT. (Arthritis Rheumatol. 2024)[4]***
  - *Population:* Patients with newly diagnosed or relapsing granulomatosis with polyangiitis (GPA) or microscopic polyangiitis (MPA) in complete remission after induction therapy. (n=135)
  - *Intervention:* 500-mg fixed-schedule rituximab infusion.
  - *Comparator:* Individually tailored regimen of rituximab.
  - *Outcome:* Plasma concentration of rituximab at 3 months and relapse. The frequency of underexposed (plasma concentration <4 μg/ml) to rituximab at 3 months was lower in fixed dose as compared to that in the tailored-infusion group (2.0% versus 18.0%; $P = 0.02$, respectively). Low rituximab plasma concentration at 3 months (CM3 <4 μg/ml) was an independent risk factor for major relapse at month 28 (odds ratio 6.56).
  - *Conclusion:* Drug level monitoring could be useful to individualize the schedule of rituximab administration within the maintenance phase.

☞

- ***Reduced-dose versus high-dose glucocorticoids added to rituximab on remission induction in ANCA-associated vasculitis: predefined 2-year follow-up study. (Ann Rheum Dis. 2024)[5]***
  - o *Population:* Patients with newly diagnosed AAV without severe glomerulonephritis or alveolar hemorrhage were studied for maintenance glucocorticoid requirements and long-term outcomes (n-140). After achieving remission, patients received the rituximab maintenance therapy (1 g/6 months).
  - o *Intervention:* Reduced-dose prednisolone (0.5 mg/kg/d) plus rituximab (375 mg/m^2/wk, 4 doses) (n-70)
  - o *Comparator:* High-dose prednisolone (1 mg/kg/d) plus rituximab (375 mg/m^2/wk, 4 doses) (n - 70)
  - o *Outcome:* Relapse at 24 months and adverse effects were assessed. At 24 months, among patients who achieved remission with the protocolised treatments, 89.7% in the reduced-dose group and 15.5% in the high-dose group discontinued prednisolone (median time to withdrawal, 150 and 375 days, respectively). Relapse occurred in 13.0% in the reduced-dose group and 7.6% in the high-dose group (p=0.311). Serious adverse events (SAEs) were less frequent in the reduced-dose group (27.5%) than in the high-dose group (46.2%) (p=0.025).
  - o *Conclusion and critical appraisal:* At 24 months, frequencies of relapse did not differ between the groups, and SAEs were less frequent in the reduced-dose group due to the lower event rate in the 6-month induction phase. However, the bias to MPO-ANCA positivity (85.8%) in the trial population should be noted.

- ***Alveolar Hemorrhage in Antineutrophil Cytoplasmic Antibody-Associated Vasculitis: Results of an International Randomized Controlled Trial. (PEXIVAS) (AJRCCM. 2024)[6]***
  - o *Population:* Patients with severe AAV (with GFR less than 50 ml/min per 1.73 m^{2}of body-surface area or DAH) participated in PEXIVAS trial (n=704)
  - o *Intervention:* PLEX, high dose glucocorticoids
  - o *Comparator:* No PLEX, standard dose glucocorticoids
  - o *Outcome:* Death rate at 3 months and 1 year and infection with and without DAH were assessed. Among those with DAH, 8/95 (8.4%) receiving PLEX died within 1 year versus 15/96 (15.6%) with no-PLEX (hazard ratio, 0.52; confidence interval [CI], 0.21-1.24), whereas 13/96 (13.5%) receiving reduced GC died versus 10/95 (10.5%) with standard GC (hazard ratio, 1.33; CI, 0.57-3.13). When ventilated, ventilator-free days were similar with PLEX versus no-PLEX and fewer with reduced GC (median, 23; IQR, 20-25) versus standard GC (median, 26; IQR, 25-28). Overall, 23/191 (12.0%) with DAH died within 1 year versus 34/513 (6.6%) without DAH.
  - o *Conclusion:* Patients with AAV and DAH differ from those without DAH. Further data are required to confirm or refute a benefit of PLEX or GC dosing on mortality.

☞

- ***Benralizumab versus Mepolizumab for Eosinophilic Granulomatosis with Polyangiitis: Multicenter, double-blind, phase 3, randomized, active-controlled noninferiority trial. (NEJM. 2024)[7]***
  - o *Population:* Adults with relapsing or refractory EGPA who were receiving standard care (n=140)
  - o *Intervention:* Benralizumab (30 mg) subcutaneously every 4 weeks for 52 weeks (n=70)
  - o *Comparator:* Mepolizumab (300 mg) subcutaneously every 4 weeks for 52 weeks (n=70)

- *Outcome:* Remission at weeks 36 and 48, accrued duration of remission, time to first relapse, oral glucocorticoid use, eosinophil count, and safety. Remission at weeks 36 and 48 was 59% in the Benralizumab group and 56% in the Mepolizumab group (P = 0.73 for superiority), showing noninferiority but not superiority of Benralizumab to Mepolizumab. The accrued duration of remission and the time to first relapse were similar in the two groups. Complete withdrawal of oral glucocorticoids during weeks 48 through 52 was achieved in 41% and 26% of the patients in Benralizumab and Mepolizumab groups respectively. The mean (±SD) blood eosinophil count at baseline was 306.0±225.0 per microliter in the benralizumab group and 384.9±563.6 per microliter in the mepolizumab group, decreasing to 32.4±40.8 and 71.8±54.4 per microliter, respectively, at week 52. Adverse events were reported in 90% of the patients in the benralizumab group and 96% of those in the mepolizumab group; serious adverse events were reported in 6% and 13%, respectively.
- *Conclusion:* Benralizumab was noninferior to Mepolizumab for the induction of remission in patients with relapsing or refractory EGPA.

DISCUSSION

Anti-neutrophil cytoplasmic antibody (ANCA) associated vasculitis (AAV) is an autoimmune condition characterized by pauci-immune vasculitis.[8] It is hypothesized that ANCA are directly pathogenic, with two major targets: Proteinase 3 (PR3) and myeloperoxidase (MPO), both enzymes present in neutrophil granules.[9] Historically, AAV is classified according to the clinical phenotypes of granulomatosis with polyangiitis (GPA, predominantly associated with PR3-ANCA), microscopic polyangiitis (MPA, predominantly associated with MPO-ANCA), and eosinophilic granulomatosis with polyangiitis (EGPA).[10] Due to an overlap in the clinical presentations and pattern of vessel involvement, these syndromes are often grouped together as ANCA-associated vasculitis.[11]

ANCA associated vasculitis is a rare disease with an estimated worldwide prevalence of 300 patients per million, whereas the reported incidence rates vary from approx. 25 per million in Europe to 33 per million in the USA.[12] The most common organ involved is the kidney with 70% to 90% of AAV of patients showing renal involvement.[13,14] In the respiratory system, AAV may involve both the upper (sinuses and ear) or the lower respiratory tracts (airways, interstitial or vascular). Patients occasionally may also have features of pleuritis.[15]

With dramatically improved prognosis and survival in the last decades, the long-term excess risk of cardiovascular and cerebrovascular diseases (CCVD) in AAV population has been increasingly recognized. A systematic review and meta-analysis observed that people with AAV had a substantial increase in risks of CCVD in general accompanied by varying degrees of most common specific types of CCVD, including myocardial infarction, heart failure, and stroke. Even after accounting for traditional cardiovascular risk factors, AAV history was associated with a significantly elevated risk of CCVD.[1]

There is a paucity of data related to AAV from the Indian subcontinent. A retrospective study, including 42 patients with GPA from western India reported an equal female-to-male proportion of patients. Pulmonary, ENT and renal involvement were common, and the study also reported high relapse rates. The authors also reported that Rituximab was an effective therapy for severe, relapsing, or refractory disease.[16]

The diagnosis of AAV is made based on a constellation of clinical, laboratory findings and imaging studies; and not simply based on one factor. The hallmark of diagnosis of AAV is the presence of necrotizing inflammation of the wall of small- and/or medium-sized vessels, which may show necrotizing granulomas (GPA) or eosinophilic infiltration (EGPA). For management purposes, it is important to classify AAV in organ/life-threatening and non-organ/ life-threatening diseases (Table 1).

Table 1: EULAR 2022 definition of organ/life threatening and non-threatening diseases[19]

Examples of potentially organ/life-threatening manifestations*	Examples of manifestations that are not immediately organ/life-threatening*
Glomerulonephritis	Nasal and paranasal disease without bony involvement (erosion) or cartilage collapse or olfactory dysfunction or deafness
Pulmonary haemorrhage	Skin involvement without ulceration
Meningeal involvement	Myositis (skeletal muscle only)
Central nervous system involvement	Non-cavitating pulmonary nodules
Retro-orbital disease	Episcleritis
Cardiac involvement	
Mesenteric involvement	
Mononeuritis multiplex	

* Non-life-threatening diseases may become life-threatening with evolution and hence must be evaluated on a case-to-case basis.

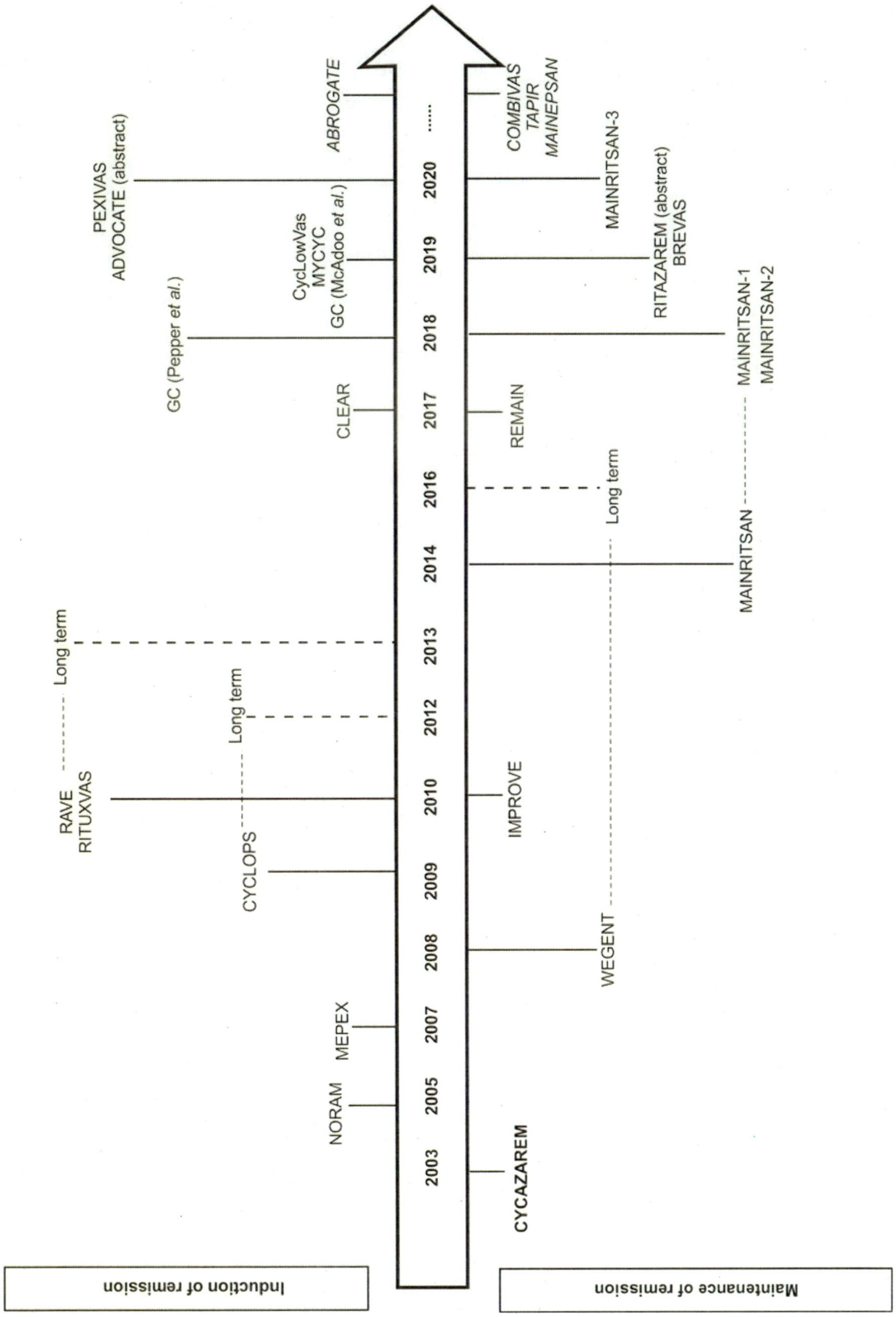

Figure 1: Hallmark trial and chronology of suggested drugs used in AAV[17]

Management

The management of AAV includes 3 phases: induction phase, maintenance phase and a follow-up phase. Relapses may occur during the maintenance or follow-up phases and require a re-induction process.

Table 2: Phases and goals of treatment of AAV	
Phase of treatment	**Goals**
Induction (3-6 months)	To control vasculitis activity
Maintenance (2 years at least)	Prevent flares Rehabilitate
Long-term follow-up	Monitor flare Manage comorbidity risks

* In case of flare at any point of time during maintenance phase, a re-induction has to be started.

Table 3: Treatment options available for the management of AAV	
Induction	**Maintenance**
Glucocorticoids	Rituximab
Rituximab	Azathioprine
Cyclophosphamide	Methotrexate
MMF	MMF
PLEX	
Avacopan	

Note: Currently, there is no evidence for the use of PLEX in DAH.

The treatment of AAV is constantly evolving and currently available treatment options are summarized in Table 3. At present, for the induction of remission in patients with life-threatening AAV, a combination of high-dose glucocorticoids with a combination of pulse cyclophosphamide or rituximab is used. MMF and methotrexate may be used as induction agents in non-life- threatening cases. Maintenance of remission is achieved with drugs like Rituximab, Azathioprine, Methotrexate and MMF.

The major limitations with some of these studies were the lack of homogeneity, and under-representation of respiratory vasculitis; thereby, inability to tailor treatment according to the organ involvement. As in other diseases, there is an unmet need for personalized medicines with AAV.

Following the results of the **ADVOCATE** trial, the C5a1R inhibitor Avacopan is poised to revolutionise steroid-sparing strategies in GPA and MPA.[18] Furthermore, post-hoc analyses of the ADVOCATE trial highlighted a greater improvement of glomerular-filtration-rate (eGFR) in patients with baseline eGFR<20ml/min and in health-related quality of life respectively, in AAV patients in the Avacopan arm compared to those in the GC arm of the trial.[2,3]

The **ADVOCATE study** included 83-85% of Caucasians, and hence, results may not apply to other populations.[18] Respiratory system involvement was seen in approximately 40% of the population, in both arms. Safety and clinical effects beyond week 52 were not addressed, highlighting the need for longer-duration trials.

Results of these studies suggest that Avacopan may be used as an adjunct (as a replacement for glucocorticoids) for remission induction in patients with ANCA-associated vasculitis. However, one should note that the safety and efficacy of Avacopan beyond 52 weeks of treatment has not been addressed.

EULAR practice guidelines for Avacopan are given below:[19]

- **Avacopan may be used along with rituximab or cyclophosphamide to reduce the overall glucocorticoid dose.**

  We concur with the same while emphasizing on paucity of long-term data with respect to Avacopan.

A study looking at the combination of high dose/low dose of glucocorticoids with Rituximab was performed.[5] The majority of the study cohort consisted of females (56-62%) and MPA (76-78%). Respiratory involvement was seen in 58-59% of the study population. The efficacy outcomes were comparable in the two groups, however, as expected, adverse effects of glucocorticoids were higher in the high-dose glucocorticoid group. Serious adverse effects (subjective) were also noted more frequently in the high-dose glucocorticoid group. These results indicate that high-dose glucocorticoids are not needed when Rituximab is used for the treatment of AAV. Concurring with same a recent meta-analysis published, which included 1145 patients, from three RCTs and two observational studies, found that low dose glucocorticoid strategy was associated with fewer infections maintaining equivalent efficacy.[20]

On the basis of the available data, we may cautiously consider reduced dose (0.5 mg/kg) glucocorticoids in combination with rituximab in select patients with non-life-threatening AAV.

EULAR practice guidelines for glucocorticoid dose are as below:[19]

- **The dose of glucocorticoids should be as per the protocol used in the PEXIVAS trial.**

  In the reduced-dose protocol, patients receive a standard weight-based dose for the first week; at the start of the second week, the dose is reduced by approximately 50%, followed by subsequent taper. At 6 months, the cumulative dose of oral glucocorticoids in the reduced-dose group was 60% less than that in the standard-dose group. After 22 weeks, the tapering is individualized.

While PLEX has been used frequently for the management of renal manifestations of AAV, meta-analysis have reported that in spite of the reduction in the risk of ESKD, there were no mortality benefits. PLEX was frequently associated with serious infections. It appears that the increased risk of serious infections has contributed as a possible cause, for the lack of effect of PLEX on mortality. Also, PLEX has no effects on remission, relapse, and health-related quality of life.

The role of plasma exchange in DAH due to AAV remains an area of interest and debate. A sub-group analysis of PEXIVAS trial found that participants with DAH differed from those without DAH in multiple ways, including baseline characteristics and a significantly increased risk of death at 30 days and 1 year.[6] The numerical differences in mortality at 3 and 12 months, in this sub-group analyses for those with DAH between the PLEX and no-PLEX groups are of unclear clinical significance because they are based on small numbers of events and not statistically significant.

On the basis of available data, PLEX may be used only for a select group of AAV. This is however currently not recommended and needs further data generation.

EULAR practice guidelines for PLEX are as below:[19]

- **Plasma exchange may be considered as part of therapy to induce remission in GPA or MPA for those with a serum creatinine >300 μmol/L (3.3 mg/dl) due to active glomerulonephritis or in those with AAV/ anti GBM Ab overlap. PLEX is not recommended in the management of diffuse alveolar hemorrhage (DAH).**

The best maintenance therapy for AAV is still not known; Rituximab, MMF and azathioprine are commonly used drugs for this purpose. Data regarding the use of Rituximab for maintenance of remission for AAV is limited. Larger studies are required to look for further options to prevent relapse, especially in the high-risk groups as mentioned earlier. Further trials should also look at the lowest possible glucocorticoid dose at which remission maintenance is possible, especially in high-risk groups.

Interindividual variability in response to immunosuppressants remains unexplored in AAV. Rituximab pharmacokinetics and pharmacodynamics as well as genetic polymorphisms could contribute to variability. A study suggested that rituximab drug level monitoring could be useful to individualize the schedule of its administration within the maintenance phase so as to minimize adverse effects of B cell depletion without compromising clinical efficacy.[4]

A network meta-analysis, published in 2021, compared the safety and efficacy of MMF, cyclophosphamide, and rituximab in patients with AAV. It looked at 6 RCTs with more than 500 patients.[21] **The analysis showed that Rituximab is the most effective remission-induction therapy for patients with AAV, followed by MMF and cyclophosphamide. However, the propensity to relapse was lowest with cyclophosphamide followed by rituximab and MMF. Rituximab also appeared as the safest option with reduced propensity for severe adverse events.**

However, these results should be interpreted cautiously as there is no head-to-head trial between these agents. **Although rituximab showed a high relapse rate, the accompanying desirable safety profile placed it as the first therapeutic choice for patients with AAV.**

The results of this meta-analysis suggest that rituximab may be used as an alternative to cyclophosphamide for induction as well as maintenance of remission in patients with AAV, especially in cases of relapsing disease.[21]

Current EULAR practice guidelines are as below:[19]

- **For induction of remission in patients with *new-onset or relapsing* GPA or MPA with *organ-threatening or life-threatening disease*, the recommended treatment is with a combination of glucocorticoids and either rituximab or cyclophosphamide. Rituximab is preferred in relapsing disease.**
- **For *non-organ-threatening or non-life-threatening* GPA or MPA, induction with a combination of glucocorticoids and rituximab is recommended. Methotrexate or mycophenolate mofetil can be considered as an alternative to rituximab in these cases.**
- **It is important to remember that non-life-threatening diseases may evolve into life-threatening forms and thereby close follow-up remains essential.**

There is a lack of head-to-head trials between various available treatment options, and as previously noted, there is a great deal of heterogeneity in the study populations. It is important to identify the risk factors of relapse, to ensure early recognition and management of the same.

Over the next 10 years, the likelihood of continued incremental progress for patients with ANCA-associated vasculitis is high. Mortality and remission rates have significantly improved over the years and attention is now to be focused on how to achieve rapid and sustained remission while minimizing treatment toxicity. Due to the disease heterogeneity as previously alluded to, further research on individualization of treatment according to disease subtype, genetic factors, and risk of relapse will be necessary to truly offer a state-of-the-art therapy.[17] Substantial leaps forward in the ability to diagnose, treat, and monitor ANCA-associated vasculitis, however, will require breakthroughs in understanding disease biology.

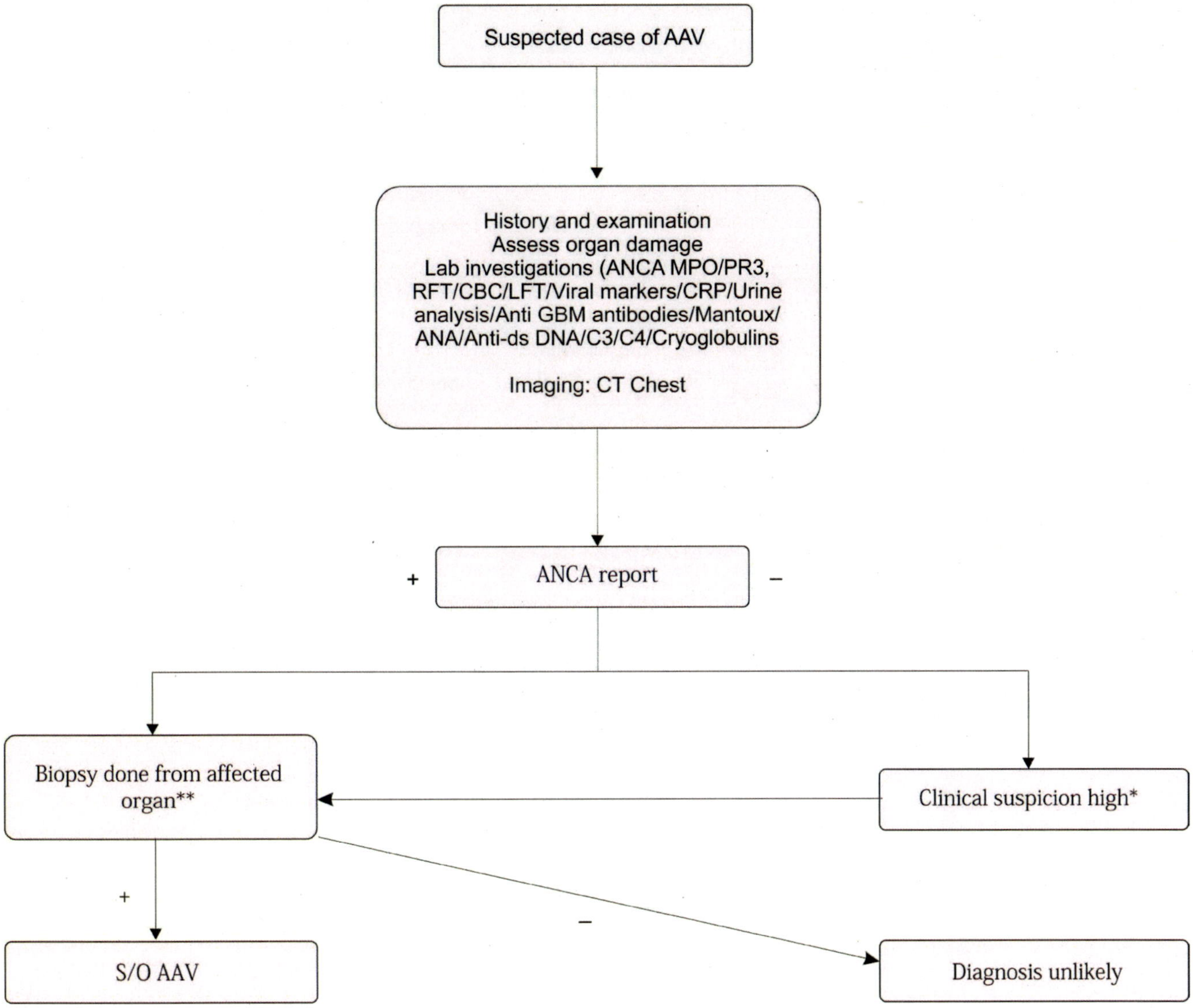

* In case of low clinical suspicion with, negative ANCA, Diagnosis is unlikely to be AAV (ANCA associated vasculitis).

** Biopsy may be contraindicated in few cases: bleeding diathesis, advanced uraemia, concurrent plasma exchange, the presence of anti-phospholipid antibodies/lupus anticoagulant or respiratory failure due to alveolar haemorrhage. In such cases, treatment is on the basis of clinical suspicion. A delayed biopsy may be considered if expected treatment response is not seen.[22]

Flowchart 1: Diagnostic Approach of ANCA Associated Vasculitis

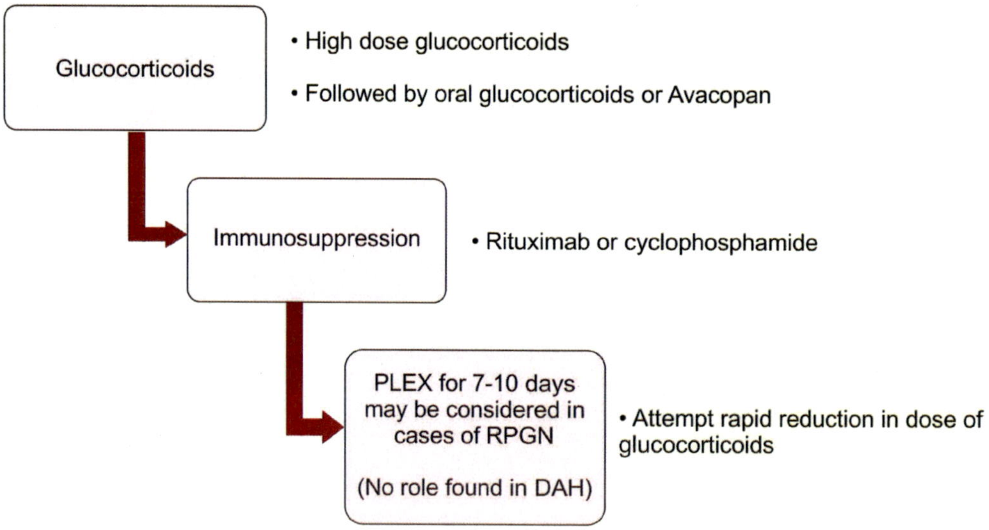

* In case of non-organ-threatening disease, mycophenolate mofetil, methotrexate or rituximab may be used for induction purposes. The rest of the approach remains the same.[17,19]

Flowchart 2: Induction of Remission in Severe/Organ-Threatening GPA/MPA: Suggested Options

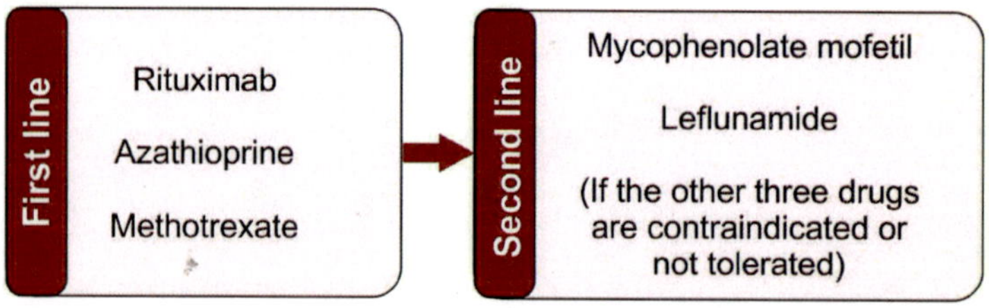

* Remission to be maintained for at least 2 years.

Flowchart 3: Maintenance of Remission in Severe/Organ-Threatening GPA/MPA: Suggested Options

REFERENCES

1. Xie W, Xiao S, Li X, Huang J, Zhang Z. Cardiovascular and cerebrovascular outcomes in anti-neutrophil cytoplasmic antibody-associated vasculitis: A systematic review with meta-analysis. Autoimmun Rev. 2024 Jun;23(6):103587. doi: 10.1016/j.autrev.2024.103587. Epub 2024 Aug 3. PMID: 39098514.

2. Strand V, Jayne DRW, Horomanski A, Yue H, Bekker P, Merkel PA; ADVOCATE Study Group. The impact of treatment with avacopan on health-related quality of life in antineutrophil cytoplasmic antibody-associated vasculitis: a post-hoc analysis of data from the ADVOCATE trial. Lancet Rheumatol. 2023 Aug;5(8):e451-e460. doi: 10.1016/S2665-9913(23)00092-9. Epub 2023 Jul 24. PMID: 38251577.

3. Geetha D, Dua A, Yue H, Springer J, Salvarani C, Jayne D, Merkel P; ADVOCATE Study Group. Efficacy and safety of avacopan in patients with ANCA-associated vasculitis receiving rituximab in a randomised trial. Ann Rheum Dis. 2024 Jan 11;83(2):223-232. doi: 10.1136/ard-2023-224816. PMID: 37979959; PMCID: PMC 10850685.

4. Khoudour N, Delestre F, Jabot-Hanin F, Jouinot A, Nectoux J, Letouneur F, Izac B, Vidal M, Guillevin L, Puéchal X, Charles P, Terrier B, Blanchet B. Association Between Plasma Rituximab Concentration and the Risk of Major Relapse in Antineutrophil Cytoplasmic Antibody-Associated Vasculitides During Rituximab Maintenance Therapy. Arthritis Rheumatol. 2023 Nov;75(11):2003-2013. doi: 10.1002/art.42556. Epub 2023 Aug 13. PMID: 37134130.

5. Furuta S, Nakagomi D, Kobayashi Y, Hiraguri M, Sugiyama T, Amano K, Umibe T, Kono H, Kurasawa K, Kita Y, Matsumura R, Kaneko Y, Ninagawa K, Hiromura K, Kagami SI, Inaba Y, Hanaoka H, Ikeda K, Nakajima H; LoVAS collaborators. Reduced-dose versus high-dose glucocorticoids added to rituximab on remission induction in ANCA-associated vasculitis: predefined 2-year follow-up study. Ann Rheum Dis. 2024 Jan 2;83(1):96-102. doi: 10.1136/ard-2023-224343. PMID: 37734880.

6. Fussner LA, Flores-Suárez LF, Cartin-Ceba R, Specks U, Cox PG, Jayne DRW, Merkel PA, Walsh M; PEXIVAS Investigators. Alveolar Hemorrhage in Antineutrophil Cytoplasmic Antibody-Associated Vasculitis: Results of an International Randomized Controlled Trial (PEXIVAS). Am J Respir Crit Care Med. 2024 May 1;209(9):1141-1151. doi: 10.1164/rccm.202308-1426OC. PMID: 38346237; PMCID: PMC11092964.

7. Wechsler ME, Nair P, Terrier B, Walz B, Bourdin A, Jayne DRW, Jackson DJ, Roufosse F, Börjesson Sjö L, Fan Y, Jison M, McCrae C, Necander S, Shavit A, Walton C, Merkel PA; MANDARA Study Group. Benralizumab versus Mepolizumab for Eosinophilic Granulomatosis with Polyangiitis. N Engl J Med. 2024 Mar 7;390(10):911-921. doi: 10.1056/NEJMoa2311155. Epub 2024 Feb 23. PMID: 38393328.

8. Kitching AR, Anders HJ, Basu N, *et al.* ANCA-associated vasculitis. Nat Rev Dis Primers. 2020;6(1):71.

9. RJ F, RS T, LA C, *et al.* Anti-neutrophil cytoplasmic autoantibodies induce neutrophils to degranulate and produce oxygen radicals in vitro. Proc Natl Acad Sci USA. 1990;87:4115–19.

10. Xiao H, Hu P, Falk RJ, *et al.* Overview of the pathogenesis of ANCA associated vasculitis. Kidney Dis (Basel). 2016;1:205–15.

11. Jennette JC, Falk RJ, Bacon PA, *et al.* 2012 revised international Chapel Hill Consensus Conference Nomenclature of Vasculitides. Arthritis Rheum. 2013; 65(1): 1- 11.

12. Watts RA, Hatemi G, Burns JC, Mohammad AJ. Global epidemiology of vasculitis. Nat Rev Rheumatol. 2022 Jan; 18(1):22-34. doi: 10.1038/s41584-021-00718-8. Epub 2021 Dec 1. PMID: 34853411; PMCID: PMC8633913.

13. Geetha D, JA J. ANCA-associated vasculitis: Core curriculum 2020. Am J Kidney Diseases. 2020;75: 124–37.

14. Scott J, Hartnett J, Mockler D, *et al.* Environmental risk factors associated with ANCA-associated vasculitis: A systematic mapping review. Autoimmun Rev. 2020;19: 102660.

15. Gómez-Puerta JA, Hernández-Rodríguez J, López-Soto A, Bosch X. Antineutrophil cytoplasmic antibody-associated vasculitides and respiratory disease. Chest. 2009 Oct;136(4):1101-1111. doi: 10.1378/chest.08-3043. PMID: 19809051.

16. Singh, Sunilkumar Rajmani; Oak, Jyotsna; Olickal, Mahin Salim. Granulomatosis with Polyangiitis: Experience of 42 Patients from a Single-Center, Tertiary Care Hospital in Mumbai. Indian Journal of Rheumatology 16(2):p 145-S151, June 2021. doi: 10.4103/injr.injr_176_20.

17. Samman KN, Ross C, Pagnoux C, Makhzoum JP. Update in the Management of ANCA-Associated Vasculitis: Recent Developments and Future Perspectives. Int J Rheumatol. 2021 Apr 8;2021:5534851. doi: 10.1155/2021/5534851. PMID: 33927768; PMCID: PMC8049818.

18. Jayne DRW, Merkel PA, Schall TJ, Bekker P; ADVOCATE Study Group. Avacopan for the Treatment of ANCA-Associated Vasculitis. N Engl J Med. 2021 Feb 18;384(7):599-609. doi: 10.1056/NEJMoa2023386. Erratum in: N Engl J Med. 2024 Jan 25;390(4):388. doi: 10.1056/NEJMx230010. PMID: 33596356.

19. Hellmich B, Sanchez-Alamo B, Schirmer JH, Berti A, Blockmans D, Cid MC, Holle JU, Hollinger N, Karadag O, Kronbichler A, Little MA, Luqmani RA, Mahr A, Merkel PA, Mohammad AJ, Monti S, Mukhtyar CB, Musial J, Price-Kuehne F, Segelmark M, Teng YKO, Terrier B, Tomasson G, Vaglio A, Vassilopoulos D, Verhoeven P, Jayne D. EULAR recommendations for the management of ANCA-associated vasculitis: 2022 update. Ann Rheum Dis. 2023 Mar 16:ard-2022-223764. doi: 10.1136/ard-2022-223764. Epub ahead of print. PMID: 36927642.

20. Alchi MB, Lever R, Flossmann O, Jayne D. Efficacy and safety of low-versus high-dose glucocorticoid regimens for induction of remission of anti-neutrophil cytoplasm antibody-associated vasculitis: a systematic review and meta-analysis. Scand J Rheumatol. 2023 Sep;52(5):564-573. doi: 10.1080/03009742.2023.2211387. Epub 2023 Jun 20. PMID: 37339385.

21. Lee YH, Song GG. Comparative efficacy and safety of rituximab, mycophenolate, and cyclophosphamide inactive antineutrophil cytoplasmic antibody-associated vasculitis: A Bayesian network meta-analysis of randomized controlled trials. Int J Clin Pharmacol Ther. 2021 Oct;59(10):645-653. doi: 10.5414/CP204024. PMID: 34338191.

22. Jordan N, D'cruz DP. Association of Lupus Anticoagulant With Long-Term Damage Accrual in Antineutrophil Cytoplasmic Antibody-Associated Vasculitis. Arthritis Care Res (Hoboken). 2016 May;68(5):711-5. doi: 10.1002/acr.22723. PMID: 26415137.

CHAPTER

6

Pulmonary Hypertension

Authors: Dr. Ruchi Sharma, Dr. Shekhar Kunal

Reviewer: Dr. Bhushan Shah

INTRODUCTION

Pulmonary hypertension (PH) is a pathophysiological disorder that encompasses a variety of clinical conditions. It is associated with a variety of cardiac and respiratory disorders. Traditionally, PH has been categorized into five different groups based on the underlying etiology and pathophysiological process. Pulmonary arterial hypertension (PAH) belongs to group I PH and comprises idiopathic, heritable, connective tissue disease-associated and those due to congenital heart diseases.

Methodology

A PubMed search was carried out with the search term {"pulmonary hypertension" OR "pulmonary arterial hypertension" OR "PH" OR "PAH"}. Articles between the period of 1st August 2023 to 1st August 2024 were reviewed. A total of 148 articles turned up during the search and were screened for relevance and research importance out of which 17 were selected for this review.

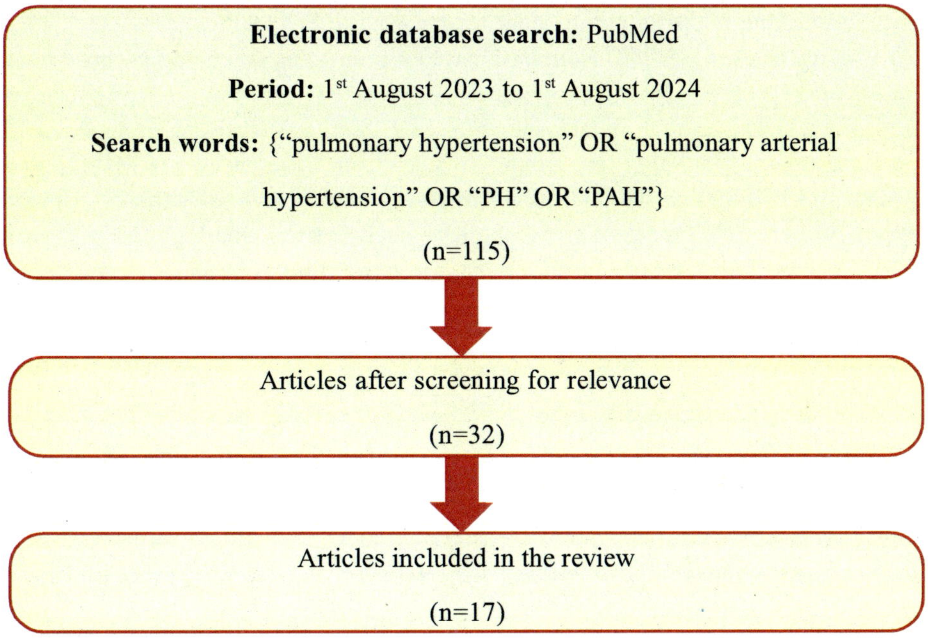

Analysis of Literature

- ***Inhaled Efficacy and safety of macitentan for pulmonary hypertension: A meta-analysis. (Clin Respir J. 2023)***[1]
  - o *Population:* Patients with pulmonary hypertension. (n=1,322)
  - o *Intervention:* Macitentan. (n=723)
  - o *Comparator:* Placebo. (n=599)
  - o *Outcome:* Macitentan effectively decreased pulmonary vascular resistance (PVR) (SMD = -0.53, 95% CI: -0.77—0.29, $p < 0.05$), cardiac index (CI) (SMD = 0.60, 95% CI: 0.37-0.83, $p < 0.05$) and N-terminal pro-brain natriuretic peptide (NT-proBNP) (SMD = -0.22, 95% CI: -0.40—0.03, $p < 0.05$). Macitentan also significantly reduced PVR (SMD = -0.58, 95% CI: -0.80—0.35, $p < 0.05$), 6-min walk distance (6WMD) (SMD = 0.33, 95% CI: 0.15-0.50, $p < 0.05$), CI (SMD = 0.48, 95% CI: 0.28-0.69, $p < 0.05$), mean pulmonary arterial pressure (mPAP) (SMD = -0.43, 95% CI: -0.64—0.23, $p < 0.05$) and NT-proBNP (SMD = -0.55, 95% CI: -1.07—0.03, $p < 0.05$) between baseline and follow-up. Adverse reactions to macitentan were mild, with headache, anemia and bronchitis.
  - o *Conclusion:* Macitentan therapy for PH is effective and safe.

- ***Treatment effects of pulmonary artery denervation for pulmonary arterial hypertension stratified by REVEAL risk score: Results from PADN-CFDA trial. (J Heart Lung Transplant. 2023)***[2]
  - o *Population:* Patients with pulmonary hypertension. (n=128)
  - o *Outcome:* In the intermediate-high-risk group, those treated with PADN (Pulmonary Artery Denervation) and PDE-5i had a greater improvement in 6 MWD from baseline to 6 months as compared to those treated with sham plus PDE-5i. From baseline to 6 months, pulmonary vascular resistance (PVR) was reduced by -6.1 ± 0.6 and -2.0 ± 0.7 Wood units following PADN plus PDE-5i and sham plus PDE-5i, respectively, along with the significant reduction of NT-proBNP in the intermediate-high-risk group. No significant differences in 6 MWD, PVR, and NT-proBNP between the PADN plus PDE-5i and sham plus PDE-5i groups among low-risk patients. Right ventricular function was equally improved by PADN treatment across the low, intermediate-, and high-risk groups. Clinical worsening was less with PADN plus PDE-5i treatment during the 6-month follow-up.
  - o *Conclusion:* In patients with pulmonary arterial hypertension, pulmonary artery denervation plus PDE-5i improved exercise capacity, NT-proBNP, hemodynamic, and clinical outcomes during the 6-month follow-up among intermediate-high risk patients.

- ***Anticoagulation in chronic thromboembolic pulmonary hypertension: A systematic review and meta-analysis (Thromb Res. 2023)***[3]
  - o *Population:* Patients with chronic thromboembolic pulmonary hypertension from 7 studies. (n=2,969)
  - o *Intervention:* Direct oral anticoagulants. (DOAC)
  - o *Comparator:* Vitamin K Agonist. (VKA)

- *Outcome:* No differences in major bleeding (RR 0.59, 95 % CI [0.34-1.02], I2 = 0 %) and all-bleeding (RR 0.87, 95 % CI [0.67-1.13], I2 = 0 %). DOAC was associated with a lower risk of mortality (RR 0.54, 95 % CI: 0.37-0.79, I2 = 5 %). Higher risk of recurrent pulmonary embolism (PE) was seen in three studies (RR 3.80, 95 % CI: [1.93-7.50], I2 = 11 %). No significant differences were noted in terms of VTE.
- *Conclusion:* DOAC compared to VKA was associated with a significantly lower mortality and higher risk of recurrent PE.

- ***Long-term safety of macitentan in patients with pulmonary hypertension: A meta-analysis of randomised controlled trials. (Eur J Clin Invest. 2023)[4]***
  - *Population:* Patients with pulmonary hypertension from 6 RCTs. (n=1,003)
  - *Intervention:* Macitentan.
  - *Comparator:* Placebo.
  - *Outcome:* Anemia (RR: 3.86, 95% CI: 2.05-7.30), headache (RR: 1.52, 95% CI: 1.02-2.26), and bronchitis (RR: 2.24, 95% CI: 1.30-3.87) were more frequent in the macitentan groups. No statistically significant difference in the proportion of patients with at least one adverse event (AE) or serious adverse event (SAE), AEs leading to discontinuation of study treatment, all-cause death, right ventricular failure (RVF), and peripheral edema between the two groups.
  - *Conclusion:* Long-term use of macitentan is safe for patients with PH, although with a higher risk of anemia, headache, and bronchitis.

- ***A Meta-analysis Assessing the Efficacy of Balloon Pulmonary Angioplasty in Resolving Chronic Thromboembolic Pulmonary Hypertension. (Altern Ther Health Med. 2023)[5]***
  - *Population:* Patients with chronic thromboembolic pulmonary hypertension (CTEPH) from 7 studies.
  - *Intervention:* Balloon pulmonary angioplasty (BPA).
  - *Comparator:* Placebo.
  - *Outcome:* BPA demonstrated a significant reduction in pulmonary arterial pressure in CTEPH patients (Mean difference (MD) = -9.80, 95% CI: -1.10 to -8.59, P < .00001). BPA also resulted in a decrease in pulmonary vascular resistance in CTEPH patients (MD = -4.70, 95% CI: -7.17 to -2.22, P = .0002). Moreover, BPA was associated with improved 6-minute walk distance of CTEPH patients (MD = 43.86, 95% CI: 26.19 to 61.53, P < .00001). Additionally, BPA led to a reduction in NT-proBNP levels in CTEPH patients (MD = -3.46, 95% CI: -10.63 to 3.71, p-value = 0.34). BPA also resulted in an improvement in the WHO functional class of CTEPH patients, with an increase in class I-II (MD = 0.28, 95% CI: 0.22 to 0.35, P < .00001) and a decrease in class III-IV (MD = 0.16, 95% CI: 0.10 to 0.26, P < .00001).
  - *Conclusion:* BPA as an alternative treatment option for CTEPH patients, leading to improvements in prognostic factors such as hemodynamics, functional ability, and biomarkers.

- ***Phase 1 Study of MK-5475, an Inhaled Soluble Guanylate Cyclase Stimulator, in Participants with Pulmonary Hypertension Associated with Chronic Obstructive Pulmonary Disease. (Int J Chron Obstruct Pulmon Dis. 2024)[6]***
  - *Population:* Patients with COPD (FEV1/FVC <0.7; FEV1 >30% predicted) and PH (mean pulmonary arterial pressure ≥25 mmHg). (n=22)
  - *Intervention:* MK-5475. Dosage: dry-powder inhaler once daily for 7 days in Part 1 (360 μg) or 28 days in Part 2 (380 μg). (n=14)

- *Comparator:* Placebo (n=8)
- *Outcome:* Nine participants were randomized in Part 1, and 14 participants in Part 2. Incidences of AEs were comparable between MK-5475 and placebo: overall (5/14 [36%] versus 5/8 [63%]), drug-related (1/14 [7%] versus 2/8 [25%]), and serious (1/14 [7%] versus 1/8 [13%]). MK-5475 caused no meaningful changes in arterial blood oxygenation or pulmonary blood volume (PBV). MK-5475 versus placebo led to numerical improvements from baseline in pulmonary vascular resistance [PVR] (-21.2% [95% CI: -35.4, -7.0] versus -5.4% [95% CI: -83.7, 72.9]), with a between-group difference in PVR less than -15% and calculated PP of 51%.
- *Conclusion:* Favorable safety profile and numerical reductions in PVR observed support further clinical development of inhaled MK-5475 for PH-COPD treatment.

- ***Randomized Trial of Macitentan/Tadalafil Single-Tablet Combination Therapy for Pulmonary Arterial Hypertension. (J Am Coll Cardiol. 2024)***[7]
  - *Population:* Adults with pulmonary arterial hypertension including treatment-naïve and prior ERA or PDE5i monotherapy-treated patients. (n=187)
  - *Intervention:* ERA macitentan and PDE5i tadalafil (M/T FDC) - once-daily, single tablet. (n=108)
  - *Comparator:*

    a) Macitentan 10 mg monotherapy. (n=35)

    b) Tadalafil 40 mg monotherapy. (n=44)
  - *Outcome:* PVR reduction with M/T FDC was significantly greater vs macitentan (29%; geometric mean ratio 0.71; 95% CL: 0.61-0.82; P < 0.0001) and vs tadalafil (28%; geometric mean ratio 0.72; 95% CL: 0.64-0.80; P < 0.0001). Three patients died in the M/T FDC arm (judged unrelated to treatment). Adverse events (AEs) leading to discontinuation, serious AEs, and those of special interest (anemia, hypotension, and edema) were more frequent with M/T FDC.
  - *Conclusion:* Macitentan and tadalafil fixed dose combination significantly improved PVR vs monotherapies in PAH patients, with a safety and tolerability profile consistent with the individual components. This study supports M/T FDC as a once-daily, single-tablet combination for initial therapy and escalation to double combination therapy in patients with PAH.

- ***Long-term inhaled treprostinil for pulmonary hypertension due to interstitial lung disease: INCREASE open-label extension study. (Eur Respir J. 2023)***[8]
  - *Population:* Patients with pulmonary hypertension due to interstitial lung disease (PH-ILD). (n=240)
  - *Intervention:* Inhaled Treprostinil. (n=119)
  - *Comparator:* Placebo. (n=121)
  - *Outcome:* Mean 6MWD at week 52 was 279.1 m and the mean change from INCREASE RCT baseline was 3.5 m (22.1m for the prior inhaled treprostinil arm and -19.5 m for the prior placebo arm); the median NT-proBNP decreased from 389 pg·mL-1 at RCT baseline to 359 pg·mL-1 at week 64; and the absolute (% predicted) mean forced vital capacity change from RCT baseline to week 64 was 51 mL (2.8%). Patients who received inhaled treprostinil versus placebo in the RCT had a 31% lower relative risk of exacerbation of underlying lung disease in the OLE (hazard ratio 0.69 (95% CI 0.49-0.97); p=0.03). Adverse events leading to drug discontinuation occurred in 54 (22.3%) patients.

- o *Conclusion:* Study supports long-term safety and efficacy of inhaled treprostinil in patients with PH-ILD, and are consistent with the results observed in the INCREASE RCT.

- ***Inhaled treprostinil in pulmonary hypertension associated with COPD: PERFECT study results. (Eur Respir J. 2024)[9]***
  - o *Population:* Patients with pulmonary hypertension (PH) accompanying COPD (PH-COPD). (n=124)
  - o *Intervention:* Inhaled treprostinil (iTRE). (n=66)
  - o *Comparator:* Placebo. (n=58)
  - o *Outcome:* The study was terminated early at the recommendation of the data and safety monitoring committee based on the totality of evidence that iTRE increased the risk of serious adverse events and suggestive evidence of an increased risk of mortality. The change in 6MWD was numerically worse with iTRE exposure than with placebo exposure.
  - o *Conclusion:* Risk-benefit observations associated with iTRE in patients with PH-COPD did not support the continuation of the PERFECT study. The results of this study do not support iTRE as a viable treatment option in patients with PH-COPD.

- ***Seralutinib in adults with pulmonary arterial hypertension (TORREY): A randomised, double-blind, placebo-controlled phase 2 trial. (Lancet Respir Med. 2024)[10]***
  - o *Population:* Patients with Pulmonary Arterial Hypertension. (n=86)
  - o *Intervention:* Seralutinib (60 mg twice daily for 2 weeks, then increased to 90 mg twice daily as tolerated). (n=44)
  - o *Comparator:* Placebo. (n=42)
  - o *Outcome:* Least squares mean change from baseline to week 24 in PVR was 21·2 dyne·s/cm5 (95% CI -37·4 to 79·8) for the placebo group and -74·9 dyne·s/cm5 (-139·7 to -10·2) for the seralutinib group. Least squares mean difference between the seralutinib and placebo groups for change in PVR was -96·1 dyne·s/cm^5 (95% CI -183·5 to -8·8; p=0·03). Most common treatment-emergent adverse event in both treatment groups was cough: 16 (38%) of 42 patients in the placebo group; 19 (43%) of 44 patients in the seralutinib group.
  - o *Conclusion:* Treatment with inhaled seralutinib significantly decreased PVR, meeting the primary endpoint of the study among patients receiving background therapy for PAH.

- ***SPECTRA Phase 2b Study: Impact of Sotatercept on Exercise Tolerance and Right Ventricular Function in Pulmonary Arterial Hypertension. (Circ Heart Fail. 2024)[11]***
  - o *Population:* Patients with pulmonary arterial hypertension. (n=21)
  - o *Intervention:* Sotatercept.
  - o *Comparator:* Placebo.

- *Outcome:* Among the 21 participants completing 24 weeks of treatment, significant improvement from baseline in peak oxygen uptake, with a mean change of 102.74 mL/min ([95% CI: 27.72-177.76]; P=0.0097). Sotatercept demonstrated improvements in secondary end points, including resting and peak exercise hemodynamics, and 6-minute walk distance versus baseline measures. Cardiac magnetic resonance imaging showed improvements from baseline at week 24 in right ventricular function.
- *Conclusion:* Clinical efficacy and safety of sotatercept demonstrated in the SPECTRA study emphasize the potential of this therapy as a new treatment option for patients with pulmonary arterial hypertension.
- *Critical analysis:* Improvements in right ventricular structure and function underscore the potential for sotatercept as a disease-modifying agent with reverse-remodelling capabilities.

- ***Pulmonary arterial hypertension treatment: An individual participant data network meta-analysis. (Eur Heart J. 2024)***[12]
  - *Population:* Patients with PAH. (n=6811)
  - *Intervention:* Network meta-analysis using individual participant data from 20 Phase III randomized clinical trials of therapy for PAH.
  - *Outcome:* Mean age of the sample was 49.2 ±15.4 years; 78.4% were female, 59.7% had idiopathic PAH, and 36.5% were on background PAH therapy. After covariate adjustment, targeting the endothelin + nitric oxide pathway {β: 43.7 m [95% confidence interval (CI): 32.9, 54.4]}, nitric oxide pathway [β: 29.4 m (95% CI: 22.6, 36.3)], endothelin pathway [β: 25.3 m (95% CI: 19.8, 30.8)], and prostacyclin pathway [oral/inhaled β: 19.1 m (95% CI: 14.2, 24.0), intravenous/subcutaneous β: 24.4 m (95% CI: 15.1, 33.7)] significantly increased 6 min walk distance at 12 or 16 weeks compared with placebo. Treatments also significantly reduced the likelihood of having clinical worsening events.
  - *Conclusion:* Drugs targeting the three traditional treatment pathways significantly improve outcomes in PAH, with significant treatment heterogeneity in patients with some comorbidities. Randomized clinical trials are warranted to identify the most effective treatment strategies in a personalized approach.

- ***Efficacy and safety of iloprost in the treatment of pulmonary arterial hypertension: A systematic review and meta-analysis. (Heart Lung. 2024)***[13]
  - *Population:* Patients with PAH from 12 studies. (n=718)
  - *Intervention:* Inhaled Iloprost.
  - *Comparator:* Control group.
  - *Outcome:* Short and prolonged treatment groups significantly improved the 6-minute walking distance (6 MWD). Mortality and clinical deterioration incidences in the iloprost group were not significantly different from those in the control group. Mean pulmonary arterial pressure (mPAP) was reduced after 3 months of iloprost RCTs and 12 months of prospective treatment. Iloprost decreased pulmonary vascular resistance (PVR) by approximately 231.29 units, significantly increased cardiac output (CO), and improved the quality of life (QoL). The main adverse reactions to iloprost treatment were cough (17 %), headache (16.4 %), and flushing (12.4 %).
  - *Conclusion:* Iloprost, either used alone or as adjuvant therapy, can enhance exercise capacity, lower hemodynamic parameters, and improve long-term outcomes.

- ***Comparative Effectiveness of Sotatercept and Approved Add-On Pulmonary Arterial Hypertension Therapies: A Systematic Review and Network Meta-Analysis. (Ann Am Thorac Soc. 2024)[14]***
    - o *Population:* Patients with PAH from 18 trials. (n=5,777)
    - o *Intervention:* Sotatercept.
    - o *Comparator:* Placebo.
    - o *Outcome:* Sotatercept reduces clinical worsening as compared with placebo (relative risk [RR], 0.21; 95% confidence interval [CI] = 0.11-0.41; with high certainty). Sotatercept probably reduces clinical worsening more, compared with add-on endothelin receptor antagonists (RR, 0.28; 95% CI = 0.14-0.55), inhaled prostanoid (RR, 40.21; 95% CI = 0.07-0.67), and prostanoid taken orally (RR, 0.32; 95% CI = 0.16-0.67; all with moderate certainty). Sotatercept probably improves 6-minute-walk distance compared with placebo (mean difference [MD], 36.89 m; 95% CI = 25.26-48.51). Sotatercept probably improves 6-minute-walk distance more than add-on endothelin receptor antagonists (MD, 18.38 m; 95% CI = 5.92-30.84) and prostanoid taken orally (MD, 25.66 m; 95% CI = 13.71-37.61) however, it did not exceed the minimal clinically important difference of 33 m (both with moderate certainty).
    - o *Conclusion:* Sotatercept is an effective add-on therapy for PAH, likely superior to many approved add-on PAH therapies in reducing clinical worsening.

- ***Effects of 5-Week Oral Acetazolamide on Incremental Cycling Exercise in Pulmonary Arterial and Chronic Thromboembolic Pulmonary Hypertension: A Randomized Placebo-Controlled, Double-Blinded, Crossover Trial. (Respiration. 2024)[15]***
    - o *Population:* Patients with pulmonary vascular disease (PVD): pulmonary arterial and distal chronic thromboembolic pulmonary hypertension (CTEPH). (n=25)
    - o *Intervention:* 5 weeks of AZA (Acetazolamide) (250 mg bid).
    - o *Comparator:* Placebo.
    - o *Outcome:* Maximum load was similar after 5 weeks of AZA versus placebo (113 ± 9 vs. 117 ± 9 watts [W]), mean difference -4 W (95% CI: -9 to 1, p = 0.138). With AZA, maximum (max)-exercise partial pressure of O_2 (PaO_2) was significantly higher by 1.1 kPa (95% CI: 0.5-1.8, p = 0.003), while arterial pH and partial pressure of CO_2 were significantly lower. The gas exchange threshold was reached at a higher load with AZA (108 ± 8 W vs. 97 ± 8 W) and was therefore delayed by 11 W (95% CI: 3-19, p = 0.013), while the ventilatory equivalent for O_2 and CO_2 were significantly higher at both the max-exercise and gas exchange threshold with AZA versus placebo
    - o *Conclusion:* AZA for 5 weeks did not significantly change maximum exercise capacity in patients with PVD despite a significant increase in PaO_2. The beneficial effects of increased blood oxygenation may have been diminished by increased ventilation due to AZA-induced metabolic acidosis and increased dyspnea.

- ***Macitentan for the treatment of inoperable chronic thromboembolic pulmonary hypertension (MERIT-1): Results from the multicentre, phase 2, randomised, double-blind, placebo-controlled study. (Lancet Respir Med. 2024)[16]***
    - o Population: Patients with chronic thromboembolic pulmonary hypertension (CTEPH). (n=80)
    - o *Intervention:* Oral macitentan (10 mg once a day). (n=40)

- *Comparator:* Placebo. (n=40)
- *Outcome:* At week 16, geometric mean PVR decreased to 71·5% of baseline in the macitentan group and to 87·6% in the placebo group (geometric means ratio 0·81, 95% CI 0·70-0·95, p=0·0098). The most common adverse events in the macitentan group were peripheral edema (9 [23%] of 40 patients) and decreased hemoglobin (6 [15%]).
- *Conclusion:* Macitentan significantly improved PVR in patients with inoperable CTEPH and was well tolerated.

- ***Randomized, Multicenter Study to Assess the Effects of Different Doses of Sildenafil on Mortality in Adults With Pulmonary Arterial Hypertension. (Circulation. 2024)***[17]
  - *Population:* Patients with PAH.
  - *Intervention:* Sildenafil at doses of 20 or 80 mg TID.
  - *Comparator:* Sildenafil at 5 mg TID dose.
  - *Outcome:* Study was halted after the first interim analysis, demonstrating noninferiority for 80 mg of sildenafil versus 5 mg. Of 385 patients enrolled across all dose groups, 78 died. The primary analysis showed a hazard ratio of 0.51 (99.7% CI, 0.22-1.21; P<0.001 for noninferiority) for overall survival comparing 80 mg of sildenafil with 5 mg. Time to clinical worsening favored 80 mg of sildenafil compared with 5 mg (hazard ratio, 0.44 [99.7% CI, 0.22-0.89]; P<0.001). Sildenafil at 80 mg improved 6-minute walk distance from baseline at 6 months compared with 5 mg (least square mean change, 18.9 m [95% CI, 2.99-34.86]; P=0.0201). No significant differences were found between 80 mg of sildenafil and 20 mg in mortality, clinical worsening, and 6-minute walk distance. Adverse event-related drug discontinuations were numerically higher with 80 mg of sildenafil.
  - *Conclusion:* Sildenafil at 80 mg was noninferior to sildenafil at 5 mg when examining all-cause mortality in adults with PAH. Secondary efficacy end points favored 80 mg of sildenafil over 5 mg.
  - *Critical analysis:* On the basis of these findings, the Food and Drug Administration recently revoked the approval of 5 mg of sildenafil for adults with PAH, reinforced 20 mg TID as the recommended dose, and now allows dose titration up to 80 mg TID, if needed.

DISCUSSION

Pulmonary hypertension (PH) is a pathophysiological disorder that may involve multiple clinical conditions and may be associated with a variety of cardiovascular and respiratory diseases. The complexity of managing PH requires a multifaceted, holistic, and multidisciplinary approach, with active involvement of patients in partnership with clinicians. **The definitions for PH are based on haemodynamic assessment by right heart catheterization (RHC).** PH is defined with a mean pulmonary artery pressure >20 mm Hg at rest. The basic structure of the classification of PH remains the same as from the 2022 ESC/ERS Guidelines for the diagnosis and treatment of PH and the proceedings of the 6th World Symposium on Pulmonary Hypertension (WSPH).[18] PH is divided into 5 groups: GROUP 1: Pulmonary arterial hypertension (PAH); GROUP 2: PH associated with left heart disease; GROUP 3: PH associated with lung diseases and/or hypoxia; GROUP 4: PH associated with pulmonary artery obstructions; GROUP 5: PH with unclear and/or multifactorial mechanisms.

Diagnosis of PH is based on clinical symptoms followed by echocardiographic features of PH. Echocardiography is recommended as the first-line, non-invasive, diagnostic investigation in suspected PH. The gold standard for diagnosis of PH is right heart catheterization. **It is recommended that RHC is performed to confirm the diagnosis of PH (especially PAH or CTEPH) and to support treatment decisions. Vasoreactivity testing is recommended in patients with Idiopathic/Heritable/ Drug-induced PAH to detect those who can be treated with high doses of a CCB. A positive response to vasoreactivity testing by a reduction in mPAP ≥10 mmHg to reach an absolute value of mPAP ≤40 mmHg with an increased or unchanged CO.**

Ventilation/perfusion or perfusion lung scan is recommended in patients with unexplained PH to assess for CTEPH. CT pulmonary angiography is also recommended in the work-up of patients with suspected CTEPH. Pulmonary function tests with DLCO are recommended in the initial evaluation of patients with PH.[18] We don't propose any change in the classification or diagnostic strategy for PH. Most of the studies regarding PAH have focused on the evaluation of treatment strategies such as the use of upfront dual combination therapy or newer drugs such as selexipag, sotatercept, macitentan etc. **The current standard of care in PAH remains as the initial combination therapy with ambrisentan and tadalafil which is recommended in the guidelines.[18] Another notable development is the introduction of fixed-dose combination tablet containing macitentan and tadalafil, which provides a more convenient daily treatment. A recent trial showed that macitentan and tadalafil fixed dose combination significantly improved PVR as compared to monotherapies in PAH patients, with a safety and tolerability profile consistent with the individual components.** The findings of the study supported the role of M/T FDC as a once-daily, single-tablet combination for initial therapy and escalation to double combination therapy in patients with PAH.[7] **This marks the first single-tablet PAH therapy and simplifies medication regimens, which could improve adherence and outcomes.** Recent advancements in pulmonary hypertension (PH) have centred on new treatments, novel therapeutic pathways, and improved approaches to patient care.

In 2024, the FDA approved Sotatercept (Winrevair), which is seen as a breakthrough because it targets the bone morphogenetic protein receptor type II (BMPR-II) pathway - a mechanism implicated in disease progression. Sotatercept is a novel, first-in-class fusion protein composed of the extracellular domain of the human activin receptor type IIA fused to the Fc domain of human IgG1. Sotatercept acts as a ligand trap for members of the TGF-β superfamily, thus restoring the balance between the growth-promoting activin growth differentiation factor pathway and the growth-inhibiting BMP pathway. This drug, administered via subcutaneous injection, aims to balance the pathways that regulate blood vessel growth in the lungs, offering hope for patients who have not responded well to existing treatments. Clinical trials, including the **PULSAR study, showed promising reductions in pulmonary vascular resistance,** a critical measure in pulmonary arterial hypertension (PAH) management, suggesting enhanced outcomes for patients with advanced disease stages. **SPECTRA phase 2 study showed that improvements in right ventricular structure and function** underscore the potential for sotatercept as a disease-modifying agent with reverse-remodeling capabilities.[11] **In a recent meta-analysis, Sotatercept was an effective add-on therapy for PAH, likely superior to many approved add-on PAH therapies in reducing clinical worsening.[14]** We therefore propose the inclusion of Sotatercept as one of the treatment modalities for patients with PAH.

Another randomized study evaluating the different doses of sildenafil in PAH found that Sildenafil at 80 mg was non-inferior to sildenafil at 5 mg when examining all-cause mortality in adults with PAH. Secondary efficacy endpoints favored 80 mg of sildenafil over 5 mg.[17] **Based on this study, the Food and Drug Administration recently revoked the approval of 5 mg of sildenafil for adults with PAH, reinforced 20 mg TID as the recommended dose, and now allows dose titration up to 80 mg TID, if needed.**

Another interventional aspect that has recently been evaluated is the role of balloon pulmonary angioplasty (BPA) in patients with inoperable CTEPH. **The Japanese investigators found BPA to be superior to medical therapy in patients with inoperable CTEPH.** Additionally, the **MERIT-1 trial** evaluated the use of macitentan in CTEPH patients and **found that macitentan significantly improved PVR in patients with inoperable CTEPH** and was well tolerated.[16]

Among patients with COPD and PH (Group 3), inhaled treprostinil did not lead to a favorable result based on the PERFCT study as a result, we do not support iTRE as a viable treatment option in patients with PH-COPD.[9] Among patients with ILD and PH, **INCREASE open-label extension study** regarding **long-term inhaled treprostinil supports the usage of long-term safety and efficacy of inhaled treprostinil in patients with PH-ILD, and are consistent with the results observed in the INCREASE RCT.**[8]

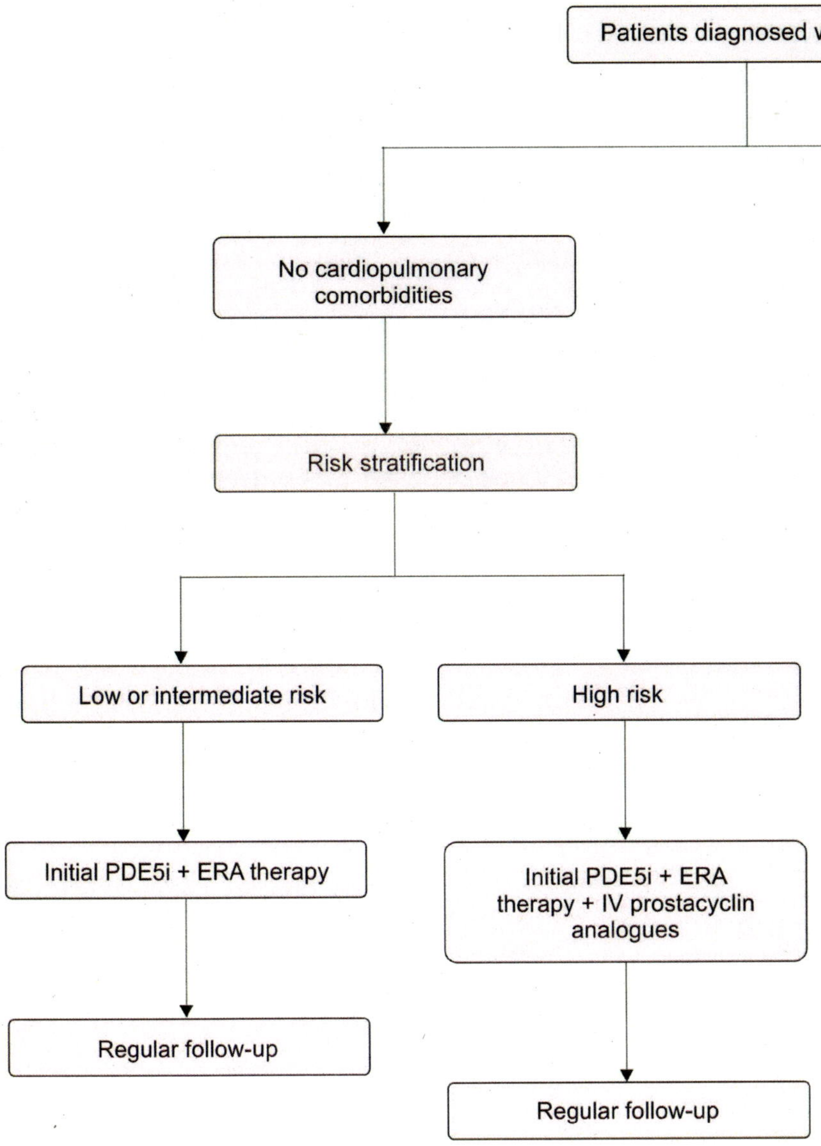

Flowchart: Pulmonary Hypertension Management

REFERENCES

1. Du D, Yuan YD. Efficacy and safety of macitentan for pulmonary hypertension: A meta-analysis. Clin Respir J. 2023 Nov;17(11):1117-1129. doi: 10.1111/crj.13621a.

2. Zhang J, Kan J, Wei Y, Zhang C, Yang Z, Gu H, Fan F, Gu H, Wang Q, Xie D, Zhang G, Guo X, Yin Y, Jin B, Zhou H, Yang Z, Wang Z, Xin Y, Zhang C, Meng L, Wang X, Zhao C, Zhang H, Yan X, Chen F, Yao C, Benza RL, Stone GW, Chen SL. Treatment effects of pulmonary artery denervation for pulmonary arterial hypertension stratified by REVEAL risk score: Results from PADN-CFDA trial. J Heart Lung Transplant. 2023 Aug;42(8):1140-1151. doi: 10.1016/j.healun.2023.03.015.

3. Ishisaka Y, Watanabe A, Takagi H, Steiger D, Kuno T. Anticoagulation in chronic thromboembolic pulmonary hypertension: A systematic review and meta-analysis. Thromb Res. 2023 Nov;231:91-98. doi: 10.1016/j.thromres.2023.10.003.

4. Wang G, Qin J, Han D. Long-term safety of macitentan in patients with pulmonary hypertension: A meta-analysis of randomised controlled trials. Eur J Clin Invest. 2023 Nov;53(11):e14059. doi: 10.1111/eci.14059. Epub 2023 Jul 1. PMID: 37392063.

5. Guo Q, Lu L, Jia B, Liu Y. A Meta-analysis Assessing the Efficacy of Balloon Pulmonary Angioplasty in Resolving Chronic Thromboembolic Pulmonary Hypertension. Altern Ther Health Med. 2023 Sep;29(6):444-448.

6. Bajwa EK, Cislak D, Kumar A, Li D, Messina EJ, Reynders T, Denef JF, Corcea V, Buch KP, Lai E, Stoch SA. Phase 1 Study of MK-5475, an Inhaled Soluble Guanylate Cyclase Stimulator, in Participants with Pulmonary Hypertension Associated with Chronic Obstructive Pulmonary Disease. Int J Chron Obstruct Pulmon Dis. 2024 May 23;19:1105-1121. doi: 10.2147/COPD.S454905.

7. Grünig E, Jansa P, Fan F, Hauser JA, Pannaux M, Morganti A, Rofael H, Chin KM. Randomized Trial of Macitentan/Tadalafil Single-Tablet Combination Therapy for Pulmonary Arterial Hypertension. J Am Coll Cardiol. 2024 Jan 30;83(4):473-484. doi: 10.1016/j.jacc.2023.10.045.

8. Waxman A, Restrepo-Jaramillo R, Thenappan T, Engel P, Bajwa A, Ravichandran A, Feldman J, Hajari Case A, Argula RG, Tapson V, Smith P, Deng C, Shen E, Nathan SD. Long-term inhaled treprostinil for pulmonary hypertension due to interstitial lung disease: INCREASE open-label extension study. Eur Respir J. 2023 Jun 29;61(6):2202414. doi: 10.1183/13993003.02414-2022.

9. Nathan SD, Argula R, Trivieri MG, Aziz S, Gay E, Medarov B, Parambil J, Raina A, Risbano MG, Thenappan T, Soto JS, Bell H, Lacasse V, Sista P, Di Marino M, Smart A, Hawkes B, Nelson E, Bull T, Tapson V, Waxman A. Inhaled treprostinil in pulmonary hypertension associated with COPD: PERFECT study results. Eur Respir J. 2024 Jun 6;63(6):2400172. doi: 10.1183/13993003.00172-2024.

10. Frantz RP, McLaughlin VV, Sahay S, Escribano Subías P, Zolty RL, Benza RL, Channick RN, Chin KM, Hemnes AR, Howard LS, Sitbon O, Vachiéry JL, Zamanian RT, Cravets M, Roscigno RF, Mottola D, Osterhout R, Bruey JM, Elman E, Tompkins CA, Parsley E, Aranda R, Zisman LS, Ghofrani HA; TORREY Study Investigators. Seralutinib in adults with pulmonary arterial hypertension (TORREY): a randomised, double-blind, placebo-controlled phase 2 trial. Lancet Respir Med. 2024 Jul;12(7):523-534.

11. Waxman AB, Systrom DM, Manimaran S, de Oliveira Pena J, Lu J, Rischard FP. SPECTRA Phase 2b Study: Impact of Sotatercept on Exercise Tolerance and Right Ventricular Function in Pulmonary Arterial Hypertension. Circ Heart Fail. 2024 May;17(5):e011227. doi: 10.1161/CIRCHEARTFAILURE.123.011227.

12. Moutchia J, McClelland RL, Al-Naamani N, Appleby DH, Holmes JH, Minhas J, Mazurek JA, Palevsky HI, Ventetuolo CE, Kawut SM. Pulmonary arterial hypertension treatment: an individual participant data network meta-analysis. Eur Heart J. 2024 Jun 1;45(21):1937-1952. doi: 10.1093/eurheartj/ehae049.

13. Zhou R, Zhao Z, Liu J, Liu M, Xie F. Efficacy and safety of iloprost in the treatment of pulmonary arterial hypertension: A systematic review and meta-analysis. Heart Lung. 2024 Mar-Apr;64:36-45. doi: 10.1016/j.hrtlng.2023.11.006.

14. Pitre T, Desai K, Mah J, Zeraatkar D, Humbert M. Comparative Effectiveness of Sotatercept and Approved Add-On Pulmonary Arterial Hypertension Therapies: A Systematic Review and Network Meta-Analysis. Ann Am Thorac Soc. 2024 Aug;21(8):1194-1203.

15. Müller J, Appenzeller P, Lichtblau M, Saxer S, Berlier C, Schneider SR, Furian M, Schwarz EI, Swenson ER, Bloch KE, Ulrich S. Effects of 5-Week Oral Acetazolamide on Incremental Cycling Exercise in Pulmonary Arterial and Chronic Thromboembolic Pulmonary Hypertension: A Randomized Placebo-Controlled, Double-Blinded, Crossover Trial. Respiration. 2024;103(3):124-133.

16. Ghofrani HA, Simonneau G, D'Armini AM, Fedullo P, Howard LS, Jaïs X, Jenkins DP, Jing ZC, Madani MM, Martin N, Mayer E, Papadakis K, Richard D, Kim NH; MERIT study investigators. Macitentan for the treatment of inoperable chronic thromboembolic

pulmonary hypertension (MERIT-1): results from the multicentre, phase 2, randomised, double-blind, placebo-controlled study. Lancet Respir Med. 2024 Apr;12(4):e21-e30. doi: 10.1016/S2213-2600(24)00027-4. PMID: 38548406.

17. Hoeper MM, Ewert R, Jansa P, Sirenko Y, Skride A, Balagtas C, Hackley S, Vogt S, Abreu P, Haughie S, Hassan T, Oudiz RJ. Randomized, Multicenter Study to Assess the Effects of Different Doses of Sildenafil on Mortality in Adults With Pulmonary Arterial Hypertension. Circulation. 2024 Jun 18;149(25):1949-1959.

18. Humbert M, Kovacs G, Hoeper MM, Badagliacca R, Berger RMF, Brida M, Carlsen J, Coats AJS, Escribano-Subias P, Ferrari P, Ferreira DS, Ghofrani HA, Giannakoulas G, Kiely DG, Mayer E, Meszaros G, Nagavci B, Olsson KM, Pepke-Zaba J, Quint JK, Rådegran G, Simonneau G, Sitbon O, Tonia T, Toshner M, Vachiery JL, Vonk Noordegraaf A, Delcroix M, Rosenkranz S; ESC/ERS Scientific Document Group. 2022 ESC/ERS Guidelines for the diagnosis and treatment of pulmonary hypertension. Eur Respir J. 2023 Jan 6;61(1):2200879.

CHAPTER 7

Pulmonary Embolism

Authors: Dr. Ruchi Sharma, Dr. Shekhar Kunal

Reviewer: Dr. Bhushan Shah

INTRODUCTION

Pulmonary thromboembolism belongs to the spectrum of diseases categorized under venous thromboembolism. This potentially life-threatening disorder has a myriad of presenting signs and symptoms. A majority of patients with pulmonary embolism (PE) often have a predisposing factor precipitating it. However, a fraction of patients lack any underlying cause leading to unprovoked PE. Evaluation of patients with PE often requires multiple diagnostic tests including clinical probability assessment. Risk stratification forms an integral component of the management of PE with anti-coagulation advocated for low-risk PE and thrombolysis in patients with high-risk PE.

Methodology

A PubMed search was carried out with the search term: {"pulmonary embolism" OR "venous thromboembolism" OR "VTE"}. Articles between the period of 1st August 2023 to 1st August 2024 were reviewed. A staggering 290 articles turned up during the search and were screened for relevance and research importance and out of which 93 were selected for this review.

Electronic database search: PubMed

Period: 1st August 2023 to 1st August 2024

Search words: {"pulmonary embolism" OR "venous thromboembolism" OR "VTE"}

(n=290)

↓

Articles after screening for relevance

(n=93)

↓

Articles included in the review

(n=16)

Analysis of Literature

Diagnostic strategy

- ***Diagnostic management of acute pulmonary embolism: A prediction model based on a patient data meta-analysis. (Eur Heart J. 2023)[1]***
    - o *Population:* Adult patients with clinically suspected PE from various clinical settings; individual patient data meta-analysis from sixteen cross-sectional or prospective studies. (n=28, 305)
    - o *Intervention:* Model-multilevel logistic regression model including ten objective candidate predictors.
    - o *Comparator:* Wells score and YEARS algorithm.
    - o *Outcome:* End-point: Diagnosis of PE confirmed by imaging at baseline or venous thromboembolism during 30 to 90-day follow-up. Final model included: age (in years), sex, previous VTE, recent surgery or immobilization, haemoptysis, cancer, clinical signs of deep vein thrombosis, inpatient status, D-dimer (in μg/L), and an interaction term between age and D-dimer. The pooled c-statistic was 0.87 (95% CI, 0.85-0.89; 95% PI, 0.77-0.93) and overall calibration was very good. The model slightly overestimated VTE probability in a lower range of estimated probabilities. Discrimination of the current model in the validation datasets was better than that of the Wells score combined with a D-dimer threshold based on age (c-statistic 0.73; 95% CI, 0.70-0.75) or structured clinical pretest probability (c-statistic 0.79; 95% CI, 0.76-0.81).
    - o *Conclusion:* The present model provides an absolute, individualized probability of PE presence in a broad population of patients with suspected PE, with very good discrimination and calibration.
    - o *Critical appraisal:* The clinical utility of the model needs to be evaluated in a prospective management or impact study

- ***PECSS: Pulmonary Embolism Comprehensive Screening Score to safely rule out pulmonary embolism among suspected patients presenting to emergency department. (BMC Pulm Med. 2023)[2]***
    - o *Population:* Adult patients with clinically suspected PE. (n=4,867)
    - o *Intervention:* Model- logistic regression model.
    - o *Comparator:* Wells score.

      End-point: Diagnosis of PE confirmed by CTPA.
    - o *Outcome:* PECSS identified seven clinical predictors (anhelation, abnormal blood pressure, in critical condition when admitted, age > 65 years and high levels of pro-BNP, CRP and UA,) strongly associated with pulmonary embolism. Patients can be safely ruled out of pulmonary embolism if PECSS ≤ 4, or if $4 <$ PECSS ≤ 6 and D-Dimer ≤ 2.5 mg/L. Compared with Wells approach, PECSS achieved lower failure rates across all pulmonary embolism severity grades.
    - o *Conclusion:* Compared to Wells score, PECSS approaches achieved lower failure rates and better compromise between sensitivity and specificity. Calculation of PECSS is easy and all predictors are readily available upon emergency department admission, making it widely applicable in clinical settings.
    - o *Critical appraisal:* Clinical utility of the model needs to be evaluated in a prospective management study.

Therapeutic strategy

- ***Oral direct thrombin inhibitors or oral factor Xa inhibitors versus conventional anticoagulants for the treatment of pulmonary embolism. (Cochrane Database Syst Rev. 2023)***[3]
  - o *Population:* Patients with pulmonary embolism from 10 RCTs. (n=13,073)
  - o *Intervention:* Oral DTIs and oral factor Xa inhibitors.
  - o *Comparator:* Conventional anticoagulants.
  - o *Outcome:* Meta-analysis showed no clear difference in the efficacy and safety of oral DTI compared with conventional anticoagulation in preventing recurrent PE (OR: 1.02, 95% CI: 0.50 to 2.04), recurrent VTE (OR: 0.93, 95% CI: 0.52 to 1.66), DVT (OR: 0.79, 95% CI 0.29 to 2.13) and major bleeding (OR 0.50, 95% CI 0.15 to 1.68).
  - o *Conclusion:* Little or no difference between DOACs and conventional anticoagulation in the prevention of recurrent PE, recurrent VTE, DVT, all-cause mortality, and major bleeding.

☞

- ***Catheter-directed thrombolysis compared with systemic thrombolysis and anticoagulation in patients with intermediate- or high-risk pulmonary embolism: systematic review and network meta-analysis. (CMAJ. 2023)***[4]
  - o *Population:* Patients with intermediate- or high-risk pulmonary embolism from 44 studies. (n=20,006 patients)
  - o *Intervention:* Catheter-directed thrombolysis (CDT).
  - o *Comparator:* Systemic thrombolysis.
  - o *Outcome:* CDT was associated with a decreased risk of death (OR: 0.43, 95% CI: 0.32-0.57), intracerebral hemorrhage (OR: 0.44, 95% CI: 0.29-0.64), major bleeding (OR: 0.61, 95% CI: 0.53-0.70) and blood transfusion (OR 0.46, 95% CI 0.28-0.77) as compared to systemic thrombolysis.
  - o *Conclusion:* With moderate certainty of evidence, the risk of death and major bleeding complications was lower with CDT than with systemic thrombolysis.

☞

- ***Comparative Efficacy and Safety of Thrombolytic Agents for Pulmonary Embolism: A Bayesian Network Meta-Analysis. (Pharmacology. 2023)***[5]
  - o *Population:* Patients with all types of acute PE: hemodynamically unstable PE (massive PE) and hemodynamically stable PE (submassive PE and low-risk PE) from 29 RCTs. (n=3,067)
  - o *Intervention:* Thrombolytic agents.
  - o *Comparator:* Heparin.
  - o *Outcome:* Mortality using thrombolytic agents (except tenecteplase) was significantly lower compared with heparin. Recurrence of PE with alteplase was significantly lower compared with heparin (RR = 0.23, 95% CI, 0.04, 0.65). Pulmonary artery systolic pressure (PASP) after using alteplase was significantly lower compared with heparin (mean difference = -11.36, 95% CI, -21.45, -1.56). Compared with heparin, the incidence of minor bleeding associated with tenecteplase was higher (RR = 3.27, 95% CI, 1.36, 7.39); compared with streptokinase, the incidence of minor bleeding associated with tenecteplase was higher (RR = 3.22, 95% CI, 1.01, 11.10).

- *Conclusion:* For patients with acute PE, four thrombolytic agents (alteplase, reteplase, streptokinase, and urokinase) appeared to be superior in efficacy compared with anticoagulants alone due to a reduction in mortality and no increase in bleeding risk. Alteplase may be a better choice because it not only reduces mortality but also reduces PE recurrence rate and treated PASP. Tenecteplase did not reduce mortality compared with anticoagulants alone and may not be a good choice of thrombolytic agent due to an increase in minor bleeding compared with streptokinase and anticoagulants alone.

- ***Thrombolytics in Cardiac Arrest from Pulmonary Embolism: A Systematic Review and Meta-Analysis. (J Intensive Care Med 2023)***[6]
  - *Population:* Patients with cardiac arrest presumed to be related to pulmonary embolism (PE) from 13 studies. (n=803)
  - *Intervention:* Intravenous thrombolysis.
  - *Comparator:* Standard care.
  - *Outcome:* Intravenous thrombolysis was associated with higher rates of ROSC (OR 2.55, 95% CI = 1.50-4.34), but without a significant difference in survival to hospital discharge (OR 1.41, 95% CI = 0.79-2.41) or bleeding complications (OR 2.21, 0.95-5.17).
  - *Conclusion:* Use of intravenous thrombolytics in cardiac arrest due to confirmed or presumed PE is associated with increased ROSC but not survival to hospital discharge or change in bleeding complications.

- ***Prevalence, Risk Factor and Clinical Characteristics of Venous Thrombus Embolism in Patients with Acute Exacerbation of COPD: A Prospective Multicenter Study. (Int J Chron Obstruct Pulmon Dis. 2023)***[7]
  - *Population:* Patients with acute exacerbation chronic obstructive pulmonary disease (COPD). (n=1580)
  - *Outcome:* Prevalence of VTE was 24.5% (387/1580) and PE was 16.8% (266/1580). VTE patients were older; had higher BMI; and longer course of COPD than non-VTE patients. History of VTE, cor pulmonale, less purulent sputum, increased respiratory rate, higher D-dimer, and higher NT-proBNP/BNP were independently associated with VTE in hospitalized patients with AECOPD. Mortality at 1-year was higher in patients with VTE than in patients without VTE (12.9% vs 4.5%, p<0.01).
  - *Conclusion:* VTE is common in COPD patients and is associated with poor prognosis.

- ***Comparison of outcomes and complications in conventional versus ultrasound-accelerated catheter directed thrombolysis for treatment of pulmonary embolism: A systematic review and meta-analysis. (Perfusion. 2023)***[8]
  - *Population:* Intermediate risk PE from 9 studies. (n=705)
  - *Intervention:* Ultrasound-accelerated catheter-directed thrombolysis (USACDT).
  - *Comparator:* Catheter-directed thrombolysis (CDT).
  - *Outcome:* No significant difference between two groups concerning pulmonary arterial systolic pressure (SMD: -0.084; 95% CI: -0.287 to 0.12; p: 0.41), RV/LV (SMD: -0.003; 95% CI: -0.277 to 0.270; p: 0.98), and Miller score (SMD: -0.345; 95% CI: -1.376 to 0.686; p: 0.51). No statistically significant differences between two groups regarding major and minor bleeding (p > .05).
  - *Conclusion:* Compared with USACDT, conventional CDT provides similar clinical and hemodynamic outcomes or safety for the treatment of pulmonary embolism without the need for very expensive technologies.

- ***Comparative Outcomes of Catheter-Directed Thrombolysis Plus Systemic Anticoagulation Versus Systemic Anticoagulation Alone in the Management of Intermediate-Risk Pulmonary Embolism in a Systematic Review and Meta-Analysis. (Am J Cardiol. 2023)***[9]
  - *Population:* Patients with intermediate-risk acute PE from 15 studies. (n=10,549)
  - *Intervention:* Catheter-Directed Thrombolysis Plus Systemic Anticoagulation (CDT + SA). (n=2,310 patients)
  - *Comparator:* Systemic Anticoagulation (SA). (n=8,239 patients)
  - *Outcome:* Compared with SA, CDT + SA was associated with significantly lower in-hospital mortality (RR 0.41, 95% CI 0.30 to 0.56, p <0.001), 30-day mortality (RR 0.34, 95% CI 0.18 to 0.67, p = 0.002), 90-day mortality (RR 0.34, 95% CI 0.17 to 0.67, p = 0.002), and 1-year mortality (RR 0.58, 95% CI 0.34 to 0.97, p = 0.04). No significant differences between the 2 cohorts in the rates of major bleeding (RR 1.39, 95% CI 0.72 to 2.68, p = 0.56), minor bleeding (RR 1.83, 95% CI 0.97 to 3.46, p = 0.06), and blood transfusion (RR 0.34, 95% CI 0.10 to 1.15, p = 0.08).
  - *Conclusion:* CDT + SA is associated with significantly lower short-term and long-term all-cause mortality, without any differences in major/minor bleeding, in patients with intermediate-risk PE.

- ***Systemic thrombolysis with newer thrombolytics vs anticoagulation in acute intermediate risk pulmonary embolism: A systematic review and meta-analysis. (BMC Cardiovasc Disord. 2023)***[10]
  - *Population:* Patients with intermediate-risk pulmonary embolism.
  - *Intervention:* Systemic thrombolysis.
  - *Comparator:* Anti-coagulation.
  - *Outcome:* No difference in in-hospital mortality (RR: 0.79; 95% CI: 0.42-1.50) or risk of major bleeding (RR:2.08;95% CI: 0.98-4.42) between systemic thrombolysis and anticoagulation. Systemic thrombolysis was associated with lower risks for vasopressor use (RR: 0.27; 95% CI: 0.11-0.64) and secondary/rescue thrombolysis (RR: 0.25; 95% CI: 0.14-0.45). Systemic thrombolysis was found to have an increased risk of intracranial hemorrhage (RR: 4.55; 95% CI: 1.30-15.9). No difference in mechanical ventilation between the two groups (RR: 0.61; 95% CI: 0.31-1.19).
  - *Conclusion:* Systemic thrombolysis had no difference in in-hospital mortality or overall risk of major bleeding versus anticoagulation however had lower risks for vasopressor use and need for secondary/ rescue thrombolysis but with an increased risk of intracranial hemorrhage.

- ***Ultrasound-assisted catheter-directed thrombolysis versus surgical pulmonary embolectomy for intermediate-high or high-risk pulmonary embolism: A randomized phase II non-inferiority trial. (Eur J Cardiothorac Surg. 2024)***[11]
  - *Population:* Patients with intermediate-high risk acute pulmonary embolism. (n=27)
  - *Intervention:* Ultrasound-assisted thrombolysis (USAT).
  - *Comparator:* Surgical pulmonary embolectomy (SPE).
  - *Outcome:* Trial was prematurely terminated due to slow enrolment. Mean age was 62.6 (SD 12.4) years, 26% were women, and 15% had high-risk PE. Mean change in RV/LV ratio was -0.34 (95% CI -0.50 to -0.18) in the USAT and -0.53 (95% CI -0.68 to -0.38) in the SPE group (mean difference: 0.152; 95% CI 0.032-0.271; Pnon-inferiority = 0.80; Psuperiority = 0.013). Mean change in Qanadli pulmonary occlusion score was -7.23 (95% CI -9.58 to -4.88) in the USAT and -11.36 (95% CI -15.27 to -7.44) in the SPE group (mean difference: 5.00; 95% CI 0.44-9.56, P = 0.032). Clinical and functional outcomes were similar between the 2 groups up to 12 months.

- *Conclusion:* In patients with intermediate-high and high-risk acute PE, USAT was not non-inferior when compared with SPE in reducing RV/LV ratio within the first 72 h. In a post hoc superiority analysis, SPE resulted in greater improvement of RV overload and reduction of thrombus burden.

- ***Treatment of acute pulmonary embolism after catheter-directed thrombolysis with dabigatran vs warfarin: Results of a multicenter randomized RE-SPIRE trial. (J Vasc Surg Venous Lymphat Disord. 2024)[12]***
  - *Population:* Patients with symptomatic high and intermediate to high PE risk after endovascular mechanical thrombus fragmentation procedure with RDT (CDT+RDT). (n=63)
  - *Intervention:* Dabigatran. (n=32)
  - *Comparator:* Warfarin. (n=31)
  - *Outcome:* Mean pulmonary artery pressure at 6-month follow-up after surgery was 24 mm Hg (interquartile range, 20.3-29.25 mm Hg) in the dabigatran group and 23 mm Hg (interquartile range, 20.0-26.3 mm Hg) in the warfarin group. Groups did not differ statistically in the deep vein thrombosis dynamics. Partial recanalization occurred in 52.0% vs 73.1% in the dabigatran and warfarin groups, respectively ($P = .15$). Complete recanalization occurred in 28.0% vs 19.2% in the dabigatran and warfarin groups, respectively ($P = .56$). No difference in major bleeding (0% vs 3.2% in the dabigatran and warfarin groups, respectively; $P = 1.00$). More non-major bleeding events in the warfarin group than in the dabigatran group (16.1% vs 0%, respectively; $p = 0.02$).
  - *Conclusion:* Dabigatran is comparable in effectiveness to warfarin. Dabigatran has greater safety in comparison with warfarin in the occurrence of all cases of bleeding in the postoperative and long-term periods.

- ***Prognostic impact of the e-TAPSE ratio in intermediate-high risk pulmonary embolism patients. (Int J Cardiovasc Imaging. 2024)[13]***
  - *Population:* Patients with acute intermediate-high-risk PE. (n=450)
  - *Intervention:* New index (Age-T index), based on age and the tricuspid annular plane systolic excursion (TAPSE).
  - *Outcome:* Receiver operating characteristic analysis established ≥ 4.9 as the optimal cut-off value for the Age-T index in predicting 30-day mortality (AUC of 0.76 ± 0.1). Sensitivity, specificity, PPV and NPV were 81.2, 85.6, 30.2 and 98.3%, respectively. Multivariate Cox regression analysis showed that an Age-T index ≥ 4.9 predicts 30-day mortality (HR: 3.24, 95% CI: 1.58-4.96, $p < 0.001$) and was also associated with a significantly higher risk of 48-h clinical deterioration (HR: 2.02, 95% CI 1.96-2.08, $p < 0.0001$) in intermediate-high risk PE patients.
  - *Conclusion:* Age-T Index appears as a useful, bed-side and non-invasive prognostic tool to identify intermediate-high risk PE patients at higher risk of death and/or 48-h clinical deterioration.

- ***Comparison of diuretics and fluid expansion in the initial treatment of patients with normotensive acute pulmonary embolism: A systematic review and meta-analysis. (Emerg Med J. 2024)[14]***
  - *Population:* Patients with normotensive acute pulmonary embolism from 4 studies. (n=452)
  - *Intervention:* Diuretics.
  - *Comparator:* Standard care.
  - *Outcome:* Patients receiving diuretics had a significant 24-hour reduction in pro-B-type natriuretic peptide (standard

mean difference of -41.97; 95% CI -65.79 to -18.15), and PASP (standard mean difference of -5.96; 95% CI -8.06 to -3.86). The intervention group had significantly higher creatinine levels (standard mean difference of 7.74; 95% CI 5.04 to 10.45).

- *Conclusion:* Furosemide appears to reduce RV dysfunction in this subset of patients.

- ***Catheter-directed thrombolysis versus thrombectomy for submassive and massive pulmonary embolism: A systematic review and meta-analysis. (Cardiovasc Revasc Med. 2024)***[15]
  - *Population:* Patients with submassive and massive pulmonary embolism from 8 studies. (n=1403)
  - *Intervention:* Catheter-directed thrombolysis.
  - *Comparator:* Thrombectomy.
  - *Outcome:* Compared to thrombectomy, CDT was associated with significantly lower in-hospital mortality (RR 0.62; 95 % CI 0.43-0.89; $p = 0.01$) and similar rates of major bleeding ($p = 0.61$), blood transfusion ($p = 0.41$), stroke ($p = 0.41$), and atrial fibrillation ($p = 0.71$). The hospital and ICU LOS, 30-day readmissions, and degree of RV/LV ratio improvement were similar between the two strategies (all $p > 0.1$). In subgroup analyses, in-hospital mortality was similar between CDT and catheter-based thrombectomy ($p = 0.48$) but lower with CDT compared with surgical thrombectomy ($p = 0.01$).
  - *Conclusion:* CDT was associated with similar in-hospital mortality compared to catheter-based thrombectomy, but lower in-hospital mortality compared to surgical thrombectomy.

- ***Direct Oral Anticoagulants vs Low-Molecular-Weight Heparin and Recurrent VTE in Patients With Cancer: A Randomized Clinical Trial. The CANVAS Trial. (JAMA. 2023)***[16]
  - *Population:* Patients with cancer and venous thromboembolism. (n=671)
  - *Intervention:* Direct oral anticoagulant (DOAC) - Rivaroxaban, apixaban, edoxaban, or dabigatran.
  - *Comparator:* LMWH.
  - *Outcome:* Primary outcome: recurrent VTE rate at 6 months. DOACs were associated with a 6.1% risk of recurrent VTE and LMWH with a 8.8% risk (reduction by 2.7% in favor of DOAC). The difference passed the non-inferiority criteria of the study. Among the major secondary criteria, risk of bleeding 5.2% with DOACs and 5.7% with LMWH. Severe adverse events were noted in 33.8% individuals on DOACs and 35.1% individuals on LMWH.
  - *Conclusion:* DOACs were non-inferior to LMWH for the prevention of recurrent VTE at 6 months.

DISCUSSION

In the past two years, the majority of trials in the field of pulmonary embolism have focused on treatment strategies. There have been a couple of studies that have focused on diagnostic strategies for pulmonary embolism. The increased awareness of venous thromboembolic disease and the ever-increasing availability of non-invasive imaging tests, mainly computed tomography (CT) pulmonary angiography (CTPA), have generated a tendency for clinicians to suspect and initiate a diagnostic workup for PE more frequently than in the past. **The current societal guidelines recommend that in suspected high-risk PE, as indicated by the presence of hemodynamic instability, bedside echocardiography or emergency CTPA (depending on availability and clinical circumstances) is recommended for diagnosis.** Based on the studies in the past two years, there is no suggested change in this recommendation.

In patients without hemodynamic instability, use of validated criteria such as the Wells or Geneva score can be used. **Recent studies have validated a newer score (Pulmonary Embolism Comprehensive Screening Score) to safely rule out pulmonary embolism among suspected patients presenting to the emergency department.**[2] Though this score performed better than the Wells Score with lower failure rates, it needs to be validated in larger cohort studies before a change in the guidelines can be recommended. It is recommended that the diagnostic strategy be based on clinical probability, assessed either by clinical judgment or by a validated prediction rule. In terms of management, risk stratification is an important component. **Initial risk stratification of suspected or confirmed PE, based on the presence of hemodynamic instability, is recommended to identify patients at high risk of early mortality.** In patients without hemodynamic instability, further stratification of patients with acute PE into intermediate- and low-risk categories is recommended. **In patients without hemodynamic instability, the use of clinical prediction rules integrating PE severity and comorbidity, preferably the PESI or sPESI, should be considered for risk assessment in the acute phase of PE**. Based on recent studies, no change in the current guidelines is advocated in terms of risk stratification.

Most of the recent studies have focused on the management of patients presenting with acute intermediate high-risk PE as this has been the gray area for the management of PE. **The major societal guidelines (European Society of Cardiology) have recommended thrombolysis as the first-line treatment strategy in the management of high-risk or hemodynamically unstable patients with pulmonary embolism.** Based on the recent data, there is no change in the guideline recommendations for acute PE. **Meanwhile, patients with low-risk or intermediate low-risk PE could be managed with anticoagulation alone**.

Among those with intermediate-high risk strict monitoring is required followed by prompt thrombolysis in case of hemodynamic instability. In terms of prognostic tools, a newer marker Age-T Index appeared to be a useful, bedside, and non-invasive prognostic tool to identify intermediate-high risk PE patients at higher risk of death and/or 48-h clinical deterioration.[13]

Regarding the management of this group, most of the data from the recent meta-analysis have shown catheter-directed thrombolysis to be a safe and effective option compared to systemic thrombolysis. There might be a change in the upcoming guidelines based on the studies in the recent past in terms of the management of intermediate-high-risk PE patients wherein CDT might be recommended. In terms of comparison between surgical embolectomy and ultrasound-assisted thrombolysis (USAT) in patients with intermediate-high and high-risk acute PE, USAT was not non-inferior.[11]

Guidelines recommend that rescue thrombolytic therapy is recommended for patients with hemodynamic deterioration on anticoagulation treatment. As an alternative to rescue thrombolytic therapy, surgical embolectomy or percutaneous catheter-directed treatment should be considered for patients with hemodynamic deterioration on anticoagulation treatment (Class IIa). Based on the findings of recent studies and meta-analysis, there might be a change from Class IIa to Class I for CDT in PE cases.

The findings of the RE-SPIRE trial showed that in the treatment of acute pulmonary embolism after catheter-directed thrombolysis with dabigatran versus warfarin, dabigatran was safe and effective.[12] **The current guidelines also recommend that when oral anticoagulation is started in a patient with PE who is eligible for a NOAC (apixaban, dabigatran,**

edoxaban, or rivaroxaban), a NOAC is recommended in preference to a VKA. NOACs are not recommended in patients with severe renal impairment, during pregnancy and lactation, and in patients with antiphospholipid antibody syndrome. No change in the guidelines is recommended in this aspect.

Conventionally, LMWH was the recommended agent for both acute management and secondary prophylaxis of cancer associated VTE. NCCN (2024) guidelines now recommend using either DOACs (apixaban, edoxaban, or rivaroxaban) or LMWH (dalteparin or enoxaparin) for non-gastroesophageal cancer. If these agents cannot be used, dabigatran (DOAC), fondaparinux, unfractionated heparin, or warfarin can be used. For gastroesophageal cancer, LMWH is still the preferred anticoagulant.

Another area where recent research has focused is the use of intravenous thrombolytics in cardiac arrest due to confirmed or presumed PE. Results showed an increased chance of return of spontaneous circulation (ROSC) however, survival to hospital discharge or change in bleeding complications did not improve. There is no change in guidelines regarding the same.

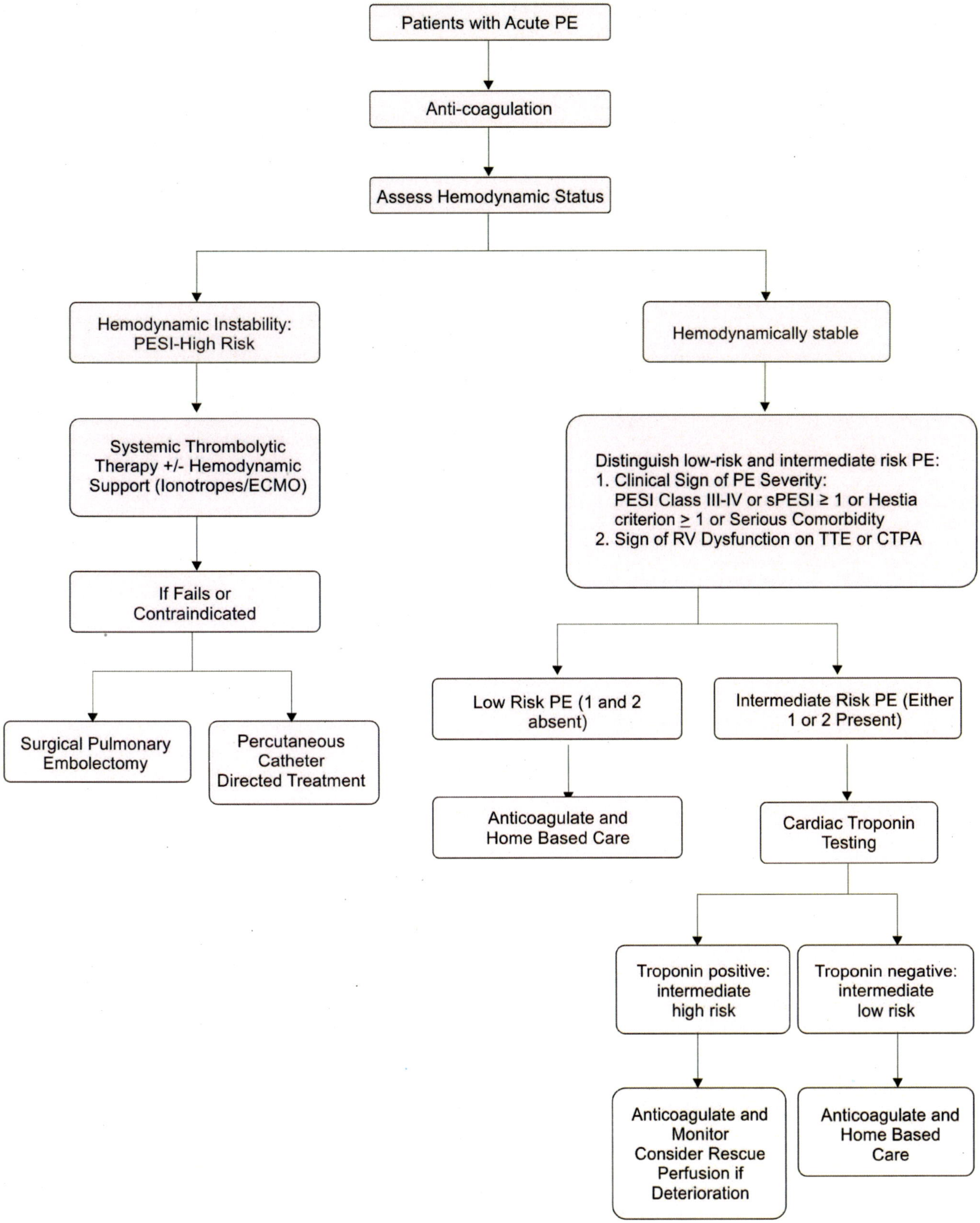

Flowchart: Pulmonary Embolism Management

REFERENCES

1. van Es N, Takada T, Kraaijpoel N, Klok FA, Stals MAM, Büller HR, Courtney DM, Freund Y, Galipienzo J, Le Gal G, Ghanima W, Huisman MV, Kline JA, Moons KGM, Parpia S, Perrier A, Righini M, Robert-Ebadi H, Roy PM, Wells PS, de Wit K, van Smeden M, Geersing GJ. Diagnostic management of acute pulmonary embolism: a prediction model based on a patient data meta-analysis. Eur Heart J. 2023 Aug 22;44(32):3073-3081. doi: 10.1093/eurheartj/ehad417.

2. Tang L, Hu Y, Pan D, Yang C, Tang C, Huang Y, Gu J, Min M, Lin X, Tong C. PECSS: Pulmonary Embolism Comprehensive Screening Score to safely rule out pulmonary embolism among suspected patients presenting to emergency department. BMC Pulm Med. 2023 Aug 7;23(1):287. doi: 10.1186/s12890-023-02580-8.

3. Li M, Li J, Wang X, Hui X, Wang Q, Xie S, Yan P, Tian J, Li J, Xie P, Yang K, Yao L. Oral direct thrombin inhibitors or oral factor Xa inhibitors versus conventional anticoagulants for the treatment of pulmonary embolism. Cochrane Database Syst Rev. 2023 Apr 14;4(4):CD010957. doi: 10.1002/14651858.CD010957.pub3.

4. Planer D, Yanko S, Matok I, Paltiel O, Zmiro R, Rotshild V, Amir O, Elbaz-Greener G, Raccah BH. Catheter-directed thrombolysis compared with systemic thrombolysis and anticoagulation in patients with intermediate- or high-risk pulmonary embolism: systematic review and network meta-analysis. CMAJ. 2023 Jun 19;195(24): E833-E843. doi: 10.1503/cmaj.220960.

5. Li HY, Wang YB, Ren XY, Wang J, Wang HS, Jin YH. Comparative Efficacy and Safety of Thrombolytic Agents for Pulmonary Embolism: A Bayesian Network Meta-Analysis. Pharmacology. 2023;108:111-126. doi: 10.1159/000527668.

6. Feltes J, Popova M, Hussein Y, Pierce A, Yamane D. Thrombolytics in Cardiac Arrest from Pulmonary Embolism: A Systematic Review and Meta Analysis. J Intensive Care Med. 2024 May;39(5):477-483. doi: 10.1177/08850666231214754. Epub 2023 Nov 30. PMID: 38037310.

7. Liu X, Jiao X, Gong X, Nie Q, Li Y, Zhen G, Cheng M, He J, Yuan Y, Yang Y. Prevalence, Risk Factor and Clinical Characteristics of Venous Thrombus Embolism in Patients with Acute Exacerbation of COPD: A Prospective Multicenter Study. Int J Chron Obstruct Pulmon Dis. 2023 May 18;18:907-917. doi: 10.2147/COPD.S410954. PMID: 37223656; PMCID: PMC10202142.

8. Farrokhi M, Khurshid M, Yarmohammadi B, Mangouri A, Alipour-Khabir Y, Alipour-Khabir S, Sargazi Moghadam N, Mosalanejad S, Nourizadeh S, Jafari S, Amani-Beni R, Hosseini-Saryazdi SM, Zarei S, Sanjarian S, Babasafari HA, Shakori Poshteh S, Masoudi N, Zahedpasha R, Kiani M, Jalalifar F, Taheri F. Comparison of outcomes and complications in conventional versus ultrasound-accelerated catheter directed thrombolysis for treatment of pulmonary embolism: A systematic review and meta-analysis. Perfusion. 2023 Sep;38(6):1123-1132. doi: 10.1177/02676591221108811. Epub 2022 Jun 20. PMID: 35724310.

9. Balakrishna AM, Kalathil RAM, Pusapati S, Atreya A, Mehta A, Bansal M, Aggarwal V, Basir MB, Kochar A, Truesdell AG, Vallabhajosyula S. Comparative Outcomes of Catheter-Directed Thrombolysis Plus Systemic Anticoagulation Versus Systemic Anticoagulation Alone in the Management of Intermediate-Risk Pulmonary Embolism in a Systematic Review and Meta-Analysis. Am J Cardiol. 2023 Oct 15;205:249-258. doi: 10.1016/j.amjcard.2023.07.170.

10. Mathew D, Seelam S, Bumrah K, Sherif A, Shrestha U. Systemic thrombolysis with newer thrombolytics vs anticoagulation in acute intermediate risk pulmonary embolism: a systematic review and meta-analysis. BMC Cardiovasc Disord. 2023 Sep 29;23(1):482. doi: 10.1186/s12872-023-03528-w.

11. Stortecky S, Barco S, Windecker S, Heg D, Kadner A, Englberger L, Kucher N. Ultrasound-assisted catheter-directed thrombolysis versus surgical pulmonary embolectomy for intermediate-high or high-risk pulmonary embolism: a randomized phase II non-inferiority trial. Eur J Cardiothorac Surg. 2024 Jul 1;66(1):ezae252. doi: 10.1093/ejcts/ezae252.

12. Gostev AA, Valiev E, Zeidlits GA, Shmidt EA, Osipova OS, Cheban AV, Saaya SB, Barbarash OL, Karpenko AA. Treatment of acute pulmonary embolism after catheter-directed thrombolysis with dabigatran vs warfarin: Results of a multicenter randomized RE-SPIRE trial. J Vasc Surg Venous Lymphat Disord. 2024 Jul;12(4): 101848. doi: 10.1016/j.jvsv.2024.101848.

13. Zuin M, Bilato C, Bongarzoni A, Zonzin P, Casazza F, Roncon L. Prognostic impact of the e-TAPSE ratio in intermediate-high risk pulmonary embolism patients. Int J Cardiovasc Imaging. 2024 Mar;40(3):467-476. doi: 10.1007/s10554-023-03010-w.

14. Febra C, Santos AR, Cabrita I, Bento J, Pacheco J, Mendes M, Isidro M, Batista R, Macedo AMAFM. Comparison of diuretics and fluid expansion in the initial treatment of patients with normotensive acute pulmonary embolism: a systematic review and meta-analysis. Emerg Med J. 2024 Feb 20;41(3):187-192. doi: 10.1136/emermed-2023-213525.

15. Ismayl M, Ismayl A, Hamadi D, Aboeata A, Goldsweig AM. Catheter-directed thrombolysis versus thrombectomy for submassive and massive pulmonary embolism: A systematic review and meta-analysis. Cardiovasc Revasc Med. 2024 Mar;60:43-52. doi: 10.1016/j.carrev.2023.10.002.

16. Schrag D, Uno H, Rosovsky R, Rutherford C, Sanfilippo K, Villano JL, et al. Direct Oral Anticoagulants vs Low-Molecular-Weight Heparin and Recurrent VTE in Patients With Cancer: A Randomized Clinical Trial. JAMA. 2023 Jun 13;329(22):1924-1933.

CHAPTER

8

Pleural Diseases

Authors: Dr. Sourabh Pahuja, Dr. Pradeep Bajad

Reviewer: Dr. Arjun Khanna

INTRODUCTION

Pleural diseases encompass a wide spectrum, spanning from localized to systemic, as well as benign to malignant conditions, affecting various medical specialties. The approach to investigating and managing pleural diseases has evolved, moving from conservative strategies to more interventional methods. Among the most challenging conditions are malignant pleural effusions, empyema, and persistent air leaks. Improved disease understanding, along with enhanced access to radio-diagnostic facilities and advanced surgical techniques, has contributed to better outcomes through timely interventions.

Methodology

A PubMed search was done using the search terms "Pleura" OR "Pleural effusion" OR "Pneumothorax". The search term was limited to Randomised Controlled Trials, Clinical trials, Systematic reviews and Meta-analysis between the 1st August 2023 to 1st August 2024. A total of 357 articles were found and assessed.

Electronic database search: PubMed

Period: 1st August 2023 to 1st August 2024

Search words: "Pleura" OR "Pleural effusion" OR "Pneumothorax"

(n=357)

↓

Articles after screening for relevance

(n=14)

Analysis of Literature

Malignant pleural effusion

- ***Talc slurry versus thoracoscopic talc insufflation for malignant pleural effusion: A systematic review and meta-analysis. (J Bras Pneumol. 2024)[1]***
  - *Population:* Patients with malignant pleural effusion from 8 studies. (n=1163)
  - *Intervention:* Talc Slurry (TS) for pleurodesis. (n=584)
  - *Comparator:* Thoracoscopic talc insufflation (TTI) for pleurodesis. (n=579)
  - *Outcome:* Pleurodesis failure rates were similar between the procedures (OR = 1.07; 95% CI: 0.56-2.06; p = 0.83); and 68% of patients had postoperative complications, which were lower in patients in the talc slurry group. Adverse effects were reported in 86 patients, including empyema (OR = 1.43; 95% CI: 0.36-5.64; p = 0.86), pain (OR = 1.22 (95% CI: 0.67-2.21; p = 0.51), and pneumonia (OR = 1.15; 95% CI: 0.30-4.46; p = 0.86).
  - *Conclusion:* Talc pleurodesis is an effective treatment for MPE.
  - *Critical appraisal:* Study had several limitations. Observational studies were analyzed and different criteria were used for evaluating success and failure rates among the studies. The type of cancer varied among the study populations.

- ***Efficacy and Safety of Indwelling Catheter for Malignant Pleural Effusions Related to Timing of Cancer Therapy: A Systematic Review. (Arch Bronconeumol. 2023)[2]***
  - *Population:* Patients of malignant pleural effusion having data regarding timing of insertion of IPC in relation to systemic chemotherapy (SCT) mentioned (i.e., before, during, or after SCT), from 10 studies. (n=2907, 3066 IPC)
  - *Outcome:* Using SCT while the IPC was in situ decreased overall mortality, increased survival time, and improved quality-adjusted survival. Timing of SCT had no effect on the risk of IPC-related infections (2.85% overall), even in immunocompromised patients with moderate or severe neutropenia (relative risk 0.98 [95%CI: 0.93-1.03] for patients treated with the combination of IPC and SCT).
  - *Conclusion:* Efficacy and safety of IPC for MPE has no relation with IPC insertion timing and ongoing chemotherapy.
  - *Critical appraisal:* Large sample size. Significant heterogeneity in studies was observed.

- ***The impact of outpatient versus inpatient management on health-related quality of life outcomes for patients with malignant pleural effusion: The OPTIMUM randomised clinical trial. (ERJ. 2024)[3]***
  - *Population:* Symptomatic patients with malignant pleural effusion. (n=142)
  - *Intervention:* Indwelling pleural catheters (IPC) with talc pleurodesis. (n=70)
  - *Comparator:* Chest drain with talc pleurodesis. (n=72)
  - *Outcome:* Global health status improved in both groups at day 30 compared with baseline. However, there was no

significant between-group difference at day 30. No significant differences were identified between groups in breathlessness and chest pain scores.

- *Conclusion:* The outpatient pathway using an IPC was not superior to inpatient treatment with a chest drain. Management choice should be based on patient preferences, acceptability of risk, social circumstances, and treatment accessibility.
- *Critical appraisal:* Multicentre, open-label randomized controlled trial. Small sample size. The main limitation is the data attrition for the primary outcome.

Pneumothorax

☞

- ***Efficacy of autologous blood patch injection for pneumothorax rate after CT-guided percutaneous transthoracic lung biopsy: A systematic review and meta-analysis. (J Cardiothoracic Surg. 2024)[4]***
  - *Population:* Iatrogenic Pneumothorax patients after CT guided percutaneous lung biopsy (CT-PTLB) from 10 studies. (n=3874)
  - *Intervention:* Injection of autologous blood patch (ABP) during biopsy needle withdrawal while doing CT guided lung biopsy
  - *Comparator:* Usual care
  - *Outcome:* ABP reduced pneumothorax (incidence: 20.0% vs. 27.9%, OR = 0.67, 95% CI = 0.48–0.66, $P < 0.001$) and chest tube insertion rate (incidence: 4.0% vs. 8.0%, OR = 0.47, 95% CI = 0.34–0.65, $P < 0.001$) after CT-PTLB.
  - *Conclusion:* ABP was effective technique in reducing the pneumothorax and chest tube insertion rate after CT-PTLB.
  - *Critical appraisal:* Publication bias & study heterogeneity was observed. Large sample size.

- ***Evaluation and Management of Primary Spontaneous Pneumothorax in Adolescents and Young Adults: A Systematic Review from the APSA Outcomes & Evidence-Based Practice Committee. (J Ped Surg. 2023)[5]***
  - *Population:* Adolescent and young adult with primary spontaneous pneumothorax from 79 studies.
  - *Outcome:* Evidence based recommendations- (1) Initial management- Initial management of adolescent and young adult primary spontaneous pneumothorax should be guided by symptoms and can include observation, aspiration, or tube thoracostomy, (2) Advanced imaging- There is no evidence of benefit for cross-sectional imaging, (3) Timing of surgery- Patients with ongoing air leak may benefit from early operative intervention within 24-48 h, (4) Operative technique- A video-assisted thoracoscopic surgery (VATS) approach with stapled blebectomy and pleural procedure should be considered., (5) Management of contralateral side- There is no evidence to support prophylactic management of the contralateral side, (6) Management of recurrence- Recurrence after VATS can be treated with repeat VATS with intensification of pleural treatment.
  - *Conclusion:* Further prospective studies are needed to better determine optimal timing of operative intervention, the most effective operation, and management of recurrence after observation, tube thoracostomy, or operative intervention.
  - *Critical appraisal:* Study did not enrol adult population. Heterogeneity was observed.

- ***Score to Predict the Occurrence of Pneumothorax After Computed Tomography-guided percutaneous transthoracic lung biopsy. (J Thorac Imaging. 2023)[6]***
  - o *Population:* Patient undergoing percutaneous transthoracic lung biopsy. (n=498)
  - o *Outcome:* Pneumothorax occurred in 124 patients (24.9%) and required drainage in 34 patients (6.8%). Pneumothorax risk factors were chronic obstructive pulmonary disease (OR [95% CI] 2.28[1.18-4.43]), several passages through the pleura (OR [95% CI] 7.71[1.95-30.48]), an anterior biopsy approach (OR [95% CI] 6.36 3.82-10.58]), skin-to-pleura distance ≤ 30 mm (OR [95% CI] 2.25[1.09-6.65]), and aerial effusion >10 mm (OR [95% CI] 9.27 [5.16-16.65]). A negative score (<73 points) predicted a probability of pneumothorax occurrence of 7.4% and late evacuation of 2.5% (OR [95% CI] respectively 0.18[0.08-0.39] and 0.15[0.04-0.55]) and suggested a reduced length of hospital stay (P=0.009).
  - o *Conclusion:* This predictive score for pneumothorax secondary to PTLB has high prognostic performance and accuracy to direct patients toward outpatient management.
  - o *Critical appraisal:* Observational type of study.

- ***Talc slurry pleurodesis in patients with secondary intractable pneumothorax: A phase 2 study. (Respir Investig. 2024)[7]***
  - o *Population:* Patient with secondary intractable pneumothorax. (n=31)
  - o *Intervention:* Talc slurry instillation via chest tube.
  - o *Outcome:* In 23 out of 28 patients, the drainage tube could be removed within 30 days of talc instillation (82.1 %, 95 % CI = 63.1-93.9), exceeding the threshold of 36.0 % (p < 0.0001). The most common event was pain (11/28 patients, 39.3 %).
  - o *Conclusion:* Talc slurry pleurodesis is effective for intractable secondary pneumothorax.
  - o *Critical appraisal:* Small sample size. Observational study, no comparator group.

☞

- ***Simple aspiration for spontaneous pneumothorax in adults: A systematic review and meta-analysis of randomized controlled trials. (Am J Emerg Med. 2024)[8]***
  - o *Population:* Patient with spontaneous pneumothorax in 10 RCTs. (n=1044)
  - o *Intervention:* Simple aspiration (SA).
  - o *Comparator:* Intercostal tube drainage (ITD).
  - o *Outcome:* Compared with the ITD group, the SA group had a significantly lower initial success rate of the procedure for the management of SP (OR 0.63, 95% CI [0.47-0.86]; P = 0.004). No significant difference in complications between the SA and ITD groups was found.
  - o *Conclusion:* Use of SA decreased the initial success rate but also decreased the duration of hospitalization and the need for operation compared with ITD. The incidence of adverse events was similar in both methods.
  - o *Critical appraisal:* Large sample size and RCT were enrolled.

- ***Bronchial Valves for Persistent Air Leak: A Systematic Review and Meta-analysis. (J Bronchology Interv Pulmonol. 2024)[9]***
  - *Population:* Patient with persistent air leak undergoing bronchial valve placement from 28 observational studies. (n=2472)
  - *Outcome:* The pooled success rate of bronchial valves in PAL was 82% (95% confidence intervals, 75 to 88; 95% prediction intervals, 64 to 92). We found a higher success rate in studies using intrabronchial valves versus endobronchial valves (84% vs. 72%) and in studies with more than 50 subjects (93% vs. 77%). However, none of the factors influenced the success rate of multivariable meta-regression. The overall complication rate was 9.1% (48/527). Granulation tissue was the most common complication reported followed by valve migration or expectoration and hypoxemia.
  - *Conclusion:* Bronchial valves are an effective and safe option for treating PAL.
  - *Critical appraisal:* Large sample size but only observational data. Heterogeneity was observed.

Intrapleural fibrinolysis

☞

- ***Surgery versus intrapleural fibrinolysis for management of complicated pleural infections: A systematic review and meta-analysis. (Respir Res. 2024)[10]***
  - *Population:* Complicated pleural infection. (n=486)
  - *Intervention:* Surgical management. (n=266)
  - *Comparator:* Intercostal drain insertion with intrapleural fibrinolysis. (n=220)
  - *Outcome:* Surgical management of complicated pleural infections was more likely to be successful than intrapleural fibrinolysis (RR 1.18; [95% CI] 1.02, 1.38) and statistically significant shorter hospital length of stay (MD: 3.85; [95% CI] 1.09, 6.62) and chest drain duration (MD: 3.42; [95% CI] 1.36, 5.48). There was no observed difference between in-hospital mortality (RR: 1.00; [95% CI] 0.99, 1.02).
  - *Conclusion:* Surgical management of complicated pleural infections results in an increased likelihood of treatment success, shorter chest drain duration, and hospital length of stay in the adult population compared with intrapleural fibrinolysis.
  - *Critical appraisal:* Significant heterogeneity & selection bias.

📖

- ***Early Video-assisted Thoracoscopic Surgery or Intrapleural Enzyme Therapy in Pleural Infection: A Feasibility Randomized Controlled Trial. The Third Multicentre Intrapleural Sepsis Trial—MIST-3. (Am J Respir Crit Care Med. 2023)[11]***
  - *Population:* Patient with pleural infection. (n=60)
  - *Intervention:*

    1) Intrapleural enzyme therapy IET. (n=19)

    2) Surgical option VATS. (n=20)
  - *Comparator:* Standard of care. (n=21)

- *Outcome:* Median times to intervention were 1.0 and 3.5 days in the IET and surgery groups, respectively (P = 0.02). Despite the difference in time to intervention, length of stay (from randomization to discharge) was similar in both intervention arms (7 d) compared with standard care (10 d) (P = 0.70). There were no significant intergroup differences in 2-month readmission and further intervention.
- *Conclusion:* IET therapy showed its benefit over early surgery. Future large sample size is required to obtain reproducible results.

☞

- ***Urokinase in the treatment of tuberculous pleurisy: A systematic review and meta-analysis. (BMC Infec Dis. 2024)***[12]
  - *Population:* Patient with tubercular pleural effusion from 29 RCTs. (n=2903)
  - *Intervention:* Intrapleural urokinase instillation. (n=1459)
  - *Outcome:* The meta-analysis results showed that, based on routine anti-tuberculosis, comparison between the treatment group treated with urokinase and the control group treated with antituberculosis alone, the time of pleural effusion absorption [MD-5.82, $P<0.00001$] and the residual pleural thickness [MD-1.31, $P<0.00001$] and pleural effusion drainage volume [MD 822.81, $P<0.00001$] were significantly different.
  - *Conclusion:* The clinical effect of urokinase is better than that of anti-tuberculous therapy alone: it can increase total pleural effusion, decrease residual pleural thickness, improve the pulmonary function, and shorten the time of pleural effusion absorption.
  - *Critical appraisal:* Large sample size and only RCTs were enrolled. Study heterogeneity was seen.

- ***Intrapleural Thrombolytics for Parapneumonic Effusion: A Network Meta-Analysis. (Curr Rev Clin Exp Pharmacol. 2024)***[13]
  - *Population:* Patients with complicated parapneumonic effusion from 16 studies.
  - *Intervention:* Intrapleural urokinase instillation.
  - *Outcome:* Compared to normal saline, a significantly less proportion of patients was referred for surgical intervention with streptokinase (0.4, 0.2 to 0.8), urokinase (0.4, 0.2 to 0.8), alteplase (0.3, 0.1 to 0.7), and alteplase + DNase (0.2, 0.1 to 0.7). Only streptokinase was observed with an increased risk of serious adverse events compared to normal saline (2.8, 1.1 to 7.1) and alteplase (6.7, 1.1 to 39.9).
  - *Conclusion:* Alteplase + DNase is likely to outperform other intrapleural therapies. streptokinase is not preferred due to the increased risk of serious adverse events.

Pleural biopsy

☞

- ***Image-Assisted Pleural Needle Biopsy or Medical Thoracoscopy: Which Method for which Patient? A Randomized Controlled Trial. (Chest. 2024)***[14]
  - *Population:* Patients with undiagnosed exudative pleural effusion. (n=228)
  - *Intervention:* Image-guided or assisted pleural biopsy. (IA-ANPB)
  - *Comparator:* Medical thoracoscopy guided pleural biopsy. (MT arm)

- *Outcome:* Patients were divided into two groups based on CT scan findings. Group 1 included patients with pleural effusion only. Group 2 included patients with pleural thickening or lesions in addition to pleural effusion. The false-negative rate was 30.3% for the IA-ANPB arm and 3.1% for the MT arm in group 1. The same rates were 11.9% for IA-ANPB and 4.7% for MT in group 2. The rate of complications between the two biopsy methods was not different (8.5% and 15.8%, respectively; P = .107).
- *Conclusion:* MT showed a high diagnostic success in all patients with pleural fluid. In patients with pleural thickening or lesion in addition to pleural effusion, image assisted pleural biopsy has same efficacy as MT.

DISCUSSION

Malignant pleural effusion (MPE)

Malignant pleural effusion (MPE) is the presence of malignant cells in pleural fluid or pleural biopsy specimens. **MPEs are primarily caused by lung cancer in men and breast cancer in women, accounting for 50–65% of all cases.**[15] The incidence of MPE has been reported to be up to 40-50% in lung cancer patients over the entire disease course.[16] While some patients may initially be asymptomatic, most eventually experience dyspnea at rest. MPE responds to chemotherapy in most cases. Treatment of MPE aims to relieve dyspnea through minimally invasive, accurate, and definitive procedures to ensure the best quality of life, minimal morbidity, and increased hospital-free days.

Role of thoracic Ultrasonography

American Thoracic Society (ATS) guidelines for MPE recommend using thoracic ultrasound to guide pleural interventions.[17] Available evidence suggests that thoracic ultrasonography-guided care for pleurodesis in patients with MPE results in shorter hospital stays than X-ray chest, which is a standard of care recommended by the British Thoracic Society guidelines for pleurodesis.[18]

Pleurodesis in Malignant pleural effusion

Pleurodesis is done as an in-patient procedure to control symptomatic recurrent malignant pleural effusion (MPE) and has a success rate of 75–80%. Management options for MPEs include thoracentesis, mechanical or chemical pleurodesis, and drainage with indwelling pleural catheters (IPCs), each method having specific advantages and disadvantages. The latest data suggest that talc slurry or talc poudrage may be offered to patients with MPE to control fluid and reduce the need for repeated procedures. The efficacy of this modality is equivalent to other pleurodesis modalities (mechanical, surgical and IPC). **BTS pleural disease guidelines have given a similar recommendation regarding talc pleurodesis (poudrage or slurry).[18]** The latest meta-analysis has shown equivalent efficacy and safety for both procedures if we compare talc slurry with thoracoscopic talc insufflation.[1]

Pain and fever is the most common complication after talc pleurodesis. The incidence of pneumonia, pneumothorax, prolonged leakage, prolonged drainage and thromboembolism is moderate. A very low likelihood of the patient developing complications like ARDS, re-expansion pulmonary edema and respiratory failure. **Like talc pleurodesis, iodopovidone is an effective agent for pleurodesis in the management of MPE, it is also safe and cheap.**

Tunnelled, indwelling pleural catheters (IPCs) have been demonstrated to manage pleural effusions, especially malignant pleural effusions effectively. IPC is a promising intervention for symptomatic MPE patients. The efficacy and safety of IPC for MPE do not vary depending on the IPC insertion timing (before, during, or after chemotherapy). **The timing of chemotherapy does not affect the risk of IPC-related infections (2.85% overall), even in immunocompromised patients with moderate or severe neutropenia. Thus, early IPC insertion is preferable in symptomatic patients.**[2] **IPC can be used as a pleurodesis modality in patients with malignant pleural effusion. However, the exact time it will take for pleurodesis is unknown,**

and IPC can be removed for only a subset of patients. Pleurodesis with IPC or ICD was compared in the latest OPTIMUM trial and reported to have similar efficacy in terms of the patient's symptom score.[3]

Pneumothorax

Management of primary spontaneous pneumothorax has shifted from interventional to conservative as far as small pneumothorax and asymptomatic cases are concerned. **The latest BTS pleural disease guidelines also recommend that conservative management be considered to treat minimally symptomatic (i.e., no significant pain or breathlessness and no physiological compromise) or asymptomatic primary spontaneous pneumothorax in adults regardless of size.**[18]

In the recent meta-analysis, the use of simple aspiration has been shown to decrease the initial success rate, but at the same time, this modality decreases the duration of hospitalization.[8]

Regarding ambulatory management of pneumothorax, guidelines state that the initial treatment of primary spontaneous pneumothorax in adults with good support can be considered in centres with available expertise and follow-up facilities. However, in patients with secondary spontaneous pneumothorax (SSP), the evidence is still insufficient to establish this as a modality of choice, especially the evidence against the use of pleural vents in SSP.

Based on a systemic review, the American Pediatric Surgical Association recommends that patients with primary spontaneous pneumothorax with ongoing air leaks may benefit from early operative intervention within 24–48 hours. A video-assisted thoracoscopic surgery (VATS) approach with stapled blebectomy and pleural procedure should be considered.[5] Talc slurry pleurodesis can be considered in intractable secondary pneumothorax with minor side effects.[7] The bronchial valve is also an effective and safe option for treating persistent air leaks.[9]

Pleural infection

Adequate drainage of infected fluid from the pleural space to achieve source control is a cornerstone of pleural infection management. **Guidelines for BTS pleural disease recommend that initial drainage of pleural infection should be undertaken using a small-bore chest tube.**[18] Small-scale data suggest that therapeutic thoracentesis can also be explored as a potential treatment option for drainage in the case of patients with pleural infection compared to chest tube insertion.[19]

Practice is shifting towards early intervention in form of surgery or intrapleural fibrinolysis. Regarding the role of intrapleural fibrinolytics in the management of pleural infection, data has shown a lot of heterogeneity. The latest evidence suggests that dual intrapleural fibrinolytic and DNase are better than individual agents alone and have some benefits regarding a lesser surgery requirement. **Even the latest guidelines indicate that a combination of tissue plasminogen activator (tPA) and DNAse should be considered to treat pleural infection, where initial chest tube drainage has ceased and leaves a residual pleural collection.**[18]

Recent study has also reported the clinical efficacy of urokinase, along with anti-tuberculous therapy (ATT) in tubercular pleural effusion. **Early urokinase with ATT can decrease residual pleural thickness, improve pulmonary function, and shorten the time of pleural effusion absorption.**[12]

Surgical management of complicated pleural infections increases the likelihood of treatment success, shorter chest drain duration, and hospital length of stay in the adult population compared with intrapleural fibrinolysis.[10] **BTS guidelines recommend surgery if there is no good response to ICD & early antibiotic therapy over intrapleural enzyme therapy if the patient is a surgical candidate. In the latest MIST–3 trials, the first RCT on early intrapleural enzyme therapy (tPA + DNase) versus early surgery in pleural infection showed no significant intergroup differences in 2-month readmission and further intervention.**[11] More extensive sample-size studies are required to assess the optimal initial management of pleural infection.

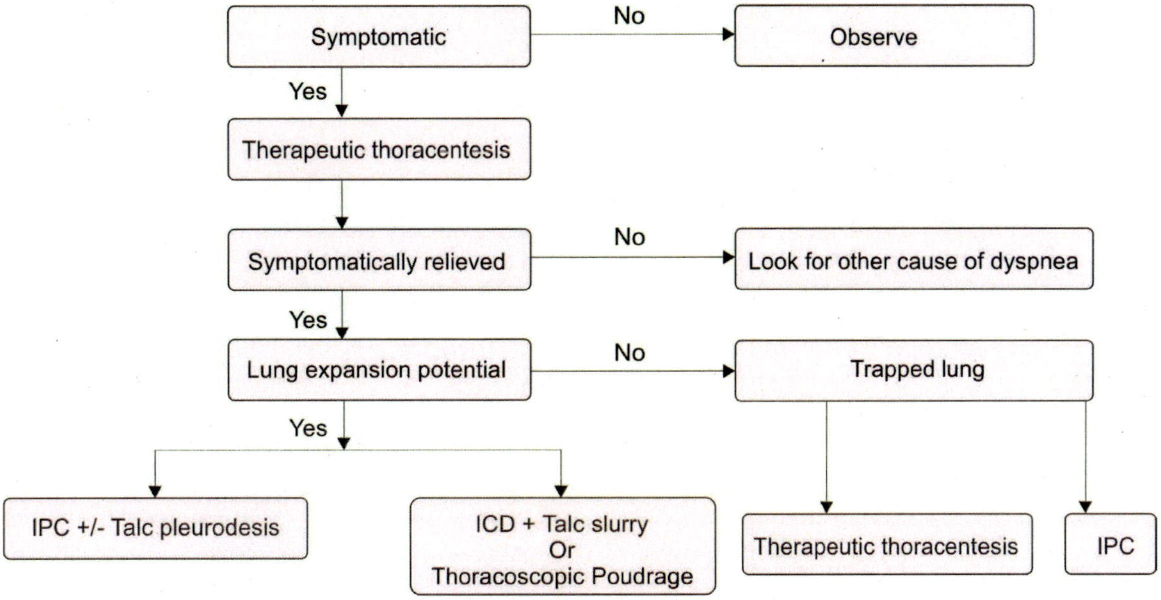

USG thorax can be used to assess the timing of removal of ICD tube
Iodopovidone can be used as an agent for chemical pleurodesis

Flowchart 1: Management of Malignant Pleural Effusion (MPE)

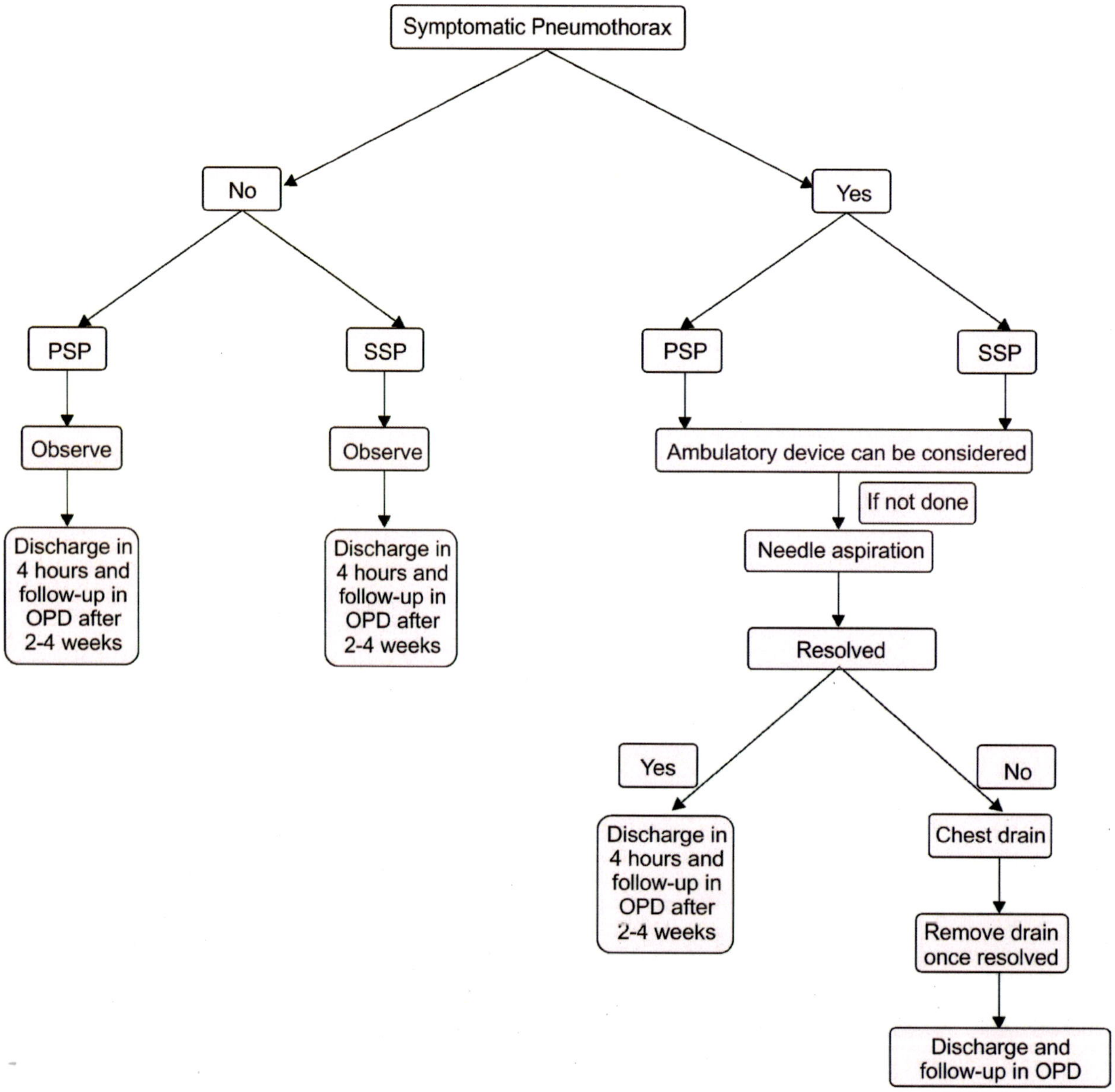

Note :

a) Short Duration observation is required, preferably in hospital.

b) Consider ICD and pleurodesis in SSP (even in the first episode).

c) Ambulatory management is conditional in SSP.

d) Hormonal therapy should be considered post surgery in catamenial pneumothorax.

PSP: Primary spontaneous Pneumothorax, SSP: Secondary spontaneous pneumothorax.

Flowchart 2: Management of Pneumothorax

REFERENCES

1. Rodrigues ALSO, Souza MEC, Moraes FCA, Lima DP, Carvalho RLC. Talc slurry versus thoracoscopic talc insufflation for malignant pleural effusion: a systematic review and meta-analysis. J Bras Pneumol. 2024 Aug 19;50(3).

2. Porcel JM, Cordovilla R, Tazi-Mezalek R, Barrios-Barreto D, Pérez-Pallarés J, Novais E Bastos H, et al. Efficacy and Safety of Indwelling Catheter for Malignant Pleural Effusions Related to Timing of Cancer Therapy: A Systematic Review. Arch Bronconeumol. 2023 Sep;59(9):566-574. English, Spanish. 37429748.

3. Sivakumar P, Fitzgerald DB, Ip H, Rao D, West A, Noorzad F, et al. The impact of outpatient *versus* inpatient management on health-related quality of life outcomes for patients with malignant pleural effusion: the OPTIMUM randomised clinical trial. Eur Respir J. 2024 Feb 8;63(2):2201215.

4. Chen X, Bian Y, Li H, Li S, Shi Z, Zhao Y, et al. Efficacy of autologous blood patch injection for pneumothorax rate after CT-guided percutaneous transthoracic lung biopsy: a systematic review and meta-analysis. J Cardiothorac Surg. 2024 Jun 14;19(1): 332.

5. Speck KE, Kulaylat AN, Baerg JE, Acker SN, Baird R, Beres AL, et al. APSA Outcomes and Evidence Based Practice Committee. Evaluation and Management of Primary Spontaneous Pneumothorax in Adolescents and Young Adults: A Systematic Review From the APSA Outcomes & Evidence-Based Practice Committee. J Pediatr Surg. 2023 Oct;58(10):1873-85.

6. Lamfichekh Y, Lafay V, Hamam J, Guillien A, Puyraveau M, Behr J, et al. Score to Predict the Occurrence of Pneumothorax After Computed Tomography-guided Percutaneous Transthoracic Lung Biopsy. J Thorac Imaging. 2023 Sep 1;38(5):315-24.

7. Watanabe T, Fukai I, Okuda K, Moriyama S, Haneda H, Kawano O, et al. Talc pleurodesis for secondary pneumothorax in elderly patients with persistent air leak. J Thorac Dis. 2019 Jan;11(1):171-176.

8. Cheng J, Ma A, Liang G. Simple aspiration for spontaneous pneumothorax in adults: A systematic review and meta-analysis of randomized controlled trials. Am J Emerg Med. 2024 Jun;80:99-106.

9. Damaraju V, Sehgal IS, Muthu V, Prasad KT, Dhooria S, Aggarwal AN, Agarwal R. Bronchial Valves for Persistent Air Leak: A Systematic Review and Meta-analysis. J Bronchology Interv Pulmonol. 2024 May 8;31(3):e0964.

10. Chang J, Indja B, King J, Chan S, Flynn CD. Surgery versus intrapleural fibrinolysis for management of complicated pleural infections: a systematic review and meta-analysis. Respir Res. 2024 Aug 24;25(1):323.

11. Bedawi EO, Stavroulias D, Hedley E, Blyth KG, Kirk A, De Fonseka D, et al. Early Video-assisted Thoracoscopic Surgery or Intrapleural Enzyme Therapy in Pleural Infection: A Feasibility Randomized Controlled Trial. The Third Multicenter Intrapleural Sepsis Trial-MIST-3. Am J Respir Crit Care Med. 2023 Dec 15;208(12):1305-15.

12. Jing W, Weng R, Lin P, Luo M. Urokinase in the treatment of tuberculous pleurisy: a systematic review and meta-analysis. BMC Infect Dis. 2024 Feb 24;24(1):258.

13. Altmann ES, Crossingham I, Wilson S, Davies HR. Intra-pleural fibrinolytic therapy versus placebo, or a different fibrinolytic agent, in the treatment of adult parapneumonic effusions and empyema. Cochrane Database Syst Rev. 2019 Oct 30;2019(10):CD002312.

14. Metintas M, Ak G, Yildirim H, Dundar E, Aydin N, Erginel S, et al. Image-Assisted Pleural Needle Biopsy or Medical Thoracoscopy: Which Method for Which Patient? A Randomýzed Controlled Trial. Chest. 2024 Aug;166(2):405-412.

15. Mongardon N, Pinton-Gonnet C, Szekely B, et al. Assessment of chronic pain after thoracotomy: a 1-year prevalence study. Clin J Pain 2011; **27**: 677–681.

16. Porcel JM, Gasol A, Bielsa S, Civit C, Light RW, Salud A. Clinical features and survival of lung cancer patients with pleural effusions. Respirology. 2015 May;20(4):654-9. doi: 10.1111/resp.12496. Epub 2015 Feb 23. PMID: 25706291.

17. Feller-Kopman DJ, Reddy CB, DeCamp MM, Diekemper RL, Gould MK, Henry T, Iyer NP, Lee YCG, Lewis SZ, Maskell NA, Rahman NM, Sterman DH, Wahidi MM, Balekian AA. Management of Malignant Pleural Effusions. An Official ATS/STS/STR Clinical Practice Guideline. Am J Respir Crit Care Med. 2018 Oct 1;198(7):839-849. doi: 10.1164/rccm.201807-1415ST. PMID: 30272503.

18. Roberts ME, Rahman NM, Maskell NA, Bibby AC, Blyth KG, Corcoran JP, et al. British Thoracic Society Guideline for pleural disease. Thorax. 2023 Jul;78 (3): 1–42.

19. Arnold DT, Tucker E, Morley A, Milne A, Stadon L, Patole S, Nava GW, Walker SP, Maskell NA. A feasibility randomised trial comparing therapeutic thoracentesis to chest tube insertion for the management of pleural infection: results from the ACTion trial. BMC Pulm Med. 2022 Aug 30;22(1):330. doi: 10.1186/s12890-022-02126-4. PMID: 36042460; PMCID: PMC9425800.

CHAPTER 9

Pulmonary Infections

Authors: Dr. Nipun Malhotra, Dr. Manu Madan, Dr. Rajnish Kaushik

Reviewer: Dr. Vidushi Rathi

INTRODUCTION

Pulmonary infections are a leading cause of morbidity and mortality, with the lung parenchyma being the most affected site, followed by other sites such as the pleura, chest wall, and lymph nodes. Pulmonary infections can be severe/life-threatening in immunocompromised hosts and the elderly. General principles in the management of these patients include imaging (computed tomography), an attempt to confirm the diagnosis by obtaining samples for microbiological diagnosis (Induced sputum, Bronchoalveolar lavage [BAL], Serological tests, Blood cultures, etc.), and initiation of appropriate medications according to clinical suspicion and de-escalation once the diagnosis is achieved.

Methodology

A PubMed search was carried out with search terms {"Aspergillosis" OR "Pneumocystis jirovecii pneumonia" OR 'Pulmonary nocardiosis" OR 'Pulmonary mucormycosis" OR 'Influenza' OR 'Community-acquired pneumonia"} Articles between the span of 1st August 2023 to 1st August 2024 were reviewed, and finally 21 were included.

Electronic database search: PubMed

Period: 1st August 2023 to 1st August 2024

Search words: {"Aspergillosis" OR "Pneumocystis jirovecii pneumonia" OR 'Pulmonary nocardiosis" OR 'Pulmonary mucormycosis" OR 'Influenza' OR 'Community acquired pneumonia"}

(n=5,494)

↓

Articles included in the review

(n=12)

Analysis of Literature

Influenza

☞

- ***Evaluation of Oseltamivir Used to Prevent Hospitalization in Outpatients With Influenza: A Systematic Review and Meta-Analysis. (JAMA Int Med. 2024)[1]***
  - o *Population:* Adults with influenza infection from 15 studies. (n=6,166)
  - o *Intervention:* Oseltamivir therapy. (n=3,373)
  - o *Comparator:* Not prescribed oseltamivir. (n=2,793)
  - o *Outcome:* Oseltamivir was also not associated with reduced hospitalization in older populations (mean age $\geq$65 years) or in patients considered at greater risk of hospitalization. Within the safety population, oseltamivir was associated with increased nausea and vomiting but not serious adverse events.
  - o *Conclusion:* Oseltamivir was not associated with a reduced risk of hospitalization but was associated with increased gastrointestinal adverse events.

☞

- ***Comparison of clinical efficacy and safety of baloxavir marboxil versus oseltamivir as the treatment for influenza virus infections: A systematic review and meta-analysis. (J Infect Chemother. 2023)[2]***
  - o *Population:* Patients admitted with influenza infection from two randomized trials and two retrospective studies. (n=2498)
  - o *Intervention:* Baloxavir marboxil.
  - o *Comparator:* Osetlamivir.
  - o *Outcome:* Among inpatients, BXM reduced mortality ($p = 0.06$) and significantly shortened hospitalization period ($p = 0.01$) compared to oseltamivir.
  - o *Conclusion:* BXM was safer and more effective in patients than oseltamivir.

Community-acquired pneumonia

Antibiotics

☞

- ***Biomarker guided antibiotic stewardship in community acquired pneumonia: A randomized controlled trial. (PLoS One. 2024)[3]***

- *Population:* Community-acquired pneumonia patients admitted in non-ICU wards. (n=468)
- *Intervention:*
  - Procalcitonin algorithm-based treatment (below 0.25 μg/L **or** a reduction to below 10% of the initial value for PCT) antibiotics were stopped. (n=156)
  - C-reactive protein algorithm-based treatment (below 100 mg/L **and** a reduction to below 50% of the initial value for CRP) antibiotics were stopped. (n=156)
- *Comparator:* Standard of care. (n=156)
- *Outcome:* The median days on antibiotics (IQR) was 7 (IQR 7-10) in the control group, 4 (IQR 3-7) in the CRP group (compared to standard care; $p < 0.001$), and 5.5 (IQR 3-9) in the PCT group ($p < 0.001$). The hazard ratio for a new prescription in patients in the PCT group compared to standard care 1.63 (CI 0.97-2.75; $p = 0.06$). No difference in time to clinical stability or length of stay was found.
- *Conclusion:* The Strategy of CRP-guided and PCT-guided treatment algorithms reduced the number of days on antibiotics in the first 30 days after hospital admission in non-ICU wards for CAP.

- ***A multicentre, randomised, double-blind, double-dummy, parallel-controlled, phase 3 clinical trial assessing the efficacy and safety of intravenous nemonoxacin malate vs. levofloxacin for community-acquired pneumonia in adult patients. (Int J Microb Agents. 2024)[4]***
  - *Population:* Community-acquired pneumonia patients. (n=525)
  - *Intervention:* Nemonoxacin 500 mg I.V. for 7-14 days. (n=349)
  - *Comparator:* Levofloxacin 500 mg I.V. for 7-14 days. (n=176)
  - *Outcome:* The clinical cure rate was 91.8% for nemonoxacin and 85.7% for levofloxacin in the modified intention to treat population ($P > 0.05$). The clinical efficacy of nemonoxacin was non-inferior to levofloxacin for treatment of CAP.
  - *Conclusion:* Nemonoxacin 500 mg IV once daily for 7-14 days is effective and safe and non-inferior to levofloxacin for treating CAP in adult patients.

- ***Clarithromycin for early anti-inflammatory responses in community-acquired pneumonia in Greece (ACCESS): A randomised, double-blind, placebo-controlled trial. (Lancet Respir Med. 2024)[5]***
  - *Population:* Community-acquired pneumonia patients. (n=278)
  - *Intervention:* Standard of care with clarithromycin. (n=139)
  - *Comparator:* Standard of care with placebo. (n=139)
  - *Outcome:* The primary composite endpoint required that patients fulfilled both of the following conditions after 72 hours (1) decrease in respiratory symptom severity score of 50% or more as an indicator of early clinical response and (2) decrease in SOFA score of at least 30% or favourable procalcitonin kinetics (defined as ≥80% decrease from baseline or procalcitonin <0·25 ng/mL), or both, as an indicator of early inflammatory response. The primary endpoint was met in 91 (68%) patients in the clarithromycin group and 51 (38%) patients in the placebo group (odds ratio [OR] 3·40 p<0·0001).
  - *Conclusion:* Adding clarithromycin to the standard of care enhances early clinical response and attenuates the inflammatory burden of community-acquired pneumonia.

Steroids

- ***Corticosteroids in Community-Acquired Bacterial Pneumonia: A Systematic Review, Pairwise and Dose-Response Meta-Analysis. (J Gen Intern Med. 2023)***[6]
  - o *Population:* Community-acquired pneumonia patients from 18 studies. (n=4661)
  - o *Intervention:* Corticosteroids.
  - o *Comparator:* Placebo.
  - o *Outcome:* Corticosteroids probably reduce the risk of requiring invasive mechanical ventilation, probably reduce intensive care unit (ICU) admission, reduce the duration of hospitalization and ICU stay. Corticosteroids may increase the risk of hyperglycemia.
  - o *Conclusion:* Corticosteroids reduce mortality in patients with more severe CAP, the need for invasive mechanical ventilation, and ICU admission.

☞

- ***Impact of different corticosteroids on severe community-acquired pneumonia: A systematic review and meta-analysis. (BMJ Open Respir Res. 2024)***[7]
  - o *Population:* Community-acquired pneumonia patients from 10 RCTs. (n=1962)
  - o *Intervention:* Corticosteroids.
  - o *Comparator:* Placebo.
  - o *Outcome:* Corticosteroids were associated with a lower rate of all-cause mortality (risk ratio (RR), 0.70 (95% CI 0.54 to 0.90)). Hydrocortisone was associated with an approximately 50% lower mortality risk (RR, 0.48 (95% CI 0.32 to 0.72)). However, dexamethasone, methylprednisolone or prednisolone were not associated with an improvement in mortality.
  - o *Conclusion:* The use of hydrocortisone, but not other types of corticosteroids, was associated with a reduction in mortality and improvement in pneumonia outcomes.

- ***Adjunct prednisone in community-acquired pneumonia: 180-day outcome of a multicentre, double-blind, randomized, placebo-controlled trial. (BMC Pulm Med. 2023)***[8]
  - o *Population:* Community-acquired pneumonia patients. (n=727)
  - o *Intervention:* Prednisolone 50 mg for 7 days. (n=361)
  - o *Comparator:* Placebo. (n=366)
  - o *Outcome:* There was no difference between groups with respect to time to death from any cause. Compared to placebo, corticosteroid-treated patients had significantly higher risks for recurrent pneumonia, (OR 2.57, p = 0.007), secondary infections (OR 1.94, p = 0.003) and new insulin dependence (OR 8.73, p = 0.041).
  - o *Conclusion:* In patients with community-acquired pneumonia, corticosteroid use was associated with an increased risk for recurrent pneumonia, secondary infections and new insulin dependence at 180 days.

- ***Hydrocortisone plus fludrocortisone for community acquired pneumonia-related septic shock: A subgroup analysis of the APROCCHSS phase 3 randomised trial. (Lancet respiratory medicine. 2024)[9]***
    - o *Population:* A pre-specified subgroup analysis of patient data in the APROCCHSS trial. All participants had septic shock. A subset of these individuals had community acquired pneumonia (CAP) while the rest did not. There were two sub-populations analyzed: CAP (n=562) and non-CAP (n=648). Both sub-populations were analyzed for intervention and comparator.
    - o *Intervention:* Intravenous hydrocortisone (50 mg every 6 hours) along with oral fludrocortisone (50 mcg) via nasogastric tube (CAP; n=361 and non-CAP; n=319).
    - o *Comparator:* Placebo (CAP; n=279 and non-CAP; n=329).
    - o *Outcome:* In the CAP sub-population, there were fewer deaths at day 90 in the hydrocortisone and fludrocortisone group (39%) compared to the placebo group (51%) with an odd ratio of 0.60 (95% confidence interval 0.70 to 1.29) favoring the intervention. However, in the non-CAP group, there were 46% deaths at day 90 in the intervention group compared to 48% in the placebo group.
    - o *Conclusion:* This pre-specified analysis of the APROCCHSS participants revealed that compared to placebo, hydrocortisone along with fludrocortisone can reduce mortality in CAP with septic shock. This benefit was not observed in septic shock due to non-CAP causes.

Diagnostic methods in pneumonia

- ***Evaluation of point-of-care multiplex polymerase chain reaction in guiding antibiotic treatment of patients acutely admitted with suspected community-acquired pneumonia in Denmark: A multicentre randomised controlled trial. (PLoS Med. 2023)[10]***
    - o *Population:* Community-acquired pneumonia patients. (n=294)
    - o *Intervention:* Point of care-Multiplex PCR testing (POC-PCR) (n=148).
    - o *Comparator:* Standard of Care (SCO) (n=146).
    - o *Outcome:* No difference in the primary outcome of prescriptions of no or narrow-spectrum antibiotics at 4-h after admission for the POC-PCR. Secondary outcomes showed that prescriptions were significantly more targeted at 4-h and more adequate at 48-h and on day 5 in the POC-PCR group. There was no difference between the groups concerning intensive care unit (ICU) admissions, readmission within 30 days, length of stay (LOS) IRR 0.82; 30-day mortality, and in-hospital mortality.
    - o *Conclusion:* POC-PCR may result in a more targeted and adequate use of antibiotics.

- ***Effect of Metagenomic Next-Generation Sequencing on Clinical Outcomes of Patients With Severe Community-Acquired Pneumonia in the ICU. A Multicenter, Randomized Controlled Trial. (Chest. 2024)[11]***
    - o *Population:* BAL fluid analysis of Severe community-acquired pneumonia patients. (n=349)
    - o *Intervention:* Metagenomic next generation sequencing (mNGS) along with conventional microbiological testing (the mNGS group) (n=179).
    - o *Comparator:* Conventional microbiological testing (CMT group) (n=170).

- *Outcome:* The time to clinical improvement was shorter with mNGS (10 days) compared to CMT alone (13 days). A higher proportion of patients had clinical improvement in the mNGS group (62%) compared to CMT alone (46.5%).
- *Conclusion:* Metagenomic next generation sequencing combined with conventional microbiological testing is associated with a shorter time to clinical improvement.
- *Critical appraisal:* The improvement in clinical status was an ordinal scale with a six-point distribution. Metagenomic NGS is an expensive technique and cost-benefit ratio is unknown. Additionally, mortality benefit was also not evaluated.

- ***Diagnostic Stewardship in Community-Acquired Pneumonia With Syndromic Molecular Testing. A Randomized Clinical Trial. (JAMA. 2024)***[12]
  - *Population:* Community-acquired pneumonia patients in the emergency department (ED) at a single center. (n=374)
  - *Intervention:* Rapid PCR testing by BioFire FilmArray Pneumonia plus panel (bioMérieux) (n=187).
  - *Comparator:* Standard of care. (n=187)
  - *Outcome:* Two primary outcomes: 1. A greater number of patients undergoing rapid PCR testing (35.3%) received pathogen-directed antimicrobials compared to those receiving standard of care (13.4%). This was an absolute reduction of 21.9 %-points. 2. The time to provide pathogen-directed antimicrobials was 34.5 hours in the rapid PCR arm compared to 43.8 hours in the standard-of-care arm.
  - *Conclusion:* Rapid PCR testing in CAP led to sooner and more targeted antimicrobial therapy.
  - *Critical appraisal:* 1. This was a single center study. 2. Cost-benefit analysis is key for expensive tests and was not evaluated in this study. 3. Standard of care testing included molecular tests. For this reason, the study more strongly favors rapid PCR testing. 4. More patients in the intervention arm received an escalation of antimicrobials compared to the control arm. This is a concern for possible antimicrobial resistance.

DISCUSSION

Influenza

Patients presenting with acute respiratory illness during flu season should be tested with point of care tests for early detection of influenza which helps in isolation of the patient. A previously published meta-analysis evaluated the usefulness of oseltamivir in outpatient treatment to avoid hospitalizations, 15 studies were analysed in the meta-analysis. Oseltamivir was not found to be associated with reduced risk of hospitalization within the ITTi (Intention to treat infected) population in the study (RR, 0.77; 95% CI, 0.47-1.27; RD, -0.14%; 95% CI, -0.32% to 0.16%). **Oseltamivir was also not associated with reduced hospitalization in older populations (mean age ≥65 years: RR, 0.99; 95% CI, 0.19-5.13) or in patients considered to be at greater risk of hospitalization (RR, 0.90; 95% CI, 0.37-2.17).** Oseltamivir was associated with increased nausea (RR, 1.43; 95% CI, 1.13-1.82) and vomiting (RR, 1.83; 95% CI, 1.28-2.63) but not serious adverse events (RR, 0.71; 95% CI, 0.46-1.08).[1]

In another meta-analysis published, **baloxavir marboxil has shown a trend toward reducing mortality and also significantly shortened hospitalization in admitted patients.**[2] In outpatients also, there were significantly lower adverse effects, shorter duration of illness, and reduced influenza viral titers and RNA loads in comparison to oseltamivir. **Similarly, in another multi-center study baloxavir might be more appropriate for influenza patients after 12-48 hours of symptom onset.**[13]

Despite the current evidence, **Oseltamivir is still the preferred agent of choice in the treatment of influenza illness, but baloxavir may be considered as an alternative in select patients.**

Community-acquired pneumonia (CAP)

Diagnosis

The use of point-of-care tests and multiplex PCR has revolutionized how we treat CAP, starting from early diagnosis of infection to targeted detection of antimicrobial resistance, and helps initiate appropriate therapy. **Recently published ERS guidelines on the treatment of CAP suggested sending a sample for multiplex PCR whenever nonstandard antibiotics are prescribed for severe CAP.**[14] Inappropriate antibiotic treatment during 48-72 hours while waiting for results for most culture-based diagnoses is associated with adverse outcomes in CAP. **The benefit of multiplex PCR testing is the ability to rapidly adjust antibiotics for unsuspected antibiotic-resistant pathogens.**

Potential harms of the use of multiplex PCR assays include cost and the inappropriate escalation of antibiotics based on a false-positive PCR result. **Data on appropriate cost-benefit analysis is not available, as most potential benefits of multiplex PCR testing have yet to consider testing costs and antibiotic acquisition costs.** A recently published RCT of 294 community-acquired pneumonia patients, found that using multiplex PCR did not lead to prescribing of narrow-spectrum antibiotics but did lead to a more targeted and more adequate prescription of antibiotics in the PCR group, but this did not lead to a significant difference in intensive care unit (ICU) admissions, readmission within 30 days, length of stay or mortality.[10] **Thus, routine use of multiplex PCR in all community-acquired pneumonia patients may not be a preferred option.**

Management

A network meta-analysis published in 2022 analyzed 12 RCTs evaluating empirical antibiotic treatment strategies for community-acquired pneumonia. **In pairwise meta-analysis, no significant differences were found among Fluoroquinolone (FQ) monotherapy, Beta lactam (BL) monotherapy and Beta lactam plus macrolide (BL-M) dual therapy for all-cause mortality, clinical success or microbiological success.** FQ monotherapy was associated with fewer adverse events compared with BL-M therapy (RR 0.80, 95% confidence interval [CI] 0.66-0.98).[15] **The network meta-analysis showed that there was no significant difference observed among FQ monotherapy, BL monotherapy and BL-M dual therapy regarding all the outcomes.**[15] However the included studies were of low quality hence a definitive recommendation could not be made.

In a meta-analysis published in 2022 of 5 RCTs which compared the efficacy of macrolides vs fluoroquinolones in treatment of atypical bacteria associated CAP, no significant differences between macrolides and fluoroquinolones were identified in rates of clinical failure of all atypical bacteria (RR = 1.57 [95% CI 0.73 to 3.38]; p = 0.251; I2 = 0%), Chlamydia pneumoniae (RR = 2.12 [95% CI 0.63 to 7.14]; p = 0.223; I2 = 0%), Mycoplasma pneumoniae (RR = 1.28 [95% CI 0.57 to 2.92]; p = 0.550; I2 = 0%), or Legionella pneumophila (RR = 0.24 [95% CI 0.02 to 2.86]; p = 0.256; I2 = 0%).[16] **ERS guidelines recommend macrolides in addition to beta-lactams for treatment of severe CAP** (conditional recommendation low quality of evidence).[14] This was based on 17 observational studies with no RCTs in the analysis. In this, a comparison of fluoroquinolones vs macrolide, in addition to beta-lactam for severe CAP was done and showed both regimens caused a significant reduction in mortality and need for ventilatory support, while mortality was significantly lower in the macrolide arm as compared to fluoroquinolone arm.[14] **Another recently published study, ACCESS study found that adding macrolides to the standard of care regimen enhances early clinical response and attenuates the inflammatory burden of community-acquired pneumonia.**[5] Thus, macrolides form an integral part of community-acquired pneumonia treatment. There is ever-growing research in the field of antibiotics, one such molecule is nemonoxacin which is non-inferior to levofloxacin.[4] But at present, more evidence is required to recommend quinolones or other newer molecules over macrolide -beta-lactam combination regimen.

Regarding de-escalation of antibiotics, ERS guidelines recommend using procalcitonin to reduce the duration of antibiotics (low quality of evidence).[14] This recommendation was based on 3 RCTs in which antibiotic treatment duration was significantly shorter in the PCT-guided group, while hospital length of stay and ICU length of stay were not different. **Limitations of using PCT levels to guide antibiotic duration are also related to an observation that PCT levels may not be elevated in bacterial co-infection in viral CAP**.[14] A recently published RCT having 3-arms, of CRP-guided therapy, procalcitonin-guided therapy, and standard of care, found that using the biomarkers does decrease the median days on antibiotics used, without affecting time to clinical stability or length of stay.[3]

ERS guidelines recommend the addition of corticosteroids in patients with severe CAP in shock (low quality of evidence).[14] **The Society for Critical Care Medicine (SCCM, 2024) guidelines also recommend using corticosteroids in severe bacterial CAP.**[17] **They made no recommendation for or against their use in hospitalized non-severe bacterial CAP individuals.** The suggested dosing is given in Table 1. However, due to common exclusion criteria of clinical trials, this recommendation does not apply to patients with viral severe CAP (influenza, SARS, and MERS), uncontrolled diabetes and for patients on corticosteroid treatment for other reasons.

The role of corticosteroids in the treatment of CAP has always been controversial, as studies have had conflicting results due to the different dosage, duration, types of steroids used and study population. In a recent meta-analysis of eighteen trials published in 2023, evaluating the effect of corticosteroids on mortality and clinical cure in CAP was analyzed.[6] **It found that corticosteroids probably reduce the risk of requiring invasive mechanical ventilation, reduce the risk of intensive care unit (ICU) admission, and reduce the duration of hospitalization and ICU stay. Another meta-analysis of ten RCTs also concluded the benefits of corticosteroids in community-acquired pneumonia and also found that amongst all steroids only hydrocortisone had a mortality benefit, decreasing mortality to 50%.**[7]

In patients with Pneumonia Severity Index risk classes IV/V, corticosteroids and antibiotic strategy resulted in USD 70587 worth of savings and an 82.6% chance of being cost-effective when compared to antibiotics alone when analyzed in the short term.[14] A study analyzing the long-term consequences of corticosteroids in community-acquired pneumonia found an increased risk for recurrent pneumonia, secondary infections, and new insulin dependence at 180 days. Thus, **corticosteroids can be given on a case-to-case basis in patients with severe pneumonia after considering its potential benefit vs risk.**

Table 1: Dosing regimens of corticosteroids in Severe Bacterial CAP. Source SCCM 2024 guidelines[17]	
	Regimen and dosing
1	**Intravenous hydrocortisone:** 200 mg once, followed by 10 mg/hr infusion for 7 days.
2	**Intravenous hydrocortisone:** 200 mg daily for 4-8 days (duration based on clinical improvement), followed by tapering of the dose to complete a total duration of 8 or 14 days. If patient is shifted out from ICU before this duration, stop hydrocortisone.
3	**Intravenous methylprednisolone:** 0.5 mg/kg every 12 hours for 7 days.
4	**Intravenous methylprednisolone:** 40 mg once, then taper over the next 20 days. 1. Days 1-7: 40 mg daily 2. Days 8-14: 20 mg daily 3. Days 15-17: 12 mg daily 4. Days 18-20: 4 mg daily These doses are to be given irrespective of whether the individual is shifted out of ICU or not. In the ICU, use continuous infusion. Once shifted out of the ICU, transition to two divided doses, either intravenous bolus or oral.

REFERENCES

1. Hanula R, Bortolussi-Courval É, Mendel A, Ward BJ, Lee TC, McDonald EG. Evaluation of Oseltamivir Used to Prevent Hospitalization in Outpatients With Influenza: A Systematic Review and Meta-Analysis. JAMA Intern Med. 2024 Jan 1;184(1):18-27. doi: 10.1001/jamainternmed.2023.0699. Erratum in: JAMA Intern Med. 2024 Jan 1;184(1):121. doi: 10.1001/jamainternmed.2023.4905. PMID: 37306992; PMCID: PMC10262060.

2. Shiraishi C, Kato H, Hagihara M, Asai N, Iwamoto T, Mikamo H. Comparison of clinical efficacy and safety of baloxavir marboxil versus oseltamivir as the treatment for influenza virus infections: A systematic review and meta-analysis. J Infect Chemother. 2024 Mar;30(3):242-249. doi: 10.1016/j.jiac.2023.10.017. Epub 2023 Oct 20. PMID: 37866622.

3. Duijkers R, Prins HJ, Kross M, Snijders D, van den Berg JWK, Werkman GM, van der Veen N, Schoorl M, Bonten MJM, van Werkhoven CH, Boersma WG. Biomarker guided antibiotic stewardship in community acquired pneumonia: A randomized controlled trial. PLoS One. 2024 Aug 20;19(8):e0307193. doi: 10.1371/journal.pone.0307193. PMID: 39163362; PMCID: PMC11335096.

4. Li Y, Zhu D, Sun S, Chang X, Cao Z, Yang Y, Fu X, Li X, Xu J, Zhu Y, Hui F, Xu X, Chen Z, Peng L, Ma Z, Mo B, Li C, Lv Y, Zhao L, Zhu G, He Y, Liu H, Chen J, Wang Y, Liang Y, Lu Y, Qin Z, Yang H, Zhang M, Wu S, Tong Z, Ye F, Xiao Z, Wang X, Qiu C, Kuang J, Huang H, Wang K, Ying K, Jin F, Lv X, Huang Y, Liu D, Wang W, Zhang Y. A multicentre, randomised, double-blind, double-dummy, parallel-controlled, phase 3 clinical trial assessing the efficacy and safety of intravenous nemonoxacin malate vs. levofloxacin for community-acquired pneumonia in adult patients. Int J Antimicrob Agents. 2024 Aug;64(2):107235. doi: 10.1016/j.ijantimicag.2024.107235. Epub 2024 Jun 6. PMID: 38851462.

5. Giamarellos-Bourboulis EJ, Siampanos A, Bolanou A, Doulou S, Kakavoulis N, Tsiakos K, Katopodis S, Schinas G, Skorda L, Alexiou Z, Armenis K, Katsaounou P, Chrysos G, Masgala A, Poulakou G, Antonakos N, Safarika A, Kyprianou M, Dakou K, Gerakari S, Papanikolaou IC, Milionis H, Marangos M, Dalekos GN, Tzavara V, Akinosoglou K, Hatziaggelaki E, Sympardi S, Kontopoulou T, Mouktaroudi M, Papadopoulos A, Niederman MS. Clarithromycin for early anti-inflammatory responses in community-acquired pneumonia in Greece (ACCESS): a randomised, double-blind, placebo-controlled trial. Lancet Respir Med. 2024 Apr;12(4):294-304. doi: 10.1016/S2213-2600(23)00412-5. Epub 2024 Jan 3. Erratum in: Lancet Respir Med. 2024 Apr;12(4):e20. doi: 10.1016/S2213-2600(24)00043-2. PMID: 38184008.

6. Pitre T, Abdali D, Chaudhuri D, Pastores SM, Nei AM, Annane D, Rochwerg B, Zeraatkar D. Corticosteroids in Community-Acquired Bacterial Pneumonia: a Systematic Review, Pairwise and Dose-Response Meta-Analysis. J Gen Intern Med. 2023 Aug;38(11): 2593-2606. doi: 10.1007/s11606-023-08203-6. Epub 2023 Apr 19. PMID: 37076606; PMCID: PMC10115386.

7. See XY, Wang TH, Chang YC, Lo J, Liu W, Choo CYW, Lee YC, Ma KSK, Chiang CH, Hsia YP, Chiang CH, Chiang CH. Impact of different corticosteroids on severe community-acquired pneumonia: a systematic review and meta-analysis. BMJ Open Respir Res. 2024 Jan 22;11(1):e002141. doi: 10.1136/bmjresp-2023-002141. PMID: 38262670; PMCID: PMC10806634.

8. Blum CA, Roethlisberger EA, Cesana-Nigro N, Winzeler B, Rodondi N, Blum MR, Briel M, Mueller B, Christ-Crain M, Schuetz P. Adjunct prednisone in community-acquired pneumonia: 180-day outcome of a multicentre, double-blind, randomized, placebo-controlled trial. BMC Pulm Med. 2023 Dec 11;23(1):500. doi: 10.1186/s12890-023-02794-w. PMID: 38082273; PMCID: PMC10712075.

9. Heming N, Renault A, Kuperminc E, Brun-Buisson C, Megarbane B, Quenot JP, et al; CRICS-TRIGGERSEP network. Hydrocortisone plus fludrocortisone for community acquired pneumonia-related septic shock: a subgroup analysis of the APROCCHSS phase 3 randomised trial. Lancet Respir Med. 2024 May;12(5):366-374.

10. Cartuliares MB, Rosenvinge FS, Mogensen CB, Skovsted TA, Andersen SL, Østergaard C, Pedersen AK, Skjøt-Arkil H. Evaluation of point-of-care multiplex polymerase chain reaction in guiding antibiotic treatment of patients acutely admitted with suspected community-acquired pneumonia in Denmark: A multicentre randomised controlled trial. PLoS Med. 2023 Nov 28;20(11): e1004314. doi: 10.1371/journal.pmed.1004314. PMID: 38015833; PMCID: PMC10684013.

11. Wu X, Sun T, He H, Xing L, Cheng Z, Geng S, et al. Effect of Metagenomic Next-Generation Sequencing on Clinical Outcomes of Patients With Severe Community-Acquired Pneumonia in the ICU: A Multicenter, Randomized Controlled Trial. Chest. 2024 Jul 25:S0012-3692(24)04863-3.

12. Markussen DL, Serigstad S, Ritz C, Knoop ST, Ebbesen MH, Faurholt-Jepsen D, et al. Diagnostic Stewardship in Community-Acquired Pneumonia With Syndromic Molecular Testing: A Randomized Clinical Trial. JAMA Netw Open. 2024 Mar 4;7(3):e240830. doi: 10.1001/jamanetworkopen.2024.0830. PMID: 38446481; PMCID: PMC10918504.

13. Cai J, Wang H, Ye X, Lu S, Tan Z, Li Z, Lin D, Qian J, Lu X, Wan J, Wang J, Ai J, Pu Y, Qu L, Wang S. Real-world effectiveness and safety of Baloxavir Marboxil or Oseltamivir in outpatients with uncomplicated influenza A: an ambispective, observational, multi-center study. Front Microbiol. 2024 Jul 23;15:1428095. doi: 10.3389/fmicb.2024.1428095. PMID: 39109213; PMCID: PMC11300241.

14. Martin-Loeches I, Torres A, Nagavci B, Aliberti S, Antonelli M, Bassetti M, Bos LD, Chalmers JD, Derde L, de Waele J, Garnacho-Montero J, Kollef M, Luna CM, Menendez R, Niederman MS, Ponomarev D, Restrepo MI, Rigau D, Schultz MJ, Weiss E, Welte T, Wunderink R. ERS/ESICM/ESCMID/ALAT guidelines for the management of severe community-acquired pneumonia. Intensive Care Med 2023 Apr 4:1–18.

15. Xu LY, Wang CC, Peng XX, Jiao Y, Zhao CZ, Zhang L, et al. Empirical antibiotic treatment strategies for community-acquired pneumonia: a network meta-analysis. J Glob Antimicrob Resist 2022;30:1–9.

16. Basilim A, Wali H, Rabaan AA, Eljaaly K. Efficacy of empiric macrolides versus fluoroquinolones in community-acquired pneumonia associated with atypical bacteria: A meta-analysis. Respir Med Re 2022;82:100931.

17. Chaudhuri D, Nei AM, Rochwerg B, Balk RA, Asehnoune K, Cadena R, et al. 2024 Focused Update: Guidelines on Use of Corticosteroids in Sepsis, Acute Respiratory Distress Syndrome, and Community-Acquired Pneumonia. Crit Care Med. 2024 May 1;52(5):e219-e233.

CHAPTER 10

Management of COVID-19

Author: Dr. Abhishek Chauhan

Reviewer: Dr. Nitesh Gupta

INTRODUCTION

The year 2020 marked a significant turning point in global history, as the world grappled with the emergence of a novel coronavirus, SARS-CoV-2, which caused the COVID-19 pandemic. This infectious disease, originating in Wuhan, China, rapidly spread across the globe, leading to unprecedented disruptions in economies, healthcare systems, and daily life. As the pandemic spread across the globe, large number of trials were conducted to understand the nature of disease and evolve management strategies. As the results from these studies are getting published, COVID-19 management guidelines by major societies have been subsequently updated to incorporate new evidence. This chapter is a humble attempt to discuss major trials and meta-analysis published over the last year.

Methodology

A PubMed search was carried out using the following search items. Articles published in English between 1st August 2023 and 1st August 2024 were reviewed. 3731 articles were screened for relevance.

Electronic database search: PubMed

Period: 1st August 2023 to 1st August 2024

Search words: ("COVID-19" OR "SARS-CoV-2") AND ("Treatment" OR "Management")

↓

Article type: Meta-Analysis, Practice guidelines, Randomised Controlled Trial

Study subjects: Humans, Adult

↓

Studies screened: 3731

↓

Studies selected: 26

Analysis of Literature

Antivirals

- ***Molnupiravir for the treatment of non-severe COVID-19: A systematic review and meta-analysis of 14 randomised trials with 34570 patients. (Journal of Antimicrobial Therapy. 2023)*[1]**
    - o *Population:* Adult patients with non-severe COVID-19. (n=34570)
    - o *Intervention:* Molnupiravir.
    - o *Comparator:* Placebo or standard care.
    - o *Outcome:* Moderate to low-certainty evidence showed that Molnupiravir was associated with a reduction in the risk of hospitalisation (RR=0.63), risk of mechanical ventilation (RR=0.37), and time to symptom resolution (mean difference = -2.91 days, 95% CI -3.66 to -2.166). Risk of hospitalization was significantly associated with higher mean age and female gender.
    - o *Conclusions:* Molnupiravir is effective in non-severe COVID-19, but the effect varied with age and gender.

☞

- ***Oral Simnotrelvir for Adult Patients with Mild-to-Moderate Covid-19. (NEJM. 2024)*[2]**
    - o *Population:* Patients with mild-to-moderate COVID-19. (n=1208)
    - o *Intervention:* Oral Simnotrelvir (750 mg) with ritonavir (100 mg) twice daily for 5 days within 72 hours of symptom onset (n=603).
    - o *Comparator:* Placebo (605).
    - o *Outcome:* Time to resolution of symptoms was significantly shorter in Simnotrelvir group (180.1 hours, 95% CI 162.1 to 201.6) as compared to placebo group (216 hours, 95% CI 203.4 to 228.1). Adverse events were higher in intervention group (29% vs 21.6%), however most of them were mild or moderate.
    - o *Conclusions:* Early administration of Simnotrelvir plus Ritonavir was effective in shortening the duration of symptoms.

☞

- ***Efficacy and Safety of 5-Day Oral Ensitrelvir for Patients With Mild-to-Moderate COVID-19: The SCORPIO-SR Randomized Clinical Trial. (JAMA Network. 2024)*[3]**
    - o *Population:* Patients with mild-to-moderate COVID-19 (n= 1821). Patients were randomized within 72 hours of disease onset into 3 groups in 1:1:1 ratio to receive Ensitrelvir 125 mg once a day (375 mg on day1) or 250mg once a day (750 mg on day 1) or placebo for 5 days.
    - o *Intervention:* Ensitrelvir 125 mg (n= 347), Ensitrelvir 250 mg. (n=340)
    - o *Comparator:* Placebo. (n=343)
    - o *Outcome:* Median time to symptom resolution was 167.9 hours (95% CI 145 to 197.6) in the 125 mg Ensitrelvir group as compared to 192.2 hours in the placebo group (192.2 hours, 95% CI 174.5-238.3). The difference in median time to symptom resolution between the groups was -24.3 hours (95% CI -78.7 to 11.7 hours). A decrease in serum HDL levels was found in Ensitrelvir group. No treatment related serious adverse events were reported.
    - o *Conclusion:* 125 mg Ensitrelvir treatment reduced the time to symptom resolution in patients treated within 72 hours of symptom onset.

- ***Molnupiravir versus favipiravir in at-risk outpatients with COVID-19: A randomized controlled trial in Thailand. (International Journal of Infectious Diseases. 2024)***[4]
  - *Population:* Patients with moderate COVID-19 and at least one factor associated with severe COVID-19 (n=977)
  - *Intervention:* Molnupiravir 800 mg twice a day for 5 days (n=487)
  - *Comparator:* Favipiravir 1800 mg (weight ≤ 90kg) or 2400 mg (weight >90kg) twice a day for one day followed by 800 mg (weight ≤90 kg) or 1000 mg (weight 90kg) twice a day for 4 days, extended to 5 additional days in case of clinical progression. (n=490)
  - *Outcome:* The primary outcomes assessed were occurrence of pulmonary involvement at day 29 (dyspnea, hypoxia, CXR findings suggestive of damage to lung parenchyma). At day 29, pulmonary involvement occurred in 0% in Molnupiravir group and 1% patients in Favipiravir group. COVID-19 related hospitalization occurred in <1% patients in Molnupiravir group and 1% in Favipiravir group. Incidence of treatment related adverse events was similar in both groups (1%)
  - *Conclusion:* Favipiravir and Molnupiravir had similar efficacy and safety profile for treatment of patients with moderate COVID-19.

- ***Efficacy and safety of antiviral treatments for symptomatic COVID-19 outpatients: Systematic review and network meta-analysis. (Antiviral Research. 2024)***[5]
  - *Population:* Patients with mild-to-moderate COVID-19. (n=1,456,523)
  - *Intervention and Comparator:* Remdesivir, Molnupiravir, Nirmatrelvir/Ritonavir.
  - *Outcomes:* Remdesivir was associated with lowest probability of hospitalization as compared to Molnupiravir and nirmatrelvir/ritonavir (P-scores 0.99, 0.26 and 0.64 respectively). Remdesivir was also found to have lowest probability of death as compared to Molnupiravir and nirmatrelvir/ritonavir (P-scores 0.90, 0.49 and 0.55 respectively). On indirect comparison, remdesivir was found to have decreased risk of hospitalization as compared to nirmatrelvir/ritonavir (RR 0.11, 95% CI 0.03-0.73) and molnupiravir (RR 0.09, 95% CI 0.02-0.40). There was no significant difference in mortality reduction and side effects.
  - *Conclusion:* Remdesivir has the highest efficacy in preventing hospitalization when compared with Molnupiravir and nirmatrelvir/ritonavir.

- ***Oral VV116 versus placebo in patients with mild-to-moderate COVID-19 in China: a multicentre, double-blind, phase 3, randomised controlled study. (Lancet Infectious Diseases. 2024)***[6]
  - *Population:* Patients with mild-to-moderate COVID-19. (n=1347)
  - *Intervention:* VV116 (Mindeudesivir)- 0.6 gm bd on day 1 followed by 0.3 gm on days 2-5. (n=674)
  - *Control:* Placebo. (n=673)
  - *Outcome:* Treatment with VV116 led to substantial reduction in time to resolution as compared with placebo (HR 1.17, 95% CI 1.04-1.33). Adverse events were similar between the groups.
  - *Conclusion:* Among patients with mild-to-moderate COVID-19, VV116 treatment leads to faster resolution of symptoms.

- ***COVID-19 Rebound After VV116 vs Nirmatrelvir-Ritonavir Treatment. (JAMA Network Open. 2024)[7]***
  - o *Population:* Adult patients with mild-to-moderate COVID-19. (n=345)
  - o *Intervention:* VV116. (n=165)
  - o *Comparator:* Nirmatrelvir-Ritonavir. (n=180)
  - o *Outcome:* There was no significant difference in rates of symptom rebound (25.6% in the VV116 group and 24.5% in the nirmatrelvir-ritonavir group) and viral load rebound (20.0% in the VV116 group and 21.7% in the nirmatrelvir-ritonavir group). Viral whole-genome sequencing of 24 rebound cases revealed the same lineage at baseline and at viral load rebound in each case.
  - o *Conclusion:* Viral load rebound and symptom rebound were both common after a standard 5-day course of treatment with either VV116 or nirmatrelvir-ritonavir.

- ***Nirmatrelvir/Ritonavir Regimen for Mild/Moderately Severe COVID-19: A Rapid Review With Meta-Analysis and Trial Sequential Analysis. (Annals of Family Medicine. 2024)[8]***
  - o *Population:* Patients with mild/moderates COVID-19. (4 RCTs, n=4070)
  - o *Intervention:* Nirmatrelvir/Ritonavir.
  - o *Control:* Placebo or no care.
  - o *Outcome:* Nirmatrelvir/ritonavir significantly decreased COVID-19 hospitalization compared with placebo/no treatment (RR = 0.17; 95% CI, 0.10-0.31; I^2 = 77.2%; 2 RCTs, 3,542 persons), but there was no significant difference for decrease of worsening severity (RR = 0.82; 95% CI, 0.66-1.01; I^2 = 47.5%; 3 RCTs, 1,824 persons), viral clearance (RR = 1.19; 95% CI, 0.93-1.51; I^2 = 82%; 2 RCTs, 528 persons), adverse events (RR = 1.41; 95% CI, 0.92-2.14; I^2 = 70.6%; 4 RCTs, 4,070 persons), serious adverse events (RR = 0.82; 95% CI, 0.41-1.62; I^2 = 0%; 3 RCTs, 3,806 persons), and all-cause mortality (RR = 0.27; 95% CI, 0.04-1.70; I^2 = 49.9%; 3 RCTs, 3,806 persons).
  - o *Conclusions:* Nirmatrelvir/Ritonavir likely prevents COVID-19 related hospitalizations in patients with mild/moderate COVID-19.

Anti-inflammatory drugs

- ***Efficacy and safety of baricitinib for the treatment of hospitalized adults with COVID19: A systematic review and meta-analysis. (European Journal of Medical Research. 2023)[9]***
  - o *Population:* Hospitalized adults with COVID-19. (n=3010)
  - o *Intervention:* Baricitinib.
  - o *Control:* Placebo or conventional therapy.
  - o *Outcome:* Fourteen-day mortality was not statistically significant between the groups (OR 0.23, 95% CI 0.03-1.84). Baricitinib decreased 28-day mortality (OR 0.60, 0.47-0.77), not including the critically ill. Baricitinib treatment led to faster recovery (mean difference -1, 95% CI -1.12 to -0.88) and shorter hospital stays (mean difference -0.80, 95% CI -0.84 to -0.76). There was no difference in infection, deep veinous thrombosis and major cardiovascular events.
  - o *Conclusions:* Baricitinib decreases mortality in non-critically ill hospitalized patients with COVID-19.

- ***Intravenous aviptadil and remdesivir for treatment of COVID-19-associated hypoxaemic respiratory failure in the USA (TESICO): A randomised, placebo-controlled trial. (Lancet Respiratory Medicine. 2023)[10]***

- o *Population:* Hospitalised adults with hypoxemic respiratory failure due to COIVD-19 within 4 days of onset of respiratory failure (n=473). Patients were randomised in 1:1:1:1 ratio to intravenous Aviptadil plus Remdesivir, aviptadil plus remdesivir with matched placebo, aviptadil matched placebo plus remdesivir or aviptadil matched placebo plus remdesivir matched placebo.
- o *Intervention:* Aviptadil 600 pmol/kg on day 1, 1200 pmol/kg on day 2 and 1800 pmol/kg on day 3 (n=231). Aviptadil was administerd as 12 hour infusion. Remdesivir 200 mg on day 1, followed by 100 mg till day 10. (n=44)
- o *Comparator:* Aviptadil matched placebo (n=230), Remdesivir matched placebo. (n=43)
- o *Outcome:* The primary outcome, assessed at day 90, was a six-category ordinal outcome: (1) at home (defined as the type of residence before hospitalisation) and off oxygen (recovered) for at least 77 days, (2) at home and off oxygen for 49–76 days, (3) at home and off oxygen for 1–48 days, (4) not hospitalised but either on supplemental oxygen or not at home, (5) hospitalised or in hospice care, or (6) dead. Mortality up to day 90 was a key secondary outcome. The odds ratio (OR) for being in a better category of the primary efficacy endpoint for aviptadil versus placebo at day 90 was 1·11 (95% CI 0·80–1·55; p=0·54). There was no significant difference in 90 day mortality.
- o *Conclusions:* Among patients with COVID-19-associated acute hypoxaemic respiratory failure, aviptadil did not significantly improve clinical outcomes up to day 90 when compared with placebo.

- ***A Risk Profile Using Simple Hematologic Parameters to Assess Benefits From Baricitinib in Patients Hospitalized With COVID-19: A Post Hoc Analysis of the Adaptive COVID-19 Treatment Trial-2. (Annals of Internal Medicine. 2024)***[11]
  - o *Population:* Hospitalized patients with COVID-19. (n=999)
  - o *Intervention:* Baricitinib + Remdesivir. (n=494)
  - o *Control:* Placebo + Remdesivir. (n=505)
  - o *Outcome:* Treatment with Baricitinib + remdesivir in the high risk quartile was associated with reduced risk for death (hazard ratio [HR], 0.38 [95% CI, 0.16 to 0.86]; *P* = 0.020), decreased progression to IMV or death (HR, 0.57 [CI, 0.35 to 0.93]; *P* = 0.024), and improved recovery rate (HR, 1.53 [CI, 1.16 to 2.02]; *P* = 0.002).
  - o *Conclusions:* Hospitalised COVID-19 patients in high risk quartile as defined by ACTT-1 risk profile have better outcomes when treated with Baricitinib and Remdesivir combination.
  - o *Critical appraisal:* This was a post hoc analysis conducted on data from ACTT-2 trial.

Steroids

- ***ACTIV-6 trial -Inhaled Fluticasone Furoate for Outpatient Treatment of Covid-19. (NEJM. 2023)***[12]
  - o *Population:* Non-hospitalised patients with COVID-19 aged more than 30 years and symptomatic for less than 7 days. (n=1407)
  - o *Intervention:* Inhaled fluticasone furoate 200 mcg daily for 14 days. (n=715)
  - o *Control:* Placebo. (n=692)
  - o *Outcome:* Treatment with inhaled fluticasone furoate for 14 days did not result in a shorter time to recovery than placebo among outpatients with COVID-19 (Hazard ratio 1.01, 95% CI 0.91 to 1.12).
  - o *Conclusion:* Inhaled fluticasone furoate doesn't shorten the time to recovery as compared with placebo.

- ***Effect of dexamethasone dose on outcomes in acute COVID-19 disease: A systematic review and meta-analysis. (Journal of Infection. 2023)***[13]

- *Population:* Adult patients with COVID-19 pneumonia treated with dexamethasone. (n=3469)
- *Intervention and comparator:* 12-24 mg/day dexamethasone (n=1775) vs 6-8 mg/day dexamethasone.
- *Outcome:* There was no significant difference in mortality between high dose and low dose dexamethasone groups (22.0% vs 20.2%, OR 1.20, 95% CI 0.86-1.67). High dose dexamethasone was associated with increased risk of hyperglycemia (23.6% vs 17.2%, p=0.0008) but not secondary infections.
- *Conclusion:* High dose dexamethasone is associated with higher risk of hyperglycemia without significant mortality benefit.
- *Critical appraisal:* This meta-analysis included 8 RCTs which compared low vs high dose dexamethasone for COVID-19. A previous meta-analysis of 20 studies including 10,155 patients[14] found that higher-dose corticosteroids probably reduce mortality (absolute risk difference, 14 fewer deaths per 1,000 [95% CI, 26 fewer to 2 fewer]; moderate certainty) and may reduce the need for mechanical ventilation (absolute risk difference, 11.6 fewer per 1,000 [95% CI, 23.2 fewer to 6.9 more]; low certainty).

Plasma

☞

- ***A controlled trial of plasma exchange compared to standard of care in the treatment of severe COVID-19 infection (COVIPLEX). (Nature Scientific Reports. 2024)***[15]
  - *Population:* Critically ill adults with severe COVID-19 associated respiratory failure, requiring supplemental oxygen or ventilator support and elevated thrombo-inflammatory markers. (n=22)
  - *Intervention:* Daily single volume plasma exchange for a minimum of 5 days. (n=11)
  - *Control:* Standard care. (n=11)
  - *Outcome:* No significant difference in reduction of inflammatory markers, severity of respiratory failure, thrombotic events or mortality. There was significant reduction in the level of thrombotic markers (Factor VIII, VWF and VWF Ag: ADAMTS 13 ratio) in the intervention arm.
  - *Conclusion:* Plasma exchange decreased the level of thrombotic markers, but it was not associated with reduction in mortality.

☞

- ***CONFIDENT trial - Convalescent Plasma for COVID-19 induced ARDS in mechanically ventilated patients. (NEJM. 2023)***[16]
  - *Population:* Adult patients with Covid-19 induce ARDS who had been on mechanical ventilation for less than 5 days .(n=475)
  - *Intervention:* Convalescent plasma with a neutralising antibody titer of at least 1:320 (n=237). Due to shortage of plasma, a titer of 1:160 was administered in 17.7% patients.
  - *Control:* Standard care. (n=238)

- *Outcome:* 28-day mortality in was found to be lower in convalescent plasma group as compared to standard care (35.4% vs 45.0%, p=0.03). This intervention was found to be beneficial in patients who were randomized within 48 hours of initiation of mechanical ventilation.
- *Conclusion:* Among patients with COVID-19 ARDS, treatment with convalescent plasma with a neutralizing antibody titer of at least 1:160 within 5 days of initiation of mechanical ventilation decreases 28-day mortality.

- ***A Randomized Controlled Study Assessing Convalescent Immunoglobulins vs Convalescent Plasma for Hospitalized Patients With Coronavirus 2019. (Clinical Infectious Diseases. 2023)***[17]
  - *Population:* High risk Covid-19 patients within 10 days of symptom onset. (n=319)
  - *Intervention:* Convalescent immunoglobulins (cIgG) 4 gm. (n=166)
  - *Comparator:* 2 high titer doses of convalescent plasma, 200 ml each on 2 consecutive days. (n=153)
  - *Outcome:* Primary endpoint was improvement on day 14 as per WHO scale. There was no significant difference between cIgG group and convalescent plasma group with respect to primary outcome (67.5% vs 67.3% respectively). At 28 days, improvement by WHO scale was higher in cIgG group as compared to convalescent plasma group (81.9% vs 70.6% respectively, 95% CI 1.9-20.7: p<0.001). Among unvaccinated patients, 84.1% patients improved in cIgG group as compared to 66.1% patients in the convalescent plasma group at day 28, p=0.024. There was no significant difference between the groups with respect to need for mechanical ventilation and mortality. Among unvaccinated patients, survival rate was higher in cIgG group (89.9% vs 77.4%) though it didn't reach statistical significance.
  - *Conclusion:* cIgG failed to reach noninferiority at day 14 but was superior to convalescent plasma at day 28, especially among unvaccinated patients.

Supportive Measures

- ***Comparison of Noninvaisve Mechanical Ventilation with High-flow Nasal cannula, Face-mask, and Helmet in hypoxemic respiratory failure in patients with COVID-19: A Randomised Controlled Trial. (Critical Care Medicine 2023)***[18]
  - *Population:* Adult patients with COVID-19 with PaO_2/FiO_2 ratio less than 300. (n=151)
  - *Intervention and comparators:* HFNC(n=47), Helmet CPAP (n=52), Face-mask CPAP. (n=52)
  - *Outcome:* The endotracheal intubation rates were 44%, 45%, and 46% (p = 0.99), and the median intubation times were 7.0, 5.5, and 4.5 days (p = 0.11) in the HFNC, face-mask CPAP, and helmet CPAP, respectively. The mortality rates were 23%, 32%, and 38% at 28 days (p = 0.24) and 43%, 38%, and 40% (p = 0.89) at 90 days for HFNC, face-mask CPAP, and helmet CPAP, respectively.
  - *Conclusion:* There was no difference in intubation rate and mortality among the three intervention groups for the COVID-19 patients with hypoxemic respiratory failure. The trial was stopped prematurely because of a decline in cases.

☞

- ***Lower vs Higher Oxygenation target and days alive without life support in COVID-19- The HOT-COVID randomized clinical trial. (JAMA 2024)***[19]
  - *Population:* Patients with COVID-19 and severe hypoxemia (requiring at least 10 L/min of oxygenation or mechanical ventilation). (n= 726)

- *Intervention and comparators:* Low oxygenation targets (PaO_2 60mm Hg) (n=365) vs High oxygenation targets (PaO_2 90 mm Hg) (n=361)
- *Outcomes:* Median number of days alive without life support (mechanical ventilation, circulatory support, or renal replacement therapy) was more in low oxygenation group (80 days vs 72 days, p=0.009). There was no significant difference in 90-day mortality (30.2% in the lower oxygenation group and 34.7% in the higher oxygenation group).
- *Conclusion:* In adult ICU patients with COVID-19 and severe hypoxemia, targeting a PaO_2 of 60 mm Hg resulted in more days alive without life support in 90 days than targeting a PaO_2 of 90 mm Hg.

- ***Therapeutic high-dose vitamin D for vitamin D deficient severe COVID-19 disease: Randomised, double-blind, placebo-controlled study (SHADE S). (Journal of Public Health 2024)***[20]
    - *Population:* Patients with moderate-to-severe COVID-19 with PaO_2/FiO_2 ratio less than 200 and vitamin D deficiency (n=90)
    - *Intervention:* Single dose 0.6 million IU Cholecalciferol. (n=45)
    - *Control:* Placebo. (n= 45)
    - *Outcome:* 25(OH)D3 levels were 12 (10–16) and 13 (12–18) ng/ml ($P = 0.06$) at baseline; and 60 (55–65) ng/ml and 4 (1–7) ng/ml by Day 7 in vitamin D and placebo groups, respectively. SOFA score at day 7 was better in Vitamin D group (3 vs 5, p=0.01), all cause 28-day mortality was lower in Vitamin D group (24% vs 44%, p=0.046).
    - *Conclusion:* High-dose vitamin D supplementation (0.6 million IU) to increase 25(OH)D > 50 ng/ml reduces mortality in moderate-to-severe COVID-19.

Vaccination

☞

- ***Immunogenicity and safety of concomitant administration of recombinant COVID-19 vaccine and quadrivalent inactivated influenza vaccine in Chinese adults: An open-label, randomized, controlled trial. (Human Vaccines and Immunotherapeutics 2024)***[21]
    - *Population:* Adults receiving COVID-19 vaccine.
    - *Intervention:* Quadrivalent influenza vaccine on the same day as COVID-19 vaccine.
    - *Comparator:* Quadrivalent influenza vaccine 14 days after COVID-19 vaccination.
    - *Outcome:* There was no significant difference in seroconversion rates of QIIV antibodies between the simultaneous and non-simultaneous groups rate (H1N1: 87.5% vs. 90.1%; H3N2: 58.1% vs. 62.0%; Yamagata: 75.0% vs. 64.5%; and Victoria: 55.1% vs. 62.8%). No significant difference in adverse events was observed between the two groups (14.2% vs. 23.5%, p = .053).
    - *Conclusion:* No immune interference or safety concerns were found for concomitant administration of COVID-19 vaccine with quadrivalent influenza vaccine in adults aged $\geq$ 18 years.

Post COVID-19 sequelae

- ***Persistence of post-COVID symptoms in the general population two years after SARS-CoV-2 infection: A systematic review and meta-analysis. (Journal of Infection. 2024)***[22]
    - *Population:* Patients with probable or confirmed infection by SARS-CoV-2, including both hospitalized and non-hospitalized patients from the general population. (n=7,912)

- *Outcome:* The most prevalent post-COVID symptoms two years after SARS-CoV-2 infection were fatigue (28.0%, 95%CI 12.0–47.0), cognitive impairments (27.6%, 95%CI 12.6–45.8), and pain (8.4%, 95%CI 4.9–12.8). Aanxiety (13.4%, 95%CI 6.3–22.5), depression (18.0%, 95%CI 4.8–36.7) and sleep disturbance (20.9%, 95%CI 5.25–43.25) were also prevalent.
- *Conclusion:* Post-COVID symptoms were present in 30% of patients 2 years after COVID-19. Fatigue, cognitive impairment and pain were the most common symptoms.

- ***Effect of Pulmonary Rehabilitation on exercise capacity, dyspnea, fatigue, and peripheral muscle strength in patients with post-COVID-19 syndrome: A systematic review and meta-analysis. (Archives of Physical Medicine and Rehabilitation. 2024)***[23]
  - *Population:* Patients with post-COVID-19 syndrome. (n=188)
  - *Intervention and comparators:* Pulmonary rehabilitation (PR) vs control; Modality of rehabilitation- face to face vs telephonic, duration of rehabilitation- 4-8 weeks vs >8 weeks.
  - *Outcome:* Pulmonary rehabilitation was associated with increased 6-minute walk distance (MD 60.56m, 40.75-80.36) and reduction in fatigue (Fatigue severity scale: -0.90 , -1.32 to -0.31) but no difference in dyspnea and muscle strength. There were no differences 4-8 weeks and more than 8 weeks pulmonary rehabilitation programs regarding exercise capacity, peripheral muscle strength and dyspnea. There were no differences between telerehabilitation and face-to-face PR regarding effects on peripheral muscle strength, dyspnea, and fatigue.
  - *Conclusion:* PR improves exercise capacity and reduces fatigue in patients with post-COVID-19 syndrome. Duration of PR (4-8 weeks vs > 8 weeks) or PR modality (telerehabilitation vs face-to-face) did not affect outcomes.

- ***Nirmatrelvir-Ritonavir and Symptoms in Adults With Post acute Sequelae of SARS-CoV-2 Infection- The STOP-PASC Randomized Clinical Trial. (JAMA Internal Medicine. 2024)***[24]
  - *Population:* Adults with moderate-to-severe PASC symptoms of 3 months or longer duration. (n=155)
  - *Intervention:* Nirmatrelvir-Ritonavir for 15 days. (n=102)
  - *Control:* Placebo-Ritonavir. (n=53)
  - *Outcome:* There was no statistically significant difference in the model-derived severity outcome pooled across the 6 core symptoms, Patient Global Impression of Severity or Patient Global Impression of Change scores, summative symptom scores at 10 weeks. There was no change from baseline to 10 weeks in PROMIS fatigue, dyspnea, cognitive function, and physical function measures.
  - *Conclusion:* Nirmatrelvir- Ritonavir did not demonstrate a significant benefit for improving select PASC symptoms.

Others

- ***COVID-19 Rapid Antigen Tests With Self-Collected vs Health Care Worker–Collected Nasal and Throat Swab Specimens. (JAMA Network Open. 2023)***[25]
  - *Population:* Individuals aged 16 years or older requesting a COVID-19 test for diagnostic or screening purposes. (n= 2674)
  - *Intervention:* Self collected nasal and throat samples for rapid antigen testing. (n=1298)
  - *Comparator:* Healthcare worker collected nasal and throat samples for rapid antigen testing. (n=1376)

    (All subjects underwent healthcare worker sampling for RT PCR)

- *Outcome:* Healthcare worker–collected throat specimens had higher mean sensitivity than HCW-collected nasal specimens for rapid antigen testing (69.4% [95% CI, 65.1%-73.6%] vs 60.0% [95% CI, 55.4%-64.5%]). Self-collected nasal specimens were more sensitive than self-collected throat specimens for rapid antigen testing (mean sensitivity, 71.5% [95% CI, 65.3%-77.6%] vs 58.0% [95% CI, 51.2%-64.7%]). Combining nasal and throat specimens increased sensitivity for HCW- and self-collected specimens by 21.4 and 15.5 percentage points, respectively, compared with a single nasal specimen.
- *Conclusion:* Adding a throat specimen to the standard practice of collecting a single nasal specimen could improve sensitivity for rapid antigen testing in healthcare and home-based settings.

- ***Risk factors for COVID-19 associated pulmonary aspergillosis: A systematic review and meta-analysis. (Lancet Respiratory Medicine. 2024)***[26]
  - *Population:* COVID-19 patients with and without covid associated pulmonary aspergillosis. (n=8,009)
  - *Outcome:* 17.5% patients were diagnosed with CAPA. Nine risk factors were identified pre-existing chronic liver disease (OR 2.56, 1.3-5.05), hematological malignancies (OR 2.47, 1.27-4.83), COPD (OR 1.92, 1.42-2.60), cerebrovascular disease (OR 1.31, 1.01-1.71) diabetes mellitus (OR 1.26, 1.04-1.53), use of mechanical ventilation (OR 2.73, 1.89-3.94), renal replacement therapy (OR 2.26, 1.76-2.90), treatment with IL-6 inhibitors (OR 2.69, 1.47-4.90), treatment with steroids (OR 1.72, 1.10-2.68).
  - *Conclusion:* Pre-existing comorbidities, steroid use, IL-6 inhibitors, mechanical ventilation and renal replacement therapies are risk factors for development of CAPA.

- ***Effects of renin-angiotensin system blockers on outcomes from COVID-19: A systematic review and meta-analysis of randomized controlled trials. (European Heart Journal. 2024)***[27]
  - *Population:* Patients with COVID-19 treated with or without RAS inhibitors. (n=3,492)
  - *Intervention and comparators:* Initiation or discontinuation of RAS blockers.
  - *Outcome:* Continuation of RAS blockers was not associated with increased risk of ICU admission (RR 0.96,95% CI 0.66-1.41), need for ventilation (RR 0.77, 05% CI 0.55-1.09), need for vasopressors (RR 0.92, 95% CI 0.58-1.44), AKI (RR 1.01, 95% CI 0.40-2.56) or thromboembolic events (RR 1.07, 95% CI 0.36-3.19). RAS blocker initiation was not associated with increased risk of ICU admission (RR 0.71, 95% CI 0.47-1.08), need for ventilation (RR 1.12 95% CI 0.91-1.38) or thromboembolic events (RR 1.20, 95% CI 0.06-23.70), although vasopressor use increased (RR=1.27, 1.02-1.57). In patients with severe/critical COVID-19, RAS blocker initiation increased the risk of all-cause death (RR1.31, 1.01-1.72).
  - *Conclusion:* ACE inhibitors and ARBs may be continued in non-severe COVID-19 infection, where indicated. Initiation of RAS blockers may be harmful in critically ill patients.

DISCUSSION

The objective while evaluating a patient with COVID-19 is to assess the severity of their symptoms, the likelihood of their condition deteriorating, and the safety of home care. This helps in determining the appropriate healthcare setting and the need for administering.

Table 1: Classification of disease severity

AIIMS/ICMR COVID-19 Guidelines	WHO Guidelines[28]	IDSA Guidelines[29]
Mild Upper respiratory tract symptoms and/or fever WITHOUT shortness of breath	**Non-severe** Absence of signs of severe or critical disease	**Mild to moderate** SpO_2>94% not requiring supplemental oxygen
Moderate Any one of: 1. Respiratory rate ≥24/min, breathlessness 2. SpO_2 90% to ≤ 93% on room air	**Severe** Oxygen saturation <90% on room air, Signs of pneumonia, Signs of severe respiratory distress	**Severe** SpO_2≤94% on room air, including patients requiring supplemental oxygen
Severe Any one of: 1. Respiratory rate >30/min, breathlessness 2. SpO_2<90% on room air	**Critical** Requires life sustaining treatment, Acute Respiratory Distress Syndrome, Sepsis, Septic shock	**Critical** Patients on mechanical ventilation and extracorporeal membrane oxygenation, including patients with end organ dysfunction as seen in sepsis/septic shock

COVID-19 specific therapy. Clinical management of COVID-19 patients is guided by disease severity. Different healthcare organizations have classified COVID-19 across a spectrum of mild to severe cases based on clinical parameters. There are differences with respect to terminology between Indian and international guidelines.

The World Health Organization guideline recommends that patients be risk-stratified to identify those who are at high, moderate or low risk of hospitalization. (Table 2)

Table 2: How to identify patients with non-severe COVID-19 at high, moderate and low risk of hospitalization.[28]
Patients at high risk (6%) of hospitalization includes those with diagnosed immunodeficiency syndromes, those who have undergone solid organ transplant and are receiving immunosuppressants, and those with autoimmune illness receiving immunosuppressants
Patients at moderate risk (3%) of hospitalization are those over 65 years, those with obesity, diabetes and/or chronic cardiopulmonary disease, chronic kidney or liver disease, active cancer, those with disabilities, and those with comorbidities of chronic disease
Patients at low risk (0.5%) of hospitalization includes those who are neither moderate nor high risk. Most patients are low risk.

Antivirals and anti-inflammatory drugs approved for treatment of COVID-19 are listed in Table 3.

Table 3: Drugs used in the management of COVID-19

Agent	Mechanism of action	Dose	Major Trials
Remdesivir	Inhibition of viral RNA transcription	**Severe COVID-19:** 200 mg on day 1, followed by 100 mg till day 10 **Non-severe COVID-19:** 200 mg on day 1 followed by 100 mg on days 2 and 3	ACTT-1 DisCoVeRy SOLIDARITY PINETREE
Molnupiravir	Inhibits RNA dependent RNA polymerase	800 mg BD for 5 days	MOVe-OUT PANORAMIC MOVe-In
Nirmatrelvir	Inhibits SARS-CoV-2 protease (3CLpro)	300 mg BD for 5 days	EPIC-HR EPIC-SR
Ritonavir	Inhibits metabolism of Nirmatrelvir	100 mg BD for 5 days	
Baricitinib	Janus Kinase inhibitor	4 mg OD till 14 days or until discharge from hospital	TACTIC-R COV-BARRIER
Tofacitinib	Janus kinase inhibitor	10 mg BD for 14 days or until discharge from hospital	STOP-COVID
Ruxolitinib	Janus Kinase inhibitor	10 mg BD for 14 days	RUXCOVID
Tocilizumab	IL-6 inhibitor	8mg/kg (up to maximum of 800 mg) single dose. Second dose can be given 12-48 hours later at the discretion of the physician	EMPACTA COVINTOC REMAP-CAP
Sarilumab	IL-6 inhibitor	400 mg, single dose	REMAP-CAP

Therapies not recommended by major guidelines- Ivermectin, Anakinra, Hydroxychloroquine, Lopinavir/Ritonavir, Famotidine, Colchicine, Sotrvimab, Casirivimib-Imdevimab.

Fluvoxamine has been approved for use by WHO and IDSA only in the settings of clinical trial.

Treatment in outpatient settings /ambulatory patients

Indian guidelines recommend home isolation for patients with mild disease. Physical distancing, indoor mask use, and strict hand hygiene are advised to limit transmission. Home pulse oximetry monitoring is recommended to guide the escalation of care if there is a worsening of the disease.

Among patients eligible for outpatient management, **COVID-19-specific treatment is recommended if they present within 5 days of symptom onset and if they are ≥50 years old and unvaccinated, ≥65 years old, immunocompromised, or have multiple comorbidities. Remdesivir and Convalescent plasma can also be used if presentation is within 8 days of symptom onset. WHO recommends initiating COVID-19 specific treatment in patients at moderate and high risk of hospitalization.** (Table 2).

Nirmatrelvir/ritonavir combination belongs to the protease inhibitor class of drugs. **Nirmatrelvir inhibits the activity of the SARS-CoV-2-3CL protease, thereby inhibiting viral replication. Ritonavir slows the metabolism of nirmatrelvir, so it remains active in the body for longer and at higher concentrations.**

In the **EPIC-HR trial**, unvaccinated adults with a high risk of severe COVID-19 were treated with Nirmatrelvir/Ritonavir. It was found that taking administration of this combination within three days of symptom onset reduced the chances of needing hospital care or dying by 89% compared to a placebo.[30] A meta-analysis of 4 RCTs and 16 real-world studies found that Nirmatrelvir/Ritonavir significantly decreased risks of hospitalization when compared with placebo (RR 0.17, CI 0.10-0.31) but there was no significant difference in all-cause mortality.[8]

The dosage of Nirmatrelvir/ritonavir needs modification in patients with renal dysfunction. For patients with moderate kidney impairment (eGFR 30 to 59 mL/min), the dose is nirmatrelvir 150 mg-ritonavir 100 mg orally twice daily for five days. Nirmatrelvir/ritonavir use is not recommended in patients with eGFR <30 mL/min.

Nirmatrelvir clearance occurs via a CYP3A4-mediated pathway, which increases the risk of potential drug interactions. Ritonavir inhibits CYP3A4, which can lead to increased blood levels of other drugs metabolized by CYP3A4, such as anticoagulants, anticonvulsants, and immunosuppressants.

In ambulatory patients with mild-to-moderate COVID-19 at high risk for progression to severe disease, the **IDSA guideline panel suggests nirmatrelvir/ritonavir initiated within five days of symptom onset at a dose of 300 mg Nirmatrelvir + 100mg Ritonavir twice a day for 5 days.**[29] **WHO guidelines recommend treatment with Nirmatrelvir/Ritonavir in patients with non-severe COVID-19 at high risk of hospitalization.**[31]

Rebound COVID-19 has been reported in patients treated with Nirmatrelvir/ritonavir. It refers to the recurrence of symptoms following initial improvement within the first few weeks following infection. It has been described in both vaccinated and unvaccinated patients. The incidence of rebound symptoms has been reported to be between 1% to 2%.[32-34] Rebound symptoms are generally mild and for patients who are at high risk of hospitalization, the potential benefits of treatment outweigh the risks of rebound.

Molnupiravir is a nucleoside analog that inhibits SARS-CoV-2 by inducing mutations in viral RNA. In the **MOVe-OUT trial**, the risk of hospitalization and death at 29 days was lower in the Molnupiravir arm by 3% (CI -5.9% to -0.1%). **The trial was stopped early due to presumed clear superiority demonstrated during interim analysis.**[35]

Further evidence for use of Molnupiravir is derived from a living network meta-analysis of 9 RCTs done by the WHO GDG.[31] **There was moderate certainty evidence to suggest that Molnupiravir decreases mortality, hospitalization, and time to symptom resolution.** A meta-analysis of 14 RCTs including 34570 patients found that Molnupiravir decreases the risk of hospitalization, decreases the risk of mechanical ventilation, and fastens symptom resolution in patients with mild COVID-19.[1]

In ambulatory patients (≥18 years) with mild-to-moderate COVID-19 at high risk for progression to severe disease who have no other treatment options, the IDSA guideline recommends Molnupiravir to be initiated within five days of symptom onset at a dose of 800mg twice a day for 5 days.[29] **WHO recommends treatment with Molnupiravir for patients with non-severe COVID-19 at high risk of hospitalization.**[31] It is not approved for use in pregnant persons and in children < 18 years of age as it may affect bone and cartilage growth. Molnupiravir carries a risk for mutagenesis in vitro for human RNAs

Remdesivir is an RNA transcriptase inhibitor and one of the earliest drugs to be approved for the treatment of COVID-19. In patients requiring oxygen supplementation, the use of remdesivir and dexamethasone was associated with significant mortality benefit decreased length of hospital stay, and faster viral clearance. In the **PINETREE trial**, the efficacy of Remdesivir was evaluated in an outpatient setting. **A 3-day course of Remdesivir reduced the risk of hospitalization to 0.7% versus 5.3% in the placebo group.**[36]

In a living network meta-analysis of 7 trials, **WHO GDG found moderate certainty evidence that Remdesivir decreased hospitalization, decreased mortality, and decreased risk of mechanical ventilation.**[31]

A network meta-analysis comparing the efficacy of antivirals in COVID-19 found that Remdesivir had the highest efficacy in preventing hospitalization when compared with Molnupiravir and nirmatrelvir/ritonavir.[5]

There are concerns regarding the hepatotoxic side effects of Remdesivir. Cardiovascular side effects like QT interval prolongation, bradycardia, and hypotension have been reported with Remdesivir. Remdesivir is safe for administration in pregnant and lactating women.[37]

Remdesivir is a therapeutic option for patients with mild COVID-19 who are at high risk of disease progression and cannot be treated with Nirmatrelvir/Ritonavir due to concerns of CYP3A4-related drug interactions.

Molnupiravir and Nirmatrelvir/Ritonavir have the convenience of oral administration whereas Remdesivir must be administered parenterally which requires additional healthcare resources. **Mindeudesivir, Simnotrelvir/Ritonavir, and Ensitrelvir are other oral antivirals that have shown efficacy in resolution of symptoms in clinical trials but it is unknown if these drugs prevent mortality.**[2,3,6] **These are yet to be incorporated in major guidelines.**

Among patients (ambulatory or hospitalized) with mild-to-moderate COVID-19 at high risk for progression to severe disease, the IDSA guidelines recommend remdesivir initiated within seven days of symptom onset at a dose of 200mg on day 1 followed by 100mg on day 2 and day 3.[29] WHO recommends a 3 -day course for treatment of non-severe COVID-19 patients at high risk of hospitalization.[31] Indian guidelines do not recommend Remdesivir for mild COVID-19.

Among patients with mild-to-moderate COVID-19, inhaled corticosteroids failed to show or exclude a beneficial effect on mortality or hospitalization. In the **ACTIV-6 trial, inhaled fluticasone did not reduce time to recovery (HR 1.01, 95% CI 0.91-1.12) or the combined rate of urgent-care/emergency department visits, hospitalizations, or death by 28 days (3.7 versus 2.1 percent; HR 1.9, 95% CI 0.8-3.5) compared with placebo.**[12] However, more than 50% of patients in this trial had received 2 doses of vaccine and the baseline risk of severe disease was low. In the open-label **PRINCIPLE trial** (n=4700) who had risk factors for severe disease ($\geq$65 years old or $\geq$50 years old with comorbidities) suggested a trend towards reduced hospitalization or death rates with inhaled steroid (Budesonide 800 mcg twice daily) compared with usual care (6.8 versus 8.8 percent; OR 0.75, 95% CI 0.55-1.03), but the **difference was not statistically significant.**[38] However, this trial included patients with presumed COVID-19 without microbiological confirmation, thereby decreasing the confidence in the findings of the study.

An older systematic review of 3 RCTs found moderate certainty evidence that inhaled corticosteroids reduced hospital admission and symptom resolution at day 14 in patients with mild COVID-19.[39]

IDSA guidelines recommend against the use of inhaled corticosteroids among patients with ambulatory mild-to-moderate COVID-19.[29]

However, **Indian guidelines recommend inhalational budesonide at a dose of 800mcg twice a day for 5 days if symptoms are persistent beyond 5 days of onset in patients who are at a high risk of progression.**

The primary mechanism of action of convalescent plasma involves the transfer of endogenously produced neutralizing antibodies from recovered patients into patients with active COVID-19 disease.

Three RCTs reported on receipt of convalescent plasma by ambulatory persons with mild COVID-19 disease.[40-42] Receipt of COVID-19 convalescent plasma was associated with a reduction in hospitalization and a trend toward a reduction in COVID-19-related hospitalizations or medically attended visits; however, the evidence remains uncertain. Among ambulatory patients with mild-to-moderate COVID-19 at high risk for progression to severe disease who have no other treatment options, the **IDSA guidelines recommend FDA-qualified high-titer COVID-19 convalescent plasma within 8 days of symptom onset if other therapeutic options are not available.**[29] **WHO guidelines recommend against the use of convalescent plasma, except in the settings of a clinical trial.**[31]

Treatment of severe and critically ill COVID-19 patients

The use of steroids in COVID-19 has been extensively studied. It significantly reduced mortality and risk of progression to mechanical ventilation in severe COVID-19 patients, but no benefit is seen in patients not requiring ventilatory support. The

RECOVERY trial is a randomized trial among hospitalized patients in the United Kingdom which compared dexamethasone 6mg once a day for 10 days against standard care.[43] 16% of patients were receiving either IMV or ECMO, 60% were receiving oxygen supplementation with or without NIV and 24% were receiving neither. Among hospitalized patients, 28-day mortality was 17% lower in the dexamethasone group. In a meta-analysis of seven trials that included 1703 critically ill patients with COVID-19, glucocorticoids reduced 28-day mortality by 8% when compared with standard care or placebo.[44] Patients not requiring respiratory support do not seem to benefit from systemic steroids.[43]

Both IDSA and WHO guidelines panels recommend dexamethasone in severe as well as critical COVID-19 patients. Indian guidelines recommend treatment with dexamethasone for both moderate and severe COVID-19 patients.

In the **SOLIDARITY trial of patients hospitalized with COVID-19, there was a small difference in overall 28-day mortality between the remdesivir group and standard care group, but it was not statistically significant.** A living network meta-analysis of 5 RCTs showed moderate certainty evidence in favor of Remdesivir concerning the reduction in the need for mechanical ventilation and low certainty evidence regarding the decrease in mortality.[31] **Treatment with Remdesivir should be initiated as early as possible in the time course of disease. Among critically ill COVID-19 patients, there was low certainty evidence for impact on mortality and mechanical ventilation.** A possible explanation for this could be that remdesivir initiation in critically ill patients on life support might have happened late after disease onset. WHO recommends Remdesivir for treatment of severe COVID-19, however, it recommends against using Remdesivir in critically ill COVID-19 patients.

The role of molnupiravir in the treatment of hospitalized COVID-19 patients was evaluated in the **MOVe-In trial**, however, the trial was terminated early after slightly higher death rates were observed in molnupiravir arm.[45]

Multiple trials have evaluated the efficacy of Janus kinase inhibitors in patients with COVID-19 owing to their anti-inflammatory effect. Treatment with baricitinib is recommended for both severe and critically ill COVID-19 patients. In the RECOVERY trial[46], baricitinib was used along with corticosteroids and IL-6 inhibitors in 2659 patients. It reduced 28-day mortality compared with usual care alone (12 versus 14 percent; RR 0.87, 95% CI 0.77-0.99) **In the ACTT-2 trial, the combination of baricitinib and remdesivir showed a trend towards lower mortality.**[47] **Corticosteroids, which are currently part of standard therapy for the management of severe COVID-19, were not used in the ACTT-2 trial.**

A systematic review of 6 RCTs (5 of which reported the use of JAK inhibitors along with corticosteroids) evaluated the efficacy of JAK inhibitors for the treatment of COVID-19.[48] Systemic JAK inhibitors probably decrease all cause mortality up to day 28 (RR 0.72, 95% CI 0.57 to 0.91; 6 studies, 11,145 participants; moderate certainty evidence), and decrease all cause mortality up to day 60 (RR 0.69, 95% CI 0.56 to 0.86; 2 studies, 1626 participants; high certainty evidence).

Further evidence for Baricitinib came from a living network meta-analysis of 4 RCTs.[31] **Baricitinib was found to decrease mortality, duration of mechanical ventilation, and hospital stay.**

Among hospitalized adults with severe COVID-19, the **IDSA panel suggests baricitinib with corticosteroids. If corticosteroids are contraindicated, the IDSA guideline panel suggests the use of baricitinib with remdesivir rather than remdesivir alone.**

Immunopathology of SARS-CoV-2 infection is characterized by elevation of proinflammatory markers. Patients with increased levels of IL-6 are at increased risk for severe disease. IL-6 inhibitors can potentially mitigate the risks of a hyperinflammatory state associated with COVID-19 infection. **An RCT of 4116 patients from the UK[49] found that adding 1 to 2 doses of Tocilizumab reduced mortality by 4%. In a meta-analysis of 27 randomized trials,[50] it was found that 28-day all-cause mortality was lower among those who received tocilizumab compared with placebo or standard of care (OR 0.83, CI 0.74-0.92).**

A living network meta-analysis of 30 RCTs found high-certainty evidence to suggest that IL-6 inhibitors decrease mortality and the need for mechanical ventilation.[31] There was low-quality evidence to suggest that IL-6 inhibitors reduce the duration of mechanical ventilation and hospitalization.

Among hospitalized adults with progressive severe or critical COVID-19 who have elevated markers of systemic inflammation (CRP ≥75 mg/dl), the IDSA guidelines recommend tocilizumab in addition to standard of care. **When tocilizumab is not available for patients who would otherwise qualify for tocilizumab, the IDSA guidelines recommend sarilumab in addition to the standard of care.**[29] **WHO guidelines also recommend treatment with IL-6 receptor blockers in patients with severe or critical COVID-19.**

WHO recommends using ruxolitinib or tofacitinib in patients with severe or critical COVID-19 only if Baricitinib or IL-6 inhibitors are not available for use.[31]

Thromboprophylaxis

There was increasing evidence of COVID-associated venous thromboembolism secondary to endothelial dysfunction, activation of coagulation cascade, platelet activation, and stasis due to prolonged immobility. **Several studies have shown a reduction in all-cause mortality or thrombotic events with therapeutic/intermediate-dose anticoagulation but with an increased risk of bleeding.**[51,52]

The American Society of Hematology (ASH) guideline suggests using prophylactic-intensity over intermediate-intensity or therapeutic-intensity anticoagulation for patients with COVID-19-related critical illness who do not have suspected or confirmed venous thromboembolism. For hospitalized patients not requiring ICU care, therapeutic-intensity anticoagulation is recommended over prophylactic-intensity anticoagulation. **The guideline recommends against using anticoagulation among outpatients or post-discharge patients who don't have any other indications for anticoagulant therapy.**[53]

Supportive measures

During the COVID-19 pandemic, awake pronging became popular due to the proven benefits of prone positioning in patients on mechanical ventilation. Prone positioning aims to improve lung mechanics and gas exchange, leading to better clinical outcomes. It may be considered for conscious, cooperative, non-intubated patients with stable heart conditions. **WHO guidelines recommend awake-prone positioning for severely ill patients hospitalized with COVID-19 requiring supplemental oxygen (including HFNO) or non-invasive ventilation.** A systematic review by WHO COVID GDG showed that awake-prone positioning possibly reduces mortality and probably reduces the need for invasive ventilation, and ICU length of stay and has little or no effect on hospital length of stay.[28]

In hospitalized patients with severe or critical COVID-19 and acute hypoxemic respiratory failure (AHRF) not needing emergent intubation, WHO guidelines recommend HFNC or CPAP, or NIV over standard oxygen therapy.[28] **The WHO COVID GDG did not make any recommendation regarding HFNO versus CPAP vs NIV due to the uncertainty of the data.**

In the **HOT COVID trial** of 726 patients, it was found that targeting a low oxygenation target (PaO_2 = 60 mm Hg) **led to more days alive without support** as compared to a high oxygenation target (PaO_2 = 90 mm Hg). However, the difference in 90-day mortality was not statistically significant.[19]

Patients with ARDS due to COVID-19 are managed as per standard ARDS protocols.

Prophylactic therapy

Pemivibart is a monoclonal antibody active against JN.1, the dominant SARS-CoV-2 variant. In March 2024, it received an emergency use approval by US FDA to prevent COVID-19 in individuals age 12 years or older (weighing at least 40 kg) who have moderate-to-severe immunocompromising conditions.[54] An ongoing randomized controlled trial (RCT) is studying pre-exposure prophylaxis (PrEP) with a single dose of 4,500 mg IV pemivibart administration in adults ≥18 years of age at increased risk of SARS-CoV-2 infection or inadequate response to COVID-19 vaccination [CANOPY trial]. Results of the effect of pemivibart in preventing symptomatic COVID infections are expected later in 2024.

Vaccines

Different platforms have been utilized to develop COVID-19 vaccines (Table 4).

Vaccination has proven effective in reducing the risk of severe COVID-19 and has been linked to a substantial decline in hospitalizations and deaths associated with the virus. Unvaccinated individuals consistently have higher rates of hospitalization and mortality from COVID-19 than vaccinated individuals.

A study of over 1 million vaccinated members of a healthcare system in USA assessed the frequency of developing a severe COVID-19 outcome after completing a primary COVID-19 vaccination.[55] The rates of severe disease (defined as hospitalization with a diagnosis of acute respiratory failure, need for noninvasive ventilation, admission to an intensive care unit including all persons requiring invasive mechanical ventilation, or death, including discharge to hospice) and death due to breakthrough COVID-19 were found to be 1.5 and 0.3 per 10,000, respectively.

A study examining over 8,000 COVID-19 deaths in the United States found that vaccination, including a bivalent booster, was significantly associated with lower mortality rates compared to no vaccination.[56] Unvaccinated individuals were 7.3 to 16.3 times more likely to die from COVID-19.

Table 4: Vaccines types and examples

Type	Description	Examples
Inactivated vaccines	Produced by growing SARS-CoV-2 in cell culture then chemically inactivating the virus. Often combined with an adjuvant to stimulate immune response.	• CoronaVac (Sinovac) • BBIBP-CorV/HBO2 (Covilo, Sinopharm [Beijing]) • Covaxin (Bharat Biotech)
Live attenuated vaccines	Produced by developing weakened versions of wild-type SARS-CoV-2 through genetic modification or growth in adverse conditions.	• COVI-VAC (Codagenix/Serum Institute of India) – in early trials
mRNA vaccines	Consist of mRNA encoding target gene. Once administered, mRNA is translated into target protein, which elicits immune response	• BNT162b2 (Pfizer-BioNTech vaccine) • mRNA-1273 (Moderna vaccine) • GEMCOVAC-19 (Gennova Biopharmaceuticals)
Vector virus vaccines	Uses a different virus (not SARS-CoV-2) as a vector or carrier that expresses the viral protein that is the intended target	• Ad26.COV2.S (Janssen/Johnson & Johnson) • ChAdOx1 nCoV-19/AZD1222 (AstraZeneca) • Gam-COVID-Vac Sputnik V (Gamaleya Institute) • Ad5-nCoV (CanSino) • DelNS1-2019-nCoV-RBD-OPT1, an intranasal flu-based RBD vaccine (University of Hong Kong) – in trials • iNCOVACC (Bharat Biotech)
Recombinant vaccines	Composed of purified viral proteins that have been expressed in one of various systems	• NVX-CoV2373 (Novavax)
DNA vaccines	Consist of plasmid DNA that contain mammalian expression promotors and the target gene, so that the target protein is expressed in the recipient	• ZyCoV-D (Cadila Healthcare)

Discontinued vaccines

Some vaccines like Covishield (SII/AstraZeneca), Ad26.COV2.S (Johnson &Johnson), monovalent mRNA-Moderna have been retracted from FDA approval or suspended by WHO. Covishield vaccine was reportedly associated with Thrombotic Thrombocytopenic Syndrome and was discontinued.

Comparison of vaccines

A network meta-analysis of 25 RCTs involving 22 vaccines showed that none of vaccines had a higher incidence of SAEs than the placebo.[57] **There were no significant differences among the various types of vaccines regarding the efficacy in preventing symptomatic SARS-CoV-2 infection, although there was a trend toward higher efficacy of the mRNA vaccines.** BNT162b2 had the highest efficacy in preventing symptomatic SARS-CoV-2 infection in adults and the elderly, whereas BIV1-CovIran had the lowest incidence of SAEs in adults. mRNA vaccines were significantly inferior in safety when compared to other vaccines.

Table 5: WHO COVID-19 vaccination recommendations

Vaccination status	Population	Recommendation
Never received a COVID-19 vaccine	All adults	1 dose[a]
	Children and adolescents with comorbidities	
	Health workers with direct patient contact	
	Pregnant persons	1 dose
	Any immunocompromised individual	2 to 3 doses[b]
Received at least 1 dose of a COVID-19 vaccine	Adults over 75 or 80 years old[c]	Revaccination 6 to 12 months after the most recent dose
	Adults over 50 or 60 years old[c] with comorbidities	
	Any individual who is immunocompromised	
	Adults over 50 or 60 years old[c]	Revaccination 12 months after the most recent dose
	Adults with comorbidities	
	Health workers with direct patient contact	
	Pregnant persons	Single dose in each pregnancy
	Healthy adults	Revaccination not routinely recommended
	Children and adolescents	

a. 2 doses required for inactivated vaccines

b. In consultation with a health worker

c. Age cut-off depending on countries

Post COVID-19 pulmonary sequelae

Lung function and radiological abnormalities have been reported in survivors of SARS-CoV-1.[58] Persistent ground glass opacities, parenchymal bands and traction bronchiectasis have been reported among survivors of COVID-19 at 1-2 years after discharge.[59] Lung function abnormalities like restrictive pattern on spirometry and diffusion impairment have been reported which show an improving trend leading to a plateau phase. **A 3 year follow up study from China reported that there was a gradual improvement in diffusing capacity of lung for carbon monoxide (DLCO) and residual lung abnormalities, however more than 30% patients continued to have persistent lung abnormalities at 3-year follow-up.**[60]

In a prospective study from Japan, 30 patients requiring ICU management for COVID-19 were treated with Nintedanib and compared with a historical control group.[61] **The primary endpoint was 28-day mortality. There was no significant difference in 28-day mortality between the groups, however length of mechanical ventilation was shorter in the nintedanib group**. Computed tomography volumetry showed that the percentages of high-attenuation areas were significantly lower in the nintedanib group at liberation from mechanical ventilation.

Trials are underway to evaluate the role of anti-fibrotics in the management of the post-covid pulmonary sequelae. **ENDOCOV-I** is a prospective trial from which is investigating the effect of nintedanib on slowing the rate of lung disease in patients who have been diagnosed with COVID-19 and have ongoing lung injury more than 30 days out from their diagnosi.[62]

Therapeutics and COVID-19: living guideline - World Health Organization (WHO)

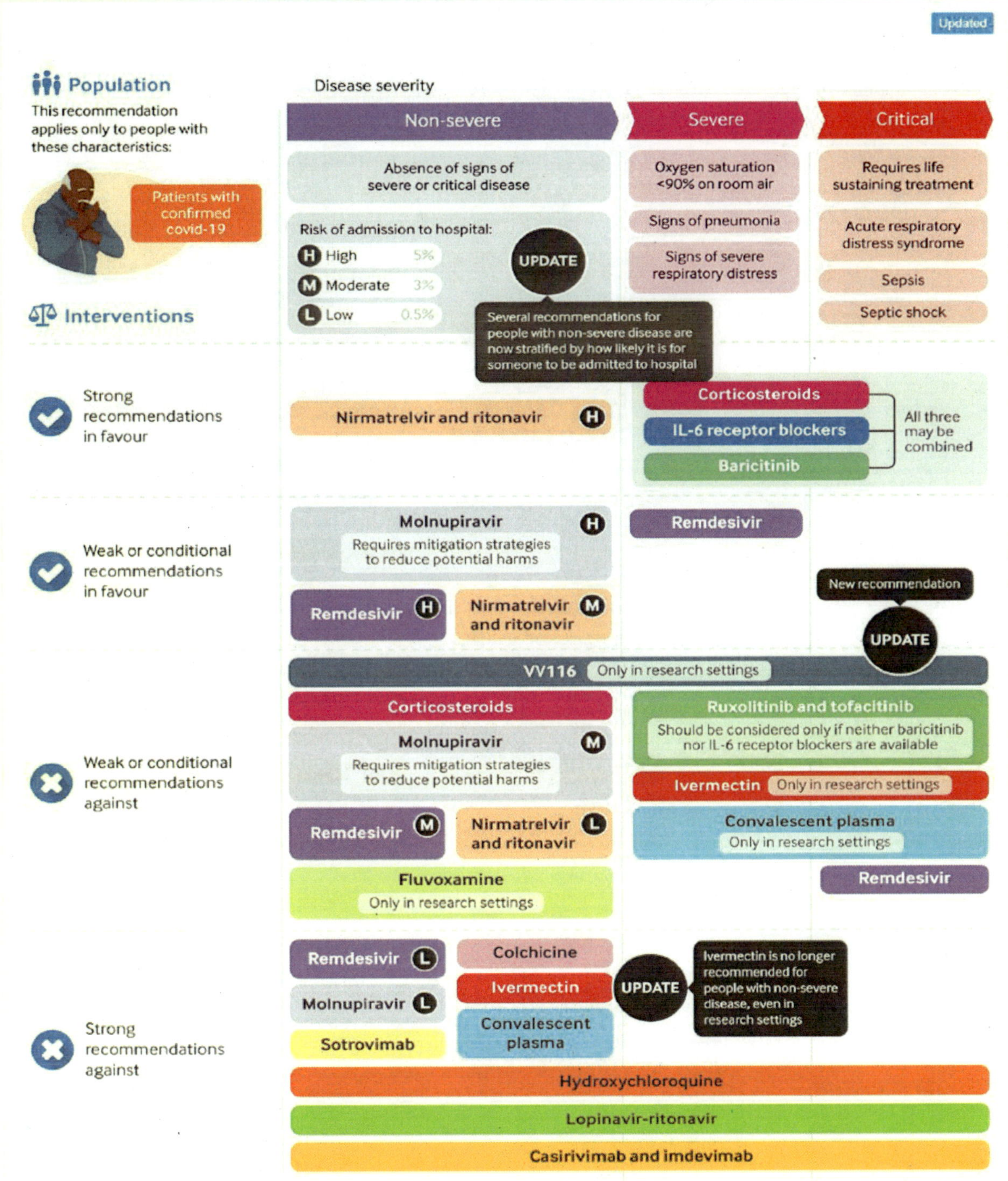

Figure 1: WHO guidelines for COVID-19 (November 2023)

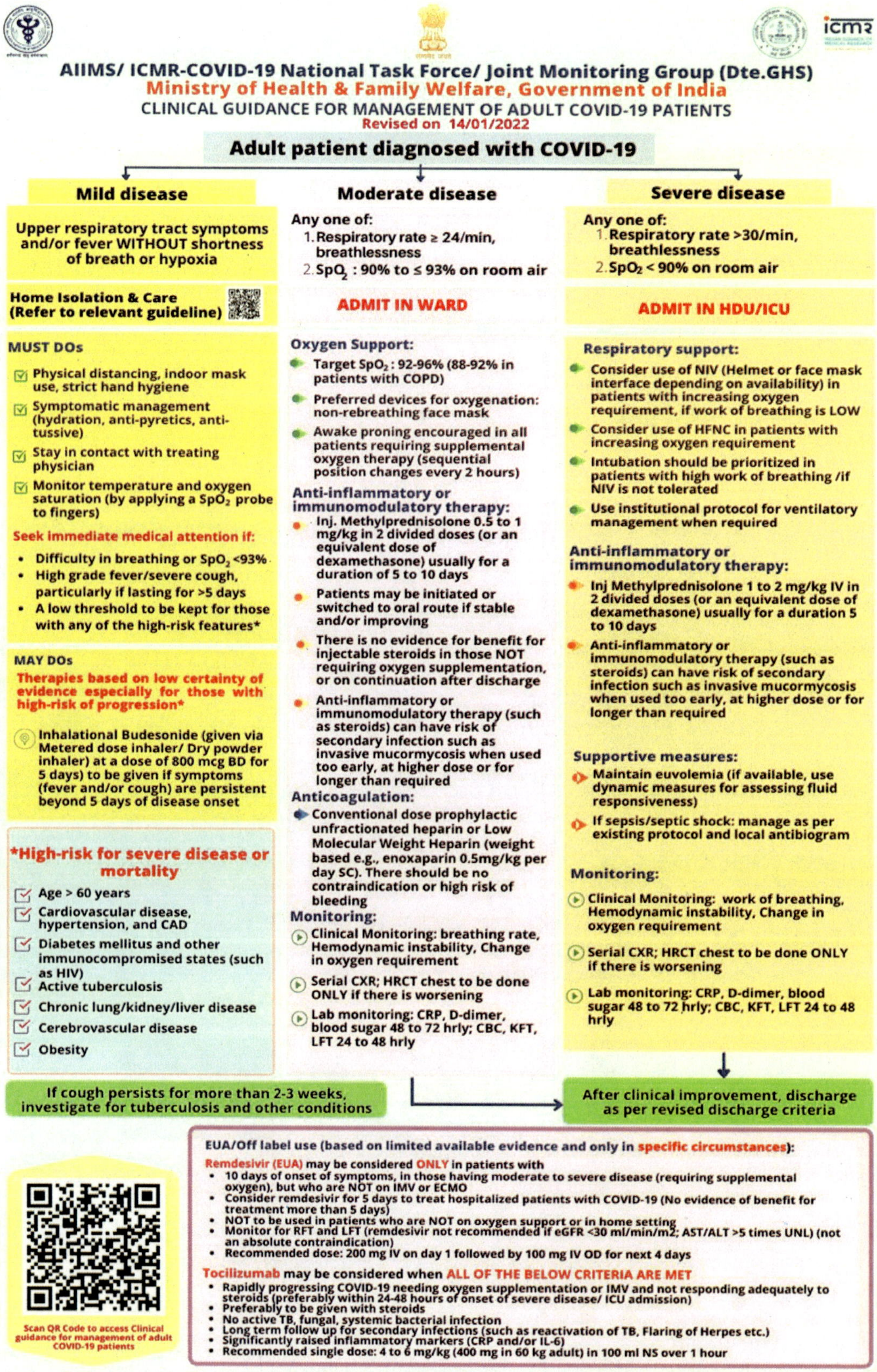

Figure 2: AIIMS-ICMR Covid-19 guidelines

REFERENCES

1. Sun M, Lai H, Huang J, Liu J, Li Y, Tian J, et al. Molnupiravir for the treatment of non-severe COVID-19: a systematic review and meta-analysis of 14 randomized trials with 34 570 patients. J Antimicrob Chemother. 2023 Sep 1;78(9):2131–9.

2. Oral Simnotrelvir for Adult Patients with Mild-to-Moderate Covid-19 | New England Journal of Medicine [Internet]. [cited 2024 Sep 3]. Available from: https://www.nejm.org/doi/full/10.1056/NEJMoa2301425

3. Yotsuyanagi H, Ohmagari N, Doi Y, Yamato M, Bac NH, Cha BK, et al. Efficacy and Safety of 5-Day Oral Ensitrelvir for Patients With Mild to Moderate COVID-19: The SCORPIO-SR Randomized Clinical Trial. JAMA Netw Open. 2024 Feb 9;7(2):e2354991.

4. Salvadori N, Jourdain G, Krittayaphong R, Siripongboonsitti T, Kongsaengdao S, Atipornwanich K, et al. Molnupiravir versus favipiravir in at-risk outpatients with COVID-19: A randomized controlled trial in Thailand. Int J Infect Dis [Internet]. 2024 Jun 1 [cited 2024 Sep 8];143. Available from: https://www.ijidonline.com/article/S1201-9712(24)00092-4/fulltext

5. Efficacy and safety of antiviral treatments for symptomatic COVID-19 outpatients: Systematic review and network meta-analysis - ScienceDirect [Internet]. [cited 2024 Sep 3]. Available from: https://www.sciencedirect.com/science/article/abs/pii/S0166354223002462?via%3Dihub

6. Fan X, Dai X, Ling Y, Wu L, Tang L, Peng C, et al. Oral VV116 versus placebo in patients with mild-to-moderate COVID-19 in China: a multicentre, double-blind, phase 3, randomised controlled study. Lancet Infect Dis. 2024 Feb 1;24(2):129–39.

7. Yang Z, Xu Y, Zheng R, Ye L, Lv G, Cao Z, et al. COVID-19 Rebound After VV116 vs Nirmatrelvir-Ritonavir Treatment: A Randomized Clinical Trial. JAMA Netw Open. 2024 Mar 13;7(3):e241765.

8. Okoli GN, Askin N, Rabbani R. Nirmatrelvir/Ritonavir Regimen for Mild/Moderately Severe COVID-19: A Rapid Review With Meta-Analysis and Trial Sequential Analysis. Ann Fam Med. 2024 Jul 1;22(4):336–46.

9. Sun J, Wang S, Ma X, Wei Q, Peng Y, Bai Y, et al. Efficacy and safety of baricitinib for the treatment of hospitalized adults with COVID-19: a systematic review and meta-analysis. Eur J Med Res. 2023 Nov 21;28(1):536.

10. Intravenous aviptadil and remdesivir for treatment of COVID-19-associated hypoxaemic respiratory failure in the USA (TESICO): a randomised, placebo-controlled trial - The Lancet Respiratory Medicine [Internet]. [cited 2024 Sep 8]. Available from: https://www.thelancet.com/journals/lanres/article/PIIS2213-2600(23)00147-9/fulltext

11. Paules CI, Wang J, Tomashek KM, Bonnett T, Singh K, Marconi VC, et al. A Risk Profile Using Simple Hematologic Parameters to Assess Benefits From Baricitinib in Patients Hospitalized With COVID-19: A Post Hoc Analysis of the Adaptive COVID-19 Treatment Trial-2. Ann Intern Med. 2024 Mar 19;177(3):343–52.

12. Boulware DR, Lindsell CJ, Stewart TG, Hernandez AF, Collins S, McCarthy MW, et al. Inhaled Fluticasone Furoate for Outpatient Treatment of Covid-19. N Engl J Med. 2023 Sep 20;389(12):1085–95.

13. Snow TAC, Arulkumaran N, Singer M, Choi SH. Effect of dexamethasone dose on outcomes in acute COVID-19 disease: A systematic review and meta-analysis. J Infect. 2023 Dec 1;87(6):490–7.

14. Pitre T, Su J, Mah J, Helmeczi W, Danho S, Plaxton W, et al. Higher-versus Lower-Dose Corticosteroids for Severe to Critical COVID-19: A Systematic Review and Dose–Response Meta-analysis. Ann Am Thorac Soc. 2023 Apr;20(4):596–604.

15. Arulkumaran N, Thomas M, Stubbs M, Prasanna N, Subhan M, Singh D, et al. A randomised controlled trial of plasma exchange compared to standard of care in the treatment of severe COVID-19 infection (COVIPLEX). Sci Rep. 2024 Jul 23;14(1):16876.

16. Convalescent Plasma for Covid-19–Induced ARDS in Mechanically Ventilated Patients | New England Journal of Medicine [Internet]. [cited 2024 Sep 3]. Available from: https://www.nejm.org/doi/full/10.1056/NEJMoa2209502

17. Maor Y, Shinar E, Izak M, Rahav G, Brosh-Nissimov T, Kessler A, et al. A Randomized Controlled Study Assessing Convalescent Immunoglobulins vs Convalescent Plasma for Hospitalized Patients With Coronavirus 2019. Clin Infect Dis. 2023 Oct 1;77(7):964–71.

18. Al Hashim AH, Al Reesi A, Al Lawati NM, Burad J, Al Khabori M, Chandwani J, et al. Comparison of Noninvasive Mechanical Ventilation With High-Flow Nasal Cannula, Face-Mask, and Helmet in Hypoxemic Respiratory Failure in Patients With COVID-19: A Randomized Controlled Trial*. Crit Care Med. 2023 Nov;51(11):1515.

19. Nielsen FM, Klitgaard TL, Siegemund M, Laake JH, Thormar KM, Cole JM, et al. Lower vs Higher Oxygenation Target and Days Alive Without Life Support in COVID-19: The HOT-COVID Randomized Clinical Trial. JAMA. 2024 Apr 9;331(14):1185–94.

20. Therapeutic high-dose vitamin D for vitamin D-deficient severe COVID-19 disease: randomized, double-blind, placebo-controlled study (SHADE-S) | Journal of Public Health | Oxford Academic [Internet]. [cited 2024 Sep 3]. Available from: https://academic.oup.com/jpubhealth/article-abstract/46/2/256/7591923? redirectedFrom=fulltext

21. Huang T, Yu J, Zhang S, Teng D, Dai D, Zhu Y, et al. Immunogenicity and safety of concomitant administration of recombinant COVID-19 vaccine and quadrivalent inactivated influenza vaccine in Chinese adults: An open-label, randomized, controlled trial. Hum Vaccines Immunother. 2024 Dec 31;20(1):2330770.

22. Fernandez-de-las-Peñas C, Notarte KI, Macasaet R, Velasco JV, Catahay JA, Ver AT, et al. Persistence of post-COVID symptoms in the general population two years after SARS-CoV-2 infection: A systematic review and meta-analysis. J Infect. 2024 Feb 1;88(2):77–88.

23. Oliveira MR, Hoffman M, Jones AW, Holland AE, Borghi-Silva A. Effect of Pulmonary Rehabilitation on Exercise Capacity, Dyspnea, Fatigue, and Peripheral Muscle Strength in Patients With Post-COVID-19 Syndrome: A Systematic Review and Meta-analysis. Arch Phys Med Rehabil. 2024 Aug 1;105(8):1559–70.

24. Geng LN, Bonilla H, Hedlin H, Jacobson KB, Tian L, Jagannathan P, et al. Nirmatrelvir-Ritonavir and Symptoms in Adults With Postacute Sequelae of SARS-CoV-2 Infection: The STOP-PASC Randomized Clinical Trial. JAMA Intern Med. 2024 Sep 1;184(9):1024–34.

25. Todsen T, Jakobsen KK, Grønlund MP, Callesen RE, Folke F, Larsen H, et al. COVID-19 Rapid Antigen Tests With Self-Collected vs Health Care Worker–Collected Nasal and Throat Swab Specimens: A Randomized Clinical Trial. JAMA Netw Open. 2023 Dec 6;6(12):e2344295.

26. Gioia F, Walti LN, Orchanian-Cheff A, Husain S. Risk factors for COVID-19-associated pulmonary aspergillosis: a systematic review and meta-analysis. Lancet Respir Med. 2024 Mar;12(3):207–16.

27. Effects of renin–angiotensin system blockers on outcomes from COVID-19: a systematic review and meta-analysis of randomized controlled trials | European Heart Journal - Cardiovascular Pharmacotherapy | Oxford Academic [Internet]. [cited 2024 Sep 3]. Available from: https://academic.oup.com/ehjcvp/article/10/1/68/7280755

28. Clinical management of COVID-19: Living guideline, 18 August 2023 [Internet]. [cited 2024 Sep 3]. Available from: https://www.who.int/publications/i/item/WHO-2019-nCoV-clinical-2023.2

29. IDSA Guidelines on the Treatment and Management of Patients with COVID-19 [Internet]. [cited 2024 Sep 3]. Available from: https://www.idsociety.org/practice-guideline/covid-19-guideline-treatment-and-management/

30. Oral Nirmatrelvir for High-Risk, Nonhospitalized Adults with Covid-19 | New England Journal of Medicine [Internet]. [cited 2024 Sep 3]. Available from: https://www.nejm.org/doi/full/10.1056/NEJMoa2118542

31. Therapeutics and COVID-19: Living guideline, 10 November 2023 [Internet]. [cited 2024 Sep 3]. Available from: https://www.who.int/publications/i/item/WHO-2019-nCoV-therapeutics-2023.2

32. Wong GLH, Yip TCF, Lai MSM, Wong VWS, Hui DSC, Lui GCY. Incidence of Viral Rebound After Treatment With Nirmatrelvir-Ritonavir and Molnupiravir. JAMA Netw Open. 2022 Dec 6;5(12):e2245086.

33. Ranganath N, O'Horo JC, Challener DW, Tulledge-Scheitel SM, Pike ML, O'Brien M, et al. Rebound Phenomenon After Nirmatrelvir/Ritonavir Treatment of Coronavirus Disease 2019 (COVID-19) in High-Risk Persons. Clin Infect Dis Off Publ Infect Dis Soc Am. 2023 Feb 8;76(3):e537–9.

34. Anderson AS, Caubel P, Rusnak JM. Nirmatrelvir–Ritonavir and Viral Load Rebound in Covid-19. N Engl J Med. 2022 Sep 14;387(11):1047–9.

35. Bernal AJ, Silva MMG da, Musungaie DB, Kovalchuk E, Gonzalez A, Reyes VD, et al. Molnupiravir for Oral Treatment of Covid-19 in Nonhospitalized Patients. N Engl J Med. 2022 Feb 9;386(6):509–20.

36. Early Remdesivir to Prevent Progression to Severe Covid-19 in Outpatients | New England Journal of Medicine [Internet]. [cited 2024 Sep 3]. Available from: https://www.nejm.org/doi/full/10.1056/NEJMoa2116846

37. Compassionate Use of Remdesivir in Pregnant Women With Severe Coronavirus Disease 2019 | Clinical Infectious Diseases | Oxford Academic [Internet]. [cited 2024 Sep 30]. Available from: https://academic.oup.com/cid/article/73/11/e3996/5919737?login=false

38. Yu LM, Bafadhel M, Dorward J, Hayward G, Saville BR, Gbinigie O, et al. Inhaled budesonide for COVID-19 in people at high risk of complications in the community in the UK (PRINCIPLE): a randomised, controlled, open-label, adaptive platform trial. The Lancet. 2021 Sep 4;398(10303):843–55.

39. Griesel[a] M, Wagner[a] C, Mikolajewska A, Stegemann M, Fichtner F, Metzendorf MI, et al. Inhaled corticosteroids for the treatment of COVID 19. Cochrane Database Syst Rev [Internet]. 2022 [cited 2024 Sep 30];2022(3). Available from: https://www.readcube.com/articles/10.1002%2F14651858.cd015125

40. Libster R, Marc GP, Wappner D, Coviello S, Bianchi A, Braem V, et al. Early High-Titer Plasma Therapy to Prevent Severe Covid-19 in Older Adults. N Engl J Med. 2021 Feb 17;384(7):610–8.

41. Korley FK, Durkalski-Mauldin V, Yeatts SD, Schulman K, Davenport RD, Dumont LJ, et al. Early Convalescent Plasma for High-Risk Outpatients with Covid-19. N Engl J Med. 2021 Nov 17;385(21):1951–60.

42. Early Outpatient Treatment for Covid-19 with Convalescent Plasma | New England Journal of Medicine [Internet]. [cited 2024 Sep 3]. Available from: https://www.nejm.org/doi/10.1056/NEJMoa2119657?url_ver=Z39.88-2003&rfr_id=ori:rid: crossref.org&rfr_dat=cr_pub%20%200pubmed

43. Dexamethasone in Hospitalized Patients with Covid-19 | New England Journal of Medicine [Internet]. [cited 2024 Sep 3]. Available from: https://www.nejm.org/doi/full/10.1056/NEJMoa2021436

44. The WHO Rapid Evidence Appraisal for COVID-19 Therapies (REACT) Working Group. Association Between Administration of Systemic Corticosteroids and Mortality Among Critically Ill Patients With COVID-19: A Meta-analysis. JAMA. 2020 Oct 6;324(13):1330–41.

45. Results Posted | Efficacy and Safety of Molnupiravir (MK-4482) in Hospitalized Adult Participants With COVID-19 (MK-4482-001) | ClinicalTrials.gov [Internet]. [cited 2024 Sep 30]. Available from: https://clinicaltrials.gov/study/NCT04575584?tab=results

46. Abani O, Abbas A, Abbas F, Abbas J, Abbas K, Abbas M, et al. Baricitinib in patients admitted to hospital with COVID-19 (RECOVERY): a randomised, controlled, open-label, platform trial and updated meta-analysis. The Lancet. 2022 Jul 30;400(10349):359–68.

47. Baricitinib plus Remdesivir for Hospitalized Adults with Covid-19 | New England Journal of Medicine [Internet]. [cited 2024 Sep 4]. Available from: https://www.nejm.org/doi/full/10.1056/NEJMoa2031994

48. Kramer[a] A, Prinz[a] C, Fichtner[a] F, Fischer AL, Thieme V, Grundeis F, et al. Janus kinase inhibitors for the treatment of COVID 19. Cochrane Database Syst Rev [Internet]. 2022 [cited 2024 Sep 30];(6). Available from: https://www.cochranelibrary.com/cdsr/doi/10.1002/14651858.CD015209/full

49. Abani O, Abbas A, Abbas F, Abbas M, Abbasi S, Abbass H, et al. Tocilizumab in patients admitted to hospital with COVID-19 (RECOVERY): a randomised, controlled, open-label, platform trial. The Lancet. 2021 May 1;397(10285):1637–45.

50. The WHO Rapid Evidence Appraisal for COVID-19 Therapies (REACT) Working Group. Association Between Administration of IL-6 Antagonists and Mortality Among Patients Hospitalized for COVID-19: A Meta-analysis. JAMA. 2021 Aug 10;326(6):499–518.

51. null null. Therapeutic Anticoagulation with Heparin in Critically Ill Patients with Covid-19. N Engl J Med. 2021 Aug 25;385(9):777–89.

52. null null. Therapeutic Anticoagulation with Heparin in Noncritically Ill Patients with Covid-19. N Engl J Med. 2021 Aug 25;385(9):790–802.

53. COVID-19 and VTE-Anticoagulation - Hematology.org [Internet]. [cited 2024 Sep 3]. Available from: https://www.hematology.org/covid-19/covid-19-and-vte-anticoagulation

54. Commissioner O of the. FDA. FDA; 2024 [cited 2024 Sep 3]. FDA Roundup: March 22, 2024. Available from: https://www.fda.gov/news-events/press-announcements/fda-roundup-march-22-2024

55. Yek C. Risk Factors for Severe COVID-19 Outcomes Among Persons Aged ≥18 Years Who Completed a Primary COVID-19 Vaccination Series — 465 Health Care Facilities, United States, December 2020–October 2021. MMWR Morb Mortal Wkly Rep [Internet]. 2022 [cited 2024 Sep 3];71. Available from: https://www.cdc.gov/mmwr/volumes/71/wr/mm7101a4.htm

56. Johnson AG. Notes from the Field: Comparison of COVID-19 Mortality Rates Among Adults Aged ≥65 Years Who Were Unvaccinated and Those Who Received a Bivalent Booster Dose Within the Preceding 6 Months — 20 U.S. Jurisdictions, September 18, 2022–April 1, 2023. MMWR Morb Mortal Wkly Rep [Internet]. 2023 [cited 2024 Sep 3];72. Available from: https://www.cdc.gov/mmwr/volumes/72/wr/mm7224a6.htm

57. Wu X, Xu K, Zhan P, Liu H, Zhang F, Song Y, et al. Comparative efficacy and safety of COVID-19 vaccines in phase III trials: a network meta-analysis. BMC Infect Dis. 2024 Feb 21;24(1):234.

58. Ng C, Chan J, Kwan T, To T, Chan Y, Ng F, et al. Six month radiological and physiological outcomes in severe acute respiratory syndrome (SARS) survivors. Thorax. 2004 Oct;59(10):889–91.

59. Carvalho CRR, Lamas C de A, Luna LAV de, Chate RC, Salge JM, Sawamura MVY, et al. Post-COVID-19 respiratory sequelae two years after hospitalization: an ambidirectional study. Lancet Reg Health – Am [Internet]. 2024 May 1 [cited 2024 Sep 8];33. Available from: https://www.thelancet.com/journals/lanam/article/PIIS2667-193X(24)00060-7/fulltext

60. Han X, Chen L, Guo L, Wu L, Alwalid O, Liu J, et al. Long-term radiological and pulmonary function abnormalities at 3 years after COVID-19 hospitalisation: a longitudinal cohort study. Eur Respir J [Internet]. 2024 Jul 1 [cited 2024 Sep 8];64(1). Available from: https://erj.ersjournals.com/content/64/1/2301612

61. Umemura Y, Mitsuyama Y, Minami K, Nishida T, Watanabe A, Okada N, et al. Efficacy and safety of nintedanib for pulmonary fibrosis in severe pneumonia induced by COVID-19: An interventional study. Int J Infect Dis. 2021 Jul 1;108:454–60.

62. ctv.veeva.com [Internet]. [cited 2024 Sep 8]. The Study of the Use of Nintedanib in Slowing Lung Disease in Patients With Fibrotic or Non-Fibrotic Interstitial Lung Disease Related to COVID-19. Available from: https://ctv.veeva.com/study/the-study-of-the-use-of-nintedanib-in-slowing-lung-disease-in-patients-with-fibrotic-or-non-fibrotic.

CHAPTER 11

Drug Sensitive Tuberculosis

Authors: Dr. Arunachalam, Dr. Murugan Natarajan

Reviewer: Dr. Jitendra Kumar Saini

INTRODUCTION

Tuberculosis is a leading global public health challenge, with high human morbidity and mortality. Until the COVID-19 pandemic, TB remained the leading cause of death from a single infectious agent, ranking above HIV/acquired immune deficiency syndrome and influenza.[1] The incidence rate of tuberculosis in India had fallen from 237 per lakh population in 2015 to 199 per lakh population in 2022, while the mortality rate had declined from 28 per lakh population in 2015 to 23 per lakh population in 2022, according to the India TB report 2024 released by the Union Health Ministry on March 27, stating that the country has set 2025 as the target for eliminating the disease.[2]

One of the goals of RNTCP when it was introduced in 1997 throughout our nation was to decrease the morbidity and mortality due to tuberculosis, and cut down the chain of transmission until TB is no longer a public health problem. The program also envisaged universal access to quality diagnosis and treatment.[3] Since then, there have been a lot of advancements in the diagnosis and treatment of tuberculosis. Rapid molecular diagnostics have reduced the turnaround time and also helped in the early identification of drug resistance. Implementing shorter regimens has helped in adherence and, in turn, led to a favourable outcome. Digital tools have helped in case management, and monitoring adherence thereby enhancing the quality of care. These efforts are augmented with Tuberculosis preventive therapy, which prevents the progression of latent TB infection to active tuberculosis.

The introduction of Artificial intelligence has transformed healthcare enhancing both diagnosis and treatment. Deep learning algorithms have helped in the analysis of chest X-rays with considerable accuracy and are a boon in resource-limited settings. They also help in predicting patients with poor outcomes at the time of diagnosis which allows health care professionals to make informed decisions about the patients.[4]

Despite all these advancements, there are deterrents to tuberculosis elimination. Undernutrition is one of them; it is not only a risk factor for TB but also leads to poor treatment outcomes, increased severity, and early TB deaths.[5] Other challenges include drug-resistant tuberculosis, HIV-TB co-infection social stigma associated with tuberculosis, and other emerging infectious diseases that steal the limelight from tuberculosis.

This introduction will provide an overview of recent advances in the diagnosis and management of drug-sensitive tuberculosis, salient programmatic updates, tuberculosis preventive therapy, and the role of artificial intelligence and nutrition in the TB care cascade which are important for achieving the WHO's sustainable development goals, 90% reduction in the number of TB deaths and an 80% reduction in the TB incidence rate (new cases per 100,000 population per year) by 2030.[6]

Methodology

A PubMed and Cochrane dataset search was done with Boolean search keywords: "Tuberculosis OR TB". Articles between the period of August 2023 to August 2024 were reviewed. Publications were limited to human studies in the English language. Initially 20,772 articles were identified. Then we systematically refined the search using the following Boolean operators and search terms "[{(tuberculosis) OR (EPTB) OR (pulmonary tuberculosis)} AND {(diagnosis) OR (treatment) OR (management) OR (chemotherapy)}]" which identified 3209 publication abstracts, which were retrieved for assessment. Out of this RCT, Systematic reviews and meta-analysis from August 2023 to August 2024 were 183. We excluded duplicate studies, while the study with a higher level of evidence and published in a high-impact journal was selected.

We finally enrolled a total of 18 studies related to drug-sensitive TB (DSTB) updates which were found eligible for practice-changing updates and likely to have an impact on upcoming treatment strategy.

Electronic database search: PubMed, Cochrane Library

Period: 1st August 2023 to 1st August 2024

Search words: [{(tuberculosis) OR (EPTB) OR (pulmonary tuberculosis)} AND {(diagnosis) OR (treatment) OR (management) OR (chemotherapy)}]

n=3,209

↓

RCT, Clinical trial, Meta-analysis & Systematic Review

n=183

↓

Articles after screening for relevance n=18

Analysis of Literature

Tuberculosis prevention

- ***High-dose, short-duration versus standard rifampicin for tuberculosis preventive treatment: A partially blinded, three-arm, non-inferiority, randomized, controlled trial. (Lancet. 2024)***[7]
  - *Population:* Participants aged 10 years or older were included if they indicated TPT according to WHO guidelines for Indonesia and Vietnam, Canadian guidelines for Canadian sites, and a positive tuberculin skin test or interferon-γ release assay. (n=1376)
  - *Intervention:* a) 20 mg/kg daily for 2 months (20 mg/kg group, n=461). b) 30 mg/kg daily for 2 months (30 mg/kg group, n=453).
  - *Comparator:* Oral rifampicin at 10 mg/kg once daily for 4 months (standard-dose group n=454).

- *Outcome:* Of the 1368 participants who were included in the modified intention to treat population, 454 were in the 10 mg/Kg group, 461 in the 20 mg/kg group, and 453 in the 30 mg/kg group. 372 (82%) in the standard-dose group, 329 (71%) in the 20 mg/kg group, and 293 (65%) in the 30 mg/kg group completed treatment. No participants in the standard-dose group, one (<1%) of 441 participants in the 20 mg/kg group, and four (1%) of 423 in the 30 mg/kg group developed grade 3 hepatotoxicity.
- *Conclusion:* 30 mg/kg daily rifampicin therapy has significantly worse safety and completion than 4 months of 10 mg/kg daily and 2 months of 20 mg/kg daily.
- *Critical appraisal:* Further studies to compare the effectiveness of weekly regimen as the convenience and cumulative dosage are minimal compared to daily therapy.

- ***Household- Versus Incentive-Based Contact Investigation for Tuberculosis in Rural South Africa: A Cluster-Randomized Trial. (Clin Infect Dis. 2023)***[8]
  - *Population:* TB contacts in 28 public primary care clinics in South Africa.
  - *Intervention:* In the incentive-based arm, both index patients and ≤10 of their close contacts (either within or outside the household) were given small cash incentives for presenting to study clinics for TB screening (n=14 clinics).
  - *Comparator:* In the household tracing strategy, study teams visited the households of consenting TB index patients, where symptom screening was done for all household contacts. A spot sputum sample was collected for TB testing from all contacts, regardless of symptoms. (n=14 clinics).
  - *Outcome:* A total of 2923 patients were started on TB treatment during the study period: 1413 during household-based tracing periods and 1510 during incentive-based tracing periods (adjusted incidence rate ratio [IRR]: 1.05; 95% CI: .97–1.13).
  - *Conclusion:* Incentive-based contact investigation for TB has similar effectiveness to traditional household-based approaches and may be a viable alternative or complementary approach to household-based investigation.
  - *Critical appraisal:* The study clinics were purposively sampled based on the burden of TB patients so the findings may not be generalized to remote clinics with low TB burden. Study clinics and patients were not blinded to allocation, so there is a possibility of resultant bias.

Diagnosis

- ***Ratios from full blood count as markers for TB diagnosis, treatment, prognosis: A systematic review. (Int J Tuberc Lung Dis. 2023)***[9]
  - *Population:* Studies done on patients with tuberculosis and control mentioning MLR (Monocyte: Lymphocyte) and NLR (Neutrophil: Lymphocyte ratio). (n=11,952)
  - *Intervention:* MLR and NLR in patients with tuberculosis.
  - *Comparator:* MLR and NLR in normal individuals.
  - *Outcome:* Increased MLR and NLR were associated with TB disease when compared to healthy controls and individuals with TB infection. MLR was shown to be prognostic for progression to TB disease and to decrease in response to TB treatment.
  - *Conclusion:* Higher MLR and NLR are associated with TB disease and could be used as easy-to-obtain, low-cost additional diagnostic biomarkers.
  - *Critical appraisal:* Most of the studies had a retrospective study design and further controlled studies are required.

- ***A systematic review and meta-analysis of circulating serum and plasma microRNAs in TB diagnosis. (BMC Infectious Diseases. 2024)***[10]
  - o *Population:* Systematic review and meta-analysis on online search of articles involving circulating miRNA among LTB, Pulmonary TB, and healthy individuals from 7 studies.
  - o *Intervention:* Participants with latent tuberculosis and active tuberculosis.
  - o *Comparator:* Healthy individuals.
  - o *Outcome:* Overall sensitivity of 81.9% (95% CI: 74.2, 87.7) and specificity of 68.3% (95% CI: 57.8, 77.2). The miRNA signature model (miR197-3p, miR-let-7e-5p, and miR-223-3p) has been shown to diagnose DR-TB with a sensitivity of 100% and specificity of 75%.
  - o *Conclusion:* miRNA biomarkers show a promising future for TB diagnostics.
  - o *Critical appraisal:* Minimal number of study articles.

- ***Oral swabs with a rapid molecular diagnostic test for pulmonary tuberculosis in adults and children: A systematic review. (The Lancet Global Health. 2024)***[11]
  - o *Population:* Participants were adults (aged 15 years or older) and children (younger than 15 years) who were evaluated for presumptive pulmonary tuberculosis. (n=3083)
  - o *Outcome:* Sensitivity on oral swabs ranged from 36% (95% CI 26–48) to 91% (80–98) in adults and 5% (1–14) to 42% (23–63) in children. Specificity ranged from 66% (95% CI 52–78) to 100% (97–100), with most studies reporting specificity of more than 90%. Meta-analysis was not performed because of sampling and testing heterogeneity.
  - o *Conclusion:* Oral swabs with molecular testing can provide accurate results for the diagnosis of pulmonary tuberculosis. The highest sensitivities in this review approach, the acceptable sensitivity range for an initial diagnostic test relative to the performance of sputum-based diagnostics, suggesting that with continued optimization, swabs could be a good sample type for tuberculosis detection.
  - o *Critical appraisal:* Future studies with a standardized protocol for comparing different aspects of oral swab collection and processing are needed to recommend it as a point-of-care diagnostic test.

Treatment

- ***Effectiveness of a comprehensive package based on electronic medication monitors at improving treatment outcomes among tuberculosis patients in Tibet: A multicentre randomized controlled trial. (The Lancet. 2024)***[12]
  - o *Population:* Participants had drug-susceptible tuberculosis and were aged 15 years or older when starting standard tuberculosis treatment. (n=278)
  - o *Intervention:* Patients received an electronic medication monitor box. The box included audio medication-adherence reminders and recorded box-opening data, which were transmitted to a cloud-based server and were accessible to healthcare providers to allow remote adherence monitoring. A linked smartphone app-enabled text, audio, and video communication between patients and healthcare providers. Patients selected a treatment supporter (often a family member) who was trained to support patients with using the electronic medication monitor and app. (n=143)
  - o *Comparator:* Patients in the control group received usual care plus a deactivated electronic medication monitor, which only recorded and transmitted box-opening data that was not made available to healthcare providers. The control group also had no access to the app or trained treatment supporters. (n=135)

- *Outcome:* In the intervention group, 87 (10%) of the 854 treatment months showed poor adherence compared with 290 (37%) of the 795 months in the control group. The corresponding adjusted risk difference for the intervention versus control was –29·2 percentage points (95% CI –35·3 to –22·2; p<0·0001). Secondary treatment outcomes such as treatment success, which was found to be 133 (94%) of the 142 individuals in the intervention arm and 98 (73%) of the 134 individuals in the control arm, with an adjusted risk difference of 21 percentage points (95% CI 12·4–29·4; p<0·0001).
- *Conclusion:* The interventions were effective at improving tuberculosis treatment adherence and outcomes in high-burden and low-resource settings.
- *Critical appraisal:* The electronic monitor medication box is an add-on cost to the treatment program with increased compliance with therapy.

- ***Efficacy and tolerability of a 4-month ofloxacin-containing regimen compared to a 6-month regimen in the treatment of patients with superficial lymph node tuberculosis: A randomized trial. (BMC Infectious Diseases. 2024)***[13]
  - *Population:* Participants were new, adult, HIV-negative, microbiologically and/or histopathologically confirmed superficial lymph node TB patients. (n=302)
  - *Intervention:* Four-month ofloxacin-containing test regimen [ofloxacin (O), isoniazid (H), rifampicin (R), pyrazinamide (Z) -2RHZO daily/ 2RHO thrice-weekly, n=152]
  - *Comparator:* Six-month thrice-weekly control regimen (2HRZE /4RH, n=150).
  - *Outcome:* Of 302 patients randomized, 298 (98.7%) were eligible for modified intention-to-treat (ITT) analysis and 294 (97%) for per-protocol (PP) analysis. The TB recurrence-free favorable response in the PP analysis was 94.0% (95% CI: 90.1–97.8) and 94.5% (95% CI: 90.8–98.2) in the test and control regimen respectively, while in the ITT analysis, it was 92.7% and 93.2%. The TB recurrence-free favourable response in the test regimen was non-inferior to the control.
  - *Conclusion:* The 4-month ofloxacin-containing regimen was found to be non-inferior and as safe as the 6-month thrice-weekly control regimen.
  - *Critical appraisal:* A single-centric study and the six-month thrice-weekly control regimen which is not the current standard of care for lymph node TB, was used as a comparator in the trial. When the study was initiated in 2012, the Revised National TB Control Programme (RNTCP) of India offered a Category-I regimen for new TB patients (2HRZE in the intensive phase and 4 HR in the continuation phase, given thrice -weekly).

- ***Efficacy and safety of an innovative short-course regimen containing clofazimine for the treatment of drug-susceptible tuberculosis: A clinical trial. (Emerging Microbes & Infections. 2023)***[14]
  - *Population:* Patients with newly diagnosed bacteriologically-confirmed pulmonary tuberculosis. (n=113)
  - *Intervention:* Four-month regimen, consisting of clofazimine, protionamide, pyrazinamide, and ethambutol. (n=56)
  - *Comparator:* Standard six-month regimen in patients with drug-susceptible tuberculosis. (n=57)
  - *Outcome:* Treatment success occurred in 41.3% (19/46) and 70.2% (33/47) of the patients who received the per-protocol and standard regimens, respectively. The unfavorable outcomes in the per-protocol regimen are due to adverse drug reactions (34.8%vs. 12.9%), primarily drug-induced hepatitis.

- *Conclusion:* The short-course regimen appeared to have inferior efficacy and a higher incidence of hepatitis.
- *Critical appraisal:* Small sample size and multivariate analysis not performed.

- ***Tuberculosis (TB) treatment challenges in TB-diabetes comorbid patients: A systematic review and meta-analysis. (Annals of Medicine. 2024)***[15]
  - *Population:* Meta-analysis and systematic review of 44 studies.
  - *Intervention:* Adult patients with the diagnosis of TB, involving both TB-diabetes mellitus type 2 (DM type 2) comorbid patients.
  - *Comparator:* Patients with the diagnosis of TB without type 2 DM.
  - *Outcome:* Pooled HR for the impact of DM on extended treatment duration and recurrence were HR 0.72, (95% CI 0.56–0.83, $p < 0.01$) and HR 0.93, (95% CI 0.70–1.04, $p = 0.08$). The pooled HR for the impact of DM on composite TB treatment outcomes was calculated as 0.76 (95% CI 0.60–0.87), $p < 0.01$ with an effect size of 41.18.
  - *Conclusion:* A negative impact of DM was found on recurrence and extended treatment duration in TB patients treated with DOTS therapy.
  - *Critical appraisal:* The glycemic control is not uniformly monitored and further studies are required involving a larger group of population and consistent methodology.

- ***Alternative Methods for Therapeutic Drug Monitoring and Dose Adjustment of Tuberculosis Treatment in Clinical Settings: A Systematic Review. (Clin Pharmacokinet. 2023)***[16]
  - *Population:* Participants were patients on first and second-line anti-tubercular drugs from 75 studies.
  - *Intervention:* Minimally invasive and lower cost tests using alternative biomatric methods (Dried blood spots, Urine, Saliva, and hair), efficacy for therapeutic drug monitoring other than serum or plasma during anti-tubercular therapy.
  - *Outcome:* Blood spots reduced the sample volume requirement and shipping costs. Urinary samples can allow point-of-care testing in high-burden settings. Saliva sampling has the advantage of minimal pre-processing requirements. Multi-analyte panels have been tested in hair with the capacity to test a wide range of drugs including their metabolites.
  - *Conclusion:* Reported data were mostly from small studies and alternative biometrics need to be qualified in large and diverse populations for the demonstrate feasibility and utility in operational settings.

- ***High rate of adverse drug reactions with a novel tuberculosis re-treatment regimen combining triple doses of both isoniazid and rifampicin. (TRIDORE STUDY) (Int J Infect Dis. 2023)***[17]
  - *Population:* Patients with rifampicin-susceptible recurrent smear-positive tuberculosis. (n=127)
  - *Intervention:* 6 Months of triple dose of Both Isoniazid and Rifampicin with a normal dose of pyrazinamide and Ethambutol 6(R3H3ZE). (n=62)
  - *Comparator:* Patients taking a normal dose of 6(HRZE). (n=65)
  - *Outcome:* Between March 2021 and February 2022, 127 consenting patients were randomly assigned to either the intervention or control arm: 62 and 65 were treated with 6R3H3ZE and 6RHZE, respectively. Of 127, 111 (87.4%) were male and the median age (interquartile range) was 37 (30-48) years. The median body mass index at enrolment was 18.1 (16.3-19.7) kg/m^2. Drug-related severe adverse events (AEs) (grade III-V) were significantly more frequent when 6R3H3ZE was used (5/62 vs 0/65, $P = 0.03$, difference weighted for site 8% [95% confidence interval: 1.0,14.3]).

- *Conclusion:* Combination of triple-dose R with triple-dose H in a re-treatment regimen for patients with Rs-TB causes excess drug-related Adverse Events.
- *Critical appraisal:* No blinding. Information bias when clinicians evaluated safety events.

- ***Examining interventions that aim to enhance TB treatment adherence in Southeast Asia: A systematic review and meta-analysis. (Indian Journal of Tuberculosis. 2024)***[18]
  - *Population:* Tuberculosis patients from across eight countries in South-East Asia. (n=7198)
  - *Intervention:* Directly observed therapy, text-message reminders, food incentives. (n=3163)
  - *Comparator:* No adherence intervention. (n=4035)
  - *Outcome:* The risk ratio, derived from the meta-analysis of eight included studies was 1.04 (95% CI 1.01,1.08; $I^2 = 29\%$), favoring the interventions over controls with little concern for heterogeneity or risk of bias. Implementing a TB treatment intervention increases the likelihood of adherence by 4%.
  - *Conclusion:* Interventions in Southeast Asia to promote TB treatment adherence were slightly more likely to report increased TB treatment completion when compared to a control group.

- ***Efficacy and safety of intrathecal dexamethasone combined with isoniazid in the treatment of tuberculous meningitis. (BMC Neurol. 2024)***[19]
  - *Population:* Adult patients aged 18 and older with suspected or diagnosed TB M. (n=1360)
  - *Intervention:*

    a) Intrathecal dexamethasone and isoniazid+ regular oral or intravenous anti-TB. (n=392)

    b) Intrathecal higher concentration dexamethasone and isoniazid+ regular oral or intravenous anti-TB. (n=319)
  - *Comparator:*

    a) Regular oral or intravenous anti-TB. (n=372)

    b) Intrathecal lower concentration dexamethasone and isoniazid+ regular oral or intravenous anti-TB. (n=277)
  - *Outcome:*

    a) For the primary outcome studied namely, efficacy, safety, and CSF findings, the efficacy was better in patients receiving adjunct intrathecal injections (RR 1.3, 95% CI 1.2-1.4, $P < 0.001$). The adverse reaction rate of intrathecal dexamethasone and isoniazid (IDI) was significantly lower than that among patients who received oral or IV anti-TB drugs alone (RR 0.59, 95% CI 0.37-0.92, $P = 0.021$). There was also a significant decrease in the CSF proteins, leucocytes, CSF pressure, and improvement of CSF chlorides, while there was no difference in the glucose enhancement.

    b) Treatment efficacy for patients receiving higher IDI doses was significantly higher than those receiving lower IDI doses (RR 1.23, 95% CI 1.14-1.33, P < 0.001). While there was minimal reduction in the protein level there was no difference in the reduction of leucocytes and glucose. The mean difference in CSF pressure in the high-dose group was with higher-dose (isoniazid 200 mg + dexamethasone 10 mg) IDI injection was 160 ± 38, and the lower-dose (isoniazid 100mg + dexamethasone 5 mg) group (230 ± 67) ($P < 0.05$). No significant difference in adverse reaction rate between the two (RR 0.82, 95%CI 0.43–1.56, P=0.544).
  - *Conclusion:* Intrathecal dexamethasone and isoniazid can be effectively integrated into the treatment regimen, potentially reducing inflammation, and improving patient prognosis compared to conventional oral or intravenous anti-TB medication.
  - *Critical appraisal:* Limited number of publications. Most of the studies were from China which might have an impact on the generalizability of the results.

- ***The effect of medication event reminder monitoring on treatment adherence of TB patients. (Int J Tuberc Lung Dis. 2023)***[20]
  - o *Population:* Participants were provided with a Medication event reminder modification device (MERM) to store their medications.
  - o *Intervention:* Medication event reminder Monitoring Device.
  - o *Comparator:* Patients on ATT without event reminder monitoring device.
  - o *Outcome:* Out of 2,142 patients screened, 798 met the criteria, and 250 were enrolled. The intervention group had a 28% lower rate of poor adherence compared to the control group. It also reduced the number of patients missing at least 14 out of 30 doses by 39% and decreased the total percentage of missed doses by 25%.
  - o *Conclusion:* MERM is effective in improving TB treatment adherence in a resource-limited environment.

- ***Four-Month High Dose Rifampicin-susceptible pulmonary tuberculosis. (NEJM. 2023)***[21]
  - o *Population:* Rifampicin-susceptible pulmonary tuberculosis. (n=672)
  - o *Intervention:* Four-Month High-Dose Rifampicin Regimens for Pulmonary Tuberculosis with 2 study regimens.

    a) Rifampicin dose was 1200mg. (n=192)

    b) Rifampicin dose 1800mg. (n=195)
  - o *Comparator:* Standard 6-month control regimen for treatment of pulmonary tuberculosis. (n=191)
  - o *Outcome:* The study looked at treatment failure and relapse rates. Favorable response rates were 93% for the control group, 90% for SR1, and 87% for SR2. The difference in risk between SR2 and the control group was 6.3 percentage points. Serious adverse events occurred in 4.0% of the control group, 4.5% of SR1, and 4.4% of SR2. Although non-inferiority was not shown.
  - o *Conclusion:* A four-month high-dose rifampicin treatment did not cause significant side effects but was not as effective as the standard six-month treatment for rifampicin-sensitive pulmonary tuberculosis.

- ***Nutritional supplementation to prevent tuberculosis incidence in household contacts of patients with pulmonary tuberculosis in India (RATIONS): A field-based, open-label, cluster-randomized, controlled trial. (Lancet. 2023)***[22]
  - o *Population:* Household contacts of 2800 patients with microbiologically confirmed pulmonary tuberculosis across 28 tuberculosis units of the National Tuberculosis Elimination Programme in four districts of Jharkhand, India. (n=10,345)
  - o *Intervention*: Nutritional Supplement to household contacts in the intervention group (14 Tuberculosis Units comprising 5621 participants).
  - o *Comparator:* Household Contacts of Tuberculosis Patients (14 Tuberculosis Units comprising 4724 participants).
  - o *Outcome:* In the intervention group, the overall incidence of tuberculosis decreased by 39% (adjusted IRR of 0·61 (95% CI 0·43–0·85; a HR 0·59 [0·42–0·83]), and the incidence of microbiologically confirmed pulmonary tuberculosis decreased by 48%.
  - o *Conclusion:* Nutritional supplementation to household contacts of microbiologically confirmed pulmonary tuberculosis reduces the incidence of tuberculosis among contacts. An estimated 30 households (111 household contacts) would need to be provided nutritional supplementation to prevent one incident of tuberculosis.

- ***Same-day testing with initiation of antiretroviral therapy or tuberculosis treatment versus standard care for persons presenting with tuberculosis symptoms at HIV diagnosis: A randomized open-label trial from Haiti.(PLOS Medicine. 2023).***[23]

    - *Population:* Adults with TB symptoms at initial HIV diagnosis at GHESKIO in Haiti. (n=500)
    - *Intervention:* Same-day treatment (same-day TB testing with same-day TB treatment if TB diagnosed; same-day ART if TB not diagnosed). (n=250)
    - *Comparator:* Adults with TB symptoms at initial HIV diagnosis receiving standard care (initiating TB treatment within 7 days and delaying ART to day 7 if TB not diagnosed). In both groups, ART was initiated 2 weeks after TB treatment. (n=250)
    - *Outcome:* The primary outcome measured was retention in care, defined as having HIV-1 RNA levels below 200 copies/mL at 48 weeks, analysed using intention-to-treat (ITT) methodology. There was no significant difference between the groups in this outcome (60.8% vs. 67.2%; risk difference: -0.06; 95% CI [-0.15, 0.02]; p = 0.14). This study suggests that a short delay in initiating ART does not seem to negatively impact outcomes.
    - *Conclusion:* For patients diagnosed with HIV who also have TB symptoms, starting treatment on the same day did not lead to better retention in care or higher rates of viral suppression.
    - *Critical appraisal:* The study was conducted in a single urban setting and the findings may not be generalizable to other settings.

- ***Standard-dose versus double-dose dolutegravir in HIV-associated tuberculosis in South Africa (RADIANT-TB): A phase 2, non-comparative, randomized controlled trial. (LANCET HIV 2023).***[24]

    - *Population*: Adults older than 18 years of age, with plasma HIV-1 RNA greater than 1000 copies per mL, CD4 count greater than 100 cells per µL, ART-naive or first-line ART interrupted, and on rifampicin-based antituberculosis therapy for less than 3 months. (n=108)
    - *Intervention:* Tenofovir disoproxil fumarate, lamivudine, and dolutegravir plus supplemental 50 mg dolutegravir 12 h later. (n=52)
    - *Comparator:* Tenofovir disoproxil fumarate, lamivudine, and dolutegravir plus matched placebo 12 h later. (n=53)
    - *Outcome:* At week 24, 83% of participants in both the supplemental dolutegravir group and the placebo group had their HIV-1 RNA levels reduced to less than 50 copies per mL. So, the rate of viral suppression was similar in both groups.
    - *Conclusion:* People with HIV-associated tuberculosis might not need to take dolutegravir twice a day.

DISCUSSION

Molecular-Based Tests for TB Diagnosis

Early and accurate diagnosis of infectious diseases is required to stop their spread and increase the chances for successful treatment. For tuberculosis (TB), even now, the traditional time-consuming culture method remains the **"gold standard"** for testing by physicians. However, **the World Health Organization (WHO) recommends using a nucleic acid amplification test (NAAT), such as the Xpert MTB/RIF, for diagnosing TB and rifampicin resistance.**[25] Some new diagnostic methods have been discovered and studied for TB diagnosis.

Role of Lipoarabinomannan (LAM) in TB Diagnosis

LAM is a 17.5-kD heat-stable glycolipid released from metabolically active or decaying TB bacilli cell walls during tuberculosis infection and detected in patients' urine. Compared to sputum, urine samples are easier to collect and store in young children, with significantly fewer infection control problems.

Approved use/Indication: **WHO has recommended using the Lateral flow urine lipoarabinomannan assay (LF-LAM) test in TB diagnosis.**[25,26]

1. *LAM in inpatient settings:* WHO strongly recommends using (LF-LAM) to assist in the diagnosis of active TB in HIV-positive adults, adolescents, and children with signs and symptoms of TB (pulmonary and extrapulmonary) or with advanced HIV disease or who are seriously ill or else irrespective of signs and symptoms of TB and with a CD4 cell count of fewer than 200 cells/mm^3.
2. *In outpatient settings*: WHO suggests using LF-LAM to assist in the diagnosis of active TB in HIV-positive adults, adolescents, and children: with signs and symptoms of TB (pulmonary and extrapulmonary) or else **irrespective of signs and symptoms of TB** and with a CD4 cell count of fewer than 100 cells/mm^3.

Tests based on the detection of mycobacterial LAM antigen in urine have emerged as potential point-of-care tests for TB. The currently available urinary LAM assays have suboptimal sensitivity and are, therefore, unsuitable as a diagnostic test for TB in all population. The LAM testing has shown around 30-70% sensitivity in pediatric populations and HIV patients with low CD4 counts. **Those who are malnourished and have severe HIV or other systemic diseases may be suitable candidates for LAM testing.** This finding supports the hypothesis that LAM is only shed into the urine of patients with active pulmonary TB in the context of glomerular dysfunction caused by HIV infection.[27,28] The polyclonal antibodies used in the test could cross-react with urinary tract pathogens, and fast-growing non-tuberculous mycobacteria leading to its lower specificity. **The Fuji LAM test has the highest sensitivity and specificity among other LAM tests.**[29] The Alere Determine TB LAM Ag (Alere LAM) test was the first commercially available LAM test with the highest sensitivity, so most of the data and studies are on this variant. However, with upcoming modifications in the LAM test, diagnostic accuracy is much more promising, even in non-HIV populations.

Fuji LAM test is a WHO-recommended test to diagnose TB in severe HIV patients. It can be used as an alternative test to diagnose TB in non-HIV patients where obtaining a sputum sample is difficult.

Role of GeneXpert

The **Xpert MTB/RIF** assay has revolutionized tuberculosis (TB) control by contributing to the rapid diagnosis of TB disease and drug resistance. The test simultaneously detects **Mycobacterium tuberculosis complex (MTBC)** and resistance to rifampin (RIF) in less than 2 hours. The Xpert MTB/RIF assay is a nucleic acid amplification (NAA) test that uses a disposable cartridge with the **GeneXpert Instrument System.**

A new updated Xpert assay, Xpert MTB/RIF Ultra, has been available for TB diagnosis and resistance detection with improved performance and faster time to result with higher sensitivity, especially in smear-negative TB cases. Both tests accurately diagnose pulmonary tuberculosis, but their role in extrapulmonary TB is poorly defined because of variable sensitivity and specificity.

The development of Xpert MTB/RIF was a major step toward improving tuberculosis and rifampicin resistance detection globally. The most recent version, Xpert MTB/RIF Ultra, attempts to further improve the limit of mycobacterial DNA detection by amplifying two different insertion sequences (IS6110 and IS1081) in a larger reaction chamber.[27] **Xpert ultra has shown higher sensitivity and lower specificity than Xpert MTB/RIF for pulmonary tuberculosis, especially in smear-negative participants and people living with HIV. In extrapulmonary cases, ultra has slightly low specificity but significantly high sensitivity, particularly in pleural effusion. Xpert MTB/Rif and Ultra both have variable sensitivity. Xpert Ultra had higher sensitivity and lower specificity for tuberculous meningitis than Xpert MTB/RIF against culture.**[30,31] Future research should acknowledge the concern associated with culture as a reference standard in paucibacillary specimens and consider ways to address this limitation. The advent of next-generation sequencing has elicited curiosity in the diagnosis of EPTB especially TB meningitis but analysis shows that mNGS had no significant advantage in diagnosing TBM compared to Xpert Ultra and Xpert. However, the specificity of all three methods was >95%, indicating a low misdiagnosis rate. It is safe to conclude that mNGS has moderate sensitivity, good specificity, and high accuracy for diagnosing TBM.[32]

In extrapulmonary TB diagnosis, Xpert Ultra has significantly higher sensitivity than Xpert, specifically in pleural effusion but low specificity is a concern for Xpert Ultra. In cerebrospinal fluid sample analysis, interpretation of Xpert ultra should be done with caution. For sputum analysis, it is recommended to use Xpert ultra over Xpert as it has higher sensitivity and near the same specificity.

A Novel, fast (within hours) culture-free diagnostic method with an ultra-sensitive enzyme-linked immunosorbent assay for the detection of live *Mycobacterium tuberculosis* with high sensitivity has also been tried. The assay has a good sensitivity, 86.9%, and excellent specificity, by distinguishing TB from non-tuberculous mycobacteria. It also has the advantage of less turnaround time for diagnosis when compared to the conventional culture methods.[33]

Treatment

Scientific basis of tuberculosis treatment for drug-sensitive tuberculosis.

The goals of tuberculosis treatment are as follows:

1. Combining different effective drugs to avoid the selection of resistant *M. tuberculosis* strains;
2. Ensuring that treatment is long enough to sterilize the tissues infected with *M. tuberculosis* and, therefore, prevent relapse.
3. Ensuring cure.

The ideal treatment regimen should contain 4 drugs, two are core, and two are companion drugs. Core drugs are those that can kill mycobacterium tuberculosis in any of its metabolic phases. **Among the 2 core drugs one should have bactericidal activity and the other should have good sterilizing activity. The role of companion drugs is to protect the action of core drugs and to avoid resistance selection.** Bactericidal drugs reduce infectiousness by quickly acting on the rapidly multiplying bacteria while sterilizing drugs act on the dormant and semidormant bacilli facilitating cure and preventing relapse. Drugs with good sterilizing activity reduce the duration of treatment. Once the bacteriological conversion happens the companion drugs can be stopped and the core drugs can continue till the treatment completion. Of the currently available antituberculosis drugs, isoniazid has the highest early bactericidal effect against rapidly growing tubercle bacilli, while rifampicin and pyrazinamide are thought to have the greatest sterilizing effects against those with spurts of metabolism and under acid inhibition, respectively.[34,35]

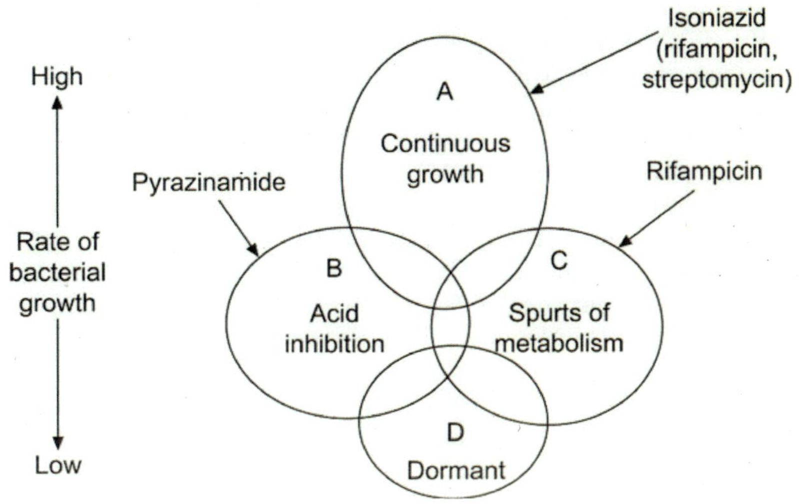

Picture depicting the metabolic phases and the drugs that act on the respective phases

Constant efforts to identify novel therapies for the treatment of tuberculosis have led to the identification of several promising drugs and drug regimens. Indian guideline for drug-sensitive TB was last updated in 2016 and led to significant changes in the treatment regimen, response assessment, and monitoring.[2,36] The last significant changes came in 2021 when it was recommended to use **sputum GeneXpert testing** for every presumptive TB case. However, treatment duration and drugs in the ATT regimen have been the same for years. The standard ATT regimen for pulmonary as well as extrapulmonary TB as per the National Tuberculosis Elimination Programme (NTEP) continues to be 2 months of HREZ followed by 4 months of HRE. With increasing yearly incidence, this is of utmost urgency that new TB management strategies are found.

World Health Organization (WHO) released the latest updated guidelines for managing DSTB in May 2022. Following were the significant changes and recommendations in treatment strategy.[36]

1. **People aged 12 years or older with drug-susceptible pulmonary TB may receive a 4-month regimen of isoniazid, rifapentine, moxifloxacin, and pyrazinamide** (conditional recommendation, moderate certainty of evidence).
2. **In children and adolescents between 3 months and 16 years of age with non-severe TB (without suspicion or evidence of MDR/RR-TB), a 4-month treatment regimen (2HRZ(E)/2HR) should be used** (strong recommendation, moderate certainty of evidence).

Centers for Disease Control and Prevention (CDC) has also recently recommended the 4-month (rifapentine-moxifloxacin) RPT-MOX regimen for treating patients aged ≥ 12 years with body weight ≥ 40 kg with pulmonary TB caused by organisms that are not known or suspected to be drug-resistant and who have no contraindications to this regimen.[37] The 4-month daily treatment regimen consists of an intensive phase of 8 weeks of daily treatment with RPT, MOX, INH, and PZA, followed by a continuation phase of 9 weeks of daily treatment with RPT, MOX, and INH. Baseline molecular drug-susceptibility testing for rapid identification of mutations associated with resistance to at least INH, PZA, RIF, and fluoroquinolones is advisable. **Phenotypic DST** should follow with a panel to include at least RIF (as surrogate for RPT), INH, PZA, and MOX as the preferred fluoroquinolone.[30] **It is to be noted that these newer regimens recommended by CDC and WHO are for a subpopulation of pulmonary tuberculosis which are non-severe, thus all cases of extrapulmonary TB should continue to be exclusively treated with the current standard ATT regimen (2HREZ/4HRE) regimen unless evidence emerges for the same.**

At present **directly observed therapy (DOT)** for tuberculosis treatment is standard practice that involves observing treatment adherence, monitoring the patient for adverse events, and providing economic support for treatment. **Based on recent evidence CDC recommends video DOT (vDOT) as equivalent to in-person DOT for persons undergoing treatment for diagnosed tuberculosis.**[38]

In recent years, new shorter-duration ATT regimens have demonstrated success while maintaining the same treatment efficacy. The new vital drugs are moxifloxacin, rifapentine, and drugs used upfront in MDR TB management. Adding moxifloxacin to the treatment regimen of pulmonary tuberculosis patients could significantly increase the sputum culture conversion rate, leading to shortening ATT to 4 months. However, it has no significant effect on the recurrence rate.[39,40] Arranging a moxifloxacin susceptibility test would be a more significant concern for highly prevalent countries. We now have quality data from about 2-4 months of ATT, which shows a similar treatment efficacy.[41] The major update is the recent short-course ATT regimen of bedaquiline and linezolid which has only two months of therapy. However, it is based on a single study data; further larger and more diverse population-based studies are required before adopting such regimens. Bedaquiline and linezolid being an important part of the MDR TB regimen, may not be feasible to use for DSTB in TB-endemic countries like India. It is uncertain whether the clinical implementation of such adaptive treatment would be feasible outside the context of a trial, as it requires careful monitoring and considerable resources that may not be available to many TB programs. Recent ongoing trials on TB drugs would discover and offer exciting new ultrashort combination regimens for drug-sensitive TB. **While recent studies may prompt the suggestion of alternative treatment regimens for tuberculosis in pediatric and adult populations, it is still important to adhere to the current national guidelines for tuberculosis treatment until new updates are adopted by national guidelines.**

Tuberculosis and Malnutrition

Almost half of the patients with severe illness with tuberculosis have undernutrition. The proportion of severe undernutrition among adults with TB was 25% in Tamil Nadu, 30% in Karnataka, and 38% in Gujarat. To address this Tamilnadu implemented a capacity-building initiative called TN-KET (Tamil Nadu Kasanoi Irapilla Thittam), where nodal inpatient care facilities were created that helps in the clinical management of very severe undernutrition in adults, in line with the guidelines in the *Inpatient Care Guide for Adults with TB Who Are Severely Ill.* Patients with tuberculosis are screened for severe illness at the time of diagnosis with the following parameters. Body mass index (BMI) less than or equal to (≤) 14.0 kg/m, BMI less than or equal to (≤) 16.0 kg/m^2 with leg swelling, Respiratory rate greater than (>) 24 per minute, Oxygen saturation less than (<) 94%, not able to stand without support (standing with support, squatting, sitting, or bedridden). If any of these is present, the patient is admitted with a special focus given to address the nutritional aspect of the patient. This scheme has been successful in reducing early TB death in many districts in Tamil Nadu.[42,43]

Tuberculosis Preventive Treatment

The National Tuberculosis Elimination Program (NTEP) released guidelines for TB preventive treatment (TPT), a significant update in TB control. **The concept and goal are to prevent the conversion of infection to disease so that the number of active cases can be reduced, leading to a decrease in TB incidence.**[44]

TPT services complement screening for active TB, infection control, prevention and care of HIV and other comorbidities and health risks, access to universal health care, social protection, and poverty alleviation. The following are the major components of the TPT program.

1. Identifying at-risk populations.
2. Diagnosis of TB infection via tuberculin skin test (TST) and interferon-gamma release assay (IGRA) test.
3. Enumerating the target population, ruling out active TB disease, and initiating TB preventive treatment.
4. Two regimens are available: three-month isoniazid plus rifapentine and six months isoniazid.

WHO's Tuberculosis preventive treatment guidelines recommended several TPT regimens for LTBI treatment including 6 or 9 months of daily isoniazid, a 3-month regimen of weekly rifapentine plus isoniazid, or a 3-month regimen of daily isoniazid plus rifampicin.[45] A 1-month regimen of daily rifapentine plus isoniazid or 4 months of daily rifampicin alone may also be offered as alternatives.[46]

To strengthen existing systems and seamlessly extend quality TB care to patients in the private sector project JEET is being jointly implemented in India by the William J. Clinton Foundation (WJCF), Centre for Health Research and Innovation (CHRI) and Foundation for Innovative New Diagnostics (FIND), under the guidance of Central TB Division (CTD) and Ministry of Health and Family Welfare (MOHFW). The project proposes to contract agencies at the district level to work closely with the patient and all patient touch points, including chemists, pharmacies, clinics, providers, hospitals, laboratories, and NTEP.[47]

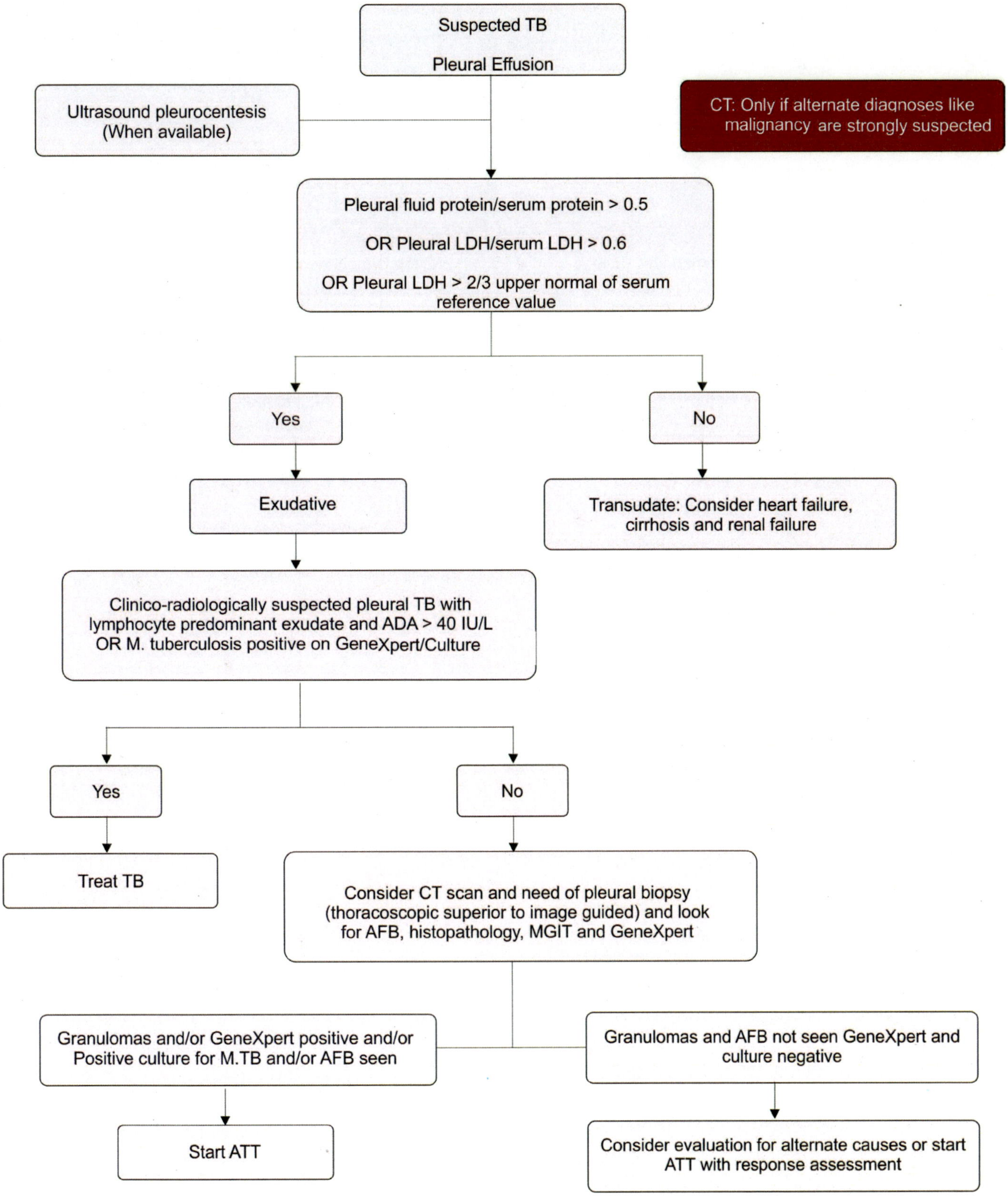

Flowchart 1: Flowchart to Diagnose Tubercular Pleural Effusion (as per Central TB Division, India)[37]

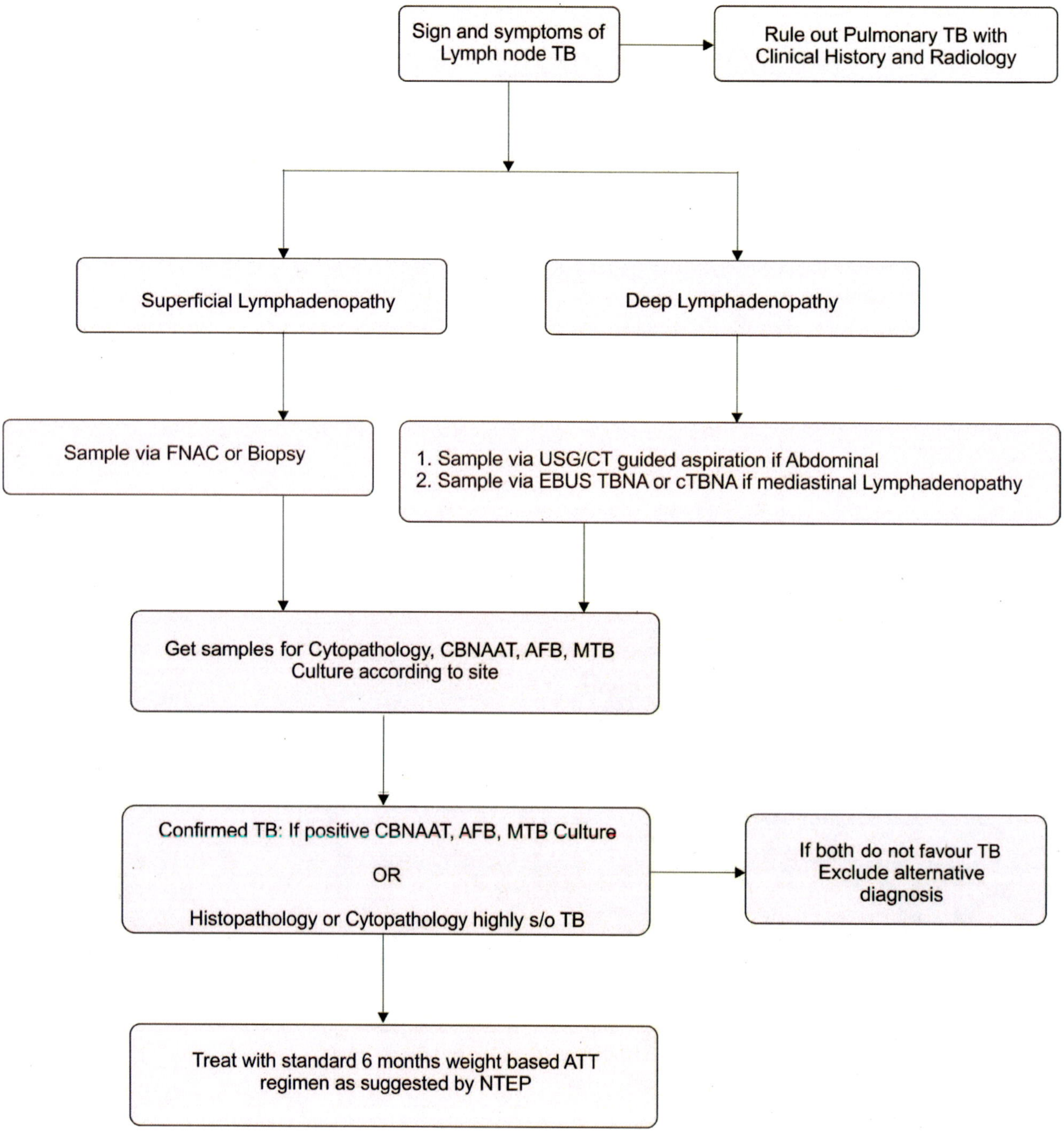

Flowchart 2: Flowchart to Diagnose TB Lymphadenitis (as per Central TB Division, India)[37]

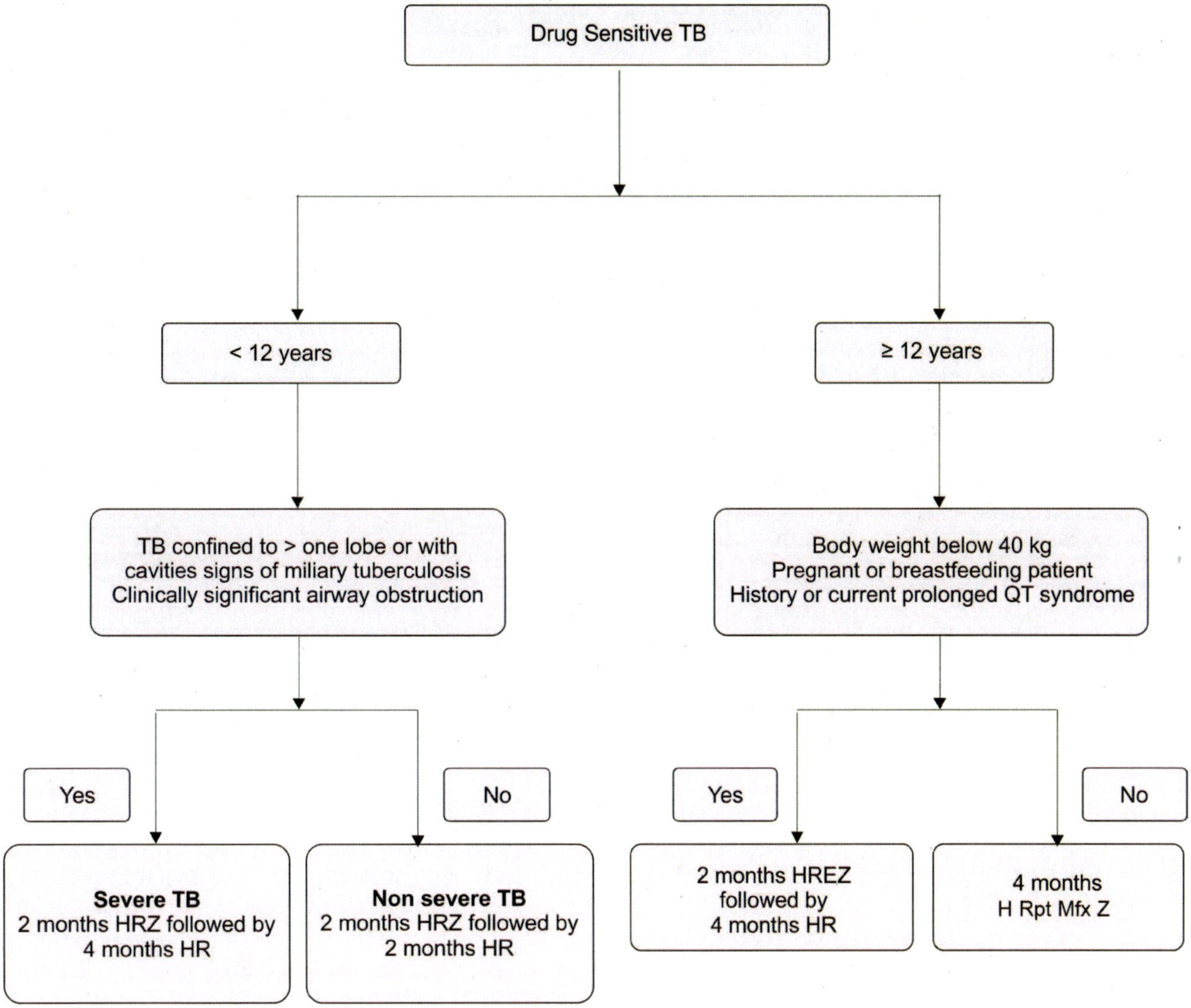

Flowchart 3: Suggested Flowchart for DSTB Treatment (as per **WHO** and CDC)

Flowchart 3: Treatment of DSTB based on recent studies. Abbreviations: H-Isoniazid, R-Rifampicin, E-Ethambutol, Z-Pyrazinamide, Rpt-Rifapentine, Mfx-Moxifloxacin. Daily dosing of Isoniazid, rifampicin, ethambutol and pyrazinamide is as per WHO and NTEP guideline.
Dose of rifapentine is 1200 mg once daily and moxifloxacin is 400 mg once a day.

All cases of extrapulmonary TB should be exclusively treated with current standard ATT regimen (2HREZ/4HRE) regimen. Standard ATT regimen for pulmonary as well as extrapulmonary TB by NTEP is 2 months HREZ followed by 4 months HRE.

* While recent studies may prompt the suggestion of alternative treatment regimens for tuberculosis in pediatric and adult populations, it is still important to adhere to the current national guidelines for tuberculosis treatment until new updates are made available.

REFERENCES

1. Health Organisation W. World TB Report, 2023. Vol. t/malaria/, January. 2023.
2. Ministry of Health and Family Welfare. India TB repeort 2023.
3. MOHFW. RNTCP [Internet]. Available from: https://dghs.gov.in/content/1358_3_RevisedNationalTuberculosis Control Programme.aspx
4. Du J, Su Y, Qiao J, Gao S, Dong E, Wang R, et al. Application of artificial intelligence in diagnosis of pulmonary tuberculosis. Chin Med J (Engl) [Internet]. 2024 Mar 5 [cited 2024 Aug 23];137(5):559–61. Available from: https://pubmed.ncbi.nlm.nih.gov/38369956/
5. Sinha P, Lönnroth K, Bhargava A, Heysell SK, Sarkar S, Salgame P, et al. Food for thought: addressing undernutrition to end tuberculosis. Lancet Infect Dis. 2021;21(10):e318–25.
6. Khanna A, Saha R, Ahmad N. National TB elimination programme - What has changed. Indian J Med Microbiol. 2023;42(January):103–7.
7. Ruslami R, Fregonese F, Apriani L, Barss L, Bedingfield N, Chiang V, et al. High-dose, short-duration versus standard rifampicin for tuberculosis preventive treatment: a partially blinded, three-arm, non-inferiority, randomised, controlled trial. Lancet Respir Med [Internet]. 2024 Jun 1 [cited 2024 Aug 23];12(6):433–43. Available from: https://pubmed.ncbi.nlm.nih.gov/38552659/
8. Hanrahan CF, Nonyane BAS, Lebina L, Mmolawa L, Siwelana T, West NS, et al. Household- Versus Incentive-Based Contact Investigation for Tuberculosis in Rural South Africa: A Cluster-Randomized Trial. Clin Infect Dis [Internet]. 2023 Apr 1 [cited 2024 Aug 19];76(7):1164–72. Available from: https://pubmed.ncbi.nlm.nih.gov/36458857/
9. Fritschi N, Vaezipour N, Buettcher M, Portevin D, Naranbhai V, Ritz N. Ratios from full blood count as markers for TB diagnosis, treatment, prognosis: a systematic review. Int J Tuberc Lung Dis [Internet]. 2023 Nov 1;27(11):822–32. Available from: https://www.ingentaconnect.com/content/10.5588/ijtld.22.0598
10. Gunasekaran H, Sampath P, Thiruvengadam K, Malaisamy M, Ramasamy R, Ranganathan UD, et al. A systematic review and meta-analysis of circulating serum and plasma microRNAs in TB diagnosis. BMC Infect Dis [Internet]. 2024 Dec 1 [cited 2024 Aug 23];24(1). Available from: https://pubmed.ncbi.nlm.nih.gov/38622570/
11. Church EC, Steingart KR, Cangelosi GA, Ruhwald M, Kohli M, Shapiro AE. Oral swabs with a rapid molecular diagnostic test for pulmonary tuberculosis in adults and children: a systematic review. Lancet Glob Heal [Internet]. 2024 Jan 1 [cited 2024 Aug 24];12(1):e45–54. Available from: https://pubmed.ncbi.nlm.nih.gov/38097297/
12. Wei X, Hicks JP, Zhang Z, Haldane V, Pasang P, Li L, et al. Effectiveness of a comprehensive package based on electronic medication monitors at improving treatment outcomes among tuberculosis patients in Tibet: a multicentre randomised controlled trial. Lancet (London, England) [Internet]. 2024 Mar 9 [cited 2024 Aug 24];403(10430):913–23. Available from: https://pubmed.ncbi.nlm.nih.gov/38309280/
13. Hissar S, Velayutham B, Tamizhselvan M, Rathinam S, Arunbabu C, Vidhya JB, et al. Efficacy and tolerability of a 4-month ofloxacin-containing regimen compared to a 6-month regimen in the treatment of patients with superficial lymph node tuberculosis: a randomized trial. BMC Infect Dis [Internet]. 2024 Dec 1 [cited 2024 Aug 24];24(1). Available from: https://pubmed.ncbi.nlm.nih.gov/39054415/
14. Zheng X, Gui X, Yao L, Ma J, He Y, Lou H, et al. Efficacy and safety of an innovative short-course regimen containing clofazimine for treatment of drug-susceptible tuberculosis: a clinical trial. Emerg Microbes Infect [Internet]. 2023 Dec 31;12(1). Available from: https://www.tandfonline.com/doi/full/10.1080/22221751.2023.2187247
15. Khattak M, Rehman A ur, Muqaddas T, Hussain R, Rasool MF, Saleem Z, et al. Tuberculosis (TB) treatment challenges in TB-diabetes comorbid patients: a systematic review and meta-analysis. Ann Med [Internet]. 2024 Dec 31;56(1). Available from: https://www.tandfonline.com/doi/full/10.1080/07853890.2024.2313683
16. Rao PS, Modi N, Nguyen NTT, Vu DH, Xie YL, Gandhi M, et al. Alternative Methods for Therapeutic Drug Monitoring and Dose Adjustment of Tuberculosis Treatment in Clinical Settings: A Systematic Review. Clin Pharmacokinet [Internet]. 2023 Mar 1 [cited 2024 Aug 24];62(3):375–98. Available from: https://pubmed.ncbi.nlm.nih.gov/36869170/
17. Souleymane MB, Kadri S, Piubello A, Tsoumanis A, Soumana A, Issa H, et al. High rate of adverse drug reactions with a novel tuberculosis re-treatment regimen combining triple doses of both isoniazid and rifampicin. Int J Infect Dis. 2023;133(2023):78–81.
18. Davis RA, Leavitt HB, Singh A, Fanouraki E, Yen RW, Bratches RW. Examining interventions that aim to enhance TB treatment adherence in Southeast Asia: A systematic review and meta-analysis. Indian J Tuberc. 2024 Jan 1;71(1):48–63.
19. Gao Y, Su J, Ma Y, Sun Y, Cui J, Jin X, et al. Efficacy and safety of intrathecal dexamethasone combined with isoniazid in the treatment of tuberculous meningitis: a meta-analysis. BMC Neurol [Internet]. 2024;24(1):1–14. Available from: https://doi.org/10.1186/s12883-024-03701-4.
20. Velen K, Nguyen TA, Pham CD, Le HT, Nguyen HB, Dao BT, et al. The effect of medication event reminder monitoring on treatment adherence of TB patients. Int J Tuberc Lung Dis [Internet]. 2023 Apr 1 [cited 2024 Aug 24];27(4):322–8. Available from: https://pubmed.ncbi.nlm.nih.gov/37035979/
21. Jindani A, Atwine D, Grint D, Bah B, Adams J, Ticona ER, et al. Four-Month High-Dose Rifampicin Regimens for Pulmonary Tuberculosis. NEJM Evid [Internet]. 2023 Aug 22 [cited 2024 Aug 18];2(9). Available from: https://pubmed.ncbi.nlm.nih.gov/38320155/
22. Bhargava A, Bhargava M, Meher A, Benedetti A, Velayutham B, Sai Teja G, et al. Nutritional supplementation to prevent tuberculosis

incidence in household contacts of patients with pulmonary tuberculosis in India (RATIONS): a field-based, open-label, cluster-randomised, controlled trial. Lancet [Internet]. 2023 Aug;402 (10402):627–40. Available from: https://linkinghub.elsevier.com/retrieve/pii/S014067362301231X

23. Dorvil N, Rivera VR, Riviere C, Berman R, Severe P, Bang H, et al. Same-day testing with initiation of antiretroviral therapy or tuberculosis treatment versus standard care for persons presenting with tuberculosis symptoms at HIV diagnosis: A randomized open-label trial from Haiti. PLoS Med [Internet]. 2023;20(6 June):1–17. Available from: http://dx.doi.org/10.1371/journal.pmed.1004246

24. Griesel R, Zhao Y, Simmons B, Omar Z, Wiesner L, Keene CM, et al. Standard-dose versus double-dose dolutegravir in HIV-associated tuberculosis in South Africa (RADIANT-TB): a phase 2, non-comparative, randomised controlled trial. Lancet HIV [Internet]. 2023;10(7):e433–41. Available from: http://dx.doi.org/10.1016/S2352-3018(23)00081-4

25. Health Organisation W. Interpretation of the third edition of WHO consolidated guidelines on tuberculosis: module 3: diagnosis: rapid diagnostics for tuberculosis detection. Vol. 46, WHO. 2024.

26. Health Organization W. WHO Policy Update Lateral flow urine LAM for the diagnosis of active TB in people living with HIV. 2019.

27. Kroidl I, Clowes P, Reither K, Mtafya B, Rojas-Ponce G, Ntinginya EN, et al. Performance of urine lipoarabinomannan assays for paediatric tuberculosis in Tanzania. Eur Respir J [Internet]. 2015 Sep;46(3):761–70. Available from: http://www.ncbi.nlm.nih.gov/pubmed/26113682

28. Sigal GB, Pinter A, Lowary TL, Kawasaki M, Li A, Mathew A, et al. A Novel Sensitive Immunoassay Targeting the 5-Methylthio-<scp>d</scp> -Xylofuranose–Lipoarabinomannan Epitope Meets the WHO's Performance Target for Tuberculosis Diagnosis. Miller MB, editor. J Clin Microbiol [Internet]. 2018 Dec;56(12). Available from: https://journals.asm.org/doi/10.1128/JCM.01338-18

29. Seid G, Alemu A, Tsedalu T, Dagne B. Value of urine-based lipoarabinomannan (LAM) antigen tests for diagnosing tuberculosis in children: systematic review and meta-analysis. IJID Reg [Internet]. 2022 Sep 1 [cited 2024 Aug 24];4:97–104. Available from: https://pubmed.ncbi.nlm.nih.gov/35880002/

30. Kohli M, Schiller I, Dendukuri N, Yao M, Dheda K, Denkinger CM, et al. Xpert MTB/RIF Ultra and Xpert MTB/RIF assays for extrapulmonary tuberculosis and rifampicin resistance in adults. Cochrane database Syst Rev [Internet]. 2021 Jan 15 [cited 2024 Aug 24];1(1). Available from: https://pubmed.ncbi.nlm.nih.gov/33448348/

31. Zifodya JS, Kreniske JS, Schiller I, Kohli M, Dendukuri N, Schumacher SG, et al. Xpert Ultra versus Xpert MTB/RIF for pulmonary tuberculosis and rifampicin resistance in adults with presumptive pulmonary tuberculosis. Cochrane database Syst Rev [Internet]. 2021 Feb 22 [cited 2024 Aug 24];2(2). Available from: https://pubmed.ncbi.nlm.nih.gov/33616229/

32. Xiang ZB, Leng EL, Cao WF, Liu SM, Zhou YL, Luo CQ, et al. A systematic review and meta-analysis of the diagnostic accuracy of metagenomic next-generation sequencing for diagnosing tuberculous meningitis. Front Immunol [Internet]. 2023 [cited 2024 Aug 24];14. Available from: https://pubmed.ncbi.nlm.nih.gov/37822937/

33. Wang WH, Takeuchi R, Jain SH, Jiang YH, Watanuki S, Ohtaki Y, et al. A novel, rapid (within hours) culture-free diagnostic method for detecting live Mycobacterium tuberculosis with high sensitivity. EBioMedicine [Internet]. 2020;60:103007. Available from: https://doi.org/10.1016/j.ebiom.2020.103007

34. Caminero JA, Scardigli A. Classification of antituberculosis drugs: A new proposal based on the most recent evidence. Eur Respir J [Internet]. 2015;46(4):887–93. Available from: http://dx.doi.org/10.1183/13993003.00432-2015

35. Mitchison D, Davies G. The chemotherapy of tuberculosis: Past, present and future. Int J Tuberc Lung Dis. 2012;16(6):724–32.

36. Organization WH. Global Tuberculosis Report 2021. [Internet]. Available from: https://www.who.int/ publications/i/item/9789240048126

37. Centers for Disease control. Treatment for TB Disease 2022 [Internet]. Available from: https://www.cdc.gov/tb/topic/treatment/tbdisease.htm

38. Mangan JM, Woodruff RS, Winston CA, Nabity SA, Haddad MB, Dixon MG, et al. Recommendations for Use of Video Directly Observed Therapy During Tuberculosis Treatment — United States, 2023. MMWR Morb Mortal Wkly Rep [Internet]. 2023 Mar 24;72(12):313–6. Available from: http://www.cdc.gov/mmwr/volumes/72/wr/mm7212a4.htm?s_cid=mm7212a4_w

39. Dorman SE, Nahid P, Kurbatova E V., Phillips PPJ, Bryant K, Dooley KE, et al. Four-Month Rifapentine Regimens with or without Moxifloxacin for Tuberculosis. N Engl J Med [Internet]. 2021 May 6 [cited 2024 Aug 24];384(18):1705–18. Available from: https://pubmed.ncbi.nlm.nih.gov/33951360/

40. Sun M, Fan J. Moxifloxacin is a safe and effective candidate agent for tuberculosis treatment: a meta-analysis of randomized controlled trials. Ann Palliat Med [Internet]. 2021 Feb;10(2):2027–35. Available from: https://apm.amegroups.com/article/view/61732/html

41. Paton NI, Cousins C, Suresh C, Burhan E, Chew KL, Dalay VB, et al. Treatment Strategy for Rifampin-Susceptible Tuberculosis. N Engl J Med [Internet]. 2023 Mar 9 [cited 2024 Aug 24];388(10):873–87. Available from: https://pubmed.ncbi.nlm.nih.gov/36808186/

42. Shewade HD, Frederick A, Kiruthika G, Kalyanasundaram M, Chadwick J, Daniel Rajasekar T, et al. The First Differentiated TB Care Model From India: Delays and Predictors of Losses in the Care Cascade. Glob Heal Sci Pract [Internet]. 2023 Apr 28 [cited 2024 Aug 24];11(2). Available from: https://pubmed.ncbi.nlm.nih.gov/37116929/

43. Shewade HD, Nagaraja SB, Vanitha B, Murthy HJD, Bhargava M, Singarajipura A, et al. Screening for Severe Illness at Diagnosis Has the Potential to Prevent Early TB Deaths: Programmatic Experience From Karnataka, India. Glob Heal Sci Pract [Internet]. 2022 Aug 1 [cited 2024 Aug 24];10(4). Available from: https://pubmed.ncbi.nlm.nih.gov/36041840/

44. Ministry of Health and Family Welfare, Government of India. Guidelines for Programmatic Management of Tuberculosis Preventive

Treatment in India. Tbc Publ [Internet]. 2021;123. Available from: https://tbcindia.gov.in

45. World Health Organisation. WHO: operational handbook on tuberculosis [Internet]. Module 1:Tuberculosis Preventive Therapy. 2024. Available from: https://apps.who.int/iris/bitstream/handle/10665/340256/9789240022614-eng.pdf

46. World Health Organisation. Interpretation of WHO consolidated guidelines on tuberculosis: Module 1: prevention: tuberculosis preventive treatment [Internet]. Available from: https://www.who.int/publications/i/item/9789240001503

47. India T. JEET [Internet]. Available from: https://tbalertindia.org/jeet/

CHAPTER 12

Management of Drug-Resistant Tuberculosis

Authors: Dr. Amitesh Gupta, Dr. Parul Mrigpuri

Reviewer: Dr. Rupak Singla

INTRODUCTION

Introduction of newer medications like bedaquiline (Bdq) and delamanid (Dlm), as well as use of repurposed drugs like linezolid (Lzd) and clofazimine (Cfz), have improved the outcome in drug resistant tuberculosis (DR-TB) patients. However, compliance to prolonged treatment duration with longer regimens and adverse drug reactions still form a major obstacle in beating the menace of DR-TB. World Health Organisation (WHO) is now laying emphasis on use of various shorter oral regimens for multi-drug resistant tuberculosis (MDR-TB) that had demonstrated good success in global trials.

Methodology

A PubMed search was done using the search terms "DR-TB" or "drug resistant tuberculosis" or "management of drug-resistant tuberculosis". The search term was limited to Randomized Control Trials and systematic reviews and meta-analyses between 1st August 2023 to 1st August 2024. A total of 70 articles were found. Of these, 58 articles were removed which were not relevant to the discussion. The remaining articles were analyzed and included for discussion. Additional useful articles were also added to facilitate the flow of the article for driving through the relevant points.

'**Electronic database search:** PubMed

Period: 1st August 2023 to 1st August 2024

Search term used:

"DR-TB" OR "Drug-resistant Tuberculosis" OR

"Management of drug-resistant Tuberculosis"

↓

Inital articles found: 70

↓

Articles excluded: 58

↓

Articles analysed: 12

Analysis of Literature

☞

1. *Pan TB regimens for drug sensitive (DS-TB) and DR-TB*

- ***Bedaquiline-pretomanid-moxifloxacin-pyrazinamide for drug-sensitive and drug-resistant pulmonary tuberculosis treatment: A phase 2c, open-label, multicentre, partially randomised controlled trial. (SimpliciTB trial) (Lancet 2024)***[1]

  - o *Population:* 18 years or older with pulmonary TB who were sputum smear positive for acid-fast bacilli. Both drug sensitive tuberculosis (DS TB) (n=303) and MDR TB (n=152) were enrolled.

  - o *Intervention:*

    a) 4 months of BPaMZ (bedaquiline 200 mg once daily for 8 weeks, followed by bedaquiline 100 mg daily for 9 weeks, together with daily pretomanid 200 mg, moxifloxacin 400 mg, and pyrazinamide 1500 mg for all 17 weeks in DS TB. (n=150)

    b) MDR-TB participants received BPaMZ for 26 weeks (bedaquiline 200 mg daily for 8 weeks, then 100 mg daily for 18 weeks, together with pretomanid 200 mg plus moxifloxacin 400 mg plus pyrazinamide 1500 mg daily for 26 weeks). (n=152)

  - o *Comparator*: Standard WHO weight-based dosing of isoniazid, rifampicin, pyrazinamide, and ethambutol for 8 weeks, followed by isoniazid and rifampicin for 17 weeks in DS TB cases. (n=153)

    End Points: The primary efficacy endpoint was time to sputum culture-negative status by 8 weeks; the key secondary endpoint was an unfavorable outcome at week 52.

  - o *Outcome:*

    a) By week 8, 84% of 145 and 47% of 148 participants were culture-negative on 4 months of BPaMZ and HRZE, respectively. 86% of participants with DR-TB receiving 6 months of BPaMZ (n=152) reached culture-negative status by week 8.

    b) At week 52, 83% of 144, 93% of 144, and 83% of 133 on 4 months of BPaMZ, HRZE, and 6 months of BPaMZ had favorable outcomes, respectively.

    c) Serious liver-related adverse events were reported by 20 participants overall. 11 (7%) among those on 4 months of BPaMZ, one (1%) on HRZE, and eight (5%) on 6 months of BPaMZ.

  - o *Conclusion:* For DS-TB, BPaMZ successfully met the primary efficacy endpoint of sputum culture conversion. The regimen did not meet the key secondary efficacy endpoint due to adverse events resulting in treatment withdrawal.

  - o *Critical appraisal:* The potential for treatment-shortening efficacy of the BPaMZ regimen is there for DS-TB (threefold) and DR-TB however the challenge is to develop regimens with BPaMZ with lower risk of severe adverse drug events.

2. *Newer shorter regimens for DR-TB*

☞

- ***Short oral regimens for pulmonary rifampicin-resistant tuberculosis (TB-PRACTECAL): An open-label, randomized, controlled, phase 2b-3, multi-arm, multicenter, non-inferiority trial. (Lancet. 2023)*** [2]
    - o *Population:* 15 years and older with pulmonary rifampicin-resistant tuberculosis. (n=552)
    - o *Intervention:* Participants were randomly assigned, in a 1:1:1:1 to receive 36-80 weeks standard care; 24 weeks oral bedaquiline, pretomanid, and linezolid (BPaL); BPaL plus clofazimine (BPaLC); or BPaL plus moxifloxacin (BPaLM).
    - o *Comparator*: 36-80 weeks standard of care.

      End Points: The primary outcome was the percentage of participants with a composite unfavourable outcome (treatment failure, death, treatment discontinuation, disease recurrence, or loss to follow-up) at 72 weeks.
    - o *Outcome*: a) Unfavourable outcomes were reported in 12% of 137 participants for whom outcome was assessable in the BPaLM group and 41% of 137 participants in the standard care group.
    - o *Conclusion:* The 24 weeks, all-oral BPaLM regimen is safe and efficacious for the treatment of pulmonary rifampicin-resistant tuberculosis.
    - o *Critical appraisal:* The findings form the basis for BPaLM becoming the preferred regimen for adolescents and adults with pulmonary rifampicin-resistant tuberculosis and has already been added to the WHO guidance for treatment of this condition in 2022.

3. *Efficacy and safety of newer drugs/repurposed drugs for management of DR-TB*

- ***Efficacy and safety of bedaquiline-containing regimens in patients of drug-resistant tuberculosis: An updated systematic review and meta-analysis. (Journal of Clinical Tuberculosis and Other Mycobacterial Diseases. 2023)*** [3]
    - o *Population*: MDR-TB/pre-extensively drug resistant (XDR) TB/XDR TB patients (confirmed after culture or drug-susceptibility testing) on bedaquiline regimens from 36 observational studies (n=9934) and 5 experimental studies (n=468). ?
    - o *Outcome:* The pooled treatment success rate in studies of patients treated with regimens containing bedaquiline only was 78.4 % (95 % CI, 74.2–82.1) and 73.6 % (95 % CI, 64.6–81.0) in studies consisting of patients who were treated with regimens containing bedaquiline and delamanid.
    - o *Conclusion:* Bedaquiline-based regimens demonstrate high rates of culture conversion and treatment success with good safety profile.

- ***The Efficacy and Safety of Bedaquiline in the Treatment of Pulmonary Tuberculosis Patients: A Systematic Review and Meta-Analysis. (Antibiotics. 2023)*** [4]
    - o *Population*: Patients with sputum positive rifampicin-resistant MDR TB patients treated with bedaquiline from 29 studies (n=23,358).
    - o *Outcome:* The use of BDQ-containing regimens demonstrated improved rates of sputum conversion at 24 weeks (RR = 1.27, 95% CI: 1.10 to 1.46) and during follow-up (RR = 1.33, 95% CI: 1.06 to 1.66). However, the use of BDQ-containing regimens was associated with increased incidences of cardiotoxicity (RR = 4.54, 95% CI: 1.74 to 11.87).
    - o *Conclusion:* BDQ-containing regimens demonstrated a higher rate of sputum culture conversion, and a higher rate of cure compared to regimens without BDQ. ECG monitoring is a must as advised by the National TB elimination programme during pre-treatment evaluation.

☞

- ***Efficacy and safety of bedaquiline and delamanid in the treatment of Drug-Resistant Tuberculosis in Adults: A systematic review and meta-analysis. (IJTB. 2024)***[5]
  - *Population:* DR-TB patients in which bedaquiline and delamanid have been added to the WHO-recommended regimen for treating drug-resistant tuberculosis from 21 studies. (n=3583)
  - *Outcome:* The delamanid-only regimen reported the highest culture conversion rate of 85%. At six months, combination therapy yielded a culture conversion rate of 82%, with bedaquiline-only regimens reporting a rate of 80%. The incidence of QTc prolongation reported in each cohort is as follows: bedaquiline 0.163 ($p < 0.001$), delamanid 0.344 ($p = 0.272$) and combined 0.340 ($p < 0.001$).
  - *Conclusion:* This article demonstrated the efficacy of delamanid and bedaquiline, and their concomitant use in the treatment of drug-resistant tuberculosis. Moreover, the use of these drugs decreased mortality in DR-TB patients and the risk of cardiotoxicity was lower with concomitant use of both bedaquiline and delamanid.

- ***Efficacy of pretomanid-containing regimens for drug-resistant tuberculosis: A systematic review and meta-analysis of clinical trials. (Narra J. 2023)***[6]
  - *Population*: DR-TB patients started on pretomanid-containing regimen, with treatment duration of six months (24 weeks) from 4 studies. (n=237)
  - *Outcome*: Pretomanid containing regimen was associated with favourable outcome with OR: 46.73; 95%CI: 11.76–185.7, $p<0.001$.
  - *Conclusion:* This meta-analysis indicates that the pretomanid-containing regimen could increase the likelihood of achieving a favorable outcome in DR-TB patients.

☞

- ***The Safety and Tolerability of Linezolid in Novel Short-Course Regimens Containing Bedaquiline, Pretomanid, and Linezolid to Treat Rifampicin-Resistant Tuberculosis: An Individual Patient Data Meta-analysis. (Clinical Infectious Diseases. 2024)***[7]
  - *Population*: MDR/RR-TB patients with additional resistance to a fluoroquinolone antibiotic or second-line injectable agent (pre-extensively drug-resistant [preXDR]-TB) or extensively drug-resistant (XDR)-TB (resistance to both a fluoroquinolone or a second-line injectable agent), who were treated with BPaL-containing regimens from 3 trials having 8 unique BPaL regimens. (n=591)
  - *Outcome:* Among patients who were randomized to a daily dose of 1200 mg linezolid, 68 of 195 (35%) experienced a grade 3–4 adverse event, compared to 89 of 396 (22%) patients receiving BPaL-containing regimens containing 600 mg linezolid.
  - *Conclusion:*Regimens containing BPaL were relatively well tolerated when they included a daily linezolid dose of 600 mg.

4. ***Effect of Diabetes mellitus on outcome of DR-TB***

- ***The impact of diabetes mellitus on the emergence of multidrug-resistant tuberculosis and treatment failure in TB-diabetes comorbid patients: A systematic review and meta-analysis. (Front Public Health. 2023)[8]***
  - o *Population:* Patients with MDR-TB from 30 studies.
  - o *Outcome:*

    a) Tuberculosis–Diabetes Mellitus (TB-DM) patients were at higher risk to develop MDR-TB as compared to TB-non-DM patients (HR 0.81, 95% CI: 0.60–0.96, $p < 0.001$)

    b) TB-DM patients were at higher risk to experience treatment failure rates as compared to TB-non-DM patients (HR 0.46, 95% CI: 0.27–0.67, $p < 0.001$).
  - o *Conclusion*: This study highlights that DM has a significant impact on development of DR-TB and also increases the failure rate among these patients. Hence, effort should be for earlier screening of MDR-TB, thorough MDR-TB monitoring, and designing proper and effective treatment strategies to prevent disease progression.

- ***Diabetes mellitus affects the treatment outcomes of drug-resistant tuberculosis: A systematic review and meta-analysis. (BMC infectious diseases. 2023)[9]***
  - o *Population:* DR-TB and multidrug-resistant TB (MDR-TB) patients from 25 studies. (n=16905)
  - o *Outcome:* The pooled odds ratio (OR) was 1.56 (95% CI: 1.24–1.96) for unsuccessful outcomes, 0.64 (95% CI: 0.44–0.94) for cured treatment outcomes, 0.63 (95% CI: 0.46–0.86) for completed treatment outcomes, and 1.28 (95% CI: 1.03–1.58) for treatment failure.
  - o *Conclusion*: This study highlights the importance of diagnosing DM in DR-TB /MDR-TB, the need to control blood sugar levels and ensure therapeutic monitoring during the treatment of DR-TB/MDR-TB patients for successful outcomes.

5. ***Bedaquiline resistance in DR-TB***

☞

- ***Baseline and treatment-emergent bedaquiline resistance in drug-resistant tuberculosis: A systematic review and meta-analysis. (ERJ. 2023)[10]***
  - o *Population:* Patients with documented bedaquiline resistance via minimum inhibitory concentration (MIC) values having at least rifampicin-resistant TB developed either during treatment or at baseline, from 14 studies. (n=9975)
  - o *Outcome:* This analysis found a pooled prevalence of baseline bedaquiline resistance of 2.4% and a pooled prevalence of treatment-emergent bedaquiline resistance of 2.1%.
  - o *Conclusion*: Highlights the need for a rapid diagnostic test to detect bedaquiline resistance to avoid the development of escalating levels of bedaquiline resistance.

6. *Effectiveness and safety of tuberculosis preventive treatment for contacts of patients with DR-TB*

☞

- ***Effectiveness and safety of tuberculosis preventive treatment for contacts of patients with multidrug-resistant tuberculosis: A systematic review and meta-analysis. (Clinical Microbiology and Infection. 2023)***[11]
    - *Population:* Contacts of patients with MDR-TB from 11 studies. (n=1105)
    - *Outcome:* The pooled relative risk for disease progression in contacts receiving TPT versus those without treatment was 0.34 (95% CI: 0.16–0.72). Subgroup analysis indicated a lower pooled relative risk for regimens based on the drug-resistance profile of the index patients with TB compared to uniform treatment regimens.
    - *Conclusion:* TPT reduces the risk of TB disease progression in contacts of patients with MDR-TB. Tailored TPT regimens based on the drug-resistance profiles of index patients may provide additional benefits.

7. *Role of Next-generation sequencing (NGS) to diagnose DR-TB*

- ***Targeted next-generation sequencing to diagnose drug-resistant tuberculosis: A systematic review and meta-analysis. (Lancet. 2024)***[12]
    - *Population*: Patients in whom NGS was used to predict drug resistance in Mycobacterium tuberculosis infections, using primary samples, reference strain collections, or cultured isolates from individuals with presumed or confirmed tuberculosis from 124 studies.
    - *Outcome*: The combined sensitivity of targeted NGS across all drugs was 94·1% (95% credible interval [CrI] 90·9–96·3) and specificity was 98·1% (97·0–98·9). Sensitivity for individual drugs ranged from 76·5% (52·5–92·3) for capreomycin to 99·1% (98·3–99·7) for rifampicin.
    - *Conclusion:* Targeted NGS demonstrates high sensitivity and specificity for detecting drug resistance across panels of tuberculosis drugs and can be performed directly on clinical samples.

DISCUSSION

Epidemiology – Global and India

Tuberculosis (TB) is responsible for causing significant morbidity and deaths globally. As per Global TB report 2024, an estimated 10.8 million individuals suffered from tuberculosis (TB) worldwide.[13] In India, the incidence of TB is approximately one-fourth of the global incidence of 10.8 million cases, that is 2.8 million cases in 2023. Out of this an estimated 400,000 people developed multidrug-resistant or rifampicin resistant TB (MDR/RR-TB) globally and 110,000 individuals were reported to have developed MDR/RR-TB in India. About 27% of the world's drug-resistant tuberculosis (DR-TB) cases were recorded in India.[13]

Definitions

Multidrug-resistant tuberculosis (MDR-TB): A TB patient, whose biological specimen is resistant to both rifampicin (R) and isoniazid (H) with or without resistance to other first-line anti-TB drugs.

Mono-resistance: A TB patient, whose biological specimen is resistant to one first-line anti-TB drug only.

Rifampicin-resistant tuberculosis (RR-TB): A TB patient, whose biological specimen is resistant to R, detected using phenotypic or genotypic methods, with or without resistance to other anti-TB drugs. It includes any resistance to R, in the form of mono-resistance, poly-resistance, MDR or Extensively drug resistance (XDR).

Poly-resistance: Resistance of the clinical isolate to more than one first-line antitubercular drugs other than both isoniazid and rifampicin is referred to as poly-resistance.

Extensively drug-resistant TB (XDR-TB): TB caused by *Mycobacterium tuberculosis* (MTB) strains that fulfil the definition of MDR/RR-TB and are also resistant to any fluoroquinolone (levofloxacin or moxifloxacin) and at least one additional Group A drug (currently to either bedaquiline or linezolid [or both])

Pre-extensively drug-resistant TB (Pre-XDR-TB): TB caused by MTB strains that fulfill the definition of MDR/RR-TB and are also resistant to any fluoroquinolone (FQ).

Diagnosis of drug resistance TB

There are two methods available to determine drug resistance/susceptibility:

Genotypic/Molecular testing for resistance: In these tests the information regarding the known gene mutations associated with drug resistance is utilized to diagnose drug resistance. Turnaround time for diagnosis is a few hours to 2–3 days only. Commonly available genotypic methods are:

a) **Xpert MTB/RIF or cartridge-based nucleic acid amplification test (CBNAAT):** This test detects the presence of Mycobacterium tuberculosis DNA. Approximately 95% of the rifampicin resistance in Mycobacterium tuberculosis is attributed to the rpoB region, which is the gene responsible for detecting the rifampicin resistance. **It has been observed that Xpert MTB/RIF has a high sensitivity for CSF, stomach aspirates, and lymph node aspirates and for pleural fluid and other extrapulmonary specimens, it is relatively low.**[14] The Xpert RIF/MTB results take two hours to give results. Xpert MTB/RIF ultra is a different variant that offers nearly 100% sensitivity for smear-positive cases and approximately 93% sensitivity for smear-negative pulmonary TB cases.[15] **Within a single test, Xpert MTB/XDR can identify mutations linked to resistance to isoniazid, fluoroquinolones, second-line injectable drugs (amikacin, kanamycin, capreomycin), and ethionamide. It takes less than 90 minutes to get the results.**[16]

b) **Truelab real-time quantitative micro-PCR system (Truenat):** Molbio Diagnostics, Goa, India, offers two chip-based micro real-time PCR NAAT products: Truenat MTB and Truenat MTB-Rif Dx, which are used for detecting tuberculosis and rifampicin resistance, respectively.[17]

c) **Line probe assay (LPA): LPA version 1 is limited to use on smear-positive samples (direct testing) or culture isolates of Mycobacterium TB (indirect testing).** There is a 72-hour turnaround time. Its benefit is that this test provides information on isoniazid resistance genes katG (high-level resistance) and inhA (low-level resistance and ethionamide resistance), in addition to the rifampicin resistance gene rpoB. LPA has a sensitivity and specificity of 95.8% and 98.4%, respectively, for identifying rifampicin resistance and 94.5% and 99.3%, respectively, for detecting isoniazid resistance, according to the WHO Interpretation and Reporting Manual 2022.[18]

d) **Patho-TB test:** The Patho-TB test is a rapid flow-through diagnostic method that detects TB bacilli on a filter. It uses antibodies raised and purified against TB bacilli, which react with a gold conjugate. The presence of bacilli is indicated by a red or pink color on the filter. **The Patho-TB test has a high reproducibility rate and can be used in conjunction with other screening tests, such as AFB microscopy**. It can be especially useful in areas with poor lab conditions.[19]

The WHO has authorized the second-line probe assay (SL-LPA) to identify resistance to second-line injectables and fluoroquinolones (FQ), two types of second-line anti-tubercular medications. Mutations in the FQ resistance genes gyrA and gyrB, as well as the SLID resistance genes rrs and eis (low-level kanamycin resistance), are detected by SL-LPA. **Smear-negative scenarios can utilize SL-LPA version 2.**[20]

Phenotypic/conventional culture and drug sensitivity testing (DST): They can be done on either

a) **Solid culture:** It is done on **Lowenstein–Jensen** and **Middlebrook 7H10/11**. The turnaround time for solid culture is up to 42 days and for DST is up to another 42 days.

b) **Liquid culture (LC):** Also called BACTEC (BD Diagnostics, Sparks, MD, USA), MGIT960 (BD Diagnostics) and BacT/ALERT (BioMerieux SA, Marcy l'Etoile, France) systems. DST and culture turnaround times typically range from three to four weeks. For DST, **MGIT is the recommended approach due to its shorter turnaround time.** It can be used for testing both the pulmonary and extra-pulmonary specimens for sensitivity to first as well as second-line anti-TB drugs. Additionally, liquid culture is utilized for long-term follow-up of patients receiving drug-resistant tuberculosis treatment and to monitor response to treatment.[21]

Gene sequencing

Targeted NGS has a lot of potential for diagnosing DR-TB quickly. Pyrosequencing, Sanger sequencing, and other methods can all be used to accomplish targeted sequencing. Nearly the whole-genome of Mycobacterium tuberculosis (MTB) can be obtained from a sample by WGS, whereas MTB sequencing data at specific genetic loci of interest can be produced using targeted NGS. However, issues with cost, integration into current laboratory workflows, technical training and skills required to utilize the technology, computational expertise, and the requirement for expert guidance regarding the management and clinical interpretation of sequencing data have impeded the uptake of these technologies for DR-TB diagnosis.[12,22,23]

Integrated drug-resistant TB algorithm (Figure 1)

Upfront NAAT is offered to all presumptive TB patients. This includes PLHIV, children, extrapulmonary TB (EP-TB), smear negative/not available (NA) with chest X-ray suggestive of TB, contacts of DR-TB patients and other vulnerable groups. **All TB patients in whom an appropriate specimen can be collected are to be offered NAAT for bacteriological confirmation of TB and RR-TB and further test for fluoroquinolone resistance using SL-LPA.**

The algorithm helps to segregate the patients based on NAAT results as RR detected or RR not detected and offer DST-guided treatment.

- **The left arm: Rifampicin resistance detected** When rifampicin resistance is detected, the patient is offered first-line (FL) and SL-LPA. **RR detected in a new case with no risk factors for DR-TB needs to be retested if only M. TB detected was very low as that could be false-positive.** While FL LPA provides information on InhA mutations associated with Eto resistance, SL-LPA provides information on resistance to Lfx, Mfx and Am. LC, DST would be set up for Z,

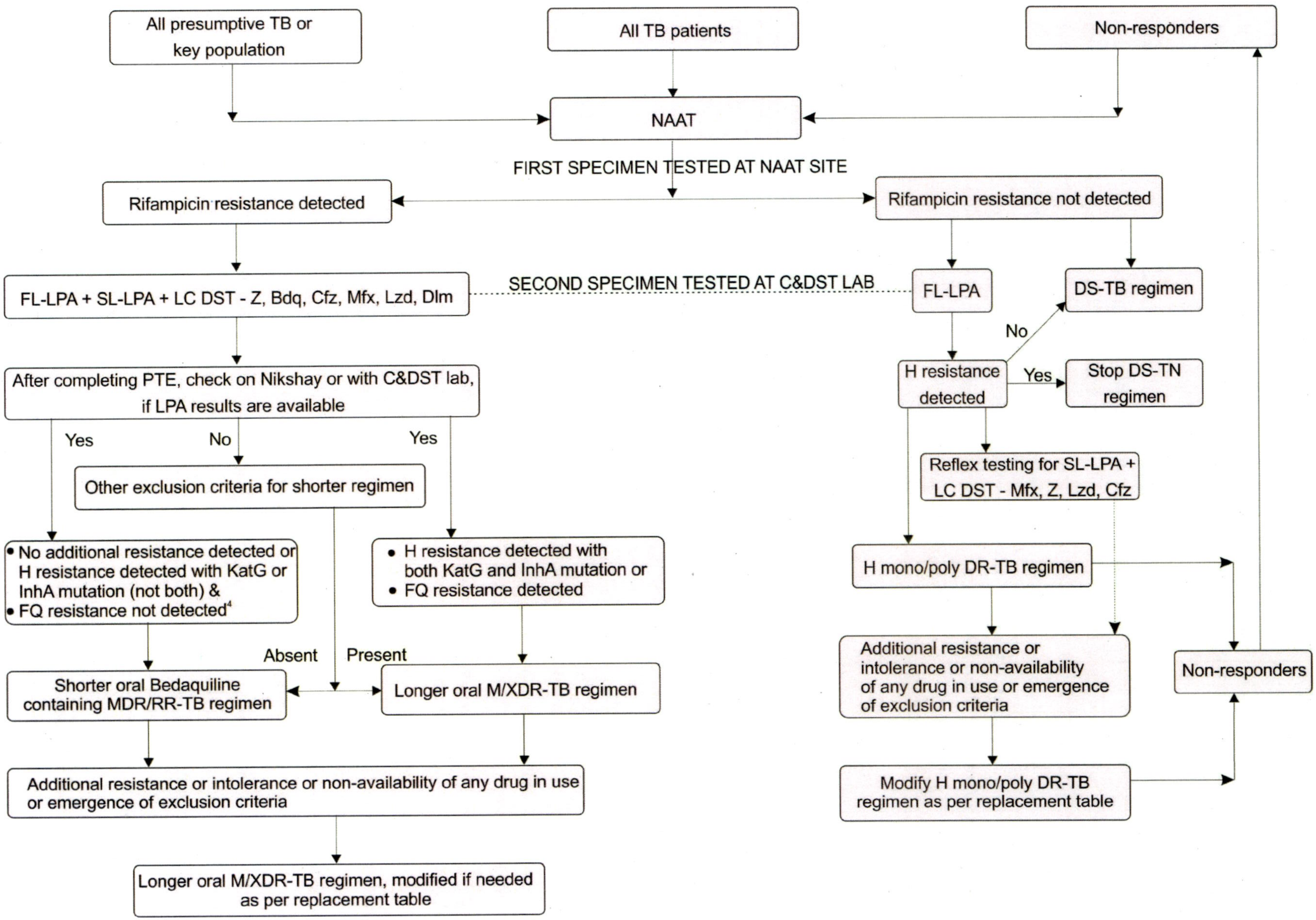

Figure 1: Integrated diagnostic and treatment algorithm for DR-TB (Adapted from Guidelines for programmatic management of drug-resistant tuberculosis in India 2021)

Mfx (if resistance detected by LPA), Lzd, Cfz*, Bdq* and Dlm* (*when available). Treatment is initiated based on the results of LPA and if required modified based on the LC DST results which would be available later. If FQ resistance is not detected and H resistance is detected due to mutations either in katG or InhA (but not both) the patient is eligible for shorter oral bedaquiline-containing MDR/RR-TB regimen. If FQ resistance is detected or H resistance is due to mutations in both katG and InhA, the patient is eligible for longer oral M/XDR-TB regimen.

o **The right arm: Rifampicin resistance not detected** When rifampicin resistance is not detected, the patient is offered FL LPA for detecting resistance to H. If H resistance is not detected, the patient is continued on a DS TB regimen. If H resistance is detected, the patient is eligible for H-mono/Poly DR-TB regimen. SL LPA will be performed for detecting resistance to FQ and LC DST will be performed for Mfx (if resistant by SL LPA), Z, Lzd and Cfz* (*when available). Treatment is initiated based on LPA results and modified based on the LC DST results which would be available later.

A second NAAT is carried out at the Culture and DST laboratory using the decontaminated deposit if there is a discrepancy in rifampicin resistance between NAAT and LPA. A microbiologist will make the final determination. Only smear-positive specimens can be subjected to direct LPA. If the smear results are negative, a culture is done, and if the culture is positive, the isolate is subjected to an indirect LPA.

What is new in diagnosis of DR-TB

WHO consolidated guidelines on tuberculosis. Module 3: Diagnosis - Rapid diagnostics for tuberculosis detection released in March 2024 has given certain recommendations for diagnosis of tuberculosis.[24]

Xpert Ultra is now recommended as an initial test for TB and rifampicin resistance in all adults and children with signs and symptoms of pulmonary TB. In children, the recommended use of Xpert MTB/RIF has been expanded to gastric aspirate, and stool. In HIV-positive adults and children with signs and symptoms of disseminated TB, Xpert MTB/RIF may be used in blood, as a diagnostic test for disseminated TB.

TB-LAMP–A commercial molecular assay, the Loopamp™ Mycobacterium tuberculosis complex (MTBC) detection kit (Eiken Chemical Company, Tokyo, Japan), is based on the loop-mediated isothermal amplification (LAMP) reaction. Referred to as TB-LAMP, this is a manual assay that requires less than 1 hour to perform and can be read with the naked eye under UV light. Because it requires little infrastructure and is relatively easy to use, **TB-LAMP is being explored as a rapid diagnostic test and an alternative to smear microscopy in resource-limited settings. TB-LAMP may be used as a replacement test for sputum-smear microscopy for diagnosing pulmonary TB in adults with signs and symptoms consistent with TB.** TB-LAMP may be used as a follow-on test to smear-microscopy in adults with signs and symptoms consistent with pulmonary TB, especially when further testing of sputum smear-negative specimens is necessary.[24]

Lateral flow urine lipoarabinomannan assay: Tests based on the detection of the lipoarabinomannan (LAM) antigen in urine have emerged as potential point-of-care tests for TB. The currently available urinary LAM assays have suboptimal sensitivity and are therefore not suitable as general diagnostic tests for TB. **However, unlike traditional diagnostic methods, they demonstrate improved sensitivity for TB diagnosis among individuals co-infected with HIV**.[24]

For targeted NGS, recommendations are that in people with bacteriologically confirmed pulmonary TB disease, targeted next-generation sequencing technologies may be used on respiratory samples to diagnose resistance to rifampicin, isoniazid, fluoroquinolones, pyrazinamide and ethambutol rather than culture-based phenotypic drug susceptibility testing. In people with bacteriologically confirmed rifampicin-resistant pulmonary TB disease, targeted NGS technologies may be used on respiratory samples to diagnose resistance to isoniazid, fluoroquinolones, bedaquiline, linezolid, clofazimine, pyrazinamide, ethambutol, amikacin and streptomycin rather than alternative to culture-based phenotypic drug susceptibility testing.[24]

Management of DR-TB

Newer Drugs

Bedaquiline (Bdq) is a diarylquinoline that specifically targets mycobacterial ATP synthase, an enzyme essential for the supply of energy to *Mycobacterium* TB. Pre-clinical, laboratory, and animal experiments have shown strong bactericidal and sterilizing activities against *M.tb*. **As per Indian guidelines Bedaquiline has been approved for children of age ≥5 years and above and weighing ≥ 15 kgs.**[22]

Delamanid (Dlm) is the first approved drug in the class of nitro-dihydro-imidazo-oxazoles for the treatment of MDR-TB. It is a bactericidal drug. **Dlm is already approved for use and available under NTEP for all irrespective of the age and weight ≥10 kgs.**[22]

As per communication by WHO in 2023, bedaquiline is now recommended for the treatment of MDR/RR-TB in adults and children of all ages. Bedaquiline and its M2 metabolite penetrate the cerebrospinal fluid of people with pulmonary TB, but the role for bedaquiline in the treatment of TB meningitis remains unclear and requires additional studies. **Bedaquiline and delamanid can be used together in people with MDR/RR-TB, including children, with careful electrocardiogram (ECG) monitoring**. Neuropsychiatric side effects, such as night terrors and disturbed sleep can happen in children treated with delamanid particularly in combination with cycloserine.[25,26]

Table 1: WHO Grouping of Drugs

GROUPS & STEPS	DRUG	
Group A:	Levofloxacin OR Moxifloxacin	Lfx Mfx
	Bedaquiline	Bdq
	Linezolid	Lzd
Group B:	Clofazimine	Cfz
	Cycloserine OR Terizidone	Cs Trd
Group C:	Ethambutol	E
	Delamanid	Dlm
	Pyrazinamide	Z
	Imipenem-cilastatin OR Meropenem	Ipm-Cln Mpm
	Amikacin (OR Streptomycin)	Am (S)
	Ethionamide OR Prothionamide	Eto Pto
	p-aminosalicylic acid	PAS

Regimens for DR-TB treatment

The standardized treatment regimen for M/XDR-TB include:

a. All oral H mono/poly DR-TB regimen.

b. Shorter RR/MDR-TB regimen which could be Bedaquiline containing oral regimen or injection containing regimen.

c. Longer oral regimen.

Table 2: Standard regimen for initiating treatment of MDR/RR TB or H mono-poly DR TB		
Regimen class	**Intensive phase**	**Continuation phase**
H mono/poly DR TB (R resistance not detected and H resistance)		
All oral H mono-poly DR TB regimen@	(6) Lfx R E Z	
MDR / RR TB		
Shorter Injection MDR TB regimen@	(4-6) Mfx^h Km/Am* Eto Cfz Z H^h E	(5) Mfx^h Cfz Z E
Shorter oral MDR TB regimen	(4–6) Bdq $_{(6\,m)}$, Lfx, Cfz, Z, E, Eto H$^{(h)}$	(5) Lfx, Cfz, Z, E
^Longer oral DR TB regimen@	(18-20) Bdq(6) Lfx Lzd# Cfz Cs	

* If the intensive phase is prolonged, the injectable agent is only given three times a week in the extended intensive phase.

\# Reduce Lzd to 300 mg/day after 6 to 8 months.

@ Pyridoxine to be given to all DR TB patients as per weight band.

All oral H mono/poly DR TB regimen is of 6 months with no separate IP/CP.

Also, w.e.f 24th March 2022, shorter injection containing MDR TB regimen has been phased out from India and only shorter oral bedaquiline-containing MDR/RR-TB regimen will be available in the entire country.

Shorter oral MDR TB regimen consists of an initial phase of 4 months that may be extended up to 6 months and a continuation phase of 5 months, giving a total duration of 9–11 months. Bdq is used for a duration of 6 months. IP should be given for at least 4 months.

As per WHO 2022 consolidated guidelines in eligible patients shorter oral Bedaquiline-containing regimen is preferred over longer oral regimen. WHO 2022 guidelines have also suggested that 4 months of ethionamide can be replaced by 2 months of linezolid.[21]

^ Longer oral regimen: Longer oral M/XDR-TB regimen is 18-20 months with no separate IP or CP. The composition of this regimen is bedaquiline (6 months or longer) – levofloxacin – *linezolid – clofazimine – cycloserine (*linezolid dose is to be reduced after 6-8 months). In XDR-TB, the treatment is to be given for 20 months.

Inclusion and Exclusion criteria for shorter MDR regimen

Inclusion criteria

1. DST based inclusion criteria

- Rifampicin resistance, either detected or inferred.
- MDR/RR-TB with H resistance detected/inferred based on InhA mutation only or based on KatG mutation only (not both).
- MDR/RR-TB with FQ resistance not detected.

2. Other inclusion criteria

- Children, aged 5 years to less than 18 years of age and weighing at least 15 kg, given their special needs, in consultation with the pediatrician.
- No history of exposure to previous treatment with second-line medicines in the regimen (Bdq, Lfx, Eto or Cfz) for more than one month (unless susceptibility to these medicines is confirmed).
- No extensive TB disease.
- No severe extra-pulmonary TB.
- Non-pregnant, non-lactating women.

Exclusion criteria

1. DST based exclusion criteria

- MDR/RR-TB patients with H resistance detected due to both KatG and InhA mutations and
- MDR/RR-TB patients with FQ resistance detected.

2. Other exclusion criteria

- If result for FL-LPA, SL-LPA and DST to Z, BDQ* and Cfz* is not available after pre-treatment.
- Evaluation is completed and it is a time to initiate the first dose of the regimen, then, exclude those with history of exposure for > 1 month to Bdq, Lfx, Eto or Cfz.
- Intolerance to any drug or risk of toxicity from a drug in shorter oral Bedaquiline containing MDR/RR-TB regimen (e.g. drug–drug interactions).
- Extensive TB disease characterized by bilateral cavitary lesions or extensive parenchymal damage on chest radiography, including the presence of cavities or bilateral disease in children under 15 years.
- Severe EP-TB, including miliary TB, TB meningitis, or central nervous system (CNS) TB. In children aged under 15 years, extrapulmonary forms of disease other than lymphadenopathy (peripheral nodes or isolated mediastinal mass without compression).
- Pregnant and lactating women and children below 5 years.

Principles of Designing a WHO recommended all oral longer MDR-TB regimen

Whenever an MDR-TB regimen is being designed the following principles should be kept in mind:

- **MDR-TB regimen should be composed of at least 4-5 drugs likely to be effective, including all drugs of group A plus 1-2 drugs from group B.** If any of the medications in groups A or B are contraindicated or not tolerated, group C medications may be utilized to accomplish the regimen. The WHO recommends starting treatment with all three Group A agents and at least one Group B agent to ensure that treatment starts with at least four TB agents likely to be effective and that at least three agents are included for rest of the treatment if Bdq is stopped. However, **NTEP guidelines recommend to start with all 5 drugs of Group A and B and continue with 4 drugs in the latter part of the regimen (beyond 6-8 months) provided the patient tolerates the drugs and to facilitate operational ease in the field.**[22]

In case of the need for replacement of any of the component(s) in the longer oral M/XDR-TB regimen, the following broad principles apply:

The drugs are replaced according to their efficacy, no demonstrable resistance, prior use, side effects profile, and background resistance to the replacement drug in the country as per the NDRS report. The regimen should preferably consist of fully oral drugs. However, in certain circumstances, injectables may have to be used for the need of efficacy and side effect profile. In situations where no replacement of any drug is required in the first 6 or 8 months of treatment in MDR-TB or XDR-TB patients, continue with at least 3 drugs after this depending on resistance, tolerability, availability, and contraindications of any one of Group A or B drugs.[21]

According to the PMDT guidelines 2021, the replacement sequence of Group C drugs for a longer oral regimen for M/XDR-TB is recommended in the order of: delamanid, amikacin, pyrazinamide, ethionamide, PAS, ethambutol, and carbapenems. When designing a regimen for M/XDR-TB patients, it is advised to combine the use of Bdq and Dlm if all five medications from Groups A and B cannot be used. In the last twelve months of treatment, Dlm and Am can not be started.[22]

Drug dosage and administration for Drug Resistant TB

The dosage of drugs varies as per weight of the patients. Adult patients (≥ 18 years) are classified in weight bands of <16 kg, 16-29 kg, 30-45 kg, 46-70 kg and >70kg.

The dosage for drugs used in various DR TB regimens by weight bands for adults are enumerated in Table 3.

Table 3: Dosage of DR TB drugs for adults

S. No	Drugs	16-29 kg	30-45 kg	46-70 kg	>70 kg
1	Rifampicin(R)[1]	300 mg	450 mg	600 mg	600 mg
2	High dose H (H^h)	300 mg	600 mg	900 mg	900 mg
3	Ethambutol(E)	400 mg	800 mg	1200 mg	1600 mg
4	Pyrazinamide(Z)	750 mg	1250 mg	1750 mg	2000 mg
5	Levofloxacin (Lfx)	250 mg	750 mg	1000 mg	1000 mg
6	Moxifloxacin (Mfx)	200 mg	400 mg	400 mg	400 mg
7	High dose Mfx (Mfx^h)	400 mg	600 mg	800 mg	800 mg
8	Bedaquiline (Bdq)	Week 0–2: Bdq 400 mg daily Week 3–24: Bdq 200 mg 3 times per week			
9	Linezolid (Lzd)	300 mg	600 mg	600 mg	600 mg
10	Clofazimine (Cfz)	50 mg	100 mg	100 mg	200 mg
11	Cycloserine (Cs)[4]	250 mg	500 mg	750 mg	1000 mg
12	Delamanid (Dlm)	50 mg twice daily (100 mg) for 24 weeks in 6-11 years of age 100 mg twice daily (200 mg) for 24 weeks for >11 years of age			
13	Imipenem/cilastatin (Ipm / Cls)[4]	1000 mg imipenem/1000 mg cilastatin twice daily			
14	Meropenem (Mpm)[4]	1000 mg three times daily (alternative dosing is 2000 mg twice daily)			
15	Amikacin (Am)[2]	500 mg	750 mg	750 mg	1000 mg
16	Capreomycin (Am)[2]				
17	Kanamycin (Km)[2]	500 mg	750 mg	750 mg	1000 mg
18	Ethionamide (Eto)[4]	375 mg	500 mg	750 mg	1000 mg
19	Na-PAS (60% weight/vol)[3,4]	10 gm	14 gm	16 gm	22 gm
20	Amoxycillin and potassium clavulanate (Amx/Clv) (In child: WHO 80 mg/Kg in 2 divided doses)	875/125 mg BD	875/125 mg BD	875/125 mg (2 morning +1 evening)	875/125 (2 morning +1 evening)
21	Pyridoxine (Pdx)	50 mg	100 mg	100 mg	100 mg

Important Trials for shortening DR-TB treatment

Many of trials have been done for the evaluating shorter treatment regimens for drug-resistant tuberculosis, with some having published their results and others nearing completion. **One such trial was the BEAT trial, which determined the effectiveness and safety of combining 2 new drugs with 2 repurposed drugs—bedaquiline, delamanid, linezolid, and clofazimine—for 24–36 weeks in adults diagnosed with pulmonary MDR-TB. After 24–36 weeks of treatment, this regimen resulted in a satisfactory favorable outcome (91%) in pulmonary MDR-TB patients with additional drug resistance. Cardiotoxicity was minimal, and myelosuppression, while common, was detected early and treated successfully.**[28]

Another trial, the **The endTB trial enrolled 754 patients using outcome-adapted randomization.** The trial evaluated five nine-month treatment regimens each experimental regimen included at least one new drug combined with up to four companion drugs. The control regimen was the local standard of care, consistent with the latest WHO recommendations, including bedaquiline and/or delamanid, when indicated.

Trial Regimens	Bedaquiline	Delamanid	Clofazimine	Linezolid	Quinolone	Pyrazinamide	Duration (months)
endTB 1	Bdq			Lzd	Mfx	Z	9
endTB 2	Bdq		Cfz	Lzd	Lfx	Z	9
endTB 3	Bdq	Dlm		Lzd	Lfx	Z	9
endTB 4		Dlm	Cfz	Lzd	Lfx	Z	9
endTB 5		Dlm	Cfz		Mfx	Z	9
Control Arm	Local SDC*						18-24

* Standard of care (SCO) control, composed according to WHO Guidelines, may include Bdq and/or Dlm

Figure 2: Five different arms in endTB trial (Adapted from endTB trial)

Regimens 1, 2, and 3 achieved favorable outcomes in 89.0%, 90.4%, and 85.2% of participants, respectively. Regimen 5 also showed a strong treatment response at 85.6% and was non-inferior to the control's 80.7%, holding promise as an alternative to patients unable to receive another regimen.[29]

The **NExT TB trial** was done to improve treatment outcomes while reducing drug toxicity and shortening the treatment duration to ~6 months in MDR-TB patients. **Participants were randomly assigned (1:1 ratio) to a ~6-month all-oral regimen that included levofloxacin, bedaquiline, and linezolid, or the standard-of-care (SOC) ≥9-month** WHO-approved injectable-based regimen. Out of a total of 93 patients enrolled 55% were human immunodeficiency virus-positive. **A favorable outcome was observed in 51% of patients compared to 22.7% in the standard-of-care arm.**[30]

A trial being done in China (Prospect Trial) is evaluating the modified STREAM regimen that replaces three group C drugs, ethambutol (EMB), pyrazinamide (PZA), and prothionamide (PTO), with more effective, two group B drugs, linezolid (LZD) and cycloserine (CS), while omitting high-dose isoniazid (INH) for confirmed INH-resistant cases. The control arm will receive a modified STREAM regimen B without high-dose INH and injectable kanamycin (KM) that incorporates experimental arm LZD and CS. The primary outcome measures the proportion of participants with favorable treatment outcomes at treatment completion (week 40), while the same measurement taken at 48 weeks post-treatment completion is the secondary outcome. The trial results are currently awaited.[31]

What is new and upcoming in DR-TB treatment

Bedaquiline, pretomanid, and linezolid make up the BPaL therapy regimen. Patients with XDR-TB or MDR-TB who did not respond to treatment or were not able to tolerate the medication were treated with BPaL. **The regimen is informed by the highly encouraging outcomes of the Nix and Zenix TB studies. Linezolid was administered at a dose of 1200 mg for the full 26-week period in the Nix-TB trial. Ninety percent of patients had a satisfactory outcome; nevertheless, the adverse effects caused by linezolid, such as peripheral neuropathy (81%) and myelosuppression (48%), frequently resulted in linezolid dose reductions or suspensions.**[32] In Zenix-TB Trial different dosages and duration of linezolid were tried. The participants were randomized to receive bedaquiline for 26 weeks (200 mg daily for 8 weeks, then 100 mg daily for 18 weeks), pretomanid (200 mg daily for 26 weeks), and daily linezolid at a dose of 1200 mg for 26 weeks or 9 weeks, or 600 mg for 26 weeks or 9 weeks. **The group that was administered a three-drug regimen, including 600 mg of linezolid for 26 weeks, experienced a reduced incidence of adverse events and fewer adjustments to the linezolid dose.**[33]

WHO Consolidated guidelines on DR-TB treatment 2022 update has recommended a shorter oral regimen for patients with multidrug-resistant tuberculosis (MDR-TB) and rifampicin-resistant tuberculosis (RR-TB), which has demonstrated positive outcomes worldwide.[21] This is based on TB-PRACTECAL randomized clinical trial and other evidence. TB-PRACTECAL is an open-label, randomized, controlled, phase II/III non-inferiority trial evaluating the safety and efficacy of 24-week regimens containing bedaquiline, pretomanid, linezolid with moxifloxacin (BPaLM) or along with clofazimine (BPaLC) in different arms to treat rifampicin-resistant tuberculosis. **Participants, 552 in number were randomly assigned, in a 1:1:1:1 ratio using variable block randomization and stratified by trial site, to receive 36–80 weeks standard care; 24-week oral bedaquiline, pretomanid, and linezolid (BPaL); BPaL plus clofazimine (BPaLC); or BPaL plus moxifloxacin (BPaLM) in stage one of the trial respectively. The standard care and BPaLM groups with 151 participants each proceeded to stage two. Unfavorable outcomes were reported in 16 (12%) of 137 participants for whom outcome was assessable in the BPaLM group and 56 (41%) of 137 participants in the standard care group.[2]**

As per WHO 2022 consolidated guidelines the 6-month BPaLM regimen, comprising bedaquiline, pretomanid, linezolid (600 mg), and moxifloxacin, may be used programmatically in place of 9-month or longer (>18 months) regimens, in patients (aged ≥14 years) with MDR/RR-TB who have not had previous exposure to bedaquiline, pretomanid and linezolid (defined as > 1-month exposure). This regimen may be used without moxifloxacin (BPaL) in the case of proven resistance to fluoroquinolones (in patients with pre-XDR-TB).[21]

The following points must be also taken into consideration while starting BPaLM/BPaL regimen as per WHO 2022 consolidated guidelines[21]

a) Adults and adolescent patients aged 14 years and older with MDR/RR-TB or with MDR/RR-TB and resistance to fluoroquinolones (pre-XDR-TB) are eligible BPaLM/BPaL irrespective of the HIV status.

b) People with confirmed pulmonary TB and all forms of extrapulmonary TB except for TB involving the CNS, osteoarticular and disseminated (miliary) TB are eligible.

c) Patients who have less than 1-month previous exposure to bedaquiline, linezolid, pretomanid or delamanid. If exposure is greater than 1 month, these regimens may still be given, if resistance to the specific medicines with such exposure has been ruled out.

d) Due to limited evidence regarding the safety of pretomanid in pregnant and breast-feeding women, these group of patients are not eligible for these regimens.

e) In case of consecutive treatment interruption (of all medicines in the regimen) of up to 2 weeks should be made up and added to the treatment duration. In case of linezolid after consecutive administration of linezolid at recommended doses (600 mg/daily) for at least 9 weeks, in case of intolerability the dose can either be adjusted down (to linezolid 300 mg/daily) or omitted (while other medicines in the regimen are continued) for a total of a maximum of 8 weeks throughout the treatment course.

These recommendations may be adopted by upcoming Indian guidelines for treatment of DR-TB. The diagnostic algorithm will also be modified as given in Figure 3. However, till these guidelines are released, it is imperative to follow programmatic guidelines for treatment of DR-TB released in 2021.

Recently WHO has released a rapid communication in August 2024 regarding newer shorter regimens for management of DR-TB based on evidence from the results of BEAT trial and endTB clinical trial in which they have given following recommendations[34]

1. **The 6-month BDLLfxC regimen, composed of bedaquiline, delamanid, linezolid (600 mg), levofloxacin, and clofazimine, may be used programmatically in place of 9-month or longer (>18 months) regimens, in all patients with MDR/RR-TB who have not had previous exposure to bedaquiline, delamanid and linezolid (defined as >1 month exposure).** BDLLfxC can be initiated without delay in case of unknown FQ-resistance at time of diagnosis of RR-TB (and may be continued with both levofloxacin and clofazimine if FQ-DST results cannot be obtained). BDLLfx is continued for FQ-sensitive TB; BDLC for FQ-resistant TB. **This regimen may be considered in patient groups who are not eligible for BPaLM/BPaL.**

2. **The use of the modified 9-month, all-oral regimens (BLMZ, BLLfxCZ, and BDLLfxZ) is preferred over currently recommended longer (18-month) regimens in patients with MDR/RR-TB who have not had previous exposure to bedaquiline, delamanid and linezolid (defined as >1-month exposure) and in whom resistance to fluoroquinolones has been excluded**. Among these regimens, using BLMZ is suggested over BLLfxCZ, and BLLfxCZ is suggested over BDLLfxZ.

Treatment Outcome

PMDT 2021 guidelines define treatment outcome of DR-TB as cured, treatment completed, treatment failed, died, or lost to follow-up.[22]

Cured: A pulmonary TB patient with bacteriologically confirmed TB at the beginning of treatment who completed treatment as recommended by the national policy with evidence of bacteriological response (with at least two consecutive cultures, taken on different occasions at least 7 days apart, found to be negative) and no evidence of treatment failed.

Treatment completed: A TB patient who completed treatment as recommended by the national policy and whose outcome does not meet the definition for cure or treatment failed.

Treatment success: The sum of cured and treatment completed is taken as treatment success.

Lost to follow-up: If a TB patient does not start the treatment or interrupts treatment for 2 consecutive months or more.

Treatment failed: A patient whose treatment regimen needs to be terminated or permanently changed to a new regimen option or treatment strategy. Reasons for the change may be no clinical and/or bacteriological response, adverse drug reactions (ADRs) or evidence of additional resistance to drugs in the regimen.

Died: A TB patient who dies before starting or during treatment.

Use of Steroids in DR-TB

In cases of respiratory insufficiency, adrenocortical insufficiency, pericardial disease, or severe CNS disease, corticosteroids may be administered. When administering steroids to a patient, it is imperative to make sure they receive an appropriate anti-TB medication at the correct dosage.[34]

Indications of Surgery

Patients with localized DR-TB disease may benefit from surgery alongside chemotherapy, particularly if the procedure is performed by a skilled surgeon and tthe patient receives optimal postoperative care.[35] When unilateral localized disease is present, surgery should be considered in the following patients:

- Lack of a bacteriological or clinical response to chemotherapy after receiving effective anti-TB medication for six to nine months.
- High degree of resistance or widespread parenchymal involvement increases the chance that treatment may fail or cause a relapse.
- Morbid complications of parenchymal disease e.g., hemoptysis, bronchiectasis, broncho-pleural fistula, or empyema; and
- Recurrence after completion of anti-TB treatment.

WHO has recommended surgical procedures such as wedge resections or lobectomy in patients with localized lesions.

Special considerations in extra pulmonary (EP) DR-TB

In EPTB cases where when there is a high index of suspicion for DR-TB, appropriate samples should be sent for MGIT culture and DST as well as molecular tests such as GeneXpert MTB/RIF assay and line probe assays before starting empiric 2nd line ATT. While making a regimen in CNS TB cases, the drugs should be selected preferably based on the following propensity of anti-TB drugs for crossing the blood-brain barrier and sensitivity pattern:[37]

a) **Drugs having good penetration ability into CSF: isoniazid, pyrazinamide, prothionamide/ethionamide, cycloserine, linezolid.**

b) **Drugs which are able to pass when meninges are inflamed: second-line injectables, and streptomycin.**

c) **Drugs with variable penetration:** fluoroquinolones.

d) **Drugs with poor penetration:** PAS and ethambutol.

e) Drugs with no data available for CNS penetration: bedaquiline, delamanid, and clofazimine.

In lymph node TB where the treatment has been started based on clinical grounds or suggestive cytology or histopathology for TB, the response to treatment should be assessed at 4 months and possible treatment failure should be considered in patients who have worsened or deteriorated after initial improvement – requires diagnostic investigations to rule out DR-TB and assess the need for a treatment change. Deterioration in the first 3 months may also be due to a paradoxical reaction.[38]

Therapeutic Drug Monitoring (TDM)

Despite receiving appropriate doses of anti-TB medicine and a dependable laboratory report indicating that the sputum is still susceptible to either rifampicin or INH, or both, some patients remain sputum smear-positive and culture-positive. In such situations, if compliance with treatment has been ensured, it is essential to investigate whether the patient is absorbing the drugs well. **Research from India and other countries has revealed that many patients exhibit low serum concentrations of anti-TB medications, particularly for rifampicin.[39,40] Patients with malnourishment and TB-HIV co-infection are also more likely to experience it.[39,41]** A study by Singla et al in India on non-responding drug-sensitive TB patients under treatment, found that in 85.3% of patients, rifampicin plasma levels were low, and in 39.1%, isoniazid plasma levels were low. Low body mass index, pulmonary tuberculosis, and disseminated tuberculosis, far-advanced disease, bilateral findings on chest X-ray, cavities, and low rifampicin levels were associated with unfavorable outcomes. **In this study, it was also seen that, in 59.6% of patients who have received ≥6 months of treatment, the outcome was favorable in whom intervention was done by augmenting the treatment regimen with three to four second-line drugs along with increasing the dose of R and H.[40]** An important issue in India is the lack of therapeutic drug monitoring (TDM) facilities.

Treatment of Contacts of DR-TB

The Guidelines on Programmatic Management of TB Preventive Treatment (PMTPT) were released in 2021.[42] These guidelines have now been implemented across India to gain and document experiences regarding feasibility, safety monitoring, and enhancement in treatment outcomes of TB preventive treatment. **Household contacts (HHC) of patients with MDR/RR-TB or H mono-resistance are at higher risk of TB infection (TBI) than contacts exposed to drug-sensitive TB, however, the risk of progression to TB disease does not differ among contacts in both groups.**

Preventive treatment among HHC of MDR-TB index patients (in whom FQ resistance has been ruled out) and among HHC of H resistant index patients (in whom R resistance has been ruled out), the target population, using 6Lfx and 4R respectively has been introduced in a phased manner for all age groups. The recommended dosages of medicines for TB preventive treatment among contacts of DR-TB index patients after ruling out active TB and confirming TBI, with treatment dosages adjusted by age and weight are given in Table 4 below.

Table 4: The recommended dosages of medicines for TB preventive treatment among contacts of DR-TB index patients (As per PMTPT guidelines)	
Regimen	**Dose by age and weight band**
Six months of daily levofloxacin (6Lfx) for contacts of R resistant FQ sensitive patients^	Age > 14 years, by body weight: < 45 kg, 750 mg/day; ≥ 45 kg, 1g/day Age < 15 years (range approx. 15–20 mg/kg/day), by body weight: • 5–9 kg: 150 mg/day • 10–15 kg: 200–300 mg/day • 16–23 kg: 300–400 mg/day • 24–34 kg: 500–750 mg/day
Four months of rifampicin daily (4R) for contacts of H resistant R sensitive patients*	Age 10 years & older: 10 mg/kg/day@ Age <10 years: 15 mg/kg/day (range, 10–20 mg)

^ 6H can be considered as the TPT regimen option for contacts of index patients with RR-TB with FQ and H sensitive, after ruling out active TB in them

* In children from 0-14 years, 4R should only be used after ruling out active TB in limited geographies/populations for evidence generation to guide future scale up for country wide implementation.

@ Maximum dose of R would be 600 mg/day.

Conclusion/End Message

- Focus on Prevention of DR-TB.
- Phenotypic tests take longer time, but good to assess response to treatment.
- Genotypic tests provide faster results.
- Newer Genotypic tests may be a game changer for early identification of Pre-XDR TB and early initiation of appropriate regimen.
- Follow Integrated diagnostic and treatment algorithm for management of DR-TB patients.
- Contacts of DR-TB need to be treated with TB preventive therapy after testing them for TB infection and ruling out active TB as per guidelines.

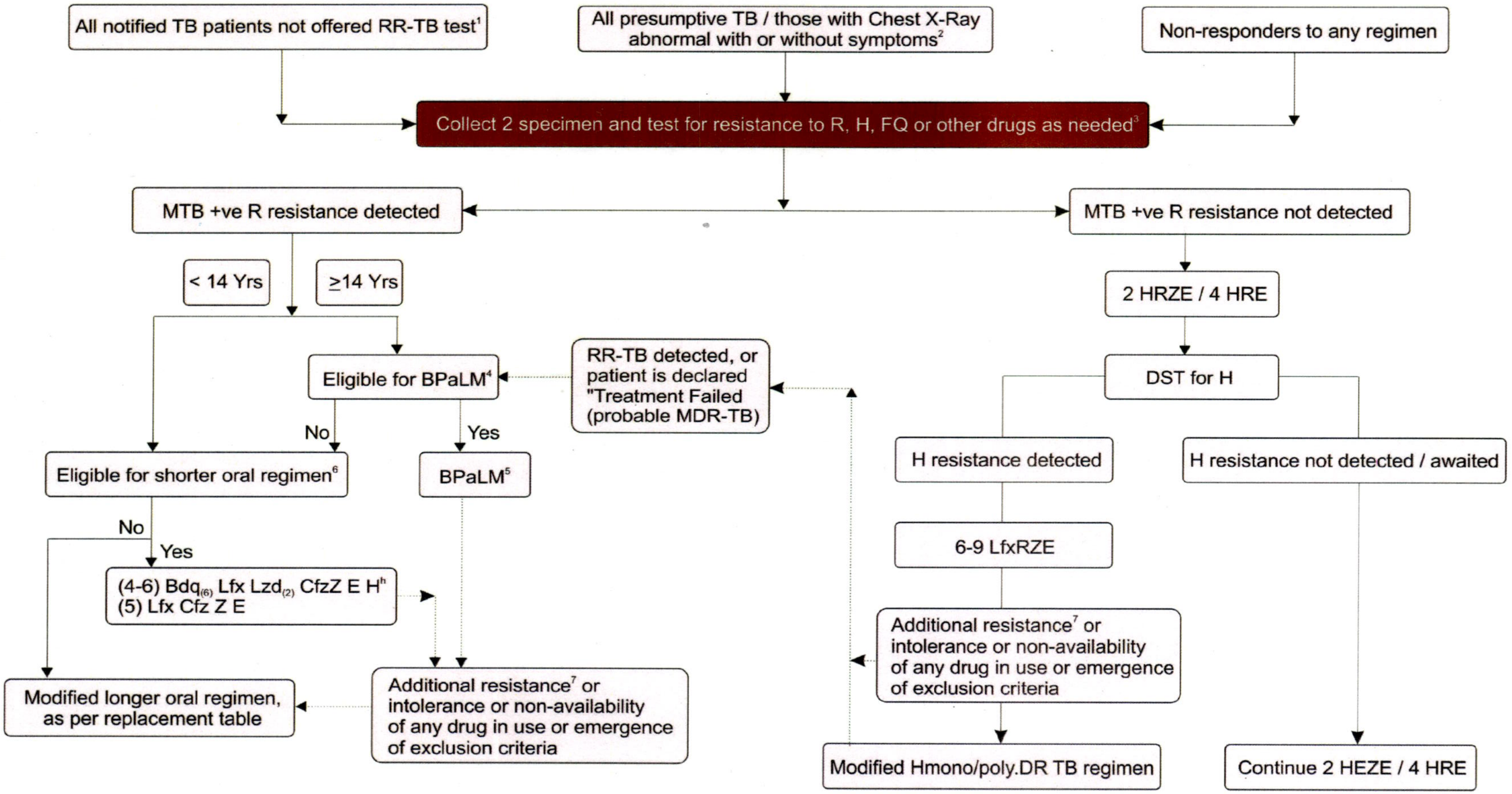

Figure 3: Proposed and updated Integrated diagnostic and treatment algorithm for Drug susceptible and resistant Tuberculosis by Guidelines for programmatic

REFERENCES

1. Cevik M, Thompson LC, Upton C, Rolla VC, Malahleha M, Mmbaga B, et al. Bedaquiline-pretomanid-moxifloxacin-pyrazinamide for drug-sensitive and drug-resistant pulmonary tuberculosis treatment: a phase 2c, open-label, multicentre, partially randomised controlled trial. The Lancet Infectious Diseases. 2024 May; S1473309924002238.

2. Nyang'wa BT, Berry C, Kazounis E, Motta I, Parpieva N, Tigay Z, et al. Short oral regimens for pulmonary rifampicin-resistant tuberculosis (TB-PRACTECAL): an open-label, randomised, controlled, phase 2B-3, multi-arm, multicentre, non-inferiority trial. The Lancet Respiratory Medicine. 2024 Feb;12(2):117–28.

3. Ur Rehman O, Fatima E, Ali A, Akram U, Nashwan A, Yunus F. Efficacy and safety of bedaquiline containing regimens in patients of drug-resistant tuberculosis: An updated systematic review and meta-analysis. Journal of Clinical Tuberculosis and Other Mycobacterial Diseases. 2024 Feb;34:100405.

4. Tong E, Wu Q, Chen Y, Liu Z, Zhang M, Zhu Y, et al. The Efficacy and Safety of Bedaquiline in the Treatment of Pulmonary Tuberculosis Patients: A Systematic Review and Meta-Analysis. Antibiotics. 2023 Aug 31;12(9):1389.

5. Ahmed SH, Haider H, Moeed A, Mahmood A, Shivani N, Shuja SH, et al. Efficacy and safety of bedaquiline and delamanid in the treatment of drug-resistant tuberculosis in adults: A systematic review and meta-analysis. Indian Journal of Tuberculosis. 2024 Jan;71(1):79–88.

6. Simanjuntak AM, Daenansya R, Afladhanti PM, Yovi I, Suyanto S, Anggraini D, et al. Efficacy of pretomanid-containing regiments for drug-resistant tuberculosis: A systematic review and meta-analysis of clinical trials. Narra J. 2023 Dec 29;3(3):e402.

7. Hasan T, Medcalf E, Nyang'wa BT, Egizi E, Berry C, Dodd M, et al. The Safety and Tolerability of Linezolid in Novel Short-Course Regimens Containing Bedaquiline, Pretomanid, and Linezolid to Treat Rifampicin-Resistant Tuberculosis: An Individual Patient Data Meta-analysis. Clinical Infectious Diseases. 2024 Mar 20;78(3):730–41.

8. Rehman AU, Khattak M, Mushtaq U, Latif M, Ahmad I, Rasool MF, et al. The impact of diabetes mellitus on the emergence of multi-drug resistant tuberculosis and treatment failure in TB-diabetes comorbid patients: a systematic review and meta-analysis. Front Public Health. 2023 Nov 16;11:1244450.

9. Xu G, Hu X, Lian Y, Li X. Diabetes mellitus affects the treatment outcomes of drug-resistant tuberculosis: a systematic review and meta-analysis. BMC Infect Dis. 2023 Nov 20;23(1):813.

10. Perumal R, Bionghi N, Nimmo C, Letsoalo M, Cummings MJ, Hopson M, et al. Baseline and treatment-emergent bedaquiline resistance in drug-resistant tuberculosis: a systematic review and meta-analysis. Eur Respir J. 2023 Dec;62(6):2300639.

11. Zhou G, Luo S, He J, Chen N, Zhang Y, Cai S, et al. Effectiveness and safety of tuberculosis preventive treatment for contacts of patients with multidrug-resistant tuberculosis: a systematic review and meta-analysis. Clinical Microbiology and Infection. 2024 Feb;30(2):189–96.

12. Van Rie A, Warren R. Time to change to next-generation sequencing for management of drug-resistant tuberculosis? The Lancet Infectious Diseases. 2024 May;S1473309924003001.

13. Global Tuberculosis Report 2024 [Internet]. [cited 2024 Nov 14]. Available from: https://www.who.int/teams/global-tuberculosis-programme/tb-reports/global-tuberculosis-report-2024.

14. World Health Organization. WHO operational handbook on tuberculosis: module 3: diagnosis: rapid diagnostics for tuberculosis detection [Internet]. 2021 update. Geneva: World Health Organization; 2021 [cited 2022 May 11]. Available from: https://apps.who.int/iris/handle/10665/342369.

15. World Health Organization. Use of Xpert MTB/RIF and Xpert MTB/RIF Ultra on GeneXpert 10-colour instruments: WHO policy statement [Internet]. Geneva: World Health Organization; 2021 [cited 2022 May 11]. Available from: https://apps.who.int/iris/handle/10665/350154.

16. Pillay S, Steingart KR, Davies GR, Chaplin M, De Vos M, Schumacher SG, et al. Xpert MTB/XDR for detection of pulmonary tuberculosis and resistance to isoniazid, fluoroquinolones, ethionamide, and amikacin. Cochrane Database Syst Rev. 2022 May 18;5(5):CD014841.

17. Jeyashree K, Shanmugasundaram D, Rade K, Gangakhedkar RR, Murhekar MV. Impact and operational feasibility of TrueNat™ MTB/Rif under India's RNTCP. Public Health Action. 2020 Sep 21;10(3):87–91.

18. Line probe assays for detection of drug-resistant tuberculosis: interpretation and reporting manual for laboratory staff and clinicians [Internet]. [cited 2024 Aug 18]. Available from: https://www.who.int/publications/i/item/9789240046665

19. Nour-Neamatollahi A, Siadat SD, Yari S, Tasbiti AH, Ebrahimzadeh N, Vaziri F, et al. A new diagnostic tool for rapid and accurate detection of Mycobacterium tuberculosis. Saudi Journal of Biological Sciences. 2018 Mar;25(3):418–25.

20. World Health Organization. The use of molecular line probe assays for the detection of resistance to second-line anti-tuberculosis drugs: policy guidance [Internet]. Geneva: World Health Organization; 2016 [cited 2022 May 11]. 42 p. Available from: https://apps.who.int/iris/handle/10665/246131

21. WHO consolidated guidelines on tuberculosis. Module 4: treatment - drug-resistant tuberculosis treatment, 2022 update [Internet]. [cited 2023 Jul 7]. Available from: https://www.who.int/publications-detail-redirect/9789240063129

22. 8368587497Guidelines for PMDT in India.pdf [Internet]. [cited 2022 May 11]. Available from: https://tbcindia.gov.in/WriteReadData/l892s/8368587497Guidelines%20for%20 PMDT%20in%20India.pdf

23. WHO issues rapid communication on use of targeted next-generation sequencing for diagnosis of drug-resistant tuberculosis [Internet]. [cited 2024 Aug 7]. Available from: https://www.who.int/news/item/25-07-2023-who-issues-rapid-communication-on-use-of-targeted-

next-generation-sequencing-for-diagnosis-of-drug-resistant-tuberculosis

24. WHO consolidated guidelines on tuberculosis: module 3: diagnosis: rapid diagnostics for tuberculosis detection, 3rd ed [Internet]. [cited 2024 Aug 18]. Available from: https://www.who.int/publications/i/item/9789240089488

25. Use of bedaquiline in children and adolescents with multidrug- and rifampicin-resistant tuberculosis: information note [Internet]. [cited 2024 Aug 18]. Available from: https://www.who.int/publications/i/item/9789240074286

26. Use of delamanid in children and adolescents with multidrug- and rifampicin-resistant tuberculosis: information note [Internet]. [cited 2024 Aug 18]. Available from: https://www.who.int/publications/i/item/9789240074309

27. Ahmad N, Ahuja SD, Akkerman OW, Alffenaar JWC, Anderson LF, Baghaei P, et al. Treatment correlates of successful outcomes in pulmonary multidrug-resistant tuberculosis: an individual patient data meta-analysis. The Lancet. 2018 Sep;392(10150):821–34.

28. Padmapriyadarsini C, Vohra V, Bhatnagar A, Solanki R, Sridhar R, Anande L, et al. Bedaquiline, Delamanid, Linezolid and Clofazimine for Treatment of Pre-extensively Drug-Resistant Tuberculosis. Clin Infect Dis. 2022 Jun 29;76(3):e938-946.

29. endTB clinical trials | endTB [Internet]. [cited 2024 Aug 18]. Available from: https://endtb.org/clinical-trial

30. Esmail A, Oelofse S, Lombard C, Perumal R, Mbuthini L, Goolam Mahomed A, et al. An All-Oral 6-Month Regimen for Multidrug-Resistant Tuberculosis: A Multicenter, Randomized Controlled Clinical Trial (the NExT Study). Am J Respir Crit Care Med. 2022 May 15;205(10):1214–27.

31. Gao J, Gao M, Du J, Pang Y, Mao G, Lounis N, et al. A pragmatic randomized controlled trial to evaluate the efficacy and safety of an oral short-course regimen including bedaquiline for the treatment of patients with multidrug-resistant tuberculosis in China: study protocol for PROSPECT. Trials. 2024 Apr 1;25(1):227.

32. Conradie F, Diacon AH, Ngubane N, Howell P, Everitt D, Crook AM, et al. Treatment of Highly Drug-Resistant Pulmonary Tuberculosis. N Engl J Med. 2020 Mar 5;382(10):893–902.

33. Conradie F, Bagdasaryan TR, Borisov S, Howell P, Mikiashvili L, Ngubane N, et al. Bedaquiline-Pretomanid-Linezolid Regimens for Drug-Resistant Tuberculosis. N Engl J Med. 2022 Sep 1;387(9):810–23.

34. Key updates to the treatment of drug-resistant tuberculosis: rapid communication, June 2024 [Internet]. [cited 2024 Aug 31]. Available from: https://iris.who.int/handle/10665/378472

35. Schutz C, Davis AG, Sossen B, Lai RPJ, Ntsekhe M, Harley YX, et al. Corticosteroids as an adjunct to tuberculosis therapy. Expert Rev Respir Med. 2018 Oct;12(10):881–91.

36. The role of surgery in the treatment of pulmonary TB and multidrug- and extensively drug-resistant TB.

37. 7702334778Training_Module_on_Extrapulmonary_TB_-_Book_24032023.pdf [Internet]. [cited 2024 Aug 31]. Available from: https://tbcindia.mohfw.gov.in/wp-content/uploads/2023/05/7702334778Training_Module_on_Extrapulmonary_TB_-_Book_24032023.pdf

38. 5585665076Index-TB-Guidelines.pdf [Internet]. [cited 2024 Aug 31]. Available from: https://tbcindia.mohfw.gov.in/wp-content/uploads/2023/05/5585665076Index-TB-Guidelines.pdf

39. Peloquin CA. Therapeutic drug monitoring in the treatment of tuberculosis. Drugs. 2002;62(15):2169–83.

40. Singla R, Gupta A, Kumar V, Padmapriyadarsini C, Tayal D, Anand S, et al. Study of risk factors and clinical management of patients with clinical non-response due to low plasma levels of anti-tubercular drugs. Monaldi Arch Chest Dis [Internet]. 2024 Jul 23 [cited 2024 Aug 7]; Available from: https://www.monaldi-archives.org/macd/article/view/3036

41. Van Tongeren L, Nolan S, Cook VJ, FitzGerald JM, Johnston JC. Therapeutic drug monitoring in the treatment of tuberculosis: a retrospective analysis. Int J Tuberc Lung Dis. 2013 Feb;17(2):221–4.

42. Guidelines for Programmatic Management of Tuberculosis Preventive Treatment in India.pdf [Internet]. [cited 2023 Jul 18]. Available from: https://tbcindia.gov.in/WriteReadData/l892s/Guidelines for Programmatic Management of Tuberculosis Preventive Treatment in India.pdf

CHAPTER 13

Sleep Related Breathing Disorders

Authors: Dr. Ganesh Narwade, Dr. Sharada Vinod Kutty, Dr. Rohit Vadala

Reviewer: Dr. Tejas Suri

INTRODUCTION

Sleep medicine is one of the important sub-specialties of Pulmonology, dealing with dedicated understanding and managing various sleep-related breathing disorders. This field is gradually gaining more public awareness because of the impact of untreated sleep disorders on the quality of life. It is increasingly being identified as one of the important conditions resulting in increased morbidity and subsequent mortality. This article reviews recent updates in the field of sleep-disordered breathing (SDB) in various diagnostic and therapeutic modalities.

Methodology

A PubMed search was carried out with the search term "sleep disordered breathing." Articles between 1st August 2023, and 1st August 2024 were reviewed. 45 articles turned up during the search, and they were screened for relevance and research significance. Out of these, 33 were selected for this review.

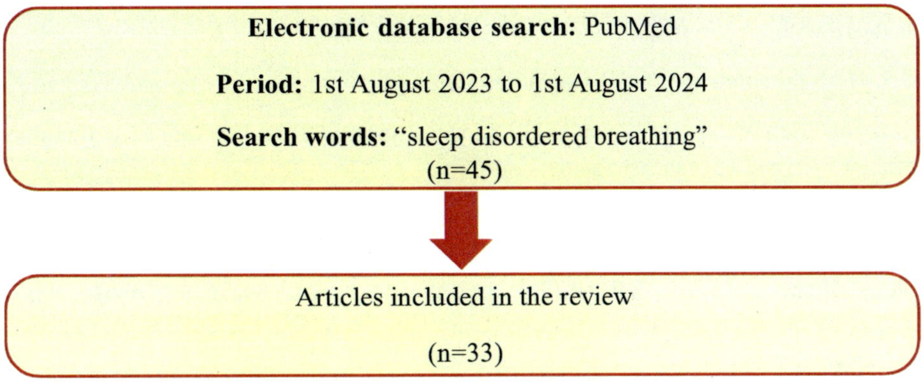

Analysis of literature

A. Diagnosis and clinical implications of sleep-disordered breathing (SDB)

- ***Maternal sleep disordered breathing and offspring growth outcome: A systematic review and meta-analysis. (Sleep Med Rev. 2024)***[1]
    - o *Population*: Pregnant females with sleep-disordered breathing from 63 manuscripts (n=67,671,110 pregnant women).
    - o *Intervention*: 31 studies used subjective methods to define sleep disordered breathing, 24 applied objective methods, while 8 used international codes. Random effect models were used to assess association between habitual snoring and obstructive sleep apnea and abnormal offspring outcomes.

- *Outcome*: Large for Gestational Age (LGA): Maternal habitual snoring (subjective methods) and obstructive sleep apnea (OSA) diagnosed by objective methods were associated with an increased risk of LGA newborns (OR 1.46; 95% CI 1.02–2.09 and OR 2.19; 95% CI 1.63–2.95, respectively). Small for Gestational Age (SGA): Maternal OSA was associated with an increased risk for SGA newborns (OR 1.28; 95% CI 1.02–1.60).

  Mean Birth weight: No significant differences in mean birth weight between newborns of mothers with and without SDB were observed.
- *Conclusion*: The systematic review and meta-analysis provide evidence that maternal sleep-disordered breathing (SDB) is associated with abnormal offspring growth outcomes.
- *Critical appraisal*: This study highlights the importance of screening and management of SDB before and during pregnancy. Data generation is required to inform standardized screening and treatment practices for the SDB and pregnancy. Future studies should investigate underlying mechanisms and whether treatment of sleep disordered breathing ameliorates neonatal growth.

- ***Sleep-Disordered Breathing and Prevalent Hypertension in Men with and Without HIV. (J Acquir Immune Defic Syndr. 2023)***[2]
  - *Population*: This study investigated the independent and interactive associations between sleep-disordered breathing (SDB), and hypertension in a cohort of men with and without HIV (n=779), with 436 living with HIV and 343 without HIV. The participants were part of the Multicenter AIDS Cohort Study (MACS).
  - *Intervention*: SDB was assessed using in-home polysomnography in 779 men (436 with and 343 without HIV). Oxygen desaturation index were used to quantify SDB severity. Hypertension (HTN) was defined as blood pressure $\geq$ 140/90mmHg. The associations between HIV, SDB, and HTN were characterized using multivariable logistic regression.
  - *Outcome*: Prevalence of Hypertension: Hypertension prevalence was 53.8% overall, with similar rates between men with HIV (52.1%) and those without (56.0%).

    Prevalence of SDB: High prevalence of SDB was noted, with 82.8% of men having an AHI $\geq$ 5 events/hour.

    Independent Association: Men with both HIV and SDB had an adjusted OR of 3.24 (95% CI: 1.62 to 6.47) for hypertension, showing no significant increase over either factor alone.
  - *Conclusion*: The study concluded that both HIV and SDB are independently associated with hypertension. However, the combination of HIV and SDB does not further elevate the risk of hypertension beyond the presence of either condition alone. These findings suggest that while SDB and HIV are significant risk factors for hypertension, their combined effect does not exacerbate the condition.
  - *Critical appraisal*: This study points to an important association between SDB and HIV infection. Both SDB and HIV infection are hypothesized to be associated with increased systemic inflammation and cardiovascular risk. With HAART and increased life spans of those with HIV, screening for comorbidities becomes significant. Further trials are needed to make recommendations.

- ***Algorithmic detection of sleep-disordered breathing using respiratory signals: A systematic review. (Physiol Meas. 2024)***[3]
  - *Population*: The reviewed studies include subjects undergoing SDB detection using various respiratory signals from 32 studies.
  - *Intervention*: Algorithms utilizing respiratory signals, including nasal airflow (NAF), oronasal airflow (OAF), thoracic respiratory effort (TRE), and abdominal respiratory effort (ARE), were evaluated.

Classification Techniques used were:

1. Threshold rule-based methods: 8 studies
2. Machine learning models: 13 studies
3. Deep learning models: 11 studies

The performance of different signal sources and classification methods (threshold rule-based, machine learning, and deep learning models) were compared.

- *Outcomes*: Signal Sources: NAF-based algorithms showed the highest average accuracy at 94.11%, outperforming other signals at 78.19%. Hypopnea detection sensitivity was modest, with a maximum of 73.34% for single-source respiratory signals.
- *Conclusions*: Multiple algorithms have been successfully applied for SDB detection. The accuracy of these algorithms is highly dependent on the choice of signal source, signal processing methods, feature selection, and model selection. TRE and ARE signals are particularly reliable for identifying various types of SDB due to the distinct patterns of chest and abdominal motion associated with different respiratory disorders.
- *Critical appraisal*: This study discussed the possible signals that can be used for SDB detection. The article emphasizes the need to develop a single respiratory signal (including contactless respiratory signal) source to improve the detection of hypopneas in addition to apneas. Larger studies are needed to validate machine learning algorithms.

- ***Sleep disordered breathing and neurobehavioral deficits in children and adolescents: A systematic review and meta-analysis. (BMC Pediatr. 2024)***[4]
  - *Population*: The study included children and adolescents aged 5 to 18 years. Data were collected from general populations and those with neurobehavioral deficits. (5 studies included in analysis)
  - *Intervention*: Full night-time polysomnography or overnight, limited-channel home cardiorespiratory recordings to diagnose sleep disordered breathing.
  - *Outcomes*: Prevalence of SDB: General population: 11% (95% CI: 2%-20%), Neurobehavioral patients: 25% (95% CI: 7%-42%).

    Risk of Neurobehavioral Deficits: Children with SDB had a threefold higher risk of neurobehavioral impairments (RR 3.24, 95% CI: 1.25-8.41). Population Attributable Fraction (PAF): 17.3%-19.8% of neurobehavioral consequences may be attributed to SDB.
  - *Conclusion*: A significant proportion of neurobehavioral consequences in children and adolescents can be attributed to sleep-disordered breathing. The findings emphasize the importance of early identification and treatment of SDB, as well as screening for SDB in patients with neurobehavioral impairments to prevent long-term consequences.
  - *Critical appraisal*: The study reveals an association of neurobehavioral deficits and SDB in children and adolescents. This is not a confirmed causal relationship since confounders are not addressed. The use of statistical formulae for PAF may overestimate the effect of SBD on neuro-behavioral deficits, even though the causality is not established. More longitudinal studies are needed to further identify this association.

☞

- ***Changes in sleep-disordered breathing from the acute to the stable phase of pulmonary embolism: The ESAET study. (Sleep Med. 2023)***[5]
  - *Population*: Hospitalized non-hypotensive acute pulmonary embolism patients. (n=111)

- *Intervention*: Sleep studies using respiratory polygraphy within 48 hours of PE diagnosis (acute phase) and another sleep study at 3 months follow-up (stable phase). Transthoracic echocardiography to look for right ventricular (RV) dysfunction and computed tomography were performed.
- *Outcome*: A total of 111 patients were included. 77 patients (69%) had RV dysfunction. AHI decreased by an average of 8.7 events/hour from the acute phase (mean AHI 24.4 events/hour) to the stable phase (mean AHI 15.7 events/hour, p=0.013). Patients with RV dysfunction showed a greater decrease in AHI (12.3/hour vs 0,43/hour).
- *Conclusion*: The study demonstrated a clinically significant transient increase in sleep-disordered breathing (SDB) during the acute phase of pulmonary embolism (PE), particularly in patients with RV dysfunction. The changes in AHI were noted to be significantly more in patients with RV dysfunction compared to those without. These findings suggest that the timing of sleep studies in PE patients should consider the phase of PE to avoid overestimation of obstructive sleep apnea (OSA) severity and unnecessary treatment.
- *Critical appraisal*: This is a clinically significant longitudinal study and speaks to the importance of timing of polysomnography in patients with acute pulmonary embolism. Larger studies are needed to validate these findings and develop standardized recommendations.

- ***Efficacy of Roncolab mobile application for diagnosing the primary sign of sleep-disordered breathing (snoring) in children. (Sleep Med. 2023)***[6]
  - *Population*: This was a single centre observational, analytical study of children screened for sleep-disordered breathing (SDB) (n=31) aged 7-11 years.
  - *Intervention*: Pediatric Sleep Questionnaire (PSQ) and use of RoncoLab mobile application to record and measure snoring intensity and frequency at home.
  - *Outcome*: Statistical analysis using Cohen's Kappa index demonstrated good agreement between RoncoLab and PSQ in diagnosing primary snoring, with a Kappa index of 0.743 ($p<0.05$). The RoncoLab app showed high sensitivity (0.92) and specificity (0.82), indicating its reliability as a diagnostic tool for primary snoring in children.
  - *Conclusion*: RoncoLab can be effectively used alongside PSQ for initial SDB screening in pediatric populations.
  - *Critical appraisal*: Although the RoncoLab app is not currently validated, it demonstrates good agreement with the PSQ, demonstrating acceptable sensitivity and specificity. Further multi-centric studies are required to validate its role in diagnosing sleep-disordered breathing in children.

- ***Should mild obstructive sleep apnea be treated? A systematic review from the standpoint of disease progression. (J Laryngol Otol. 2023)***[7]
  - *Population*: OSA patients from 17 longitudinal studies and 1 randomized controlled trial (RCT). (n=5777)
  - *Intervention*: The study investigated the progression of untreated obstructive sleep apnea and evaluated whether mild obstructive sleep apnea should be treated from the standpoint of disease progression.
  - *Outcomes*: AHI and RDI Changes: In mild OSA patients, the mean pre-study AHI was 5.21, and post-study AHI was 8.03 over a median follow-up of 53.1 months. This corresponds to an increase of 0.0531 events/hour per month. In moderate to severe OSA patients, the mean pre-study AHI was 28.9, and post-study AHI was 30.3 over a median follow-up of 57.8 months. This corresponds to an increase of 0.0235 events/hour per month.
  - *Conclusion*: While mild OSA shows some progression over time, it does not typically advance to moderate or severe OSA within the observed period. The rate of progression in mild OSA patients is slower and tends to plateau over

time. Patients aged under 60 and with a lower BMI are more likely to show disease progression. The findings suggest that treating mild OSA may not be necessary solely to prevent disease progression, but treatment decisions should still be guided by symptoms and quality of life improvements.

- o *Critical appraisal*: This study suggests that mild OSA may be followed up without PAP therapy. However, this study follows AHI changes over time and also reports that a lower BMI is associated with disease progression.

- ***Normal multiple sleep latency test values in adults: A systematic review and meta-analysis. (Sleep Med. 2023)***[8]
  - o *Population*: Healthy adults from 100 studies (n=4058). Participants with known sleep disorders, medical conditions, psychiatric conditions, or those who were night shift workers were excluded.
  - o *Intervention*: Multiple Sleep Latency Test (MSLT) performed in healthy adults to determine the normative value for mean sleep latency (MSL).
  - o *Outcomes*: Normative MSL Values: For the earlier definition of sleep onset, the pooled MSL was 11.7 minutes (95% CI: 10.8–12.6; 95% PI: 5.2–18.2). For the later definition of sleep onset, the pooled MSL was 11.8 minutes (95% CI: 10.7–12.8; 95% PI: 7.2–16.3).
  - o *Conclusion*: The study established updated normative values for mean sleep latency in healthy adults using the MSLT. It found no significant associations between MSL and most demographic or methodological variables, except for a negative association with AHI.
  - o *Critical appraisal*: The study aims to establish normative values for MSLT in a healthy adult population. Further insights are needed on the impact of age on MSL and also the impact of sleep disordered breathing during overnight polysomnography performed the night before MSLT.

- ***Prevalence of obstructive sleep apnea (OSA) among preschool aged children in the general population: A systematic review. (Sleep Med Rev. 2024)***[9]
  - o *Population*: Untreated pediatric obstructive sleep apnea (OSA) is associated with significant co-morbidities affecting behavior, neurocognitive development, endocrine & metabolic health. This review evaluated the presence of OSA among pre-school aged children. Children from thirty studies (n=33,842) included.
  - o *Intervention*: Pre-school aged children from 31 studies included. 7 studies confirmed OSA using objective methods following initial screening for habitual snoring with only 2 studies (n=82/4575) using PSG to confirm OSA while the other 5 studies (n=449/2486) implemented insensitive objective recording methods to confirm disease. The remaining studies used questionnaires to evaluate OSA.
  - o *Outcomes*: Prevalence Rates: Studies using polysomnography (PSG) reported OSA prevalence ranging from 0.7% to 6.4%.

    Studies using home sleep apnea testing (HSAT) reported OSA prevalence ranging from 0.9% to 13.0%. Studies using validated sleep questionnaires (VSQ) reported higher prevalence rates, ranging from 3.3% to 42.2%, with recent studies showing an increase to as high as 20.4%.

    Studies using non-validated sleep questionnaires (NVSQ) reported OSA prevalence ranging from 0.6% to 20.1%, with significant variability due to differences in questionnaire sensitivity and definitions of snoring and habitual snoring.
  - o *Conclusion*: The prevalence of obstructive sleep apnea in preschool-aged children varies widely depending on the methodology and criteria used. There was high heterogeneity in study methodologies of available data. Recent studies suggest an increase in prevalence rates, potentially linked to factors such as rising obesity rates and increased air pollution. The findings underscore the need for standardized diagnostic criteria and the use of objective testing to accurately assess the prevalence of OSA in young children.

- *Critical appraisal*: This study establishes the increasing prevalence of SDB in younger individuals. While multiple risk factors have been postulated, further studies are needed to understand the pathophysiology and management pathways.

☞

- ***Sleep and sleep disorders during pregnancy and postpartum: The Life-ON study. (Sleep Med. 2024)***[10]
  - *Population*: Multicentric, prospective study among pregnant women and postpartum women to assess sleep and sleep disorders.
  - *Intervention*: Home polysomnography was performed among pregnant women (n=439) between 23rd and 25th week of pregnancy and sleep-related questionnaires at 9 points in time during pregnancy and 6 months postpartum.
  - *Outcomes*: Sleep Quality (PSQI): Poor sleep quality was reported by 34% in the first trimester, 46% in the third trimester, and 71% in the first month postpartum.

    Insomnia: Insomnia prevalence increased to 31.5% in the third trimester and peaked at 34.4% immediately after delivery, dropping to 15.9% by 7 weeks postpartum.

    Excessive Daytime Sleepiness (ESS): EDS was reported by 46.9% of women at least once, peaking at 30.3% in the first trimester and decreasing to 13% at 6 months postpartum. EDS showed weak correlation with insomnia and poor sleep quality but not with respiratory disturbance index (RDI) or periodic limb movements (PLMS).

    Restless Legs Syndrome (RLS): RLS prevalence was 25%, peaking in the third trimester.

    Polysomnographic Data: 24% of women slept less than 6 hours, and 30.6% had a sleep efficiency below 80%. SDB (RDI≥5) was found in 4.2% of women, with a positive correlation with BMI.

    Periodic Limb Movements (PLMS): 45% of women had a PLMS index higher than 5, with a significant correlation with RLS.
  - *Conclusion*: The Life-ON study highlights the high prevalence of sleep disorders during pregnancy and postpartum, with significant variations across different trimesters and postpartum periods. Poor sleep quality, insomnia, EDS, and RLS are common, with the highest disturbances occurring around delivery. Routine assessment of sleep disturbances in the perinatal period is necessary for early detection and clinical management.
  - *Critical appraisal*: This study reports the burden of SDB in pregnancy and provides a foundation for future randomized controlled trials to develop treatment protocols in this special population.

☞

- ***Clinical Characteristics of Primary Snoring vs Mild Obstructive Sleep Apnea in Children: Analysis of the Pediatric Adenotonsillectomy for Snoring (PATS) Randomized Clinical Trial. (JAMA Otolaryngol Head Neck Surg. 2024)***[11]
  - *Population*: Multi-center, single-blind, randomized trial conducted at 6 academic sleep centers. Children aged 3.0 to 12.9 years who were candidates for adenotonsillectomy (AT) due to polysomnography-diagnosed mild obstructive sleep-disordered breathing (n=459) were included.
  - *Intervention*: A combination of clinical characteristics was assessed to differentiate children with primary snoring with mild OSA.
  - *Outcomes*: Demographic Characteristics: Median age: 6.0 years, Gender: 50.1% female, Obesity prevalence: 19.2%. Racial/Ethnic Distribution: 26.4% Black, 16.4% Hispanic, 51.5% White, 5.7% other.

Black race (OR 2.08; 95% CI 1.32-3.30), obesity (OR 1.80; 95% CI 1.12-2.91), and high urinary cotinine levels (>5 μg/L) (OR 1.88; 95% CI 1.15-3.06) were significantly associated with mild OSA.

- *Conclusion*: The study concluded that primary snoring and mild OSA in children are difficult to distinguish based solely on clinical characteristics without the use of polysomnography. These findings suggest that the decision to perform adenotonsillectomy should not rely solely on clinical characteristics and that polysomnography remains essential for accurate diagnosis and treatment planning in pediatric obstructive sleep-disordered breathing.
- *Critical appraisal*: The study reports use of polysomnography for diagnosing & planning treatment of pediatric obstructive sleep-disordered breathing rather than clinical characteristics in this specific population.

- ***Association between sleep apnea and risk of cognitive impairment and Alzheimer's disease: a meta-analysis of cohort-based studies. (Sleep Breath. 2024)***[12]
  - *Population*: Patients diagnosed with SDB/OSA through various methods, including at-home polysomnography, self-report questionnaires, and ICD codes from 15 studies.
  - *Outcomes*: Risk of Cognitive Impairment and Dementia: The overall pooled analysis showed that patients with SDB/OSA had a significantly higher risk of cognitive impairment and/or all-cause dementia (HR 1.52, 95% CI: 1.32–1.74) compared to patients without SDB/OSA. When considering only studies that diagnosed SDB based on polysomnography, the association with all-cause cognitive impairment was weaker (HR 1.32, 95% CI: 1.00–1.74).
  - *Conclusion*: The findings suggest a potential association between SDB/OSA and an increased risk of cognitive impairment and dementia, including Alzheimer's disease. However, the strength of this association varies depending on the diagnostic method used, with objective assessments like polysomnography showing a somewhat weaker relationship.
  - *Critical appraisal*: Of the 15 studies, 5 used questionnaires/self-reported symptoms. This study needs cautious interpretation since pooling together studies with the diagnosis of SDB based on polysomnography revealed a weaker association for all-cause cognitive impairment. This necessitates longitudinal studies for improved understanding.

- ***Influence of Impaired Diffusing Capacity and Sleep-disordered Breathing on Nocturnal Hypoxemia and Health Outcomes in Men with and without Human Immunodeficiency Virus. (Ann Am Thorac Soc. 2024)***[13]
  - *Population*: Multi-center cohort study among adult patients, with and without HIV infection (n=544).
  - *Intervention*: DLCO and home-based polysomnography (n=544) were performed to measure SDB-related hypoxemia among adult men with or without HIV. Multi-variable regression models characterized associations between DLCO and SDB-related hypoxemia. Structural equation models were used to assess associations of impaired DLCO & SDB-related hypoxemia measures with prevalent hypertension & type 2 diabetes mellitus.
  - *Outcomes*: Nocturnal Hypoxemia: Participants with severe SDB (AHI $\geq$ 30 events/h) and impaired DLCO had higher total sleep time with $SpO_2 < 90\%$ (T90), higher average desaturation, lower nadir SpO_2, and lower average SpO2 during sleep compared to those with preserved DLCO.

    Health Outcomes: Higher T90 was associated with higher odds of prevalent hypertension (OR 1.39, 95% CI 1.14-1.70) and type 2 diabetes (OR 1.25, 95% CI 1.07-1.46).
  - *Conclusion*: Impaired DLCO in individuals with severe SDB was significantly associated with increased nocturnal hypoxemia, as well as higher prevalence of hypertension and type 2 diabetes.
  - *Critical appraisal*: This is an interesting study that looks at the association of SDB and impaired DLCO. The study assessed sleep only for one night. This is potentially underestimating night-to-night variability in SDB severity, particularly in those with mild diseases. The patient cohort does not include women. The subgroups with moderate/severe reductions in DLCO were limited.

B. PAP therapy

- ***Adaptive servo-ventilation for sleep-disordered breathing in patients with heart failure with reduced ejection fraction (ADVENT-HF): A multicenter, multinational, parallel-group, open-label, phase 3 randomized controlled trial. (Lancet Respir Med. 2024)***[14]

    - *Population*: Adult patients with HFrEF (LVEF $\leq 45\%$) and SDB (AHI ≥ 15 events/hour) stabilized on optimal medical therapy were included. The trial was conducted at 49 hospitals across nine countries. (n=731)
    - *Intervention*: Standard optimal treatment plus ASV.
    - *Comparator*: Standard optimal treatment alone.
    - *Outcomes*: Primary Outcome: The primary composite outcome included the cumulative incidence of all-cause mortality, first admission to hospital for cardiovascular reasons, new onset atrial fibrillation or flutter, and delivery of an appropriate cardioverter-defibrillator shock. Over a mean follow-up period of 3.6 years, ASV did not significantly affect the primary composite outcome (180 events in the control group vs 166 in the ASV group; hazard ratio [HR] 0.95, 95% CI 0.77-1.18; p=0.67). For OSA, the HR for all-cause mortality was 1.00 (0.68-1.46; p=0.98) and for CSA was 0.74 (0.44-1.23; p=0.25). No safety issue related to ASV use was identified.

      Secondary Outcomes: All-Cause Mortality: No significant difference (88 deaths in the control group vs. 76 in the ASV group; HR 0.89, 95% CI 0.66-1.21; p=0.47).

      Cardiovascular Hospitalizations: No significant effect (138 first admissions in control vs. 142 in ASV; HR 1.06, 95% CI 0.84-1.33; p=0.65). AHI and Sleep Quality: ASV significantly reduced AHI (mean reduction of 34.2 events/hour), improved oxygen saturation levels, and reduced arousal frequency. Quality of Life: Improvements in the Minnesota Living with Heart Failure Questionnaire (MLHFQ) scores and Epworth Sleepiness Scale (ESS) scores were observed in the ASV group. NYHA Class demonstrated significant improvements at 1 and 2 years in the ASV group.
    - *Conclusion*: The ADVENT-HF trial concluded that ASV treatment in patients with heart failure and reduced ejection fraction did not significantly improve the primary composite outcome or mortality. However, ASV effectively eliminated sleep-disordered breathing, leading to improvements in sleep quality, health-related quality of life, and symptoms of sleep-disordered breathing and heart failure. No safety issue was noted with ASV use in the study population.
    - *Critical appraisal*: This study utilized peak flow targeted ASV. The device used is different from the RESMED device used in the SERVE-HF trial. The SERVE HF trial only included patients with CSA, whereas this trial included both CSA and non-sleepy OSA. This trial shows that ASV may be safe in HFrEF and it could be a valuable addition to the treatment options in patients with SDB and reduced LVEF. However, larger multi-centered studies are needed to validate this data.

- ***Current treatment strategies in managing side effects associated with domiciliary positive airway pressure (PAP) therapy for patients with sleep disordered breathing: A systematic review and meta-analysis. (Sleep Med Rev. 2023)***[15]
    - *Population*: Adult patients receiving domiciliary PAP therapy for SDB from 36 studies.
    - *Intervention*: Various strategies to manage side effects were investigated, including:
        - Heated Humidification (HH): Using water chambers to humidify air.
        - Nasal Sprays/Douches: Hyaluronate and saline for nasal inflammation.
        - Chin Straps: Devices to reduce mouth leak.

- Different Interfaces: Nasal masks, oronasal masks, nasal pillows, and customized interfaces.
- Dressings: Used to prevent pressure ulcers.

o *Outcomes*: PAP Therapy Compliance: No significant differences were found between interventions in terms of hours of use per night.

Epworth Sleepiness Score (ESS): No significant differences were observed between different interventions.

Residual Apnea-Hypopnea Index (AHI): No clinically meaningful differences were noted between various interventions.

o *Conclusion*: The systematic review and meta-analysis concluded that while various interventions are used to manage side effects of PAP therapy, there is limited evidence supporting their effectiveness in improving clinical outcomes such as PAP compliance, ESS, residual AHI, or interface leak. Heated humidification (HH) might help manage nasal symptoms and mucosal inflammation, but its routine use remains debated.

o *Critical appraisal*: This review was limited by study heterogeneity, particularly for outcome measures. Patient demographics were not reported, making it challenging to generalize the findings to a broader clinical population. This review highlights the need for generating evidence supporting effective treatment strategies to manage side effects of positive airway pressure therapy.

- ***Adherence to continuous positive airway pressure for the treatment of obstructive sleep apnea in neurodegenerative diseases: A systematic review. (Sleep Med Rev. 2023)***[16]

o *Population*: OSA patients with neurodegenerative diseases from 17 studies,8 studies on Alzheimer's disease (AD), and/or mild cognitive impairment (MCI), 6 studies on Parkinson's' disease (PD), 3 studies on Multiple system atrophy (MSA).

o *Intervention*: PAP therapy, primarily CPAP, with adherence defined variably across studies (e.g., >4 hours/night for ≥ 70% of nights).

o *Outcomes:*

1. Adherence Rates:

   AD/MCI: Adherence rates ranged from 28% to 61% across study durations of 3 weeks to 3.3 years.

   PD: Attrition rates ranged from 8% to 75%, with adherent patients using their device for 3.27 to 5.12 hours/night over study durations of 6 weeks to 12 months.

   MSA: Acceptance rates of 69% to 72%, with average nightly use of 4.42 to 6.18 hours.

2. Predictors of Adherence:

   AD/MCI: Younger age, white race, better initial CPAP confidence, being married were associated with higher adherence. APOE4 positive and unmarried individuals were more likely to abandon CPAP.

   PD: Longer disease duration, worse motor symptoms, poor sleep quality, lower percentage of REM sleep, non-white race, and female sex were linked to lower adherence. Lower education levels also predicted higher attrition rates.

   MSA: Increased disease severity and the presence of floppy epiglottis were associated with poorer adherence.

3. Impact on Outcomes:

   AD/MCI: Improvement in excessive daytime sleepiness, depressive symptoms, sleep quality, daily activities, and some aspects of cognition in adherent patients. Caregiver satisfaction also improved.

   PD: Improved daytime sleepiness, anxiety symptoms, sleep architecture, and global non-motor symptoms with PAP adherence. Mixed results on cognitive function improvements.

MSA: Adherent patients showed better sleep quality and improved vigilance. No significant difference in survival time between treated and untreated individuals.

- *Conclusion*: PAP therapy can benefit patients with neurodegenerative diseases by improving sleep quality, daytime symptoms, and some cognitive functions. However, adherence is challenging, with high attrition rates and various barriers affecting different patient groups. Strategies to improve adherence should be personalized, considering predictors like age, disease severity, race, and initial patient confidence in using CPAP.
- *Critical appraisal*: This systematic review recognizes several potential barriers to adherence to PAP therapy. Further studies are required to standardize the definition of long-term adherence to PAP therapy and to thereby assess interventions that can improve adherence in this patient population.

- ***Effects of Adaptive Servo-Ventilation on Quality of Life: The READ-ASV Registry. (Ann Am Thorac Soc. 2024)***[17]
  - *Population*: Prospective multicenter European READ-ASV registry evaluating the effects of first time ASV therapy on disease-specific quality of life. Central sleep apnea with or without OSA who were prescribed ASV therapy (n=801) were included.
  - *Intervention*: ASV therapy was prescribed in adults with CSA with or without OSA (n=801).
  - *Outcomes*: Primary Outcome: Quality of Life (FOSQ Score): The median FOSQ score significantly increased from baseline by +0.8 points (IQR -0.2 to 2.2; $P < 0.001$) after 12 months of ASV therapy. Significant improvements were observed particularly in symptomatic participants (FOSQ score < 17.9 and/or ESS score > 10) with an increase of +1.69 points (IQR 0.38 to 3.05).

    Secondary Outcome: Daytime Sleepiness (ESS Score): The median ESS score significantly decreased from baseline by -2.0 points (IQR -5.0 to 0.0; $P < 0.001$).
  - *Conclusion*: ASV therapy was associated with significant improvements in disease-specific quality of life and reductions in daytime sleepiness, especially in individuals with pronounced sleep-disordered breathing symptoms before therapy initiation. These improvements support the use of ASV as an effective treatment option for patients with CSA and/or OSA.
  - *Critical appraisal*: This data provides real-world information regarding ASV usage and QoL. 'However, since this is registry data, it is purely observational and is inherently susceptible to potential biases.

C. Surgical interventions

- ***Adenotonsillectomy for Snoring and Mild Sleep Apnea in Children: A Randomized Clinical Trial. (JAMA. 2023)***[18]
  - *Population*: Children with snoring and mild sleep apnea. (n=459)
  - *Intervention*: Adenotonsillectomy within four weeks after randomization.
  - *Comparator*: Watchful waiting and provided supportive care.
  - *Outcomes*: Primary Outcomes: Executive Function: Measured by the Behavior Rating Inventory of Executive Function

(BRIEF) Global Executive Composite (GEC) T score. There were no significant differences between the two groups (difference, -0.96 points [95% CI, -2.66 to 0.74]; P=0.27).

Attention: Measured by the Go/No-go (GNG) test d-prime signal detection score, with no significant group differences (difference, 0.05 [95% CI, -0.18 to 0.27]; P=0.68).

- o *Conclusion*: Early adenotonsillectomy in children with mild SDB did not significantly improve executive function or attention at 12 months. However, it did result in improved secondary outcomes, including behavior, symptoms, quality of life, and blood pressure. The findings suggest that while adenotonsillectomy may not impact cognitive outcomes, it can have beneficial effects on other health and quality-of-life measures for children with mild SDB.
- o *Critical appraisal*: While this was a well-conducted study, masking of caregivers was not feasible, and thereby secondary outcomes such as behavior/symptoms/QoL may suffer from a reporting bias.

- ***Changes in behavioral and cognitive abilities after rapid maxillary expansion in children affected by persistent snoring after long-term adenotonsillectomy: A non controlled study. (Am J Orthod Dentofacial Orthop. 2024)***[19]
  - o *Population*: Children with persistent snoring after adenotonsillectomy. The children were divided into two groups based on their obstructive apnea-hypopnea index (OAHI):

    Primary Snoring (PS) group: OAHI < 1. (n=13)

    Obstructive Sleep Apnea (OSA) group: OAHI $\geq$1. (n=11)
  - o *Intervention*: Rapid maxillary expansion (RME).
  - o *Outcomes*:
    1. Polysomnographic (PSG) Parameters:

       No significant changes in apnea-hypopnea index (AHI) or obstructive AHI (OAHI) post-RME.

       No significant differences between groups in terms of PSG parameter changes.
    2. Behavioral and Neurocognitive Parameters:

       Significant improvements in the "Somatic" and "Aggressiveness" domains of the Child Behavior Checklist (CBCL) in the OSA group ($p < 0.05$).

       No significant pre- and post-RME changes in other cognitive functions, except for visuospatial function, which showed improvement in the OSA group.
    3. Quality of Life (QOL):

       Significant decreases in PSQ and OSA-18 scores post-RME, indicating improved QOL in both groups ($p < 0.001$).
  - o *Conclusion*: Rapid maxillary expansion (RME) improved behavioral parameters and quality of life in children with persistent snoring and SDB after adenotonsillectomy, particularly in those with obstructive sleep apnea (OSA). While RME did not significantly change PSG parameters, it effectively reduced symptoms and enhanced behavioral outcomes. The study suggests that RME can be a beneficial treatment for children with SDB refractory to adenotonsillectomy. However, larger studies with control groups are needed to substantiate these findings.
  - o *Critical appraisal*: This study highlights the importance of symptom control in the management of OSA as opposed to only targeting AHI. However, there is a need for larger controlled trials.

- ***Relationship of ankyloglossia and obstructive sleep apnea: systematic review and meta-analysis. (Sleep Breath. 2024)***[20]
  - o *Population*: Children diagnosed with OSAS and healthy children from 6 studies. (n=451)

- *Intervention*: The primary intervention was the assessment of ankyloglossia in children diagnosed with OSAS. Various methods were used to evaluate the presence of a short lingual frenulum, including direct measurement and assessment of tongue mobility.
- *Outcomes*: Prevalence and Association: The meta-analysis revealed a statistically significant association between a short lingual frenulum and OSAS, with an odds ratio of 3.051 (95% CI: 1.939 to 4.801). A high-arched palate was also significantly associated with OSAS, with an odds ratio of 12.304 (95% CI: 6.141 to 24.653).

  Risk Factors: The studies highlighted that a shortened lingual frenulum might contribute to abnormal orofacial development, increasing upper airway resistance and susceptibility to airway collapsibility during sleep. Ankyloglossia and high-arched palates were identified as significant risk factors for pediatric OSAS.
- *Conclusion*: The findings suggest that children with a short lingual frenulum are at a higher risk of developing OSAS. Early diagnosis and intervention for ankyloglossia could potentially reduce the risk of developing sleep-disordered breathing in children.
- *Critical appraisal*: The studies included in the review are all observational in nature. This secondary analysis of preexisting data reveals associations between ankyloglossia and OSAS. Further directions would include trials to identify risk factors and treatment pathways (surgical or non-surgical).

- ***The role of overnight pulse oximetry in risk stratification of pediatric sleep disordered breathing in a district general hospital. (Int J Pediatr Otorhinolaryngol. 2024)***[21]
  - *Population*: Children with sleep-disordered breathing (SDB) were referred for overnight pulse oximetry over an eighteen-month period. (n=200)
  - *Intervention*: Use of overnight pulse oximetry to risk stratify patients and determine the need for post-operative monitoring following adenotonsillectomy.
  - *Comparator*: A comparison was made with the national recommendations and other risk stratification methods like polysomnography.
  - *Outcome*: The study found that overnight pulse oximetry was commonly used but often led to unnecessary inpatient stays due to its limitations in accurately predicting post-operative complications. The majority of patients had normal to mild disease based on McGill scores from pulse oximetry, and none of the patients developed major respiratory complications postoperatively.
  - *Conclusion*: Overnight pulse oximetry is not an accurate predictor of post-operative respiratory complications and results in unnecessary inpatient stays.
  - *Critical appraisal*: This is a retrospective observational study which reiterates the inaccuracy of routine pulse oximetry in the assessment of SDB.

D. Pharmacotherapy and other interventions

- ***The impact of intranasal corticosteroids (INS) in a prospective cohort of children with sleep disordered breathing. (Int J Pediatr Otorhinolaryngol. 2024)***[22]
  - *Population*: Children with sleep-disordered breathing (n=568). Most children (87%) had a history of atopic conditions such as allergic rhinitis, asthma, and eczema.
  - *Intervention*: 51% of the children underwent a trial of INS (either 50 microg Mometasone or 27.5 microg Fluticasone furoate) for six weeks.
  - *Comparator*: Children who did not undergo INS treatment (49%).

- *Outcomes*: Symptom Improvement: In the INS group, the mean OSA-5 score decreased significantly from 8.2 to 5.5 ($p < 0.0001$). Improvement was reported in 56% of children.

  Surgery Rates: The surgery rate was significantly lower in the INS group (38%) compared to the non-INS group (56%, $p < 0.001$).

  Symptom Burden: Children with higher initial OSA-5 scores (11–15) showed the greatest reduction in surgery rates with INS (54% surgery rate with INS vs. 88% without).
- *Conclusion*: Intranasal corticosteroids significantly improved symptoms of sleep-disordered breathing in children, leading to a substantial reduction in the need for surgical intervention. The INS treatment effectively reduced OSA-5 scores and minimized surgery rates, demonstrating a valuable alternative to surgical management for pediatric SDB patients.
- *Critical analysis*: In this study, since the control group included patients who were referred for surgery, the surgery rates are likely to be higher by the population characteristics. Surgery avoidance rates would be a more important outcome. The effects of INS were not found to be associated with atopic status, whereas 87% of the population had a history of atopy. One needs to address the physiological basis of improvement in non-atopic patients who received INS. It would also be necessary to look at measures such as the number needed to treat in a non-atopic population with SDB and whether the study is adequately powered to make this assessment.

☞

- ***Effects of exercise on sleep in children with overweight/obesity: A randomized clinical trial. (Obesity [Silver Spring]. 2024)***[23]
  - *Population*: Overweight/obesity. (n=109 children)
  - *Intervention*: The exercise program consisted of aerobic and resistance training 3 to 5 days per week for 20 weeks, with sessions lasting 90 minutes each, including warm-up, aerobic exercise, resistance exercise, and cool-down periods. Device assessed sleep outcomes were measured using wrist-worn actigraphy at baseline, 10th week and post intervention for 7 consecutive days & SDB was measured via pediatric sleep questionnaire.
  - *Comparison*: Usual lifestyle without any additional exercise intervention.
  - *Outcomes*: Wake After Sleep Onset (WASO) Time: The exercise training program resulted in a significant reduction in WASO time by 10.8 minutes/day ($p = 0.040$).

    Acute Effects: No significant differences were found in sleep outcomes for the nights following exercise sessions compared to non-exercise days.
  - *Conclusion*: The 20-week exercise training program significantly reduced wake after sleep onset time in children with overweight/obesity but did not have a significant effect on other sleep outcomes or sleep-disordered breathing. These findings support the promotion of exercise programs to improve sleep quality in children with overweight/obesity. However, further research is needed, particularly in children with poorer baseline sleep health, to fully understand the potential benefits of exercise on sleep.
  - *Critical appraisal*: This study informs the benefit of exercise on SDB. This is a therapeutic modality that can be extrapolated to adult populations, while correcting for possible chronic illnesses.

☞

- ***Sacubitril/valsartan has an underestimated impact on the right ventricle in patients with sleep-disordered breathing, especially central sleep apnoea syndrome. (Arch Cardiovasc Dis. 2024)***[24]

- *Population*: Prospective, observational, multi-centric study to evaluate impact of sacubitril/valsartan (S/V) on right ventricular function in patients with SDB. Symptomatic heart failure with reduced ejection fraction (HFrEF) and SDB. (n=101).

  Central-SDB (41.5%), Obstructive-SDB (22.9%), No-SDB (35.6%).
- *Intervention*: Patients were evaluated by echocardiography and nocturnal ventilatory polygraphy which allowed patients to be divided into- central-SDB, obstructive-SDB and no-SDB. Patients received S/V therapy, with doses adjusted over three months.
- *Outcomes*: Right Ventricular Function: Overall, there was an increase in TAPSE by +1.32 ± 4.74 mm (P = 0.024) and a decrease in sPAP by –3.1 ± 10.91 mmHg (P = 0.048). The central-SDB group showed the greatest improvement in RV function with an increase in TAPSE of +2.1 ± 4.9 mm (P = 0.045) and a reduction in sPAP of –8.4 ± 9.7 mmHg (P = 0.001).

  Left Ventricular Function: The entire population showed a decrease in LV end-diastolic diameter by –2.55 ± 6.56 mm (P = 0.001) and an increase in cardiac output by +0.10 (–0.50; 1.70) L/min (P = 0.118). LVEF increased significantly by +1% (0%; 7%) (P < 0.001), with the central-SDB group showing a +2.00% increase (P = 0.001).
- *Conclusion*: Sacubitril/valsartan (S/V) significantly improved right ventricular function in patients with heart failure and sleep-disordered breathing after three months of treatment, with the most pronounced benefits observed in patients with central sleep apnea syndrome. These findings highlight the potential of S/V in enhancing cardiac function in this patient population, particularly targeting those with central sleep apnea.
- *Critical appraisal*: This is an observational study and carries the inherent biases of the same. One of the significant limitations is that the patient population did not receive SGLT2 inhibitors despite cardiac failure. Due to previous data suggesting negative outcomes with ASV, the patients with reduced LVEF and significant CSA were not initiated on the same. This study, while positive in outcome, needs further randomized controlled trials before it informs treatment protocols.

- ***Patient-reported outcomes with hypoglossal nerve stimulation for treatment of obstructive sleep apnea: A systematic review and meta-analysis. (Eur Arch Otorhinolaryngol. 2023)***[25]

  - *Population*: OSA patients from 34 studies (n= 3785) with a mean follow-up of 11.8 ± 12.2 months.
  - *Intervention*: Hypoglossal nerve stimulation (HNS) therapy involves the electrical stimulation of the hypoglossal nerve to activate upper airway dilator muscles, thereby reducing airway obstruction during sleep.
  - *Outcomes*: Daytime Sleepiness (ESS): The pooled effect showed a 4.59-point improvement in the Epworth Sleepiness Scale (ESS) score (Z = 42.82, p < .001).

    Daytime Functioning (FOSQ): The Functional Outcomes of Sleep Questionnaire (FOSQ) showed a pooled effect size of 2.84 points improvement (Z = 28.38, p < .001).

    Sleep Quality (PSQI): The Pittsburgh Sleep Quality Index (PSQI) showed a mean improvement of 1.77 points (Z = 2.53, p = .010), although it did not reach the minimal important difference (MID) of 4.0 points.
  - *Conclusion*: Hypoglossal nerve stimulation (HNS) therapy significantly improves patient-reported outcomes for individuals with obstructive sleep apnea (OSA). It effectively reduces daytime sleepiness, enhances daytime functioning, and improves sleep quality, though the improvement in sleep quality did not meet the minimally important difference threshold. Patient satisfaction with HNS therapy is high (91% of patients were satisfied with HNS therapy, 92% would choose it again, and 94% would recommend it), and many patients prefer it over previous treatments.
  - *Critical appraisal*: This paper mostly includes observational data. While the emphasis is on patient-reported improvement in sleepiness and satisfaction, there is no data on patient demographics, adverse events, and treatment complications with HNS therapy. This data would impact the real-life outcomes of HNS.

☞

- ***The effect of cognitive behavioral therapy for insomnia in people with comorbid insomnia and sleep apnea: A systematic review and meta-analysis. (J Sleep Res. 2023)***[26]
    - *Population*: Comorbid insomnia and sleep apnea (COMISA) from 21 studies. (n=1040)
    - *Intervention*: Cognitive Behavioral Therapy for Insomnia (CBTi) interventions included multi-component CBTi, stimulus control therapy, sleep restriction therapy, relaxation therapy, and cognitive therapy for insomnia. These interventions were delivered in various formats such as face-to-face, tele-health, self-guided online or text-based, group CBTi, eBook CBTi, and blended delivery methods.
    - *Comparator*: Various control conditions including sleep education controls, PAP adherence programs, and surgical interventions for OSA.
    - *Outcomes*: Insomnia Severity (ISI): A meta-analysis of nine primary studies measuring the Insomnia Severity Index (ISI) indicated that CBTi was associated with a large improvement in insomnia severity (Hedges' g = -0.89, 95% CI -1.35, -0.43).

      PAP Therapy Acceptance and Adherence: CBTi was found to potentially increase rates of PAP acceptance and use in patients with COMISA.

      Daytime Functioning and Mental Health: Improvements in daytime sleepiness, anxiety, depression, and overall mental health were reported in several studies.

      Quality of Life: Improvements in quality of life and functional outcomes were noted following CBTi intervention.
    - *Conclusion*: CBTi is an effective treatment for insomnia symptoms in individuals with comorbid insomnia and sleep apnea (COMISA). It significantly reduces insomnia severity and may enhance acceptance and adherence to PAP therapy. The review suggests the need for implementation programs to integrate COMISA management pathways in sleep clinics worldwide.
    - *Critical appraisal*: Due to the wide range of studies included, there may be a difference in effect size between various studies. Further research is needed to understand the specific symptoms of insomnia and OSA that would respond to CBTi. There is also a need to identify individual characteristics and predict subgroups (amongst those with COMISA) who may better respond to treatment.

☞

- ***DAHOS Study: Efficacy of dapagliflozin in treating heart failure with reduced ejection fraction and obstructive sleep apnea syndrome - A 3-month, multicenter, randomized controlled clinical trial. (Eur J Clin Pharmacol. 2024)***[27]
    - *Population*: Prospective, multi-center, randomized controlled trial. Patients with an average left ventricular ejection fraction (LVEF) of less than 40% and an apnea-hypopnea index (AHI) greater than 15. (n=107)
    - *Intervention*: Received optimized heart failure therapy along with standard-dose dapagliflozin over 3 months.
    - *Comparator*: Received only optimized heart failure therapy over 3 months.
    - *Outcomes*: Primary Outcome: AHI Reduction: Significant improvement in AHI was observed in the dapagliflozin group compared to the control group.

      Secondary Outcomes: Oxygen Desaturation Index (ODI): Improvement in ODI and other sleep parameters such as longest apnea duration and time spent with $SpO_2 < 90\%$ were noted in the dapagliflozin group.

Cardiac Function: Significant improvements in LVEF and reductions in left ventricular end-diastolic diameter and NT-proBNP levels were observed.

Inflammatory Markers: Reduction in CRP and IL-6 levels were significant in the dapagliflozin group but not in the control group.

Quality of Life: Improvements in quality of life scores (Minnesota Living with Heart Failure Questionnaire and EQ-5D-3L), and daytime sleepiness (Epworth Sleepiness Scale) were significant in the dapagliflozin group.

Body Mass Index (BMI): BMI was significantly reduced in the treatment group.

- *Conclusion*: Dapagliflozin, in addition to optimized heart failure therapy, significantly improves both cardiac and sleep-related outcomes in patients with HFrEF and OSAS. It shows promise as a potential treatment for improving sleep parameters and reducing inflammation in this patient population.
- *Critical appraisal*: Emerging research has shown that SGLT2 inhibitors improve ventilation, in addition to its cardiovascular and glycemic effects. This study reports improvement in polysomnographic and pathophysiological effects of SDB in patients with HFrEF.

- ***Tirzepatide for the treatment of Obstructive Sleep Apnea and Obesity. The SURMOUNT-OSA trial. (N Engl J Med. 2024)***[33]

  - *Population*: Patients with OSA who were not receiving treatment with PAP therapy at baseline were enrolled in trial 1 (n=234), and those who were receiving PAP therapy at baseline were enrolled in trial 2 (n=235). AHI at least 15 events per hour (mean-50), BMI at least 30kg/m^2. No type 1 or type 2 diabetes.
  - *Intervention*: Maximum tolerated dose of Tirzepatide (10 or 15mg) for 52 weeks.
  - *Comparator*: Placebo for 52 weeks.
  - *Outcomes*: Primary Outcome: Change in AHI from baseline to 52 weeks.

    Secondary Outcomes: Percent change in AHI and body weight and changes in hypoxic burden, patient- reported sleep impairment & disturbance, high sensitivity C-reactive protein, and systolic blood pressure at 52 weeks.

    In trial 1, the mean change in AHI at week 52 was -25.3 events per hour with Tirzepatide vs 5.3 events per hour with placebo. In trial 2, the mean change in AHI at week 52 was -29.3 events per hour with Tirzepatide and -5.5 events per hour with placebo. Significant improvements in key secondary endpoints were observed with Tirzepatide as compared with placebo. The most common adverse events were mostly mild to moderate gastrointestinal symptoms.
  - *Conclusion*: Among patients with moderate-to-severe obstructive sleep apnea and obesity, Tirzepatide reduced AHI, body weight, hypoxic burden, hsCRP concentration & systolic blood pressure & improved sleep-related patient-reported outcomes.
  - *Critical appraisal*: This randomized clinical trial examines the effect of Tirzepatide in moderate-to-severe OSA leading to improvement in sleep quality & weight reduction. Larger prospective multicentre studies to validate the results of this study. Long-term cardiovascular outcomes were not assessed and also the effect of Tirzepatide in overweight or normal body mass index is not known.

E. Miscellaneous

- ***Sleep-disordered breathing is related to retinal vein occlusion: A meta-analysis. (Medicine [Baltimore]. 2023)***[28]
    - o *Population*: Retinal vein occlusion from seven observational studies (1 retrospective cohort and 6 case-control studies). (n=36,628)
    - o *Outcome*: The meta-analysis found a significant association between SDB and RVO with a risk ratio (RR) of 1.92 (95% CI: 1.60-2.30, P < .001).

      Studies that adjusted for age and sex found an RR of 2.17 (95% CI: 1.50-3.13, P < .001), and those with additional adjustments for comorbidities found an RR of 1.78 (95% CI: 1.42-2.25, P < .001).
    - o *Conclusion*: There is a significant association between sleep-disordered breathing and retinal vein occlusion in adults.
    - o *Critical appraisal*: While the study has used various statistical methods to ensure the robustness of results, there are limitations. The studies included are observational in nature. Therefore, one may hypothesize that SDB and RVO have similar pathophysiological pathways and may be associated with each other. However, prospective research is needed to better understand this relationship.

- ***Vagal nerve stimulator-associated sleep-disordered breathing secondary to vagal-induced laryngospasm in pediatric populations: Case presentation and systematic review. (Int J Pediatr Otorhinolaryngol. 2023)***[29]
    - o *Population*: Patients who underwent Vagal Nerve Stimulation (VNS) implantation for treatment-resistant epilepsy from seven studies (n=104)
    - o *Outcomes*: Primary Outcomes: Prevalence of SDB: 36% of pediatric patients with VNS implantation developed SDB.

      Diagnosis: Polysomnography identified mild SDB in 49% of cases, moderate SDB in 21%, and severe SDB in 30%.

      Pathogenesis: SDB in these patients was attributed to vagal-induced laryngospasm and vocal cord adduction during VNS stimulation, resulting in obstructive sleep events.

      Secondary Outcomes: Symptom Presentation: Nighttime symptoms included snoring, frequent arousals, parasomnias, intermittent stridor, insomnia, gasping, and apneas. Daytime symptoms included sleepiness, noisy breathing, and hyper somnolence.

      Management: VNS Settings Adjustment: Lowering VNS output current intensity and modifying stimulation parameters resolved or improved SDB symptoms.

      Non-Invasive Treatments: CPAP and BPAP were effective in some cases. Medications like nasal steroids and montelukast were used for milder cases.

      Surgical Interventions: Adenoidectomy and lingual tonsillectomy were performed in cases with anatomical obstructions contributing to SDB.
    - o *Conclusion*: VNS-associated SDB is a significant complication in pediatric patients with VNS implants for epilepsy. Diagnosis is typically made through polysomnography, with a clear correlation between VNS stimulation and obstructive sleep events. Adjustments to VNS settings are the primary treatment strategy, although non-invasive positive pressure therapies and surgical interventions may be necessary for some patients. Pre-implantation polysomnography is recommended to identify and manage pre-existing SDB.
    - o *Critical appraisal*: SDB is evolving as a significant complication of VNS in refractory epilepsy. This review reaffirms the current understanding. However, the way forward includes research to decipher specific risk factors that may be associated

with the development of SDB in patients receiving VNS. Further exploration is needed to standardize pathways to perform DISE, polysomnography, and management of SDB in this patient population.

- ***Is exposure to chemical pollutants associated with sleep outcomes? A Systematic review. (Sleep Med Rev. 2023)***[30]
    - o *Population*: Diverse populations exposed to various chemical pollutants.

      Specific subgroups analyzed: pediatric populations (related to secondhand smoke), Gulf War veterans, and individuals exposed to metals, pesticides, and air pollutants from 204 studies.
    - o *Outcomes*:

      Air Pollution: Mixed results, with many studies indicating that exposure to PM and NO_2 is associated with poor sleep quality and disturbances.

      Gulf War and Conflict-Related Exposures: Consistently associated with poor sleep quality and increased incidence of insomnia.

      Metals (e.g., Aluminum, Mercury): Linked to insomnia and difficulties in sleep maintenance.

      Pesticides: Generally associated with poorer sleep quality.

      Secondhand Smoke (SHS): Particularly in children, SHS exposure is linked to insomnia and SDB.

      Case Reports/Series: Predominantly focused on metal exposures, showing a consistent association with insomnia and impaired sleep quality.
    - o *Conclusion*: Chemical pollutants have a significant but varied impact on sleep health. The review indicates suggestive evidence linking exposure to pollutants such as particulate matter, pesticides, and metals to adverse sleep outcomes. Future research should prioritize understanding the biological mechanisms, developmental impacts, and effects on marginalized populations to address sleep health disparities. Addressing environmental pollution is crucial for improving public health, particularly in terms of sleep outcomes.
    - o *Critical appraisal*: This review is limited by the heterogeneity of the pollutants studied and the sleep outcome measurements across various studies. The symptoms and exposures are mostly self-reported/questionnaire based. While this review does inform associations between specific exposures and SDB, objective data is required.

- ***Assessment of the gut microbiota of children with obstructive sleep apnea syndrome: A systematic review. (Sleep Med. 2024)***[31]
    - o *Population*: Children diagnosed with OSAS from 5 studies. (n=451).
    - o *Outcomes*: Children with OSAS had lower microbiota diversity and different bacterial compositions compared to healthy children. Specific bacterial changes included an increase in the phylum Proteobacteria and families Enterobacteriaceae and Erysipelotrichaceae, which have pro-inflammatory properties. There was a reduction in bacteria such as Faecalibacterium and Agathobacter, which are important for maintaining intestinal health. Increased levels of Bifidobacterium and Bacteroidetes were also observed in children with OSAS. Variations in microbiota were linked to sleep disruption, suggesting that OSAS may trigger inflammatory pathways leading to gut dysbiosis.
    - o *Conclusion*: The review concluded that children with obstructive sleep apnea syndrome (OSAS) have significantly different gut microbiota compositions compared to healthy children. The differences include both a decrease in beneficial bacteria and an increase in bacteria associated with inflammation. These findings highlight the potential link between sleep disorders and gut health in children.
    - o *Critical appraisal*: The available evidence suggests that SDB may lead to gut dysbiosis. However, the possibility of a bidirectional relationship and impact on management is yet to be understood.

- ***A novel TASK channel antagonist nasal spray reduces sleep apnea severity in physiological responders: a randomized, blinded, trial. (Am J Physiol Heart Circ Physiol. 2024)***[32]
    - o *Population*: Patients with OSA, defined by an apnea-hypopnea index (AHI) of 47 ± 26 events per hour, were included in the study. Participants had no severe insomnia and were not excessively sleepy. (n=10)
    - o *Intervention*: BAY2586116 nasal spray (160 µg), the same nasal spray with restricted nasal breathing (using chinstrap or mouth tape). "BAY2586116 nasal spray is a TASK 1/3 potassium channel antagonist, in reducing the severity of obstructive sleep apnea (OSA) in physiological responders."
    - o *Comparison*: Placebo.
    - o *Outcome*: Physiological responders were defined a priori as those who had improved upper airway collapsibility (critical closing pressure ≥ 2 cmH2O) with BAY2586116 nasal spray.

      Primary Outcome: AHI Reduction: In physiological responders, the BAY2586116 nasal spray significantly reduced AHI from 36 ± 12 to 28 ± 11 events/h compared to placebo (P = 0.03). However, there was no significant overall difference in AHI between the groups when including non-responders.
    - o *Conclusion*: BAY2586116 nasal spray showed potential in reducing the severity of obstructive sleep apnea (OSA) in individuals who exhibit physiological improvement in upper airway collapsibility. The study highlighted a significant reduction in AHI and ODI, along with lower morning blood pressure in responders. These findings suggest that TASK 1/3 potassium channel antagonism could be a promising therapeutic target for treating OSA in selected patients.
    - o *Critical appraisal*: This study reveals a promising therapeutic target in SDB. The current study utilizes endotyping as an approach to treatment. The primary outcome chosen here is the AHI response. However, there is a paradigm shift to looking at non-AHI parameters in the management of SDB. With this background, further studies would require to be adequately powered to look at not just the AHI response, but also the cardiovascular outcomes and residual sleepiness in patients who receive such treatments.

DISCUSSION

A. Diagnosis and clinical implications of sleep-disordered breathing (SDB)

Sleep-disordered breathing (SDB) is a significant cause of morbidity and mortality worldwide. The common types of SDB include OSA, central sleep apnea (CSA), obesity hypoventilation syndrome (OHS), and the overlap syndrome of OSA and chronic obstructive pulmonary disease (COPD). In-lab polysomnography is the gold standard diagnostic test for OSA. The diagnostic landscape of sleep-disordered breathing is ever-changing with research and evidence generation. Western studies show that OSA prevalence is 9–13% of the general population.[34, 35] In India, Udwadia et al. have estimated the prevalence of OSA in the urban Indian population as 7.5%[36] whereas a prevalence of 13.5% was noted by Sharma et al.[37] A South Indian study published in 2018 reported the prevalence of OSA by AHI criteria was 3.74%.[38] All these studies use AHI as a basis for diagnosis and severity classification of OSA. A recently published meta-analysis showed that the prevalence of OSA in Indian adults was 11%, with a male preponderance of 14%.[39]

The diagnosis and clinical implications of sleep-disordered breathing (SDB) encompass a wide range of patient populations and health outcomes. With increasing research in the arena of maternal OSA, there is new information emerging concerning sleep disorders and possible maternal-fetal outcomes. **The Life-ON study revealed a high prevalence of sleep disorders during pregnancy and postpartum, with significant variations across different trimesters and postpartum periods.[10] Maternal SDB has further been associated with adverse offspring growth outcomes.**

In adult populations, Punjabi et al. demonstrated independent associations between SDB and hypertension in both HIV-positive and HIV-negative individuals, underscoring the cardiovascular impact of SDB.[2] This information is valuable since HIV infection itself increases cardiovascular risks. A systematic review by Yang et al. emphasized the importance of respiratory signal analysis in SDB detection, showcasing the potential of algorithmic approaches for diagnosis.[3] This data heralds the age of machine-based learning and artificial intelligence. Further, **the RoncoLab mobile application demonstrated good agreement with the Pediatric Sleep Questionnaire for diagnosing primary snoring in children. This shows potential as a screening tool for SDB in pediatric populations.[6] As sleep physicians, embracing technological advancements and leveraging artificial intelligence to improve the diagnostic pathways to sleep-disordered breathing.**

The prevalence of OSA in preschool-aged children varies widely depending on the methodology and criteria used, with recent studies suggesting an increase in prevalence rates.[9] In a study of pediatric populations, Zhang et al. found that a significant proportion of neurobehavioral consequences could be attributed to SDB, underscoring the importance of suspicion, early identification, and treatment.[4] This new data is especially important to avoid mislabeling correctible conditions as pure neurobehavioral issues. Another study performed in the pediatric populations was the Pediatric Adenotonsillectomy for Snoring (PATS) trial. **On analyzing data from the (PATS) trial it was found that primary snoring and mild OSA in children are difficult to distinguish based solely on clinical characteristics, emphasizing the importance of polysomnography for accurate diagnosis.[11]**

Does SDB have an association with pulmonary embolism? Sleep-disordered breathing (SDB) in acute pulmonary embolism (PE) shows significant improvement from the acute to stable phase, particularly in patients with right ventricular dysfunction. The **ESEAT study** demonstrated the importance of timing when conducting sleep studies in PE patients to avoid overestimating obstructive sleep apnea (OSA) severity.[5] Impaired diffusing capacity of the lung for carbon monoxide (DLCO) in individuals with severe SDB was significantly associated with increased nocturnal hypoxemia and a higher prevalence of hypertension and type 2 diabetes.[13] These studies attempted to look at the consequences of SDB and attempted to improve the diagnostic accuracy of SDB in an individual with acute illness.

A systematic review found that mild OSA shows slow progression over time, with patients under 60 and those with lower BMI is more likely to show disease progression. This suggests that treatment decisions for mild OSA should be guided by symptoms and quality of life improvements rather than solely to prevent disease progression.[7] This also speaks to the importance of individualizing treatment approaches while understanding population-based data. To better understand population metrics, a meta-analysis established updated normative values for mean sleep latency in healthy adults using the Multiple Sleep Latency Test (MSLT), finding no significant associations between mean sleep latency and most demographic or methodological variables, except for a negative association with apnea-hypopnea index.[8] A meta-analysis of cohort-based studies suggested a potential association between SDB/OSA and an increased risk of cognitive impairment and dementia, including Alzheimer's disease. However, the strength of this association varied depending on the diagnostic method used.[12]

These studies collectively highlight the complexities of SDB across different populations and conditions, emphasizing the need for accurate diagnosis and consideration of various factors in treatment decisions. Our review emphasizes the importance of evolving associations of SDB with comorbidities across ages. There is a need for further studies and specific research questions to help formulate individualized diagnostic pathways.

B. PAP therapy

Positive airway pressure (PAP) remains the primary therapy for most patients with sleep-disordered breathing. Several PAP devices are available: continuous positive airway pressure (CPAP), auto-titrating positive airway pressure (APAP), bi-level positive airway pressure (BPAP), auto-titrating bi-level positive airway pressure (Auto-BPAP) and adaptive servo-ventilation (ASV).

CPAP is the first-line therapy for patients with severe OSA, obesity hypoventilation syndrome and central sleep apnea with HFrEF.[40] CPAP improves daytime sleepiness, blood pressure, and sleep-related quality of life and reduces motor vehicle accidents. APAP detects and responds to changes in upper airway flow or resistance in real-time and adjusts the delivery of PAP.[41] **It is recommended in patients with uncomplicated OSA, and it has a limited role in complicated OSA. APAP cannot distinguish between central & obstructive apnea and large mask leaks, and it should not be used in patients with co-morbid medical conditions that could potentially affect their respiratory patterns.**[40]

A systematic review and meta-analysis published in 2019 looked at the treatment of adult OSA with PAP therapy. **Based on a meta-analysis, the use of auto-adjusting PAP did not result in clinically significant differences in patient outcomes as compared to continuous PAP therapy.**[40] **BPAP provides IPAP during inspiration & EPAP during expiration. The tidal volume delivered is proportional to the difference between IPAP and EPAP. It is used in patients who are intolerant to CPAP or require high CPAP pressures, OSA with concurrent respiratory disease, and obesity hypoventilation who have failed CPAP therapy.**[43]

Auto-BPAP adjusts the EPAP to hold the airway open while maintaining a fixed pressure support. No objective outcomes studies show that BPAP therapy improves adherence when compared with CPAP therapy for patients with uncomplicated OSA.[40] ASV is based on servo control which refers to feedback control mechanism and pressure changes that are proportional to the inspiratory effort. It is used in patients with Cheyne-Stokes breathing, central sleep apnea, and those with ventilatory control stability.[44] **SERVE-HF trial showed that the use of ASV in patients with reduced ejection fraction (<45%) resulted in more risk of cardiovascular death despite effective control of central sleep apnea.**[4] **The ADVENT-HF trial investigated the use of adaptive servo-ventilation (ASV) in patients with heart failure and reduced ejection fraction (HFrEF) who also had SDB.**[14] **While ASV effectively eliminated SDB and improved sleep quality and quality of life, it did not significantly improve the primary composite outcome or mortality.** This builds on previous research, suggesting that while ASV can address sleep symptoms, its impact on cardiovascular outcomes in HFrEF patients remains limited. The results of this trial are positive compared to the previously mentioned SERVE-HF trial.

In addition to the available modes of PAP therapy, several customization features have been developed and are now available in modern PAP therapies. These include volume-assured pressure support (VAPS), expiratory pressure relief (EPR), auto-ramp, and smart start along with the use of several types of interfaces (nasal, oro-nasal & full-face masks including nasal pillow & cradle). **VAPS is primarily preferred in sleep disorders associated with hypoventilation namely, neuromuscular diseases, obesity hypoventilation syndrome, and overlap syndrome. It senses the changes in respiratory flow and proportionally adjusts the positive pressure during inhalation (IPAP/PS) to reach a respiratory target (expiratory tidal volume/ alveolar**

ventilation).[46] EPR has been developed to improve comfort and compliance in OSA patients. It provides a small pressure drop during the later stages of inspiration and the beginning part of expiration. It is provided as a routine feature in most devices.

Management of side effects associated with positive airway pressure (PAP) therapy was explored in a systematic review by Mansell et al.[15] The review found limited evidence supporting the effectiveness of various interventions in improving clinical outcomes such as PAP compliance, sleepiness scores, or residual apnea-hypopnea index. **Heated humidification showed some promise in managing nasal symptoms, but its routine use remains debated.** Adherence to PAP therapy in patients with neurodegenerative diseases was examined in a systematic review by Lajoie et al.[16] The review found varying adherence rates across different conditions, with multiple factors influencing adherence. **While PAP therapy showed benefits in improving sleep quality and some cognitive functions, high attrition rates were observed.** This underscores the need for personalized strategies to improve adherence in these complex patient populations. Previous studies have looked at ways to improve PAP adherence which forms a huge challenge to treatment. However, the review of previous studies highlights the ongoing challenge of optimizing PAP therapy adherence and effectiveness.[47-49]

The READ-ASV registry provided real-world data on the effects of ASV therapy on quality of life in patients with central sleep apnea (CSA) and/or obstructive sleep apnea (OSA).[17] The study found significant improvements in disease-specific quality of life and reductions in daytime sleepiness after 12 months of ASV therapy, particularly in symptomatic participants. **This supports the use of ASV as an effective treatment option for patients with CSA and/or OSA, especially when focusing on quality-of-life outcomes. The ISAACC study was a randomized controlled study that evaluated the effect of OSA and its treatment with CPAP on the prevalence of cardiovascular events in patients with acute coronary syndrome (ACS). It showed that the presence of OSA was not associated with an increased prevalence of cardiovascular events among ACS patients and treatment with CPAP did not significantly reduce this prevalence.**[50]

Our review highlights the complexities of treating SDB across different patient populations with varying needs. While positive airway pressure therapies, including ASV, can effectively improve sleep quality and symptoms, their impact on long-term cardiovascular outcomes in certain populations (e.g., HFrEF patients) may be limited. Additionally, adherence to therapy remains a significant challenge, particularly in patients with neurodegenerative diseases. There is a need for long-term studies to better understand the impact of these therapies on cardiovascular outcomes and disease progression in various patient populations. We are also in urgent need of innovative strategies to improve adherence to PAP therapy, especially in complex patient groups.

C. Surgical interventions

Surgery is usually reserved as a second-line therapy for obstructive sleep apnea (OSA). **This is usually an option in patients with OSA who cannot adhere to continuous positive airway pressure (CPAP) or as adjunctive therapy along with CPAP or an oral appliance.** Surgery is rarely indicated as primary therapy in adults and is rarely a cure for OSA. However, **surgery may be considered as a first-line therapy among the pediatric OSA population** (e.g., Adenotonsillectomy).[51]

In general, factors that may increase the likelihood of achieving a low AHI post-operatively, include lower baseline AHI, lower body mass index (BMI), and less complex obstruction.[52,53] However, the pathophysiology of sleep-related breathing disorders may not be accurately mirrored in the AHI variations. **Uvulo-palato-pharyngoplasty (UPPP) and its variants are the most common surgical procedures for OSA since complex upper pharyngeal obstruction is the most common anatomic airway abnormality.** UPPP frequently improves both the physiologic abnormality of OSA and clinical symptoms, but the degree of polysomnographic benefit as evidenced by the apnea-hypopnea index (AHI) is variable, and cures are rare. **Upper airway stimulation via an implantable neuro-stimulator is also a promising treatment of the upper and lower pharyngeal airway in selected patients.**[54,55] Nowadays, **there is a preference for combining palatal and tongue surgeries (multi-level surgery) to enlarge or stabilize the upper airway and has shown effectiveness in patients with OSA when conventional device treatment has failed. A recently published SAMS trial conducted among adults with moderate or severe OSA in whom conventional therapy had failed, combined palatal and tongue surgery, compared with medical management, reduced the number of apnea and hypopnea events and patient-reported sleepiness at 6 months.**[56]

The PATS (Pediatric Adenotonsillectomy Trial for Snoring) randomized clinical trial investigated the effects of early adenotonsillectomy versus watchful waiting in children with mild SDB.[11] While the study found no significant improvement in executive function or attention at 12 months post-surgery, it revealed improvements in secondary outcomes such as behavior, symptoms, quality of life, and blood pressure. **This suggests that while adenotonsillectomy may not directly impact cognitive outcomes in mild SDB cases, it can have beneficial effects on long-term health and quality-of-life measures.**

For children with persistent snoring after adenotonsillectomy, Bariani et al. explored the use of rapid maxillary expansion (RME).[19] This study demonstrated improvements in behavioral parameters and quality of life, in children with obstructive sleep apnea (OSA). **Although RME did not significantly change polysomnographic parameters, it effectively reduced symptoms and enhanced behavioral outcomes. This highlights the potential of RME as a secondary intervention for children with refractory SDB after adenotonsillectomy.** Camañes-Gonzalvo et al. conducted a systematic review and meta-analysis examining the relationship between ankyloglossia (short lingual frenulum) and OSA in children.[20] Their findings revealed a significant association between a short lingual frenulum and OSAS, with an odds ratio of 3.051. This suggests that ankyloglossia could be an important risk factor for pediatric OSA and underscores the potential value of early diagnosis and intervention for ankyloglossia in reducing the risk of developing sleep-disordered breathing.

A study by Yuen et al.[21] investigated the role of overnight pulse oximetry in risk stratification for postoperative respiratory complications in pediatric SDB. **Their retrospective analysis found that overnight pulse oximetry was not an accurate predictor of postoperative respiratory complications and often led to unnecessary inpatient stays. This study challenges the routine use of pulse oximetry for risk stratification in pediatric SDB cases and suggests the need for more refined assessment methods.**

Collectively, these studies highlight the complexity of managing pediatric SDB and the ongoing need for evidence-based approaches. While adenotonsillectomy remains a primary intervention, its benefits may be more pronounced in quality-of-life measures than in cognitive outcomes for mild cases. For refractory cases, additional interventions like RME show promise. The identification of risk factors such as ankyloglossia opens up new avenues for early intervention and prevention. However, these studies also underscore the limitations of current diagnostic and risk stratification methods, particularly in predicting post-operative complications. This suggests a need for more accurate and comprehensive assessment tools to guide treatment decisions and post-operative care in pediatric SDB cases.

Future research should focus on developing more targeted interventions based on individual risk factors, refining diagnostic and risk stratification methods, and conducting larger, long-term studies to better understand the impact of various treatments on both short-term symptoms and long-term developmental outcomes in children and adults with SDB.

D. Pharmacotherapy and other interventions

The pharmaco-therapeutic measures in SDB have been inconsistent thus far.[57] Within the brainstem, serotonin (5-HT) acts to modulate respiratory circuitry and ventilatory behavior.[58] Further studies as discussed highlight the important role that noradrenergic and muscarinic processes have on upper airway function during sleep and the potential for pharmacotherapy to target these mechanisms to treat OSA. There is experimental work that suggests a role of newer targets like potassium receptors which may help improve upper airway tone.[59-63]

Due to the concerns with PAP therapy as previously discussed, newer modalities for treatment are being explored. **Intranasal corticosteroids (INS) have shown promising results in managing pediatric SDB. A large observational cohort study by Rowe et al. demonstrated that INS treatment significantly improved symptoms and reduced the need for surgical intervention in children with SDB.** The study reported a decrease in mean OSA-5 scores from 8.2 to 5.5 ($p < 0.0001$) and lower surgery rates (38% vs. 56%, $p < 0.001$) in the INS group compared to the non-INS group. It was noted that the effectiveness of INS was not influenced by atopic status, suggesting potential benefits for a broader patient population.[22]

Exercise interventions have also been explored as a potential treatment for SDB, particularly in children who are overweight or obese. **Torres-Lopez et al. conducted a randomized clinical trial examining the effects of a 20-week exercise program**

on sleep outcomes. While the intervention significantly reduced wake-after-sleep onset (WASO) time by 10.8 minutes/ day (p = 0.040), it did not significantly impact total sleep time, sleep efficiency, or SDB as measured by the Pediatric Sleep Questionnaire. These findings suggest that exercise may have some benefits for sleep quality in this population, but its effects on SDB may be limited.[23]

In the realm of pharmacological interventions, Cardelli et al. investigated the impact of sacubitril/valsartan (S/V) on right ventricular function in patients with chronic heart failure and SDB. The study found significant improvements in right ventricular function, particularly in patients with central sleep apnea syndrome. Notable outcomes included an increase in TAPSE by +2.1 ± 4.9 mm (P = 0.045) and a reduction in sPAP by 8.4 ± 9.7 mmHg (P = 0.001) in the central-SDB group.[24] Similarly, the DAHOS study by Xie et al. explored the efficacy of dapagliflozin in treating heart failure with reduced ejection fraction (HFrEF) and OSA. This randomized controlled trial demonstrated significant improvements in both cardiac and sleep-related outcomes, including reductions in AHI, improvements in oxygen desaturation index, and enhancements in cardiac function and quality of life measures. **These findings suggest that dapagliflozin[27] and sacubitril/valsartan[24] may help expand the armamentarium in managing cardiac function in patients with comorbid heart failure/ HFrEF and SDB.** Other methods like hypoglossal nerve stimulation and Cognitive behavioral therapy have been studied to attempt improvement in PAP adherence.

Hypoglossal nerve stimulation (HNS) has been emerging as a promising alternative for obstructive sleep apnea (OSA). A systematic review and meta-analysis by Braun et al. examined patient-reported outcomes with HNS therapy. The analysis revealed significant improvements in daytime sleepiness (4.59-point reduction in ESS score, $p < .001$) and daytime functioning (2.84-point improvement in FOSQ score, $p < .001$). Additionally, high levels of patient satisfaction and preference over previous PAP therapy were reported, suggesting HNS as a viable alternative for OSA management.[25] **For patients with comorbid insomnia and sleep apnea (COMISA), cognitive behavioral therapy for insomnia (CBTi) has shown effectiveness.** Sweetman et al.'s systematic review and meta-analysis found that CBTi was associated with a large improvement in insomnia severity (Hedges' g = -0.89, 95% CI -1.35, -0.43). The therapy also showed potential in increasing PAP acceptance and adherence, as well as improving daytime functioning and mental health outcomes.[26] **The SURMOUNT-OSA trial showed that among participants with moderate-to-severe obstructive sleep apnea and obesity, Tirzepatide given once weekly led to significant greater reduction in the apnea-hypopnea index at 52 weeks than placebo.[33] This randomized clinical trial however excluded patients who were diabetics & those who were overweight or with normal mass index patients.**

In conclusion, these studies present a diverse range of treatment options for SDB and related conditions, from pharmacological interventions to behavioral therapies and device-based treatments. Clinicians should consider these emerging treatments when managing patients with SDB, taking into account individual patient characteristics and co-morbidities.

E. Miscellaneous

The studies reviewed offer insights into how SDB intersects with other health conditions and how novel treatments are evolving. A meta-analysis by Zhang et al. explored the relationship between SDB and retinal vein occlusion (RVO). The analysis of seven observational studies involving over 36,000 adults revealed a significant association between SDB and RVO, with an overall risk ratio (RR) of 1.92 (95% CI: 1.60-2.30, $P < .001$).[27] While these findings underscore a potential shared pathophysiological mechanism between SDB and RVO, the observational nature of the included studies suggests that prospective research is needed to establish causality.

Sharma et al. provided a systematic review of SDB associated with vagus nerve stimulator (VNS) implantation in children. Their review, which included seven studies with 104 pediatric patients, found that 36% developed VNS-associated SDB. The pathogenesis was linked to vagal-induced laryngospasm and vocal cord adduction, resulting in obstructive sleep events.[29] This review highlights the importance of pre-implantation assessment and ongoing monitoring of SDB in pediatric patients with VNS. This review also informs clinicians regarding potential for iatrogenic symptoms. Further research should focus on identifying specific risk factors and standardizing diagnostic and management approaches. Wallace et al. conducted a systematic review to assess the impact of chemical pollutants on sleep outcomes. **The review highlighted that exposure to pollutants such as particulate matter (PM), nitrogen dioxide (NO_2), and secondhand smoke (SHS) is associated with poorer sleep quality**

and disorders, including insomnia and SDB.[30] The evidence for metals and pesticides also indicated negative effects on sleep. However, the review noted significant variability in pollutant types and sleep outcome measurements, and much of the data relied on self-reports. Objective measures and further studies are needed to clarify these associations and to understand the biological mechanisms linking pollution with sleep disturbances. This data gains further importance as climate change and air pollution continue to become major killers around the world. Valentim da Silva et al. reviewed studies assessing gut microbiota in children with obstructive sleep apnea syndrome (OSAS). **They found that children with OSAS had reduced microbiota diversity and increased pro-inflammatory bacteria, alongside decreased beneficial bacteria.**[31] **These findings highlight the need for further research to explore the causality and potential for therapeutic interventions targeting gut microbiota.**

Osman et al. evaluated the efficacy of BAY2586116, a TASK 1/3 potassium channel antagonist nasal spray, in treating obstructive sleep apnea (OSA).[32] In their randomized, blinded trial, the nasal spray significantly reduced the apnea-hypopnea index (AHI) and oxygen desaturation index (ODI) in physiological responders. The study suggests that TASK channel antagonism could be a promising therapeutic approach for OSA, particularly in patients who demonstrate physiological improvement in upper airway collapsibility. However, the study's small sample size and the need to assess broader outcomes, such as cardiovascular effects and residual sleepiness, call for larger trials to validate these results and explore their clinical applicability. It is important to keep in mind that AHI improvements alone may not suggest a clinical response.

This review highlights the complexity of sleep-disordered breathing and its multifaceted interactions with age, gender, comorbidities, and environmental factors. The studies reviewed provide valuable insights into these associations and emerging therapeutic options. Continued research is crucial to enhance our understanding and management of SDB, particularly through prospective studies and the development of targeted/personalized treatment approaches. Algorithms 1 and 2 summarizes the choice of diagnostic sleep study in a patient with suspected OSA and practical approach to choosing PAP therapy in various sleep disorders.

Algorithm 1: An algorithm for the choice of diagnostic sleep study in a patient with suspected OSA

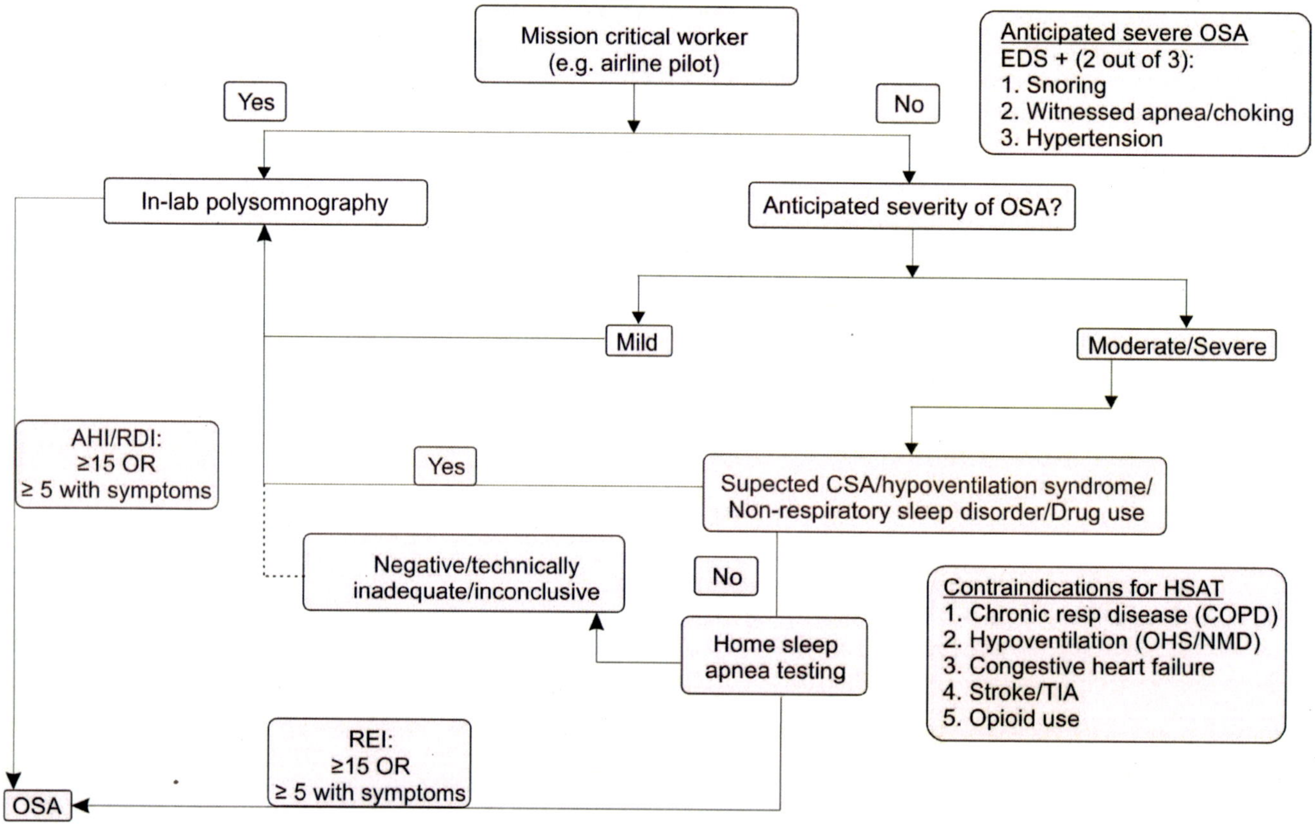

AHI, apnea - hypopnea index; COPD, chronic obstructive pulmonary disease; CSA, central sleep apnea; EDS, excessive daytime sleepiness; OHS, obesity hypoventilation syndrome; OSA, obstructive sleep apnea; RDI, respiratory disturbance index; REI, respiratory event index; TIA, transient ischemic attack

Algorithm 2: A simplified practical approach to choosing PAP therapy in various sleep disorders

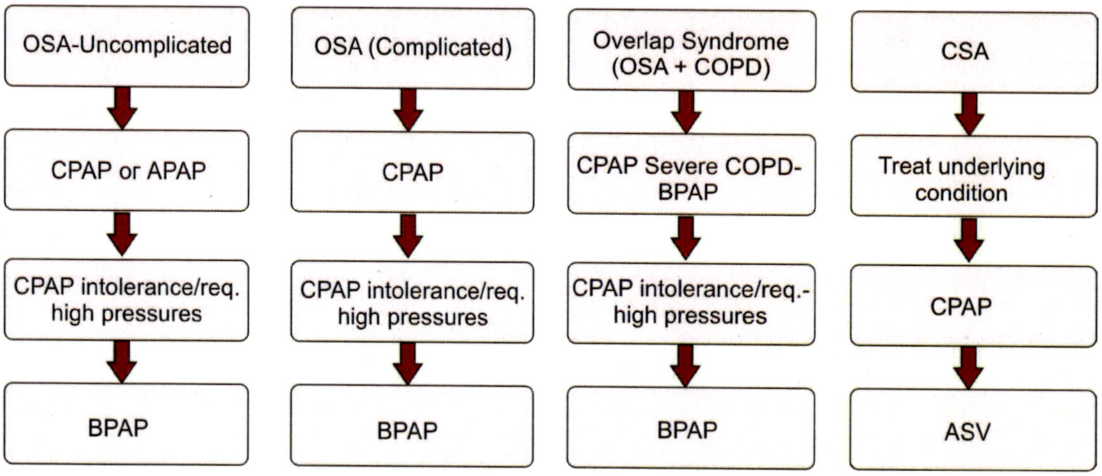

REFERENCES

1. Sanapo L, Hackethal S, Bublitz MH, Sawyer K, Garbazza C, Nagasunder A, Gonzalez M, Bourjeily G. Maternal sleep disordered breathing and offspring growth outcome: A systematic review and meta-analysis. Sleep Med Rev. 2024 Feb;73:101868. doi: 10.1016/j.smrv.2023.101868. Epub 2023 Nov 1. PMID: 37956482; PMCID: PMC11000747.

2. Punjabi NM, Brown TT, Abreu AR, Aurora RN, Patel SR, Stosor V, Cho JH, D'Souza G, Wallace D, Margolick JB. Sleep-Disordered Breathing and Prevalent Hypertension in Men With and Without HIV. J Acquir Immune Defic Syndr. 2023 Dec 1;94(4):349-354. doi: 10.1097/QAI.0000000000003276. PMID: 37643405; PMCID: PMC10824508.

3. Yang L, Ding Z, Zhou J, Zhang S, Wang Q, Zheng K, Wang X, Chen L. Algorithmic detection of sleep-disordered breathing using respiratory signals: a systematic review. Physiol Meas. 2024 Mar 21;45(3). doi: 10.1088/1361-6579/ad2c13. PMID: 38387048.

4. Zhang W, Shen Y, Ou X, Wang H, Liu S. Sleep disordered breathing and neurobehavioral deficits in children and adolescents: a systematic review and meta-analysis. BMC Pediatr. 2024 Jan 20;24(1):70. doi: 10.1186/s12887-023-04511-2. PMID: 38245707; PMCID: PMC10799548.

5. García-Ortega A, Oscullo G, Mañas-Baena E, Cano-Pumarega I, Gómez-Olivas JD, Bekki A, Beauperthuy T, Barbero E, García-Sánchez A, Inglés M, Mompeán S, Calvillo P, Jiménez-Aguilella JJ, Navarrete J, Cerveró A, Jiménez D, Martínez-García MÁ; ESAET investigators. Changes in sleep-disordered breathing from the acute to the stable phase of pulmonary embolism: The ESAET study. Sleep Med. 2023 Dec;112:88-95. doi: 10.1016/j.sleep.2023.10.003. Epub 2023 Oct 10. PMID: 37837824.

6. Aragón-Villalba G, Munoz-Quintana G, Rubin de Celis GN, Torres-Hortelano JM, Espinosa de Santillana IA. Efficacy of Roncolab mobile application for diagnosing the primary sign of sleep-disordered breathing (snoring) in children. Acta Odontol Latinoam. 2023 Dec 31;36(3):150-155. doi: 10.54589/aol.36/3/150. PMID: 38345276; PMCID: PMC10867856.

7. Fong PY, Tay ZY, Soh RY, Fook SMC, Li HH, Phua CQ. Should mild obstructive sleep apnoea be treated? A systematic review from the standpoint of disease progression. J Laryngol Otol. 2023 Aug;137(8):828-839. doi: 10.1017/S0022215122002419. Epub 2022 Nov 16. PMID: 36380495.

8. Iskander A, Jairam T, Wang C, Murray BJ, Boulos MI. Normal multiple sleep latency test values in adults: A systematic review and meta-analysis. Sleep Med. 2023 Sep;109:143-148. doi: 10.1016/j.sleep.2023.06.019. Epub 2023 Jun 29. Erratum in: Sleep Med. 2023 Oct;110:179. doi: 10.1016/j.sleep.2023.08.001. PMID: 37442016.

9. Magnusdottir S, Hill EA. Prevalence of obstructive sleep apnea (OSA) among preschool aged children in the general population: A systematic review. Sleep Med Rev. 2024 Feb;73:101871. doi: 10.1016/j.smrv.2023.101871. Epub 2023 Nov 7. PMID: 37976758.

10. Manconi M, van der Gaag LC, Mangili F, Garbazza C, Riccardi S, Cajochen C, Mondini S, Furia F, Zambrelli E, Baiardi S, Giordano A, Rizzo N, Fonti C, Viora E, D'Agostino A, Cicolin A, Cirignotta F; Life-ON Study Group; Group of Milan (Italy); Aquilino D, Barassi A, Del Giudice R, Fior G, Gambini O, Giordano B, Martini A, Serrati C, Stefanelli R, Scarone S, Canevini M, Fanti V, Stein HC, Marconi AM; Group of Turin (Italy); Raimondo E, Viglietta E; Group of Bologna (Italy); Santoro R, Simonazzi G, Bianconcini A; Group of Lugano (Switzerland); Meani F, Piazza N, Filippakos F, Gyr T. Sleep and sleep disorders during pregnancy and postpartum: The Life-ON study. Sleep Med. 2024 Jan;113:41-48. doi: 10.1016/j.sleep.2023.10.021. Epub 2023 Nov 11. PMID: 37984016.

11. Mitchell RB, Cook K, Garetz S, Tapia IE, Elden LM, Kirkham EM, Shah J, Otteson T, Zopf D, Amin R, Ishman S, Baldassari CM, Chervin RD, Hassan F, Naqvi K, Wang R, Redline S. Clinical Characteristics of Primary Snoring vs Mild Obstructive Sleep Apnea in Children: Analysis of the Pediatric Adenoton-sillectomy for Snoring (PATS) Randomized Clinical Trial. JAMA Otolaryngol Head Neck Surg. 2024 Feb 1;150(2):99-106. doi: 10.1001/jamaoto.2023.3816. PMID: 38095903; PMCID: PMC10722386.

12. Tian Q, Sun J, Li X, Liu J, Zhou H, Deng J, Li J. Association between sleep apnoea and risk of cognitive impairment and Alzheimer's disease: a meta-analysis of cohort-based studies. Sleep Breath. 2024 May;28(2):585-595. doi: 10.1007/s11325-023-02934-w. Epub 2023 Oct 20. PMID: 37857768.

13. Raju S, Siddharthan T, McCormack MC, Patel SR, Kunisaki KM, D'Souza G, Cho JH, Stosor V, Morris A, Margolick JB, Brown TT, Punjabi NM. Influence of Impaired Diffusing Capacity and Sleep-disordered Breathing on Nocturnal Hypoxemia and Health Outcomes in Men with and without Human Immunodeficiency Virus. Ann Am Thorac Soc. 2024 Jul;21(7):1085-1093. doi: 10.1513/AnnalsATS.202309-757OC. PMID: 38498872; PMCID: PMC11284323.

14. Bradley TD, Logan AG, Lorenzi Filho G, Kimoff RJ, Durán Cantolla J, Arzt M, Redolfi S, Parati G, Kasai T, Dunlap ME, Delgado D, Yatsu S, Bertolami A, Pedrosa R, Tomlinson G, Marin Trigo JM, Tantucci C, Floras JS; ADVENT-HF Investigators. Adaptive servo-ventilation for sleep-disordered breathing in patients with heart failure with reduced ejection fraction (ADVENT-HF): a multicentre, multinational, parallel-group, open-label, phase 3 randomised controlled trial. Lancet Respir Med. 2024 Feb;12(2):153-166. doi: 10.1016/S2213-2600(23) 00374-0. Epub 2023 Dec 21. PMID: 38142697.

15. Mansell SK, Devani N, Shah A, Schievano S, Main E, Mandal S. Current treatment strategies in managing side effects associated with domiciliary positive airway pressure (PAP) therapy for patients with sleep disordered breathing: A systematic review and meta-analysis. Sleep Med Rev. 2023 Dec;72:101850. doi: 10.1016/j.smrv.2023.101850. Epub 2023 Sep 23. PMID: 37812972.

16. Lajoie AC, Gu Y, Lim A, Benedetti A, Kaminska M. Adherence to continuous positive airway pressure for the treatment of obstructive sleep apnea in neurodegenerative diseases: A systematic review. Sleep Med Rev. 2023 Oct;71:101836. doi: 10.1016/j.smrv.2023.101836. Epub 2023 Aug 9. PMID: 37586145.

17. Arzt M, Munt O, Pépin JL, Heinzer R, Kübeck R, von Hehn U, Ehrsam-Tosi D, Benjafield AV, Woehrle H. Effects of Adaptive Servo-Ventilation on Quality of Life: The READ-ASV Registry. Ann Am Thorac Soc. 2024 Apr;21(4):651-657. doi: 10.1513/AnnalsATS.202310-908OC. PMID: 38241012.

18. Redline S, Cook K, Chervin RD, Ishman S, Baldassari CM, Mitchell RB, Tapia IE, Amin R, Hassan F, Ibrahim S, Ross K, Elden LM, Kirkham EM, Zopf D, Shah J, Otteson T, Naqvi K, Owens J, Young L, Furth S, Connolly H, Clark CAC, Bakker JP, Garetz S, Radcliffe J, Taylor HG, Rosen CL, Wang R; Pediatric Adenotonsillectomy Trial for Snoring (PATS) Study Team. Adenotonsillectomy for Snoring and Mild Sleep Apnea in Children: A Randomized Clinical Trial. JAMA. 2023 Dec 5;330(21):2084-2095. doi: 10.1001/jama.2023.22114. PMID: 38051326; PMCID: PMC10698619.

19. Bariani RCB, Bigliazzi R, Medda MG, Micieli APR, Tufik S, Fujita RR, de Mello CB, Moreira GA. Changes in behavioral and cognitive abilities after rapid maxillary expansion in children affected by persistent snoring after long-term adenotonsillectomy: A noncontrolled study. Am J Orthod Dentofacial Orthop. 2024 Mar;165(3):344-356. doi: 10.1016/j.ajodo.2023.10.011. Epub 2023 Dec 21. PMID: 38142392.

20. Camañes-Gonzalvo S, Montiel-Company JM, Paredes-Gallardo V, Puertas-Cuesta FJ, Marco-Pitarch R, García-Selva M, Bellot-Arcís C, Casaña-Ruiz MD. Relationship of ankyloglossia and obstructive sleep apnea: systematic review and meta-analysis. Sleep Breath. 2024 Jun;28(3):1067-1078. doi: 10.1007/s11325-024-03021-4. Epub 2024 Mar 13. PMID: 38478208; PMCID: PMC11196303.

21. Yuen HS, Sandeman J, Hone R. The role of overnight pulse oximetry in risk stratification of paediatric sleep disordered breathing in a district general hospital. Int J Pediatr Otorhinolaryngol. 2024 Feb;177:111869. doi: 10.1016/j.ijporl.2024.111869. Epub 2024 Jan 11. PMID: 38266379.

22. Rowe KS, Pinczower GD, Nixon GM, Kubba H. The impact of intranasal corticosteroids in a prospective cohort of children with sleep disordered breathing. Int J Pediatr Otorhinolaryngol. 2024 Mar;178:111899. doi: 10.1016/j.ijporl.2024.111899. Epub 2024 Feb 20. PMID: 38402717.

23. Torres-Lopez LV, Migueles JH, Cadenas-Sanchez C, Bendtsen M, Henriksson P, Mora-Gonzalez J, Löf M, Chaput JP, Ortega FB. Effects of exercise on sleep in children with overweight/obesity: a randomized clinical trial. Obesity (Silver Spring). 2024 Feb;32(2):281-290. doi: 10.1002/oby.23945. Epub 2023 Dec 19. PMID: 38112235.

24. Cardelli LS, Magaldi M, Agullo A, Richard G, Nogue E, Berdague P, Galiner M, Georger F, Picard F, Prunet E, Molinari N, Bourdin A, Jaffuel D, Roubille F. Sacubitril/valsartan has an underestimated impact on the right ventricle in patients with sleep-disordered breathing, especially central sleep apnoea syndrome. Arch Cardiovasc Dis. 2024 Jun-Jul;117(6-7):409-416. doi: 10.1016/j.acvd.2024.04.003.Epub 2024 May 18. PMID: 38811278.

25. Braun M, Stoerzel M, Wollny M, Schoebel C, Ulrich Sommer J, Heiser C. Patient-reported outcomes with hypoglossal nerve stimulation for treatment of obstructive sleep apnea: a systematic review and meta-analysis. Eur Arch Otorhino-laryngol. 2023 Oct;280(10):4627-4639. doi: 10.1007/s00405-023-08062-1. Epub 2023 Jun 24. PMID: 37354340; PMCID: PMC10477259.

26. Sweetman A, Farrell S, Wallace DM, Crawford M. The effect of cognitive behavioural therapy for insomnia in people with comorbid insomnia and sleep apnoea: A systematic review and meta-analysis. J Sleep Res. 2023 Dec;32(6):e13847. doi: 10.1111/jsr.13847. Epub 2023 Mar 5. PMID: 36872072.

27. Xie L, Li S, Yu X, Wei Q, Yu F, Tong J. DAHOS Study: Efficacy of dapagliflozin in treating heart failure with reduced ejection fraction and obstructive sleep apnea syndrome - A 3-month, multicenter, randomized controlled clinical trial. Eur J Clin Pharmacol. 2024 May;80(5):771-780. doi: 10.1007/s00228-024-03643-3. Epub 2024 Feb 22. PMID: 38386021.

28. Zhang JT, Cui S, Li Q, Li JR, Zhang YF, Zheng YH. Sleep-disordered breathing is related to retinal vein occlusion: A meta-analysis. Medicine (Baltimore). 2023 Oct 13;102(41):e35411. doi: 10.1097/MD.0000000000035411. PMID: 37832067; PMCID: PMC10578690.

29. Sharma S, Nouri MN, St-Laurent A, Wiedermann J. Vagal nerve stimulator-associated sleep disordered breathing secondary to vagal-induced laryngospasm in pediatric populations: Case presentation and systematic review. Int J Pediatr Otorhino-laryngol. 2023 Oct;173:111701. doi: 10.1016/j.ijporl.2023.111701. Epub 2023 Aug 25. PMID: 37643554.

30. Wallace DA, Gallagher JP, Peterson SR, Ndiaye-Gueye S, Fox K, Redline S, Johnson DA. Is exposure to chemical pollutants associated with sleep outcomes? A systematic review. Sleep Med Rev. 2023 Aug;70:101805. doi: 10.1016/j.smrv.2023.101805. Epub 2023 Jun 16. Erratum in: Sleep Med Rev. 2023 Dec;72:101853. doi: 10.1016/j.smrv.2023.101853. PMID: 37392613; PMCID: PMC10528206.

31. da Silva LMAV, Assunção WG, Bento VAA, Sachi VP, Colombo FE, Ique MMA, Faria BMA, Bertoz APM. Assessment of the gut microbiota of children with obstructive sleep apnea syndrome: A systematic review. Sleep Med. 2024 Aug;120:56-64. doi: 10.1016/j.sleep.2024.06.002. Epub 2024 Jun 12. PMID: 38878352.

32. Osman AM, Toson B, Naik GR, Mukherjee S, Delbeck M, Hahn M, Muller T, Weimann G, Eckert DJ. A novel TASK channel antagonist nasal spray reduces sleep apnea severity in physiological responders: a randomized, blinded, trial. Am J Physiol Heart Circ Physiol. 2024 Mar 1;326(3):H715-H723. doi: 10.1152/ajpheart.00541.2023. Epub 2024 Jan 12. PMID: 38214905.

33. Malhotra A, Grunstein RR, Fietze I, Weaver TE, Redline S, Azarbarzin A, Sands SA, Schwab RJ, Dunn JP, Chakladar S, Bunck MC, Bednarik J; SURMOUNT-OSA Investigators. Tirzepatide for the Treatment of Obstructive Sleep Apnea and Obesity. N Engl J Med. 2024 Jun 21. doi: 10.1056/NEJMoa 2404881. Epub ahead of print. PMID: 38912654.

34. Kim Y, Koo YS, Lee HY, et al. Can continuous positive airway pressure reduce the risk of stroke in obstructive sleep apnea patients? A systematic review and meta-analysis. PLoS ONE 2016; 11: e0146317

35. Peppard PE, Young T, Barnet JH, et al. Increased prevalence of sleep-disordered breathing in adults. Am J Epidemiol 2013; 177: 1006–1014.

36. Udwadia ZF, Doshi AV, Lonkar SG, Singh CI. Prevalence of sleep-disordered breathing and sleep apnea in middle-aged urban Indian men. Am J Respir Crit Care Med. 2004; 169:168–73

37. Sharma SK, Kumpawat S, Banga A, Goel A. Prevalence and risk factors of obstructive sleep apnea syndrome in a population of Delhi, India. Chest. 2006; 130:149–56

38. Pinto AM, Devaraj U, Ramachandran P, Joseph B, D'Souza GA. Obstructive Sleep Apnea in a rural population in South India: Feasibility of health care workers to administer level III sleep study. Lung India. 2018 Jul-Aug; 35(4):301-306. doi: 10.4103/lungindia.lungindia_433_17. PMID: 29970768; PMCID: PMC603438

39. Suri TM, Ghosh TS, Mittal S, Hadda V, et al. Prevalence of Obstructive Sleep Apnea in India: A systematic review and meta-analysis. AJRCCM-conference. 2023; 207:1. https://doi.org/10.1164/ajrccm-conference.2023.207.1_MeetingAbstracts.A5840

40. Patil SP et al. Treatment of Adult Obstructive Sleep Apnea with Positive Airway Pressure: An American Academy of Sleep Medicine Clinical Practice Guideline. J Clin Sleep Med. 2019 Feb 15;15(2):335-343

41. Selim B, Ramar K. Sleep-Related Breathing Disorders: When CPAP Is Not Enough. Neurotherapeutics. 2021 Jan; 18(1):81-90.

42. Farre R, et al. Response of automatic continuous positive airway pressure devices to different sleep breathing patterns: a bench study. Am J Respir Crit Care Med 2002; 166(4): 469–73.

43. Roux F, Hilbert J. Continuous positive airway pressure: new generations. Clinics in chest medicine, vol. 24; 2003. p. 315–42

44. Remmers J, et al. Remotely controlled mandibular protrusion during sleep predicts therapeutic success with oral appliances in patients with obstructive sleep apnea. Sleep. 2013; 36(10):1517–25. doi: 10.5665/sleep.3048.

45. M Cowie, Holger W, Karl W, et al. Adaptive servo-ventilation for central sleep apnea in systolic heart failure. New England journal of medicine.2015; 373:1095-1105.

46. Selim B, Ramar K. Advanced positive airway pressure modes: adaptive servo ventilation and volume assured pressure support. Expert Rev Med Devices.2016; 13(9):839-51

47. Chen LY, Chen YH, Hu SW, et al. In search of a better CPAP interface: A network metaanalysis comparing nasal masks, nasal pillows and oro-nasal masks. Journal of Sleep Research. 2022;31(6):e13686

48. H Fox, T Bitter, et al. Automatic positive airway pressure for obstructive sleep apnea in heart failure with reduced ejection fraction: A randomized controlled pilot study. Clinical Research in Cardiology. 2021; 110(7):983-992.

49. Hu Y, Zhang Z, Fang F, et al. Effects of heated humidification on positive airway pressure side effects in patients with obstructive sleep apnoea: a meta-analysis. Sleep & Breathing. 2022; 27(1):67-75.

50. Sánchez-de-la-Torre M, Sánchez-de-la-Torre A, Bertran S, Abad J, Duran-Cantolla J, Cabriada V, Mediano O, Masdeu MJ, Alonso ML, Masa JF, Barceló A, de la Peña M, Mayos M, Coloma R, Montserrat JM, Chiner E, Perelló S, Rubinós G, Mínguez O, Pascual L, Cortijo A, Martínez D, Aldomà A, Dalmases M, McEvoy RD, Barbé F; Spanish Sleep Network. Effect of obstructive sleep apnoea and its treatment with continuous positive airway pressure on the prevalence of cardiovascular events in patients with acute coronary syndrome (ISAACC study): a randomised controlled trial. Lancet Respir Med. 2020 Apr;8(4):359-367. doi: 10.1016/S2213-2600(19)30271-1. Epub 2019 Dec 12. PMID: 31839558.

51. Llombart M, Chiner E, Gómez-Merino E, Andreu A, Pastor E, Senent C, Camarasa A, Signes-Costa J. Síndrome de apneas-hipopneas durante el sueño en población infantil: diferencias en su expresión entre niños con hipertrofia amigdalar y con enfermedad concomitante [Sleep apnea-hypopnea syndrome in a pediatric population: differences between children with tonsillar hypertrophy and those with concomitant disease]. Arch Bronconeumol. 2007 Dec;43(12): 655-61. Spanish. doi: 10.1016/s1579-2129(07)60151-7. PMID: 18053542.

52. Sher AE, Schechtman KB, Piccirillo JF. The efficacy of surgical modifications of the upper airway in adults with obstructive sleep apnea syndrome. Sleep. 1996 Feb;19(2):156-77. doi: 10.1093/sleep/19.2.156. PMID: 8855039.

53. Friedman M, Ibrahim H, Bass L. Clinical staging for sleep-disordered breathing. Otolaryngol Head Neck Surg. 2002 Jul; 127(1):13-21. doi: 10.1067/mhn.2002.126477. PMID: 12161725

54. Randerath WJ, Verbraecken J, Andreas S, Bettega G, Boudewyns A, Hamans E, Jalbert F, Paoli JR, Sanner B, Smith I, Stuck BA, Lacassagne L, Marklund M, Maurer JT, Pepin JL, Valipour A, Verse T, Fietze I; European Respiratory Society task force on non-CPAP therapies in sleep apnoea. Non-CPAP therapies in obstructive sleep apnoea. Eur Respir J. 2011 May;37(5):1000- 28. doi: 10.1183/09031936.00099710. Epub 2011 Mar 15. PMID: 21406515.

55. Stuck BA, Ravesloot MJL, Eschenhagen T, de Vet HCW, Sommer JU. Uvulopalatopharyngoplasty with or without tonsillectomy in the treatment of adult obstructive sleep apnea - A systematic review. Sleep Med. 2018 Oct; 50:152-165. doi: 10.1016/j.sleep.2018.05.004. Epub 2018 May 12. PMID: 30056286

56. Stuart M, Simon C, Peter G, et al. Effect of Multi-level upper airway surgery vs medical management on the apnea- hypopnea index and patient reported daytime sleepiness among patients with moderate or severe obstructive sleep apnea. The SAMS randomized controlled trial. JAMA. 2020; 324(12):1168-1179

57. Aurora RN, Chowdhuri S, Ramar K, Bista SR, Casey KR, Lamm CI, Kristo DA, Mallea JM, Rowley JA, Zak RS, Tracy SL. The treatment of central sleep apnea syndromes in adults: practice parameters with an evidence-based literature review and meta-analyses. Sleep 35: 17– 40, 2012. doi: 10.5665/sleep.1580.

58. Richerson GB. Serotonergic neurons as carbon dioxide sensors that maintain pH homeostasis. Nat Rev Neurosci 5: 449–461, 2004. doi: 10.1038/nrn1409

59. Aishah A, Lim R, Sands SA, Taranto-Montemurro L, Wellman A, Carberry JC, Eckert DJ. Different antimuscarinics when combined with atomoxetine have differential effects on obstructive sleep apnea severity. J ApplPhysiol (1985). 2021 May 1; 130(5):1373-1382.

doi: 10.1152/japplphysiol.01074.2020. Epub 2021 Mar 18. Erratum in: J ApplPhysiol (1985). 2023 Jan 1; 134(1):84. PMID: 33734828; PMCID: PMC8424567.

60. Lim R, Messineo L, Grunstein RR, Carberry JC, Eckert DJ. The noradrenergic agent reboxetine plus the antimuscarinic hyoscine butylbromide reduces sleep apnoea severity: a double-blind, placebo-controlled, randomised crossover trial. J Physiol. 2021 Sep; 599(17):4183-4195. doi: 10.1113/JP281912. Epub 2021 Jul 14. PMID: 34174090.

61. Osman AM, Mukherjee S, Altree TJ, Delbeck M, Gehring D, Hahn M, Lang T, Xing C, Muller T, Weimann G, Eckert DJ. Topical Potassium Channel Blockage Improves Pharyngeal Collapsibility: A Translational, Placebo-Controlled Trial. Chest. 2023 Apr; 163(4):953-965. doi: 10.1016/j.chest.2022.11.024. Epub 2022 Nov 24. PMID: 36435266.

62. Thomson LDJ, Landry SA, Joosten SA, Mann DL, Wong AM, Cheung T, Adam M, Beatty CJ, Hamilton GS, Edwards BA. A single dose of noradrenergic/serotonergic reuptake inhibitors combined with an antimuscarinic does not improve obstructive sleep apnoea severity. Physiol Rep. 2022 Aug; 10(16):e15440. doi: 10.14814/phy2.15440. PMID: 36029192; PMCID: PMC9419 156.

63. Altree TJ, Aishah A, Loffler KA, Grunstein RR, Eckert DJ. The norepinephrine reuptake inhibitor reboxetine alone reduces obstructive sleep apnea severity: a double-blind, placebo-controlled, randomized crossover trial. J Clin Sleep Med. 2023 Jan 1; 19(1):85-96. doi: 10.5664/jcsm.10256. PMID: 36004739; PMCID: PMC9806793.

CHAPTER 14

Respiratory Critical Care

Authors: Dr. Naren Chandra, Dr. Gyanendra Agrawal

Reviewer: Dr. Saurabh Mittal

INTRODUCTION

Respiratory Critical Care has advanced over a period of years. The therapeutic and diagnostic algorithm of ARDS has changed over years paving way for newer definition, it also stresses the diagnosis being made in remote centers. Newer extracorporeal therapies are coming into the management path.

ICU acquired infections can cause significant morbidity and mortality. VAP develops at least 48 hours after endotracheal intubation. VAP bundle is a set of individual components and it must be implemented together to achieve significantly better results.

The role of non-invasive ventilation in respiratory failure is increasing because of ease of use and better tolerability. Long-term oxygen supplementation for at least 15 hours a day improves survival however there were some unanswered questions on risk of hospitalization and death, thus necessitating further research studies. This chapter includes the newer updates in Respiratory Critical Care (excluding COVID-19).

Methodology:

A PubMed search was done using the search terms "Respiratory distress syndrome" OR "ARDS" OR "Respiratory insufficiency" OR "Severe Pneumonia" OR "CAP" OR "NIV" or "Non-invasive ventilation" OR "ECMO" OR "EC-CO_2R" OR "Bronchoscopy in ICU". The search term was limited to Randomized Controlled Trials, Clinical trials, Systematic reviews and Meta-analysis between August 2023 to August 2024. A total of 792 articles were found and assessed.

Electronic database search: PubMed

Period: 1st August 2023 to 1st August 2024

Search words: "Respiratory distress syndrome" OR "ARDS" OR "Respiratory insufficiency" OR "Severe Pneumonia" OR "CAP" OR "NIV" OR "Non-invasive ventilation" OR "ECMO" OR "EC-CO_2R" OR "Bronchoscopy in ICU"

(n=792)

↓

Articles after screening for relevance- significant / practice changing

(n=13)

- ***Individualized, short-term course antibiotics treatment versus usual long-course treatment for ventilator-associated pneumonia (REGARD -VAP); A Multicentric, individualized randomized, open-label, non-inferiority trial. (Lancet Resp Med. 2024)[1]***
  - *Population:* Adults (age>18 years) who met the US Centre for Disease Control and Prevention National Healthcare Safety Network criteria (respiratory signs and symptoms compatible with pneumonia, mechanical ventilation for 48 hours or longer, and new radiological changes) for VAP. (Nepal, Thailand, and Singapore). (n=461)
  - *Intervention:* Short course treatment refers to $\leq$7 days and as short as 3-5 days. (n=232).
  - *Comparator:* Usual course of antibiotics - $\geq$8 days, with precise duration determined by primary clinicians). (n=229).
  - *Outcome and conclusion*: The outcome was defined by defervescence for 48 hours, stable blood pressure without ionotropic support; and discontinue antibiotics within 7 days of treatment. Individualized, short-course antibiotic treatment for VAP was non-inferior to longer-duration antibiotic treatment in terms of 60-day mortality, and pneumonia recurrence and was associated with substantially reduced antibiotic use and side effects.
  - *Critical appraisal:* Individualized, short-course antibiotic treatment for VAP could help to reduce the burden of antibiotic resistance in ICU assessed by case to case. It excluded patients with SOFA Score > 11 points (corresponding to in-hospital mortality of 80 %), immunocompromised patients (CD4 <200 cells/ mm^3, corticosteroids >0.5 mg/kg per day for 30 days, chemotherapy in the past 3 months, or solid organ or hematopoietic stem cell transplant or had other infections requiring a longer duration of antibiotics (Tuberculosis, Fungal infections, antibiotics meant for chronic suppression of chronic infections, or chronic obstructive lung disease). So, the data does not apply to these populations.

☞

- ***Prevention of ventilator-associated pneumonia through care bundles: A systematic review and meta-analysis. (J Intensive Med. 2023)[2]***
  - o *Population:* Critically ill patients from 36 studies including 116,873 mechanically ventilated (MV) participants met the inclusion criteria. A total of 84,031 participants underwent care bundles for VAP prevention. (n= 84,031)
  - o *Outcome and conclusion:* The most reported component of the ventilator bundle was head-end-bed elevation (n = 83,146), followed by oral care (n = 80,787). Implementing ventilator care bundles reduced the number of VAP episodes (OR = 0.42, 95% CI: 0.33, 0.54) and the duration of MV (MD = –1.24, 95% CI: –2.30, –0.18) in adult ICUs. Their application in combination with educational activities seemed to improve clinical outcomes. However, the data regarding mortality was inconclusive.
  - o *Critical appraisal:* VAP bundles can be implemented but measures to be taken for strict compliance must be ensured. In this study, there was varied compliance. Significant heterogeneity was seen. Subgroup analysis evaluation was not able to be performed as some studies were underpowered.

- ***Inhaled Amikacin to Prevent Ventilator-Associated Pneumonia. (NEJM. 2023)[3]***
  - o *Population:* Critically ill adults who had been undergoing invasive mechanical ventilation for at least 72 hours. (n=847)
  - o *Intervention:* Inhaled Amikacin at a dose of 20 mg per kilogram of ideal body weight once daily for 3 days. (n=417)
  - o *Comparator:* Placebo for 3 days (0.9% saline). (n=430)
  - o *Conclusion:* Among patients who had undergone mechanical ventilation for at least 3 days, a subsequent 3-day course of inhaled Amikacin reduced the burden of ventilator-associated pneumonia during 28 days of follow-up. (15% Vs 22%, p = 0.004)

- *Critical appraisal:* The study excluded patients having >96 hours of ventilation (long-term on ventilator) and severe AKI. The duration of mechanical ventilation was comparable in both the groups (median - 9 days) which doesn't correlate in ideal scenario. Also, the study was not adequately powered to look into patient-centered outcomes – death, length of hospital stay, or ICU stay.

☞

- ***Impact of different corticosteroids on severe community-acquired pneumonia: A systematic review and meta-analysis. (BMJ. 2024)[4]***
  - *Population:* Severe community-acquired pneumonia patients from 10 RCTs. (n=1962)
  - *Outcome:* Corticosteroids were associated with a lower rate of all-cause mortality (Risk Ratio (RR) - 0.70 (95% CI, 0.54 to 0.90). When stratified into different corticosteroid types, hydrocortisone was associated with an approximately 50% lower mortality risk (RR, 0.48 (95% CI 0.32 to 0.72).
  - *Conclusion:* The use of hydrocortisone, but not other types of corticosteroids, was associated with a reduction in mortality and improvement in pneumonia outcomes among patients hospitalized with severe CAP.
  - *Critical appraisal:* Severe CAP had varied inclusion and exclusion criteria in studies. The route and dose of steroids varied with significant heterogeneity.

☞

- ***Lung Ultrasonography (LUS) Accuracy for Diagnosis of Adult Pneumonia: Systematic Review and Meta-Analysis. (Adv. Resp Med. 2024)[5]***
  - *Population:* Adult pneumonia patients from 29 studies. (n=6702)
  - *Outcome and conclusion:* LUS has high diagnostic accuracy in adult pneumonia. Its contribution could form an optimistic clue in future updates considering this condition. It has a sensitivity and specificity of 94% and 96%, respectively, with an area under the SROC (summary receiver operating characteristic) curve of 0.98 according to Chavez et al. Another study from Hu et al. obtained a DOR (diagnostic odds ratio) of 509.99 and an area under the SROC curve of 0.99 (though this study predominantly – pediatric population).
  - *Critical appraisal:* LUS has varied advantages- can be preferred in children, has better reproducibility, avoids radiation exposure, has less turn-around time and the disadvantages are less reliable in obese patients and has significant interobserver variations.

- ***Lung ultrasound score (LUS) and in-hospital mortality of adults with acute respiratory distress syndrome: a meta-analysis. (BMC Resp Med. 2024)[6]***
  - *Population:* ARDS patients. (n=1022)
  - *Outcome:* In the study, 343 patients (33.6%) died during hospitalization. The pooled results suggested that the LUS score at admission was higher in non-survivors as compared to survivors (standardized mean difference = 0.73, 95% confidence interval [CI]: 0.55 to 0.91, $p < 0.001$). Moreover, a high LUS score at admission was associated with a higher risk of in-hospital mortality of patients with ARDS (risk ratio: 1.44, 95% CI: 1.14 to 1.81, $p = 0.002$).
  - *Conclusion:* The findings suggest that a high LUS score at admission may be associated with a high risk of in-hospital mortality of patients with ARDS.

- ***High-Flow Nasal Cannula Oxygen Therapy versus Non-Invasive Ventilation in patients at very high risk for extubating failure: A systematic review of randomized controlled Trials. (PLOS one. 2024)***[7]
    - o *Population:* Intubated patients from 11 studies. Population was from Asia/ Europe with age group 40-85 years and duration of MV ranging 4 -25 days. (n=2666)
    - o *Outcome:* Compared to NIV, HFNC also improved tolerance, comfort, and fewer complications, such as airway care interventions. However, NIV with active humidification may be more effective than HFNC in avoiding reintubation in patients who are at extremely high risk for extubating failure.
    - o *Conclusion:* NIV with active humidification may be more effective than HFNC in avoiding reintubation in patients who are at extremely high risk for extubating failure. In comparison, HFNC improved tolerance, comfort, and fewer complications such as airway care interventions.
    - o *Critical appraisal:* Small number of studies/ publication bias. Extubation failure risk was not clearly defined in many studies and was not standardized.

☞

- ***Incidence of noninvasive ventilation failure and mortality in patients with acute respiratory distress syndrome: A systematic review and proportion meta-analysis. (BMC Pul Med. 2024)***[8]
    - o *Population:* ARDS patients from 90 studies. (n=5847)
    - o *Outcome:* The pooled incidence of NIV failure was 48%. In patients with mild, moderate, and severe ARDS, the pooled incidence of NIV failure was 30% (n = 819, 95% CI: 21–39%), 51% (n = 1332, 95%CI: 43–60%), and 71% (n = 525, 95%CI: 62–79%), respectively. In patients with pulmonary ARDS, it was 45% (n = 2687, 95%CI: 39–51%). However, it was 30% (n = 802, 95%CI: 21–38%) in those with extrapulmonary ARDS. In patients with immunosuppression, the incidence of NIV failure was 62% (n = 806, 95%CI: 50–74%). However, it was 46% (n = 5041, 95%CI: 41–50%) in those without immunosuppression, the pooled incidence of ICU mortality was 29% (n = 2363, 95%CI: 22–36%) and that of hospital mortality was 33% (n = 2927, 95% CI: 27–40%).
    - o *Conclusion:* Nearly half of patients with ARDS experience NIV failure. The incidence of NIV failure increases with increasing ARDS severity. NIV failure is more commonly seen in Pulmonary ARDS, the Immunosuppressed subgroup.

- ***Comparison of prognosis between extracorporeal CPR (ECPR) and conventional CPR (CCPR) for patients in cardiac arrest: A systematic review and meta analysis. (BMC Emerg Med. 2024)***[9]
    - o *Population:* Cardiac arrest patients from 3 RCTs and 14 cohort studies. (n=1,67,728)
    - o *Outcome:* They found that ECPR can significantly improve good neurological prognosis (RR 1.82, 95%CI 1.42–2.34) and survival rate (RR 1.51, 95%CI 1.20 –1.89).
    - o *Conclusion:* This meta-analysis indicated that ECPR had significantly better effects on good neurological prognosis and survival rate than CCPR, especially in patients with IHCA (Inside hospital cardiac arrest). However, more high-quality studies are needed to explore the role of ECPR in patients with OHCA (Out of hospital cardiac arrest).

- ***Extracorporeal carbon dioxide removal (EC-CO_2R) for patients with acute respiratory failure: A systematic review and meta-analysis. (Ann Med. 2023)***[10]

  Population: Acute respiratory failure patients due to COPD and ARDS, from 4 RCTs and 5 observational studies. (n=1173)

- *Outcome:* Pooled analyses of related studies showed no significant difference in overall mortality between EC-CO_2R and control group, neither in RCTs targeted ARDS or acute hypoxic respiratory failure patients (RR 1.05, 95% CI 0.83 to 1.32) nor in studies targeted patients with ARF secondary to COPD (RR 0.80, 95% CI 0.58 to 1.11).
- *Conclusion:* There was no significant beneficial effect of EC-CO_2R therapy on mortality. EC-CO_2R was associated with a longer length of hospital stay and with lower intubation, tracheotomy rates, and shorter mechanical ventilation days in ARF patients with COPD (data from observational studies).
- *Critical appraisal:* Heterogeneity was seen in outcomes.

☞

- ***Effects of extracorporeal CO_2 removal (EC-CO_2R) on gas exchange and ventilator settings: A systematic review and meta analysis. (Crit care. 2024)***[11]
  - *Population:* Respiratory failure patients from 49 studies (Subgroups- ARDS, COPD –AE, Lung transplant (LTx) patients either on NIV/IMV). (n=1672)
  - *Outcome:* EC-CO_2R was associated with a significant decrease in $PaCO_2$, plateau pressure, and tidal volume and an increase in pH across all patient groups, In ARDS and lung transplant patients, the PaO_2/ FiO_2 ratio increased significantly while ventilator settings were variable.
  - *Conclusion:* EC-CO_2R effectively reduces $PaCO_2$ and acidosis allowing for less invasive ventilation (ARDS, Lung transplant patients it predominantly improves gas exchange / protective ventilation, COPD subgroup- it avoids intubation, facilitate weaning and reduction of $PaCO_2$) The findings suggest that in hypercapnic patients suffering from AE-COPD or during bridging to LTX, higher extraction devices may be superior regarding their effects on plateau pressure and especially the more pronounced effect on respiratory rate, which could contribute to a reduction of overinflation in patients with obstructive lung diseases. However, it has effects on longer ICU and hospital stay at adverse events rate -19%.
  - *Critical appraisal:* Heterogeneity seen. In Hypercapnic respiratory failure, more RCTs are needed on EC-CO_2R. Even in the COPD subgroup, it did not include severe COPD cases. EC-CO_2R was associated with a high rate of serious adverse events. Based on existing evidence, EC-CO_2R cannot be recommended for ARDS outside of clinical trials.

- ***Extracorporeal Carbon Dioxide Removal (EC-CO_2R) to Avoid Invasive Ventilation During Exacerbations of Chronic Obstructive Pulmonary Disease: VENT-AVOID Trial – A Randomized Clinical Trial. (Am J Respir Crit Care. 2024)***[12]
  - *Population:* COPD exacerbation patients from 41 US institutions. (n=113)
  - *Intervention:* Standard of care with venovenous EC-CO_2R (NIV stratum: n=26; IMV stratum: n=32)
  - *Comparator:* Standard of care alone (NIV stratum: n=22; IMV stratum: n=33).
  - *Outcome:* The trial was stopped early because of slow enrollment and 113 subjects of the planned sample size of 180. There was no significant difference in the median VFD-5 (ventilator-free days in 5 days of post-randomization) between the arms controlled by strata (P = 0.36).
  - *Conclusion:* In subjects with exacerbation of COPD, the use of EC-CO_2R compared with standard care did not improve VFD-5.

DISCUSSION

Diagnosis of Acute Respiratory Distress Syndrome (ARDS)

A New Global Definition of Acute Respiratory Distress Syndrome[13] was developed

The goal was to develop a definition that would

1) Identify patients with the currently accepted conceptual framework for ARDS.

2) **Facilitate rapid ARDS diagnosis for clinical care and research.**

3) **Be applicable in resource-limited settings.**

4) Be useful for testing specific therapies.

5) Be practical for communicating with patients and caregivers.

Criteria for ARDS

The diagnostic evaluation is focused on identifying ARDS and its cause. A thorough history and clinical examination are required. All patients with suspected ARDS should have a chest radiograph and it is also essential to exclude cardiogenic pulmonary edema. The criteria for ARDS are mentioned in Table 1.

Table 1: CRITERIA FOR A DIAGNOSIS OF ARDS[13]
Criteria That Apply to Specific ARDS Categories

	Non intubated ARDS	Intubated ARDS	Modified Definition for Resource-Limited Settings
Oxygenation	PaO_2:FiO_2 $\leq$ 300 mm Hg or SpO_2: FiO_2 $\leq$ 315 (if SpO_2 $\leq$ 97%) on HFNO with flow of $\geq$ 30 L/min or NIV/CPAP with at least 5cm H_2O end-expiratory pressure	• **Mild:** 200 < PaO_2: FiO_2 $\leq$ 300 mm Hg or 235 < SpO_2:FiO_2 $\leq$ 315 (if SpO_2 $\leq$ 97%) • **Moderate:** 100 < PaO_2: FiO_2 $\leq$ 200 mm Hg or 148 < SpO_2: FiO_2 $\leq$ 235 (if SpO_2 $\leq$ 97%) • **Severe:** PaO_2: FiO_2 $\leq$ 100 mm Hg or SpO_2:FiO_2 $\leq$ 148 (if SpO_2 $\leq$ 97%)	• SpO_2: FiO_2 $\leq$ 315 (if SpO_2 $\leq$ 97%) Neither positive end-expiratory pressure nor a minimum flow rate of oxygen is required for diagnosis in resource-limited settings.

Management of ARDS

Ventilator strategies

Regarding management, mechanical ventilation remains the cornerstone for managing ARDS patients. In a metanalysis by Yamamoto et al, low tidal volume ventilation showed the pooled risk ratio for 28-day mortality was 0.79 (CI - 0.66 - 0.94, I^2= 43%)[14], thus ATS guidelines also recommend low tidal volume ventilation (4-8ml/kg predicted body weight with Pplat $\leq$ 30 cm H_2O) compared to larger tidal volumes as they have mortality benefit.[15]

Role of NIV in ARDS: In an RCT, patients (mild ARDS) treated with NIV had improved oxygenation but didn't lower the rates of intubation (10% vs 9.2 %, p = 0.706) while the use of NIV in patients with severe ARDS is associated with high mortality rates (4.9% vs 3.1%, p = 0.721).[16] NIV failure rates can be attributed to multiple reasons- the severity of ARDS (more severe ARDS is associated with increased failure rates), etiology of ARDS (Pulmonary is more severe than extrapulmonary), NIV mask (better tolerance in helmet subgroup) and in immuno-compromised population.[8] Thus, NIV may be tried in mild ARDS (case to case basis, hemodynamically stable with frequent evaluation).

Prone ventilation: Prone ventilation is reserved as a rescue therapy, it has shown a mortality benefit as seen in PROSEVA trial. Data from PROSEVA trial showed that proning for at least 16 consecutive hours had decreased all-cause mortality (16% in prone vs 32.8 % in supine [p <0.001]).[17] **Implementing early in the course of ARDS (within the first 36 hours) is preferred.[15] ATS strongly recommends prone positioning in moderate to severe ARDS (PaO_2:$FiO_2 \leq$ 150mmHg and PEEP $\geq$ 5 cm H_2O).**[15]

Role of neuromuscular blockers (NMBA): The **ACURASYS trial** showed a significant reduction in mortality in patients with moderate to severe ARDS treated with cisatracurium[18] while the data from ROSE trial showed that there was no mortality benefit associated with NMBA use at 90 days regardless of ARDS severity or duration.[19] However, a recent metanalysis from Torbic et al showed that early use of neuromuscular blockers improves oxygenation at 48 hours and 72 hours (p =0.01 and p = 0.03 respectively), reduces the incidence of ventilator-induced lung injury, decreases 28-day mortality (RR- 0.71, 95% CI, 0.52 -0.98), but doesn't improve 90-day mortality.[20] **ATS has given conditional recommendation in favor of neuromuscular blockade (early and severe ARDS).**[15]

Steroids in ARDS: In the **DEXA ARDS trial**, patients with moderate-severe ARDS it was shown that dexamethasone improved the number of ventilator-free days (mean difference of 4.8 days, 95% C.I -2.57-7.03, p<0.0001) and decreases all-cause mortality at day 60 (21% vs 36% in steroids vs control group, p<0.0047).[21] **The 2017 guidelines SCCM / ESICM recommends steroids in moderate-severe ARDS. ATS offers a conditional recommendation for corticosteroids in patients with ARDS (regardless of severity).**[15]

Optimum PEEP in ARDS: No major trials have compared important clinical outcomes such as mortality or ventilator-free days and none have shown superiority among different approaches (titration based on compliance, P-V curves, driving pressures, stress index, transpulmonary pressures, imaging like CT, electrical impedance tomography, ultrasound). At present, there is no gold standard way to determine the optimal peep.

NIV

The Official ERS/ ATS clinical practice guidelines – NIV for acute respiratory failure strongly recommends NIV in acute hypercapnic respiratory failure due to acute exacerbation of COPD, Acute respiratory failure from acute cardiogenic pulmonary edema.[22] In a metanalysis, patients with acute hypoxemic respiratory failure (AHRF) population (which included a population of acute hypoxemic respiratory failure of different etiologies like pneumonia and immunocompromised population), NIV application was associated with a lower risk of tracheal intubation compared to conventional oxygen therapy (8/44 vs 24/ 39, p <0.001).[23] NIV with helmet and HFNC are promising strategies to avoid tracheal intubation in the acute hypoxemic respiratory failure population.[23]

The development of pressure ulcers is a common side effect of NIV that negatively affects the patient's comfort and tolerance, often leading to NIV failure and adverse outcomes. The ROTA-USE STUDY will determine whether a protocolized rotational approach can reduce the incidence, number, and severity of pressure ulcers in NIV-treated patients. It is a pragmatic, open label, multi center, randomized controlled clinical trial on the rotational use of interfaces *vs* standard of care in patients treated with noninvasive positive pressure ventilation for acute hypercapnic respiratory failure: the ROTA-tional-USE of interface STUDY (**ROTA-USE STUDY),**[24] results from the study may answer questions about rotation use of masks for prevention of pressure ulcers.

HFNC

ERS task force suggests the use of HFNC over conventional oxygen therapy in patients with acute hypoxemic respiratory failure.[25] HFNC has been routinely employed in situations like post- extubation support, postoperative respiratory failure, preoxygenation during intubation. But NIV is to be preferred over HFNC in cases at high risk of extubation failure/ COPD and acute hypercapnic respiratory failure. In a study by Nava-Stefano et al, the patients who are high risk of extubation failure were defined as follows - patients who had hypercapnia, congestive heart failure, ineffective cough and excessive tracheobronchial secretions, more than one failure of a weaning trial, more than one comorbid condition, and upper airway obstruction.[26] However, HFNC has also been used in these groups of patients, but the **current ERS guidelines still suggest NIV to be preferred over HFNC in patients who are high risk of extubation failure.[22]**

Ventilator-Associated Pneumonia

Prevention: Common components included in VAP bundle- **elevation of the head end of bed (30-45 degrees), daily sedation interruption and assessment of readiness to extubate, use of subglottic secretion drainage (SSD), avoidance of scheduled ventilator circuit changes. The main impact lies in the prevention of aspiration, patient positioning, subglottic drainage, and selective decontamination of the oropharyngeal tract.** As per a review published by Tran et al, chlorhexidine has less evidence on efficacy and increased mortality.[27] **The SHEA/IDSA guideline recommends daily oral care with toothbrushing.**

The data on the role of antibiotics in the prevention of VAP is less. In an RCT by Dahyot- Fizelier et al, patients with TBI (Traumatic brain injury at risk of VAP), Ceftriaxone 2g IV single dose, within 2 hours of intubation had lower rates of VAP within seven days.[28] However further studies are required to look into the role of antibiotics in VAP prevention.

Treatment: The Antibiotic selection to be decided on the local antibiogram with emphasis on broad spectrum MDR gram negative bacilli coverage (MDR risk factors: IV antibiotic use within 90 days, septic shock at the time of VAP, ARDS preceding VAP, more than 5 days of hospitalization prior to occurrence of VAP, acute renal replacement therapy prior to VAP onset)[29]. The antibiotics against MRSA (methicillin resistant staphylococcus aureus) to be considered in patients with treatment in a unit/ with >10 to 20 % prevalence of methicillin resistant S. aureus isolates or if prevalence of MRSA is not known or known colonization with and /or prior isolation of MRSA on culture from anybody site.[29] **ERS/ESICM/ESCMID/ALAT society suggests 7-8 days course of antibiotics course in VAP without immunodeficiency, cystic fibrosis, empyema, lung abscess, cavitation or necrotizing pneumonia and with good clinical response to therapy.[30]** Individualized, short-course antibiotic treatment for VAP could help to reduce the burden of antibiotics in ICU assessed by case to case, however more studies are required.

Intubation strategies

In the practice guidelines for difficult airway management by ASA, there are multiple practice settings and interventions aimed at preoxygenation and airway management.[31]

Role of NIV in Preoxygenation

In preoxygenation for critically ill patients, the best method for critically ill undergoing intubation is unclear. In an RCT by Gibbs KW et al, preoxygenation with NIV resulted in a lower incidence of hypoxemia during intubation than preoxygenation with an oxygen mask.[32] Thus, NIV can be used for preoxygenation during intubation on case-to-case basis.

Video assisted laryngoscopy may have improved first pass rate, reduced airway trauma and oxygen desaturation as compared to direct laryngoscopy. Video laryngoscope blade are of two types: Macintosh – style and hyperangulated blades. Hyperangulated videolaryngoscope blades provide a better glottis view. Video-assisted laryngoscopy (VAL) with D blade resulted in an increased percentage of glottis opening visible (89 vs 54 percent, p value <0.001) increased first attempt intubation success (97% vs 67 %, p value <0.001) and lower rates of failed intubation (1% vs13%, p value- 0.002). Thus, hyperangulated blades may help in intubation of patients with difficult airways.[33]

Role of Lung ultrasound in ICU

The role of lung ultrasound in ICU is increasing. It can be an essential tool for rapid diagnosis and monitoring in ICU and is time saving. The VAP rate in ICU is alarming. Lung ultrasound may play an important role in early detection of VAP. In a study by Chavez et al, lung ultrasound has a sensitivity and specificity of 94% and 96%, respectively, with an area under the SROC (summary receiver operating characteristic) curve of 0.98.[34] Point of care should be implemented in all ICU with daily screening of patients as it has has better reproducibility, avoids radiation exposure, and has less turn-around time. The disadvantages are as follows, it is less reliable in obese patients and has significant interobserver variations.[35]

Steroids in Severe CAP

Several RCTs have investigated the use of adjunctive corticosteroids in mortality benefit in Severe CAP.

ESCAPE (Extended steroid use in CAP) and Santeon – CAP (Dexamethasone in CAP) - Both trials did not improve the mortality risk.[36] In CAPE COD trial (Community-acquired pneumonia-evaluation of corticosteroids) Hydrocortisone reduces all-cause mortality in ICU (steroid arm 28-day mortality – 6.2% vs 11.9 % in placebo, p = 0.006). The results of CAPE COD (population included Severe CAP (without septic shock) suggest the use of hydrocortisone within 24 hours of the development of severe CAP and also steroids are effective in viral pneumonias (except influenza).[37] **SCCM (Society of Critical Care Medicine) guideline suggests steroid use for adult patients hospitalized with severe bacterial CAP only** but steroids are also effective in viral pneumonias (less evidence in Influenza subgroup). Different regimens are being tried hydrocortisone (200 mg IV/ day for 4- 8 days then taper for a total duration of 8-14 days/ 200 mg once dose then 10 mg/hr IV infusion for 7 days), methylprednisolone (0.5 mg/kg every 12 hr for 7 days).[38] More studies are required on the optimal dose of steroids/type and duration.

Extracorporeal life support

Extracorporeal membrane oxygenation (ECMO): The indications are refractory ARDS (ATS suggests VV – ECMO in Severe ARDS) bridge to lung transplant, Post lung transplant period. CESAR trial showed that referral to an ECMO center for ECMO had improved outcomes (study pitfalls- many patients didn't receive ECMO). EOLIA trial showed ECMO has no significant difference in 60-day mortality in comparison with conventional mechanical ventilation. **Data suggests ECMO had a lower risk of treatment failure, a lower risk of renal replacement therapy, and ECMO arm had less proning.**[39] **ESICM guidelines suggest ECMO early in the course of severe ARDS. (PaO_2:FiO_2 <80 or pH <7.25 with $pCO_2 \geq 60$).**

Recent studies are on prone position during ECMO for successful weaning. The PRONECMO trial showed that prone positioning did not significantly reduce time to successful weaning. However further studies are ongoing.[40]

Extracorporeal carbon-di-oxide removal ($ECCO_2R$): The indications include refractory hypercapnic respiratory failure and ARDS (as a strategy to facilitate lung protective ventilation). **Data from SUPERNOVA trial (included moderate ARDS patients) showed that use of $ECCO_2R$ to facilitate ultra-protective ventilation was feasible.**[41] Observational data suggests $EC\text{-}CO_2R$ was associated with a longer length of hospital stay, with lower intubation and tracheotomy rates, and shorter mechanical ventilation days in ARF patients with COPD, but no mortality benefit.[39] So there are not enough data to support routine use.

Management of patients with neuromuscular weakness

Recently chest guidelines had developed an algorithm for management of patients with neuromuscular weakness for initiation of NIV (if they fit into Pulmonary function test / Symptomatic / ABG / PSG criteria).[42] An individualized approach has been developed in patients with neuromuscular disease, which emphasizes on diverse subgroup of disorders and parameters.[42]

1. ***Pulmonary Function Test criteria (PFT):*** FVC <80 % predicted with symptoms or FVC <50% predicted without symptoms, MIP <60 cm H_2O or MEP < 40 H_2O, PCF <270 L/min for age more than 12 years.

   PCF <5th percentile for age <12 years, SNIP < 70/ <60 cm H_2O in male / female patients respectively.

   (***Abbreviations:*** MIP- maximal inspiratory pressure, MEP – maximal expiratory pressure, PCF–peak cough flow, SNIP–sniff nasal inspiratory pressure).

2. ***Arterial blood gas criteria (ABG):*** $SpO_2 \leq 90\%$ for $\geq 2\%$ of sleep time, $PaCO_2$ > 45 mmHg.
3. ***Polysomnography criteria (PSG):*** Adults: AHI> 5 events/ hr, $SpO_2 \leq 88\%$ for at least 5 min continuously.

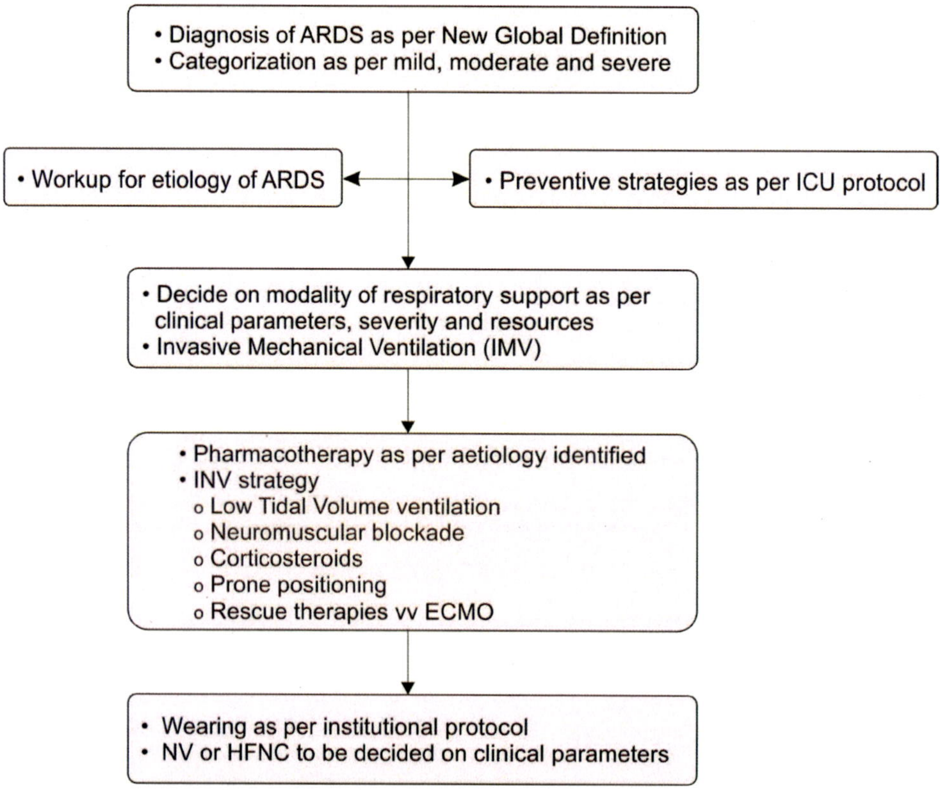

Flowchart: The Management Strategy in ARDS

REFERENCES

1. Mo Y, Booraphun S, Li AY, Domthong P, Kayastha G, Lau YH, Chetchotisakd P, Limmathurotsakul D, Tambyah PA, Cooper BS; REGARD-VAP investigators. Individualised, short-course antibiotic treatment versus usual long-course treatment for ventilator-associated pneumonia (REGARD-VAP): a multicentre, individually randomised, open-label, non-inferiority trial. Lancet Respir Med. 2024 May;12(5): 399-408. doi: 10.1016/S2213-2600(23)00418-6. Epub 2024 Jan 22. PMID: 38272050.

2. Martinez-Reviejo R, Tejada S, Jansson M, Ruiz-Spinelli A, Ramirez-Estrada S, Ege D, Vieceli T, Maertens B, Blot S, Rello J. Prevention of ventilator-associated pneumonia through care bundles: A systematic review and meta-analysis. J Intensive Med. 2023 Jun 14;3(4):352-364. doi: 10.1016/j.jointm.2023.04.004. PMID: 38028633; PMCID: PMC10658042.

3. Ehrmann S, Barbier F, Demiselle J, Quenot JP, Herbrecht JE, Roux D, Lacherade JC, Landais M, Seguin P, Schnell D, Veinstein A, Gouin P, Lasocki S, Lu Q, Beduneau G, Ferrandiere M, Plantefève G, Dahyot-Fizelier C, Chebib N, Mercier E, Heuzé-Vourc'h N, Respaud R, Gregoire N, Garot D, Nay MA, Meziani F, Andreu P, Clere-Jehl R, Zucman N, Azaïs MA, Saint-Martin M, Gandonnière CS, Benzekri D, Merdji H, Tavernier E; Reva and CRICS-TRIGGERSEP F-CRIN Research Networks. Inhaled Amikacin to Prevent Ventilator-Associated Pneumonia. N Engl J Med. 2023 Nov 30;389(22):2052-2062. doi: 10.1056/NEJMoa2310307. Epub 2023 Oct 25. PMID: 37888914.

4. See XY, Wang TH, Chang Y, *et al.* Impact of different corticosteroids on severe community-acquired pneumonia: a systematic review and meta-analysis, *BMJ Open Respiratory Research* 2024;11: e002141. doi: 10.1136/bmjresp-2023-002141.

5. Desai, D.; Shah, A.B.; Dela, J.R.C.; Mugibel, T.A.; Sumaily, K.M.; Sabi, E.M.; Mujamammi, A.H.; Malafi, M.E.; Alkaff, S.A.; Alwahbi, T.A.; et al. Lung Ultrasonography Accuracy for Diagnosis of Adult Pneumonia: Systematic Review and Meta-Analysis. *Adv. Respir. Med.* 2024, *92*, 241-253.

6. Wang, D., Qi, Y. Lung ultrasound score and in-hospital mortality of adults with acute respiratory distress syndrome: a meta-analysis. *BMC Pulm Med* 24, 62 (2024). https://doi.org/10.1186/s12890-023-02826-5.

7. Cannula Oxygen Therapy versus Non-Invasive Ventilation in patients at very high risk for extubating failure: A systematic review of randomized controlled trials. PLoS One. 2024 Apr 3;19(4):e0299693. doi: 10.1371/journal.pone.0299693. PMID: 38568930; PMCID: PMC10990192.

8. Wang, J., Duan, J. & Zhou, L. Incidence of noninvasive ventilation failure and mortality in patients with acute respiratory distress syndrome: a systematic review and proportion meta-analysis. *BMC Pulm Med* 24, 48 (2024). https://doi.org/10.1186/s12890-024-02839-8.

9. Zhong H, Yin Z, Wang Y, Shen P, He G, Huang S, Wang J, Huang S, Ding L, Luo Z, Zhou M. Comparison of prognosis between extracorporeal CPR and conventional CPR for patients in cardiac arrest: a systematic review and meta-analysis. BMC Emerg Med. 2024 Jul 27;24(1):128. doi: 10.1186/s12873-024-01058-y. PMID: 39068383; PMCID: PMC11282673.

10. Zhou Z, Li Z, Liu C, Wang F, Zhang L, Fu P. Extracorporeal carbon dioxide removal for patients with acute respiratory failure: a systematic review and meta-analysis. Ann Med. 2023 Dec;55(1):746-759. doi: 10.1080/07853890.2023.2172606. PMID: 36856550; PMCID: PMC9980035.

11. Stommel AM, Herkner H, Kienbacher CL, Wildner B, Hermann A, Staudinger T. Effects of extracorporeal CO_2 removal on gas exchange and ventilator settings: a systematic review and meta-analysis. Crit Care. 2024 Apr 30;28(1):146. doi: 10.1186/s13054-024-04927-x. PMID: 38693569; PMCID: PMC11061932.

12. Duggal A, Conrad SA, Barrett NA, Saad M, Cheema T, Pannu S, Romero RS, Brochard L, Nava S, Ranieri VM, May A, Brodie D, Hill NS; VENT-AVOID Investigators. Extracorporeal Carbon Dioxide Removal to Avoid Invasive Ventilation During Exacerbations of Chronic Obstructive Pulmonary Disease: VENT-AVOID Trial - A Randomized Clinical Trial. Am J Respir Crit Care Med. 2024 Mar 1;209(5):529-542. doi: 10.1164/rccm.202311-2060OC. PMID: 38261630.

13. Matthay MA, Arabi Y, Arroliga AC, Bernard G, Bersten AD, Brochard LJ, Calfee CS, Combes A, Daniel BM, Ferguson ND, Gong MN, Gotts JE, Herridge MS, Laffey JG, Liu KD, Machado FR, Martin TR, McAuley DF, Mercat A, Moss M, Mularski RA, Pesenti A, Qiu H, Ramakrishnan N, Ranieri VM, Riviello ED, Rubin E, Slutsky AS, Thompson BT, Twagirumugabe T, Ware LB, Wick KD. A New Global Definition of Acute Respiratory Distress Syndrome. Am J Respir Crit Care Med. 2024 Jan 1;209(1):37-47. doi: 10.1164/rccm.202303-0558WS. PMID: 37487152; PMCID: PMC10870872.

14. Yamamoto, R., Okazaki, S.R., Fujita, Y. *et al.* Usefulness of low tidal volume ventilation strategy for patients with acute respiratory distress syndrome: a systematic review and meta-analysis. *Sci Rep* 12, 9331 (2022). https://doi.org/10.1038/s41598-022-13224-y

15. Qadir N, Sahetya S, Munshi L, Summers C, Abrams D, Beitler J, Bellani G, Brower RG, Burry L, Chen JT, Hodgson C, Hough CL, Lamontagne F, Law A, Papazian L, Pham T, Rubin E, Siuba M, Telias I, Patolia S, Chaudhuri D, Walkey A, Rochwerg B, Fan E. An Update on Management of Adult Patients with Acute Respiratory Distress Syndrome: An Official American Thoracic Society Clinical Practice Guideline. Am J Respir Crit Care Med. 2024 Jan 1;209(1):24-36. doi: 10.1164/rccm.202311-2011ST. PMID: 38032683; PMCID: PMC10870893.

16. Du, K. Noninvasive ventilation in patients with acute respiratory distress syndrome. *Crit Care* 23, 358 (2019). https://doi.org/10.1186/s13054-019-2666-4

17. Albert R.K., Keniston A., Baboi L., Ayzac L., Guerin C. Prone position-induced improvement in gas exchange does not predict

improved survival in the acute respiratory distress syndrome. Am J Respir Crit Care Med. 2014;189(4):494–496. doi: 10.1164/rccm.201311-2056LE

18. Papazian L, Forel J-M, Gacouin A, et al. Neuromuscular blockers in early acute respiratory distress syndrome. *N Engl J Med* 2010;363: 1107-1116.

19. Parhar KKS, Solverson K, Zochios V. Early neuromuscular blockade in acute respiratory distress syndrome: to personalize or paralyze? J Thorac Dis. 2019 Dec;11 (12):5701-5705. doi: 10.21037/jtd.2019.12.101. PMID: 32030306; PMCID: PMC6988024.

20. Torbic H, Krishnan S, Harnegie MP, Duggal A. Neuromuscular Blocking Agents for ARDS: A Systematic Review and Meta-Analysis. Respir Care. 2021 Jan;66(1):120-128. doi: 10.4187/respcare.07849. Epub 2020 Aug 25. PMID: 32843506.

21. Villar J, Ferrando C, Martínez D, Ambrós A, Muñoz T, Soler JA, Aguilar G, Alba F, González-Higueras E, Conesa LA, Martín-Rodríguez C, Díaz-Domínguez FJ, Serna-Grande P, Rivas R, Ferreres J, Belda J, Capilla L, Tallet A, Añón JM, Fernández RL, González-Martín JM; dexamethasone in ARDS network. Dexamethasone treatment for the acute respiratory distress syndrome: a multicentre, randomised controlled trial. Lancet Respir Med. 2020 Mar;8(3):267-276. doi: 10.1016/S2213-2600(19) 30417-5. Epub 2020 Feb 7. PMID: 32043986.

22. Rochwerg B, Brochard L, Elliott MW, Hess D, Hill NS, Nava S, Navalesi P Members Of The Steering Committee, Antonelli M, Brozek J, Conti G, Ferrer M, Guntupalli K, Jaber S, Keenan S, Mancebo J, Mehta S, Raoof S Members Of The Task Force. Official ERS/ATS clinical practice guidelines: noninvasive ventilation for acute respiratory failure. Eur Respir J. 2017 Aug 31;50(2):1602426. doi: 10.1183/13993003.02426-2016. PMID: 28860265.

23. Aswanetmanee, P., Limsuwat, C., Maneechotesuwan, K. *et al.* Noninvasive ventilation in patients with acute hypoxemic respiratory failure: a systematic review and meta-analysis of randomized controlled trials. *Sci Rep* **13**, 8283 (2023). https://doi.org/10.1038/s41598-023-35323-0

24. Vaschetto R, Gregoretti C, Scotti L, De Vita N, Carlucci A, Cortegiani A, Crimi C, Mattei A, Scala R, Rocca E, Longhini F, Cammarota G, Misseri G, Dal Molin A, Scolletta S, Nava S, Maggiore SM, Navalesi P. A pragmatic, open-label, multi-center, randomized controlled clinical trial on the rotational use of interfaces vs standard of care in patients treated with noninvasive positive pressure ventilation for acute hypercapnic respiratory failure: the ROTAtional-USE of interface STUDY (ROTA-USE STUDY). Trials. 2023 Aug 13;24(1):527. doi: 10.1186/s13063-023-07560-1. PMID: 37574558; PMCID: PMC10424342.

25. Oczkowski S, Ergan B, Bos L, Chatwin M, Ferrer M, Gregoretti C, Heunks L, Frat JP, Longhini F, Nava S, Navalesi P, Ozsancak Uðurlu A, Pisani L, Renda T, Thille AW, Winck JC, Windisch W, Tonia T, Boyd J, Sotgiu G, Scala R. ERS clinical practice guidelines: high-flow nasal cannula in acute respiratory failure. Eur Respir J. 2022 Apr 14;59(4):2101574. doi: 10.1183/13993003.01574-2021. PMID: 34649974.

26. Nava S, Gregoretti C, Fanfulla F, Squadrone E, Grassi M, Carlucci A, Beltrame F, Navalesi P. Noninvasive ventilation to prevent respiratory failure after extubation in high-risk patients. Crit Care Med. 2005 Nov;33(11):2465-70. doi: 10.1097/01.ccm. 0000186416. 44752.72. PMID: 16276167.

27. Tran K, Butcher R. Chlorhexidine for Oral Care: A Review of Clinical Effectiveness and Guidelines [Internet]. Ottawa (ON): Canadian Agency for Drugs and Technologies in Health; 2019 Jan 25. Available from: https://www.ncbi. nlm.nih.gov/books/NBK541430

28. Ceftriaxone to prevent early ventilator-associated pneumonia in patients with acute brain injury: a multicentre, randomised, double-blind, placebo-controlled, assessor-masked superiority trial; Dahyot-Fizelier, ClaireDAHYOT-FIZELIER, Claire et al.-The Lancet Respiratory Medicine, Volume 12, Issue 5, 375 – 385.

29. Kalil AC, Metersky ML, Klompas M, Muscedere J, Sweeney DA, Palmer LB, Napolitano LM, O'Grady NP, Bartlett JG, Carratalà J, El Solh AA, Ewig S, Fey PD, File TM Jr, Restrepo MI, Roberts JA, Waterer GW, Cruse P, Knight SL, Brozek JL. Management of Adults With Hospital-acquired and Ventilator-associated Pneumonia: 2016 Clinical Practice Guidelines by the Infectious Diseases Society of America and the American Thoracic Society. Clin Infect Dis. 2016 Sep 1;63(5):e61-e111. doi: 10.1093/cid/ciw353. Epub 2016 Jul 14. Erratum in: Clin Infect Dis. 2017 May 1;64(9):1298. doi: 10.1093/cid/ciw799. Erratum in: Clin Infect Dis. 2017 Oct 15;65(8):1435. doi: 10.1093/cid/cix587. Erratum in: Clin Infect Dis. 2017 Nov 29;65(12): 2161. doi: 10.1093/cid/cix759. PMID: 27418577; PMCID: PMC4981759.

30. Torres A, Niederman MS, Chastre J, Ewig S, Fernandez-Vandellos P, Hanberger H, Kollef M, Li Bassi G, Luna CM, Martin-Loeches I, Paiva JA, Read RC, Rigau D, Timsit JF, Welte T, Wunderink R. International ERS/ESICM/ESCMID/ALAT guidelines for the management of hospital-acquired pneumonia and ventilator-associated pneumonia: Guidelines for the management of hospital-acquired pneumonia (HAP)/ventilator-associated pneumonia (VAP) of the European Respiratory Society (ERS), European Society of Intensive Care Medicine (ESICM), European Society of Clinical Microbiology and Infectious Diseases (ESCMID) and Asociación Latinoamericana del Tórax (ALAT). Eur Respir J. 2017 Sep 10;50(3):1700582. doi: 10.1183/13993003.00582-2017. PMID: 28890434.

31. Practice Guidelines for Management of the Difficult Airway An Updated Report by the American Society of Anesthesiologists Task Force on Management of the Difficult Airway - Anesthesiology, V 118, No 2.

32. Noninvasive Ventilation for Preoxygenation during Emergency Intubation Kevin W. Gibbs et alN Engl J Med 2024;390:2165-2177: DOI: 10.1056/NEJMoa 2313680, VOL. 390 NO. 23.

33. Köhl, V., Wünsch, V.A., Müller, M.-C., Sasu, P.B., Dohrmann, T., Peters, T., Tolkmitt, J., Dankert, A., Krause, L., Zöllner, C. and Petzoldt, M. (2024), Hyperangulated vs. Macintosh videolaryngo-scopy in adults with anticipated difficult airway management: a randomised controlled trial. Anaesthesia, 79: 957-966. https://doi.org/10.1111/anae.16326.

34. Chavez MA, Shams N, Ellington LE, Naithani N, Gilman RH, Steinhoff MC, Santosham M, Black RE, Price C, Gross M, Checkley W. Lung ultrasound for the diagnosis of pneumonia in adults: a systematic review and meta-analysis. Respir Res. 2014 Apr

23;15(1):50. doi: 10.1186/1465-9921-15-50. PMID: 24758612; PMCID: PMC4005846.

35. Raheja R, Brahmavar M, Joshi D, Raman D. Application of Lung Ultrasound in Critical Care Setting: A Review. Cureus. 2019 Jul 25;11(7):e5233. doi: 10.7759/cureus.5233. PMID: 31565634; PMCID: PMC6758979.

36. Meduri GU, Shih MC, Bridges L, Martin TJ, El-Solh A, Seam N, Davis-Karim A, Umberger R, Anzueto A, Sriram P, Lan C, Restrepo MI, Guardiola JJ, Buck T, Johnson DP, Suffredini A, Bell WA, Lin J, Zhao L, Uyeda L, Nielsen L, Huang GD; ESCAPe Study Group. Low-dose methylprednisolone treatment in critically ill patients with severe community-acquired pneumonia. Intensive Care Med. 2022 Aug;48(8):1009-1023. doi: 10.1007/s00134-022-06684-3. Epub 2022 May 13. PMID: 35723686; PMCID: PMC9208259.

37. Dequin PF, Meziani F, Quenot JP, Kamel T, Ricard JD, Badie J, Reignier J, Heming N, Plantefève G, Souweine B, Voiriot G, Colin G, Frat JP, Mira JP, Barbarot N, François B, Louis G, Gibot S, Guitton C, Giacardi C, Hraiech S, Vimeux S, L'Her E, Faure H, Herbrecht JE, Bouisse C, Joret A, Terzi N, Gacouin A, Quentin C, Jourdain M, Leclerc M, Coffre C, Bourgoin H, Lengellé C, Caille-Fénérol C, Giraudeau B, Le Gouge A; CRICS-TriGGERSep Network. Hydrocortisone in Severe Community-Acquired Pneumonia. N Engl J Med. 2023 May 25;388(21):1931-1941. doi: 10.1056/NEJMoa 2215145. Epub 2023 Mar 21. PMID: 36942789.

38. Chaudhuri D, Nei AM, Rochwerg B, Balk RA, Asehnoune K, Cadena R, Carcillo JA, Correa R, Drover K, Esper AM, Gershengorn HB, Hammond NE, Jayaprakash N, Menon K, Nazer L, Pitre T, Qasim ZA, Russell JA, Santos AP, Sarwal A, Spencer-Segal J, Tilouche N, Annane D, Pastores SM. 2024 Focused Update: Guidelines on Use of Corticosteroids in Sepsis, Acute Respiratory Distress Syndrome, and Community-Acquired Pneumonia. Crit Care Med. 2024 May 1;52(5):e219-e233. doi: 10.1097/CCM.0000000000006172. Epub 2024 Jan 19. PMID: 38240492.

39. Combes, A., Peek, G.J., Hajage, D. *et al.* ECMO for severe ARDS: systematic review and individual patient data meta-analysis. *Intensive Care Med* **46**, 2048–2057 (2020). https://doi.org/10.1007/s00134-020-06248-3

40. Giani, M., Papazian, L. & Grasselli, G. Prone positioning during extracorporeal membrane oxygenation for severe acute respiratory distress syndrome. Pro. *Intensive Care Med* **50**, 944–946 (2024). https://doi.org/10.1007/s00134-024-07449-w

41. McNamee JJ, Gillies MA, Barrett NA, et al. Effect of Lower Tidal Volume Ventilation Facilitated by Extra-corporeal Carbon Dioxide Removal vs Standard Care Ventilation on 90-Day Mortality in Patients With Acute Hypoxemic Respiratory Failure: *JAMA*. 2021;326(11): 1013–1023. doi:10.1001/jama.2021.13374

42. Respiratory management of patient with neuromuscular weakness Khan , Akram et al Chest volume 164, Issue 2, 393-413.

CHAPTER

15

Critical Care Medicine (Non-Pulmonary)

Authors: Dr. Kshitij Chatterjee, Dr. Jonathan Scheel, Dr. Jasmin Chovatiya, Dr. Sudeshna Ghosh, Dr. Caleb Bonds, Dr. Roshan Roy, Dr. Sukhdev Singh, Dr. Prasad Nadendla, Dr. Deny Sung

Reviewer: Dr. A.J. Mahendran

INTRODUCTION

Critically ill patients admitted in the ICU tend to have a complex pathophysiology, with multiple intertwined organ system involvement. Our current practice is based on a combination of prior landmark trials and pathophysiological-based rationales. In this chapter, we summarize some recent high-yield trials that significantly add to the practice of Critical Care Medicine- either by challenging current paradigms, providing solid evidence for current practices, or introducing newer therapies/strategies for managing common ICU conditions.

Methodology

Articles from multiple journals published between 1st August, 2023 and 1st August, 2024 were reviewed to form an index of articles relevant to critical care medicine. Based on our review of these, articles with high clinical impact were selected for further analysis. The order of the articles was then rearranged to facilitate the flow of pertinent topics and arranged by the primary organ system studied.

Airway management

- ***Effect of Noninvasive Airway Management of Comatose Patient's With Acute Poisoning: A Randomized Clinical Trial (NICO Trial). (JAMA. 2023)***[1]
  - o *Population:* Acute poisoning adult patients with GCS less than nine across 21 emergency rooms and one ICU in France. (n=225)
  - o *Intervention:* Intubation withheld unless emergency criteria met. (n=116)
  - o *Comparator:* Decision to intubate left to treating physician. (n=109)
  - o *Outcome:* A Conservative intubation strategy resulted in lower median ICU stay and median length hospital stay without leading difference in mortality or rates of adverse events.
  - o *Conclusion:* A conservative intubation strategy amongst patients suffering from suspected acute poisoning with GCS <9 led to improved composite outcome of in-hospital death, length of ICU stay, and length of hospital stay.
  - o *Critical appraisal:* Unblinded study may have led to biases. The composite outcome is largely attributable to length of ICU stay as there were no deaths in either group. The study also excluded patients intoxicated with single reversible substance, either opioids or benzodiazepines- limiting its generalizability.

- ***Noninvasive Ventilation for Preoxygenation during Emergency intubation (PREOXI Trial). (NEJM. 2024)***[2]
  - o *Population:* Critically ill adult patients across 7 emergency departments and 17 ICUs in the US. (n=1301)
  - o *Intervention:* Preoxygenation with noninvasive ventilation (NIV), expiratory pressure of at least 5 cm H_2O, inspiratory pressure of at least 10 cm H_2O, and an FiO_2 of 100%. (n=624)
  - o *Comparator:* Preoxygenation with nonrebreather mask or bag-mask device without manual ventilation using a flow rate of least 15 liter/minute. (n=637)
  - o *Outcome:* Hypoxemia, defined as a SpO_2 less than 85% after anesthesia until two minutes after intubation, occurred a statistically significant higher amount in the oxygen-mask group compared to the NIV group. There was also a higher cardiac arrest rate in the oxygen-mask group while no differences in aspiration were observed.
  - o *Conclusion:* Preoxygenation with NIV among critically ill adults undergoing tracheal intubation resulted in lower rates of hypoxemia and cardiac arrest compared to oxygen-mask.
  - o *Critical appraisal:* Patients were excluded if clinician determined use of either oxygenation device was contraindicated which may have led to selection bias. Real-life barriers for resources and cost, are likely to exist.

- ***Video Laryngoscopy vs Direct Laryngoscopy for Endotracheal Intubation in the Operating Room: A Cluster Randomized Clinical Trial. (JAMA. 2024)***[3]
  - o *Population:* Adult patients undergoing elective or emergent cardiac, thoracic, or vascular surgical procedures requiring intubation at a single US academic hospital. (n=8429 procedures)
  - o *Intervention:* Initial intubation attempt utilized video laryngoscopy (VL). (n=4413)
  - o *Comparator:* Initial intubation attempt utilized direct laryngoscopy (DL). (n=4016)
  - o *Outcome/conclusion:* More than one intubation attempt was required in a statistically significant higher amount in the DL arm (7.6%) compared to the VL arm (1.7%). Intubation failure was also significantly higher in the DL group while adverse events like dental or airway injuries were similar.
  - o *Critical appraisal:* 85% of the patient population was limited to elective surgical cases questioning applicability to critically ill patients. This was a single center study which bottlenecked the patient population. Patient positioning was not protocolized either, which may have been a confounding factor not accounted for.

- ***Automatic Mechanical Ventilation vs Manual Bag Ventilation During CPR A Pilot Randomized Controlled Trial. CAVE-I Trail. (Chest. 2024)***[4]
  - o *Population:* Patients with medical out of hospital cardiac arrest (OHCA) arriving in the emergency room (ER) requiring CPR and ACLS. Randomization was done in the ER. (n=60)
  - o *Intervention:* Airway management using a mechanical ventilator with continuous mandatory ventilation mode at a rate of 10 breaths per minute, tidal volume: 500 mL (male) and 450 mL (female), I:E=1:1, PEEP=5 cm water, flow trigger: off, FiO_2=100%, alarms: pressure 70 cm water. (n=30)
  - o *Comparator:* Airway management using conventional manual bag (ambu-bag), at a rate of 10 times per minute. (n=4016)
  - o *Outcome:* Rate of return of spontaneous circulation was 56.7% in intervention arm compared to 43.3% in control arm. The difference was not statistically significant (p=0.44). There was also no significant difference between the two groups for pH, pCO_2, pO_2, HCO_3, or lactate.

- o *Conclusion:* This pilot study showed that mechanical ventilation may be an alternative to Ambu-bag ventilation during CPR. The trial failed to show a significant difference. However, it did not show that the intervention was worse than the control. A larger RCT and more refined mechanical ventilation settings may be required to create sufficient evidence.

DISCUSSIONS

Non-invasive ventilation in poisoning

Airway management in acute poisoning patients is debated and lack of robust evidence prevents strong guiding recommendations.[5] Prior to the NICO trial, there was some weak evidence to suggest early intubation can reduce aspiration.[6] In alignment with this and concern for aspiration, a commonly utilized maxim reads, "GCS less than 8, intubate." The NICO trial calls such generalized management strategy into questions, at least for acute poisoning patients without obvious need for a definitive airway device. With these results, the treating clinicians would have more confidence in assessing each of these patients individually, delaying intubation if close monitoring deemed appropriate, and performing intubation if patient decompensates.

Non-invasive ventilation for preoxygenation

Endotracheal intubation of critically ill patients is a high-risk procedure with excess morbidity and mortality.[7] Minimizing the occurrence of hypoxemia has been the subject of many studies focusing on preoxygenation. These have revealed several strategies including the use of bag valve mask between induction and laryngoscopy and high flow nasal cannula before and during intubation to reduce hypoxemia.[8,9] With PREOXI trial, NIV can be firmly added atop this list of strategies for preoxygenation and there can be more confidence in avoiding aspiration. Some ventilators have dual use, functioning as NIV for preoxygenation and invasive ventilator post intubation, which may make this change in practice easier.

Choice of device (video vs direct) for intubation

Limiting the apneic period and intubation attempts are paramount to avoiding adverse events related to intubation. There has been much debate on VL vs DL in terms of first pass success and outcomes. The DEVICE trial showed improved first pass success with VL in critically ill patients.[10] A recent Cochrane review showed improved safety outcomes with VL.[11] The trend is shifting towards using VL to improve first pass success and minimize adverse events in critically ill patients.

CARDIOVASCULAR

- ***Outcomes in High-Risk Pulmonary Embolism Patients Undergoing FlowTriever Mechanical Thrombectomy or Other Contemporary Therapies: Results From the FLAME Study. (Circ Cardiovasc Interv. 2023)***[12]
  - o *Population:* Hemodynamically unstable patients with high-risk Pulmonary Embolism. (n=115)
  - o *Intervention:* FlowTriever Mechanical Thrombectomy. (n=53)
  - o *Comparator:* Standard Treatment (Systemic or catheter directed thrombolysis, anticoagulation alone). (n=61)
  - o *Outcome/Conclusion:* The primary end point was an in-hospital composite of all-cause mortality, bailout to an alternate thrombus removal strategy, clinical deterioration, and major bleeding. The primary end point occurred much less in intervention arm compared to the standard arm. In-hospital mortality occurred in 1/53 (1.9%) patients in the FlowTriever Arm and in 18/61 (29.5%) patients in the Context Arm.
  - o *Critical appraisal:* This is a small study that was non-randomized with promising results for the use of FlowTriever mechanical thrombectomy in high-risk PE patients. The study protocol did not dictate a specific treatment for PE, so treatment selection was at the discretion of the treating physician. Non-randomization and the relatively smaller size of this study makes it difficult to generalize.

- ***Microaxial Flow Pump or Standard Care in Infarct-Related Cardiogenic Shock (DanGer Shock study). (NEJM. 2024)***[13]
  - o *Population:* Patients with STEMI and Cardiogenic Shock. (n=355)
  - o *Intervention:* Micro-axial Flow Pump Group. (n=179)
  - o *Comparator:* Standard Care Group. (n=176)
  - o *Outcome/Conclusion:* The routine use of a micro axial flow pump with standard care in the treatment of patients with STEMI-related cardiogenic shock led to a lower risk of death from any cause at 180 days than standard care alone.
  - o *Critical appraisal:* Although the trial had its limitations as it is not feasible to blind the device, the outcome was significantly positive when compared to previous studies.[14-16] Although there were increased rates of adverse events questioning the safety of microaxial flow pump, the overall mortality benefit was a positive change towards the use of these devices in this population.

☞

- ***Restrictive or Liberal Transfusion Strategy in Myocardial Infarction and Anemia (MINT. trial). (NEJM. 2023)***[17]
  - o *Population:* Adults >18 years with STEMI and NSTEMI with hemoglobin level <10g/dL. (n=3504)
  - o *Intervention:* Liberal strategy transfusion to maintain hemoglobin level at or above 10g/dL until time of hospital discharge or 30 days. (n=1755)
  - o *Comparator:* Restrictive strategy group (Transfusion was permitted but not required when the hemoglobin level was less than 8 g per deciliter and was strongly recommended when the level was less than 7 g per deciliter or when anginal symptoms were not controlled with medications. (n=1749)
  - o *Outcome:* The primary outcome was a composite of recurrent myocardial infarction or death at 30 days. The primary outcome occurred in 16.9% patients in restrictive strategy group compared to 14.5% in liberal strategy group ($p = 0.07$).
  - o *Conclusion:* A liberal transfusion strategy did not significantly reduce the risk of recurrent myocardial infarction or death at 30 days.

Pulmonary embolism

The most recent guidelines for managing high-risk pulmonary embolism (PE) emphasize rapid intervention and advanced supportive care. Diagnosis often involves clinical evaluation and imaging, typically with computed tomography pulmonary angiography (CTPA) complemented by ultrasonography.[18-20] Immediate systemic thrombolysis, with agents such as tissue plasminogen activator (tPA), is recommended for patients with high-risk PE who are experiencing severe hemodynamic compromise/shock or severe right ventricular dysfunction.[20] In cases where thrombolysis is contraindicated or ineffective, surgical or catheter-based interventions may be necessary. Hemodynamic support, including the use of vasopressors and inotropes, is crucial for stabilizing blood pressure and improving cardiac output. Advanced mechanical support, such as ECMO, may be necessary for patients with refractory shock. Intensive monitoring in an ICU setting is essential to manage severe cases and monitor for complications. A multidisciplinary team approach involving cardiologists, pulmonologists, interventional radiologists, and intensivists is recommended to ensure comprehensive care. Although more studies are needed to conclude its safety and efficacy, the results from the FLAME study point towards an increased utility of thrombectomy in high-risk PE patients.[12] Several studies demonstrate safety in both massive and submassive pulmonary embolism with positive outcomes.[21] Larger studies are needed for conclusive evidence and further refine patient selection guidelines. None the less, addition of this new data further points towards increasing utility of mechanical thrombectomy in patient with high-risk PE. One study to look out for in the coming future would be the FlowTriever All-Comer Registry for Patient Safety and Hemodynamics (FLASH) study.

Cardiogenic shock in Acute Myocardial Infarction (AMI)

The management of cardiogenic shock following acute myocardial infarction (AMI) involves prompt diagnosis and treatment to improve outcomes.[22-24] Early recognition of shock is critical, characterized by tissue hypoperfusion and signs of end-organ dysfunction. Reperfusion therapy, primarily through primary percutaneous coronary intervention (PCI), is crucial for restoring myocardial blood flow. Inotropic and vasopressor medications are used to stabilize blood pressure and improve cardiac output. For patients with persistent shock despite PCI, advanced mechanical circulatory support devices, such intra-aortic balloon pumps (IABP) or extracorporeal membrane oxygenation (ECMO) may be necessary for severe cases. Careful fluid management is essential to balance resuscitation needs and avoid overload. Post-acute care includes intensive monitoring, long-term medication management, and multidisciplinary support.

The DanGer Shock study had positive findings that can help guide further studies. Although the use of microaxial flow pumps during severe cardiogenic shock in patients with acute MI has slowly made its way into standard practice, this is the first trial demonstrating mortality benefit. Unlike IMPELLA-STIC trial[14] that demonstrated no benefit and an increased risk of harm from use of IMPELLA 5.0, the DanGer Shock study showed that there is indeed benefit in the use of micro-axial flow pumps with careful patient selection.[13]

Transfusion strategies in Myocardial infarction

In patients with Acute MI and anemia, the MINT trial adds to previous studies such as REALITY, showing no significant improvement with liberal transfusion strategies.[17,25] However, in the current as well as previous trials, potential harms of these strategies cannot be fully excluded.

SEPSIS AND INFECTIOUS DISEASES

- ***Cefepime vs Piperacillin-Tazobactam in Adults Hospitalized With Acute Infection: The ACORN Randomized Clinical Trial. (JAMA. 2023)***[26]
  - *Population:* Adults with infection where clinician initiated an order for antipseudomonal antibiotics within 12 hours of presentation to the hospital in ED or ICU. (n=2511)
  - *Intervention:* Cefepime. (n=1214)
  - *Comparator:* Piperacillin-Tazobactam. (n=1297)
  - *Outcome/Conclusion:* Highest stage of AKI or death by day 14 was analyzed as the primary outcome. Piperacillin-tazobactam did not increase the risk of AKI or death among hospitalized patients. There was an increased risk of neurological dysfunction among the cefepime group.
  - *Critical appraisal:* This was a single center study and was unblinded. The median time patients received either medication was 3 days, but outcomes were measured up to 14 days which makes it difficult to say if the antibiotics were even playing a role at that point.

- ***Landiolol and Organ Failure in Patients with Septic Shock: The STRESS-L Randomized Clinical Trial. (JAMA. 2023)***[27]
  - *Population:* Adults admitted to the ICU with septic shock and tachycardia (HR $\geq$95/min) requiring > 0.1mcg/kg/min norepinephrine for >24 hours. (n=126)
  - *Intervention:* Landiolol. (n=63)
  - *Comparator:* Standard care. (n=63)
  - *Outcome/Conclusion:* Use of landiolol showed no improvement in organ function or mortality.

- *Critical appraisal:* The trial was stopped prematurely as it was unlikely to demonstrate benefit and due to concern for possible harm resulting in a small study population with n=126. Variable modalities for cardiac monitoring were used. The study used a SOFA score as the primary end point.

- ***Inhaled Amikacin to Prevent Ventilator-Associated Pneumonia (AMIKINHAL trial). (NEJM. 2023)***[28]
  - *Population:* Patients >18 years who were mechanically ventilated for at least 72 hours. (n=847)
  - *Intervention:* Inhaled Amikacin. (n=417)
  - *Comparator:* Placebo. (n=430)
  - *Outcome/Conclusion:* The study found a significant reduction in ventilator associated pneumonia in patients who received a 3-day course of inhaled amikacin.
  - *Critical appraisal:* Despite efforts to define VAP, there is a subjective nature to the diagnosis with no one definitive test. In addition to this they included confirmed VAP but also possible or definitive VAP which is ambiguous. The exclusion criteria omitted patients with severe AKI without renal replacement therapy, CKD, and tracheostomy which reduces its generalizability.

Antipseudomonal coverage

In patients with sepsis and factors predisposing to infections with Pseudomonas aeruginosa, empiric antipseudomonal coverage is recommended until microbiological date is available for targeted therapy. Local antibiograms should be used to direct empiric therapy. Some indications for adding empiric antipseudomonal coverage include:

- Immunocompromised state, neutropenia, organ transplant
- Burns, puncture wounds
- Structural lung disease (Cystic Fibrosis, Bronchiectasis)
- Patients with invasive devices
- Previous infection with Pseudomonas
- Hospital-acquired Pneumonia or Ventilator-associated pneumonia with prior IV antibiotic use within 90 days

Cefepime and Piperacillin-Tazobactam are the common choices for antipseudomonal coverage in critically ill patients. Previous evidence from several retrospective studies claimed that Piperacillin-Tazobactam was nephrotoxic, and these studies created a narrative surrounding the drug's nephrotoxicity.[29] Since then it has been shown that empiric broad spectrum antibiotics including vancomycin and Piperacillin-Tazobactam does have higher incidence of creatinine defined AKI but no significant changes in other biomarkers such as cystatin C, BUN, dialysis, or mortality when compared to vancomycin and cefepime combination.[30] The ACORN trial demonstrated that the rate of kidney injury between the Piperacillin-Tazobactam and Cefepime groups were similar. Cefepime has been associated with neurotoxicity which was seen with higher incidence in this group.[26]

Beta blockers in septic shock

Prior to the STRESS-L trial, several studies posed similar question about beta blocker use in septic shock. These prior studies found a varying degree of improvement in clinical outcomes and mortality.[31-32] Most prior studies were small with no large scale RCTs. The STRESS-L trial's findings differ from prior studies as it found no improvement in organ function or mortality.[27] This question warrants further investigation with large scale RCTs given the mixed evidence.

Prophylactic antibiotics

In this AMIKAINHAL study, amikacin reduced VAP, but we must consider several factors. Positive sputum cultures can be misconstrued with VAP. Despite the significant reduction in VAP per study definition, there was no significant difference in ventilator free days, so there is lack of therapeutic validation. In addition, the percent reduction in VAP between the two groups is very high but the number needed to treat makes it less applicable. Issues with feasibility, the required number needed to treat, and likelihood of development of multidrug resistant organisms bring into question whether it is practical to prophylactically treat all mechanically ventilated patients with inhaled antibiotics.

Hepatology/Gastrointestinal

- ***Antibiotics with or without Rifaximin for Acute Hepatic Encephalopathy in Critically Ill Patients with Cirrhosis: A Double-Blind, Randomized Controlled (ARiE) Trial. (Am J Gastroenterol. 2024)***[33]
    - *Population:* Adults with overt hepatic encephalopathy (HE) and cirrhosis admitted to ICU (n=184; Crossover in 5 patients)
    - *Intervention:* Rifaximin (550mg BID) + broad spectrum antibiotics. (n=92)
    - *Comparator:* Broad spectrum antibiotics alone. (n=92)
    - *Outcome/Conclusion:* No significant difference between the groups in resolution (or 2 grade reduction) of HE (primary outcome). No significant difference in time to resolution of HE, in-hospital mortality, incidence of nosocomial infection, and change in endotoxin levels (secondary outcomes). However, in a subgroup analysis, there was a statistically significant improvement in mortality for the intervention group in patients with decompensated cirrhosis.
    - *Critical appraisal:* Although this was a double-blind randomized controlled trial (RCT), it was done in a single center. The lack of a placebo group increases the risk for bias.

- ***Tranexamic Acid in Upper Gastrointestinal Bleed in Patients with Cirrhosis: A Randomized Controlled Trial. (Hepatology. 2024)***[34]
    - *Population:* Patients with advanced liver cirrhosis (Child-Turcotte-Pugh Class B and C) and upper gastrointestinal bleeding (UGIB). (n=600)
    - *Intervention:* Tranexamic acid (TXA) infusion. (n=300)
    - *Comparator:* Placebo. (n=300)
    - *Outcome/Conclusion:* Statistically significant improvement in bleeding control by day 5 and decreased rebleeding by week 6 with use of TXA. Statistically significant failure of initial bleeding control by day 5 and rebleeding by week 6 was seen in the placebo group for patients undergoing endoscopic interventions, especially if it was their first time. There is a small decrease in total hospital length of stay in the patients that survived. However, there was no difference in mortality by day 5 and week 6.
    - *Critical appraisal:* One of this trial's weaknesses is that it was a single center RCT. The mortality rate appears to have included all causes of mortality, and so mortality could have been from the natural progression of liver disease, infections, etc., and not specifically from hemorrhage. The separation of causes of mortality could have brought more insight into this issue.

☞

- ***Stress Ulcer Prophylaxis during Invasive Mechanical Ventilation (REVISE trial). (NEJM. 2024)*[35]**
  - o *Population:* ≥18 years of age undergoing invasive mechanical ventilation in the ICU. (n=4821)
  - o *Intervention:* Pantoprazole 40 mg intravenous daily for 5 days. (n=2417)
  - o *Comparator:* Placebo. (n=2404)
  - o *Outcome/Conclusion:* There was significant reduction in upper GI bleed in the intervention group compared to placebo group, no difference was noted in all-cause mortality among the two groups
  - o *Critical appraisal:* This was a multicenter, double blinded RCT with good internal and external validity, inclusion criteria with robust data and wide range of subgroup analysis.

Hepatic encephalopathy

Current guidelines from the Society of Critical Care Medicine (SCCM) suggest the use of rifaximin as an adjunctive therapy with nonabsorbable disaccharide (e.g. lactulose) in critically ill patients with overt hepatic encephalopathy. These suggestions are conditional recommendations with a low quality of evidence.[36] The literature on rifaximin's benefit appears to be mixed. A meta-analysis showed that rifaximin reduced mortality and increased recovery from HE.[37] However, a second meta-analysis showed that rifaximin alone had some overall benefit and no mortality benefit, but there was a decreased risk in overall mortality and a beneficial effect in HE when used in conjunction with nonabsorbable disaccharides.[38] Although the specifics are unclear, the addition of rifaximin appears to have some benefit in certain populations and little negative adverse reactions.

Upper gastrointestinal bleeding

The current management of acute upper gastrointestinal bleeding (UGIB) relies on multipronged approach of stabilization, resuscitation, and control of bleeding. Initial management includes blood product transfusion or volume resuscitation. In the absence of hemodynamic instability, literature favors restrictive transfusion strategies, targeting a hemoglobin of greater than 7 g/dL.[39-40] The American College of Gastroenterology (ACG) Guidelines recommend that patients admitted to the hospital with UGIB undergo endoscopy within 24 hours of presentation. High dose proton pump therapy is recommended for 3 days after successful endoscopic hemostatic therapy. For patients with recurrent bleeding after endoscopic therapy, guidelines suggest repeat endoscopy rather than surgery or transcatheter arterial embolization.[39] Embolization is recommended for patients with bleeding ulcers who fail endoscopic therapy. The ACG guidelines do not address role of TXA. The European Society of Gastrointestinal Endoscopy (ESGE) guidelines do not recommend the use of TXA in non-variceal UGI bleed.[41]

The above trial by Kumar et al. showed that there could be some benefit in the use of tranexamic acid in patients with cirrhosis and UGIB in reducing rebleeding risk. This contrasts with the HALT-IT trial, which was a large, international, double-blind, placebo-controlled trial that investigated the benefit of tranexamic acid use in acute GI bleeding.[42] The HALT-IT trial did not show any improvements in overall mortality and mortality due to bleeding. The HALT-IT trial also showed no difference in death due to bleeding within 5 days between UGIB, LGIB, and variceal bleed. The HALT-IT trial also showed no significant difference in all-cause mortality at 28 days, and re-bleeding (at 24 hours, 5 days, and 28 days).[42] In summary, these two trials did not show any mortality benefit in using tranexamic acid in this setting.

Stress ulcer prophylaxis

Previously, SUP-ICU (2018) has shown that PPI significantly reduced upper GI bleeding and there was no increase in mortality, *C. difficile* infection or pneumonia.[43] However, with PEPTIC trial in 2020 which compared PPIs vs H2 blockers for GI prophylaxis there were apprehensions about increased mortality with PPI use at 90 days (not reaching statistical significance).[44] As shown above, The REVISE trial demonstrated that PPIs are safe and had no significant effect on mortality.

ENDOCRINOLOGY

- ***Tight Blood-Glucose Control without Early Parenteral Nutrition in the ICU (TGC-FAST trial). (NEJM. 2024)***[45]
  - o *Population:* ≥18 years of age admitted to ICU. (n=9230)
  - o *Intervention:* Tight glucose control, 80-110 mg/dL. (n=4608)
  - o *Comparator:* Liberal glucose control, insulin was started only when blood glucose>215 (n=4622). In both groups parenteral nutrition was withheld for 1 week.
  - o *Outcome/Conclusion:* There was no difference in length of ICU stay or 90-day mortality rate between the two groups

Glycemic control in ICU

TGC-Fast large multicenter RCT with good internal validity, however, it lacks external validity. 1% of patients in tight glycemic control developed severe hypoglycemia (<40 mg/dL). It is extremely difficult to achieve in real world scenario as the insulin delivery was controlled by computer driven algorithm. Also, there was no difference in secondary outcomes which includes infection. In many institutions, especially developing countries, where resources are scarce, tighter glucose control can lead to higher rates of adverse events than reported in the trial. It is better to liberalize glucose control and follow individualized patient centered approach, based on clinical scenarios.

NEUROLOGY

- ***Trial of Early Minimally Invasive Removal of Intracerebral Hemorrhage (ENRICH trial). (NEJM. 2024)***[46]
  - o *Population:* Patients with Acute Intracerebral Hemorrhage of 30-80ml. (n=300)
  - o *Intervention:* Surgical Removal of Hematoma and Medical Management. (n=150)
  - o *Comparator:* Medical Management of Hematoma. (n=150)
  - o *Outcome/Conclusion:* Surgical removal of hematomas within 24 hours increased functional outcomes at 180 days compared to medical management alone based upon a modified Rankin functional scale with scores of 0.458 in the surgical group and 0.374 in the control group (difference of 0.084 at 95% confidence interval of 0.005 to 0.163).
  - o *Critical appraisal:* Early procedural intervention appears to be favorable in improving function at 180 days. However, in subgroup analysis these results were mostly found in groups with lobular hemorrhage, while patients with basal ganglia hemorrhage had no statistically significant improvement. Selection criteria was changed partway through enrollment resulting in increased selection of patients with lobar hemorrhages. Patients with <30ml or >80ml hemorrhages or extension into substantial or intraventricular spaces were excluded. These selection biases may have impacted the combined 180 day modified Rankin scores and limit application to clinical practice.

- ***Efficacy of Haloperidol to Decrease the Burden of Delirium in Adult Critically Ill Patients: The EuRIDICE Randomized Clinical Trial. (Crit Care. 2023)***[47]
  - o *Population:* ICU patients with acute delirium. (n=132)
  - o *Intervention:* Haloperidol. (n= 65)

- *Comparator:* Placebo. (n= 67)
- *Outcome/Conclusion:* Haloperidol does not reduce ICU delirium and coma free days compared to placebo. There were some indications that delirium associated events such as self-extubating or removal of indwelling devices as well as requirement of benzodiazepines may be reduced in the treatment group. Adverse drug related events appeared similar.
- *Critical appraisal:* The trial was stopped before its completion due to primary end point futility. Secondary outcomes indicated a possible reduction in agitation events, but confidence intervals for some included possible harm as well. Medication was titrated and administered based upon nursing assessments of RASS and Intensive Care Delerium Screening Checklist which may lead to observer bias.

- ***Adjunctive Dexamethasone for Tuberculous Meningitis in HIV-Positive Adults (ACT-HIV trial). (NEJM. 2023)***[48]
  - *Population:* Adults with HIV and Tuberculous Meningitis. (n=520)
  - *Intervention:* Dexamethasone and standard treatment. (n=263)
  - *Comparator:* Placebo and Standard Treatment. (n=257)
  - *Outcome/Conclusion:* Death at 12 months were similar between groups (hazard ratio of 0.85 with 95% confidence interval of 0.66 to 1.10). The addition of dexamethasone to standard tuberculous meningitis therapy for patients with HIV did not result in 12 month mortality benefits. Furthermore, secondary outcomes such as incidence of immune reconstitution inflammatory syndrome in the first 6 months were similar as well.
  - *Critical appraisal:* The trial had a relatively small sample size. It was also noted that across the trial around 25% of patients had received glucocorticoids outside of the trial parameters themselves. Another thing to consider is that patients were largely from resource limited regions, many of them with advanced HIV/AIDS and low CD4 counts.

- ***Liberal or Restrictive Transfusion Strategy in Patients with Traumatic Brain Injury (HEMOTION trial). (NEJM. 2023)***[49]
  - *Population:* Critically ill patients with moderate or severe traumatic brain injury and anemia. (n=742)
  - *Intervention:* Transfusions initiated at a hemoglobin level of ≤10 g/dL (liberal strategy). (n=371)
  - *Comparator:* Transfusions initiated at ≤7 g/dL (restrictive strategy). (n=371)
  - *Outcome:* Primary: Unfavorable outcome as assessed by the Glasgow-outcome scale-extended score at 6 months - occurred in 68.4% individuals in the liberal strategy compared to 73.5% in the restrictive strategy, absolute difference of 5.4% in favor of liberal strategy. Secondary outcomes: mortality, functional independence, quality of life, and depression at 6 months: there were no consistent differences in any of these outcomes.
  - Conclusion: Liberal transfusion of red-cells in moderate to severe traumatic brain injury did not reduce the risk of unfavorable neurologic outcomes at 6 months compared to restrictive transfusion.
  - *Critical appraisal:* Blinding was not feasible for this trial as the treating teams were aware of the cut-off for transfusion strategy. The two groups were not balanced at baseline; with relatively more severe patients in the restrictive group and this may have affected outcomes.

☞

- ***Tenecteplase for Ischemic Stroke at 4.5 to 24 Hours without Thrombectomy. (NEJM. 2024)***[50]
  - *Population:* Patients with large vessel occlusion of the middle cerebral artery or internal carotid artery who had not undergone endovascular thrombectomy. (n=516)
  - *Intervention:* Tenecteplase (0.25 mg/kg, maximum 25 mg), at 4.5 to 24 hrs (n=264)

- *Comparator:* Standard medical treatment (with antiplatelet drugs alone), at 4.5 to 24 hrs. (n=252)
- *Outcome:* The incidence of rescue endovascular thrombectomy was similar in the groups. Compared to standard treatment, the intervention with tenecteplase resulted in a higher percentage of patients with the modified Rankin score of 0 or 1 at 90 days (33% vs 24.2%, p=0.03). Mortality was 13.3% with tenecteplase and 13.1% with standard treatment. The incidence of symptomatic intracranial hemorrhage was 3% with tenecteplase and 0.8% with standard treatment.
- *Conclusion:* Patients with large vessel occlusive stroke not undergoing endovascular thrombectomy, had less disability, similar mortality, and a higher incidence of intracranial hemorrhage with tenecteplase compared to standard treatment.
- *Critical appraisal:* Blinding was not feasible for this trial. The effect size of the intervention at 4.5-24 hours was similar to tenecteplase within 3 hours, however, it was smaller than endovascular thrombectomy. More RCTs are required for evaluation of this intervention. This trial showed that in the subset of patients with large vessel occlusive stroke who are unable to receive endovascular thrombectomy, tenecteplase may be a better alternative to antiplatelet therapy for disability reduction, but not mortality reduction, and at the cost of a greater intracranial hemorrhage risk.

☞

- ***Dual Antiplatelet Treatment up to 72 Hours after Ischemic Stroke. INSPIRES RCT. (NEJM. 2023)***[51]
  - *Population:* Patients with mild ischemic stroke or high-risk transient ischemic attack (TIA) presumed to be of atherosclerotic origin. Only patients who had not undergone thrombolysis or thrombectomy were included in the trial. (n=6100)
  - *Intervention:* Within 72 hours of onset of symptoms: Oral clopidogrel (300 mg on first day followed by 75 mg once daily till 90th day) and aspirin (100-300 mg on first day followed by 100 mg once daily till 21st day. (n=3050)
  - *Comparator:* Within 72 hours of onset of symptoms: Oral placebo plus aspirin (100-300 mg on first day followed by 100 mg once daily till 21st day. (n=3050)
  - *Outcome:* There were fewer patients who had a new stroke in the intervention group (7.3%) compared to the control group (9.2%); with a hazard ratio of 0.79 (p=0.008) in favor of the intervention. Moderate to severe bleeding occurred in 0.9% patients in the intervention group and 0.4% in the control group (hazard ratio: 2.08, p=0.03).
  - *Conclusion:* Patients with mild ischemic stroke or high-risk TIA presumed to be atherosclerotic origin had a lower risk of new stroke at 90 days with a combination of clopidogrel and aspirin compared to aspirin alone, but at the cost of higher risk of moderate-to-severe bleeding.
  - *Critical appraisal:* The benefit of using clopidogrel-aspirin combination to lower the risk of recurrent stroke was previously known if initiated within the first 24 hours of onset. This RCT found the benefit of this combination at an extended period of initiation (=within 72 hours of onset). However, this is applicable only in mild ischemic stroke or high-risk TIA. Patients with cardioembolic stroke, moderate or severe stroke, and any stroke with thrombectomy or thrombolysis were not included in the trial.

Spontaneous intracerebral hemorrhage

Management of spontaneous intracerebral hemorrhage (ICH) begins with rapid diagnosis using CT or MRI and a thorough neurological assessment.[52,53] Blood pressure should be controlled aggressively, aiming for a target systolic pressure below 140-160 mmHg to prevent further bleeding. For patients on anticoagulants, prompt reversal of these medications is necessary. Surgical interventions, including decompression or hematoma evacuation, may be required for large hemorrhages or deteriorating conditions. Monitoring and managing intracranial pressure (ICP) is crucial for severe cases, using head elevation, hyperosmolar therapy (such as hypertonic saline or mannitol) to help control elevated ICP. Supportive care includes managing blood glucose, prophylaxis for seizures in the appropriate context, and prevention of further complications. Early rehabilitation is essential for functional recovery, and secondary prevention often involves managing risk factors like hypertension. A multidisciplinary team approach is essential for comprehensive care and optimal outcomes.

Previous trials have had varied results on the impact of procedural intervention for spontaneous intracerebral hemorrhage with most trending towards minimal or non-statistically significant differences. The Intraoperative Stereotactic Computed Tomography-Guided Endoscopic Surgery or ICES trial showed possible functional outcome benefits from procedural interventions within 48 hours of onset.[54] Meanwhile the efficacy and safety of minimally invasive surgery with thrombolysis in intracerebral hemorrhage evacuation or MISTIE III trial showed no benefits for moderate to large bleeds between medical of procedural intervention.[55] The ENRICH trial discussed above indicates that for smaller bleeds, specifically for lobar hemorrhages, early minimally invasive hematoma removal improved the functional outcomes.

Delirium in ICU

Delirium is an acute change in the mental status of a patient, and it is commonly seen in the ICU. It can be characterized as either hyperactive, hypoactive, or mixed delirium. When a sudden change in a patient's mentation is observed, reversible causes should be identified first. Some of the more common reversible causes include infection, medication, hypoglycemia, metabolic, etc. A thorough history, physical exam, labs, and imaging should be obtained to ascertain the cause. Prevention and treatment of the underlying cause are the main treatments of ICU delirium, such as: frequent re-orientation, early mobilization, good sleep schedule etc. Minimizing sedatives, especially benzodiazepines is helpful in prevention of delirium. If needed for agitation, patient or staff safety, pharmacological interventions can be used, such as: Haloperidol, Quetiapine, Olanzapine, Dexmedetomidine etc.[56]

Multiple trials have looked at the use of antipsychotics in the ICU for acute onset delirium management given the preponderance of acute neurological changes in critically ill patients. Of these trials most indicate a lack of improvement in delirium itself. The Haloperidol and Ziprasidone for Treatment of Delerium in Critical Illness trial in 2018 did not show any significant differences between placebo and treatment groups in regard to delirium free days.[57] The Haloperidol for the treatment of Delerium in ICU patients trial in 2022 looked at 90 day mortality and found no statistical difference.[58] The EuRIDICE trial described above assessed not only the outcome of delirium free days but also focused on the secondary agitation related outcomes which could impact patient morbidity during ICU stay. The use of antipsychotics did not change delirium free days but may reduce risk of secondary agitation outcomes. Patients who are at high risk from secondary agitation events such as self-extubation or accidental removal of hemodynamic support device could possibly benefit. However, further studies are needed to assess these outcomes.

Dexamethasone in tubercular meningitis

Glucocorticoids have frequently been used in the past to treat patients with tuberculosis meningitis. The Dexamethasone for the Treatment of Tuberculous Meningitis in Adolescents and Adults study in 2004 found mortality benefit for patients who received steroids alongside standard therapy.[59] However, there was some confounding on the response in patients with HIV. Patients with advanced HIV disease are at risk for inflammatory response from immune reconstitution during initiation of therapy and have high mortality rates. The Elevated Cerebrospinal Fluid Cytokine Levels in Tuberculous Meningitis Predict Survival in Response to Dexamethasone study in 2021 indicated that mortality outcomes were associated with inflammatory response and that pretreatment cytokine levels in cerebral spinal fluid could indicate response and benefit from steroids.[60] As such, the ACT-HIV trial assessed if this increased risk of inflammatory response in HIV patients could be limited by using steroids which had previously been shown to possibly confer improved mortality. However, this study indicates that HIV patients with advanced disease may not benefit from dexamethasone as much as immunocompetent patients.

REFERENCES

1. Freund Y, Viglino D, Cachanado M, et al. Effect of Noninvasive Airway Management of Comatose Patients With Acute Poisoning: A Randomized Clinical Trial. JAMA. 2023;330(23):2267. doi:10.1001/jama.2023.24391

2. Gibbs KW, Semler MW, Driver BE, et al. Noninvasive Ventilation for Preoxygenation during Emergency Intubation. N Engl J Med. 2024;390(23):2165-2177. doi:10.1056/NEJMoa2313680

3. Ruetzler K, Bustamante S, Schmidt MT, et al. Video Laryngoscopy vs Direct Laryngoscopy for Endotracheal Intubation in the Operating Room: A Cluster Randomized Clinical Trial. JAMA. 2024;331(15): 1279. doi:10.1001/jama.2024.0762

4. Shin J, Lee HJ, Jin KN, et al. Automatic Mechanical Ventilation vs Manual Bag Ventilation During CPR: A Pilot Randomized Controlled Trial. Chest. 2024 Aug;166(2):311-320.

5. Orso D, Vetrugno L, Federici N, D'Andrea N, Bove T. Endotracheal intubation to reduce aspiration events in acutely comatose patients: a systematic review. Scand J Trauma Resusc Emerg Med. 2020;28(1):116. doi:10.1186/s13049-020-00814-w

6. Eizadi-Mood N, Saghaei M, Alfred S, et al. Comparative evaluation of Glasgow Coma Score and gag reflex in predicting aspiration pneumonitis in acute poisoning. Journal of Critical Care. 2009;24(3):470.e9-470.e15. doi:10.1016/j.jcrc.2008.08.008

7. Cabrini L, Landoni G, Baiardo Redaelli M, et al. Tracheal intubation in critically ill patients: a comprehensive systematic review of randomized trials. Crit Care. 2018;22(1):6. doi:10.1186/s13054 017-1927-3

8. Casey JD, Janz DR, Russell DW, et al. Bag-Mask Ventilation during Tracheal Intubation of Critically Ill Adults. N Engl J Med. 2019;380(9):811-821. doi:10.1056/NEJMoa1812405

9. Sjöblom A, Broms J, Hedberg M, et al. Pre oxygenation using high flow nasal oxygen vs. tight facemask during rapid sequence induction. Anaesthesia. 2021;76(9):1176-1183. doi:10.1111/anae.15426

10. Prekker ME, Driver BE, Trent SA, et al. Video versus Direct Laryngoscopy for Tracheal Intubation of Critically Ill Adults. N Engl J Med. 2023;389(5):418-429. doi:10.1056/NEJMoa2301601

11. Hansel J, Rogers AM, Lewis SR, Cook TM, Smith AF. Videolaryngoscopy versus direct laryngoscopy for adults undergoing tracheal intubation. Cochrane Anaesthesia Group, ed. Cochrane Database of Systematic Reviews. 2022;2022(4). doi:10.1002/14651858.CD011136.pub3

12. Silver MJ, Gibson CM, Giri J, et al. Outcomes in High-Risk Pulmonary Embolism Patients Undergoing FlowTriever Mechanical Thrombectomy or Other Contemporary Therapies: Results From the FLAME Study. Circ: Cardiovascular Interventions.2023;16(10). doi:10.1161/CIRCINTERVENTIONS.123.013406

13. Møller JE, Engstrøm T, Jensen LO, et al. Microaxial Flow Pump or Standard Care in Infarct-Related Cardiogenic Shock. N Engl J Med. 2024;390(15):1382-1393. doi:10.1056/NEJMoa2312572

14. Bochaton T, Huot L, Elbaz M, et al. Mechanical circulatory support with the Impella® LP5.0 pump and an intra-aortic balloon pump for cardiogenic shock in acute myocardial infarction: The IMPELLA STIC randomized study. Archives of Cardiovascular Diseases. 2020;113(4):237-243. doi:10.1016/j.acvd.2019.10.005

15. Ouweneel DM, Eriksen E, Sjauw KD, et al. Percutaneous Mechanical Circulatory Support Versus Intra-Aortic Balloon Pump in Cardiogenic Shock After Acute Myocardial Infarction. Journal of the American College of Cardiology. 2017;69(3):278-287. doi:10.1016/j.jacc.2016.10.022

16. Seyfarth M, Sibbing D, Bauer I, et al. A Randomized Clinical Trial to Evaluate the Safety and Efficacy of a Percutaneous Left Ventricular Assist Device Versus Intra-Aortic Balloon Pumping for Treatment of Cardiogenic Shock Caused by Myocardial Infarction. Journal of the American College of Cardiology. 2008;52(19):1584-1588. doi:10.1016/j.jacc.2008.05.065

17. Carson JL, Brooks MM, Hébert PC, et al. Restrictive or Liberal Transfusion Strategy in Myocardial Infarction and Anemia. N Engl J Med. 2023;389(26):2446-2456. doi:10.1056/NEJMoa2307983

18. Giri J, Sista AK, Weinberg I, et al. Interventional Therapies for Acute Pulmonary Embolism: Current Status and Principles for the Development of Novel Evidence: A Scientific Statement From the American Heart Association. Circulation. 2019;140(20). doi:10.1161/CIR.0000000000000707

19. Konstantinides SV, Meyer G, Becattini C, et al. 2019 ESC Guidelines for the diagnosis and management of acute pulmonary embolism developed in collaboration with the European Respiratory Society (ERS). European Heart Journal. 2020;41(4):543-603. doi:10.1093/eurheartj/ehz405

20. Stevens SM, Woller SC, Baumann Kreuziger L, et al. Executive Summary. Chest. 2021;160(6):2247-2259. doi:10.1016/j.chest.2021.07.056

21. Tu T, Toma C, Tapson VF, et al. A Prospective, Single-Arm, Multicenter Trial of Catheter-Directed Mechanical Thrombectomy for Intermediate-Risk Acute Pulmonary Embolism. JACC: Cardiovascular Interventions. 2019;12(9):859-869. doi:10.1016/j.jcin.2018.12.022

22. Naidu SS, Baran DA, Jentzer JC, et al. SCAI SHOCK Stage Classification Expert Consensus Update: A Review and Incorporation of Validation Studies. Journal of the Society for Cardiovascular Angiography & Interventions. 2022;1(1):100008. doi:10.1016/j.jscai.2021.100008

23. Vahdatpour C, Collins D, Goldberg S. Cardiogenic Shock. JAHA. 2019;8(8):e011991. doi:10.1161/JAHA.119.011991

24. Byrne RA, Roșsello X, Coughlan JJ, et al. 2023 ESC Guidelines for the management of acute coronary syndromes. European Heart Journal. 2023;44(38):3720-3826. doi:10.1093/eurheartj/ehad191

25. Ducrocq G, Gonzalez-Juanatey JR, Puymirat E, et al. Effect of a Restrictive vs Liberal Blood Transfusion Strategy on Major Cardiovascular Events Among Patients With Acute Myocardial

Infarction and Anemia: The REALITY Randomized Clinical Trial. JAMA. 2021;325(6):552. doi:10.1001/jama.2021.0135.

26. Qian ET, Casey JD, Wright A, et al. Cefepime vs Piperacillin Tazobactam in Adults Hospitalized With Acute Infection: The ACORN Randomized Clinical Trial. JAMA. 2023;330(16):1557. doi:10.1001/jama.2023.20583.

27. Whitehouse T, Hossain A, Perkins GD, et al. Landiolol and Organ Failure in Patients With Septic Shock: The STRESS-L Randomized Clinical Trial. JAMA. 2023;330(17):1641. doi:10.1001/jama.2023.20134.

28. Ehrmann S, Barbier F, Demiselle J, et al. Inhaled Amikacin to Prevent Ventilator-Associated Pneumonia. N Engl J Med. 2023;389(22):2052 2062. doi:10.1056/NEJMoa2310307.

29. Jensen JUS, Hein L, Lundgren B, et al. Kidney failure related to broad-spectrum antibiotics in critically ill patients: secondary end point results from a 1200 patient randomised trial. BMJ Open. 2012;2(2):e000635. doi:10.1136/bmjopen-2011-000635.

30. Miano TA, Hennessy S, Yang W, et al. Association of vancomycin plus piperacillin–tazobactam with early changes in creatinine versus cystatin C in critically ill adults: a prospective cohort study. Intensive Care Med. 2022;48(9):1144-1155. doi:10.1007/s00134-022-068110.

31. Lescroart M, Pequignot B, Kimmoun A, Klein T, Levy B. Beta blockers in septic shock: What is new? J Intensive Med. 2022;2(3):150-155. doi:10.1016/j.jointm.2022.01.004.

32. Hasegawa D, Sato R, Prasitlumkum N, et al. Effect of Ultrashort Acting β-Blockers on Mortality in Patients With Sepsis With Persistent Tachycardia Despite Initial Resuscitation. Chest. 2021;159(6):2289-2300. doi:10.1016/j.chest.2021.01.009.

33. Kulkarni AV, Avadhanam M, Karandikar P, et al. Antibiotics With or Without Rifaximin for Acute Hepatic Encephalopathy in Critically Ill Patients With Cirrhosis: A Double-Blind, Randomized Controlled (ARiE) Trial. Am J Gastroenterol. 2024;119(5):864-874. doi:10.14309/ajg.0000000000002575.

34. Kumar M, Venishetty S, Jindal A, et al. Tranexamic acid in upper gastrointestinal bleed in patients with cirrhosis: A randomized controlled trial. Hepatology. 2024;80(2):376-388. doi:10.1097/HEP.0000000000000817.

35. Cook D, Deane A, Lauzier F, et al. Stress Ulcer Prophylaxis during Invasive Mechanical Ventilation. N Engl J Med. 2024;391(1):9-20. doi:10.1056/NEJMoa2404245.

36. Nanchal R, Subramanian R, Alhazzani W, et al. Guidelines for the Management of Adult Acute and Acute-on-Chronic Liver Failure in the ICU: Neurology, Peri-Transplant Medicine, Infectious Disease, and Gastroenterology Considerations. Critical Care Medicine. 2023;51(5):657-676. doi:10.1097/CCM.0000000000005824.

37. Kimer N, Krag A, Møller S, Bendtsen F, Gluud LL. Systematic review with meta analysis: the effects of rifaximin in hepatic encephalopathy. Aliment Pharmacol Ther. 2014;40(2):123-132. doi:10.1111/apt.12803.

38. Zacharias HD, Kamel F, Tan J, Kimer N, Gluud LL, Morgan MY. Rifaximin for prevention and treatment of hepatic encephalopathy in people with cirrhosis. Cochrane Hepato-Biliary Group, ed. Cochrane Database of Systematic Reviews. 2023;2023(7). doi:10.1002/14651858.CD011585.pub2.

39. Laine L, Barkun AN, Saltzman JR, Martel M, Leontiadis GI. ACG Clinical Guideline: Upper Gastrointestinal and Ulcer Bleeding. Am J Gastroenterol. 2021;116(5):899-917. doi:10.14309/ ajg.000000 0000001245.

40. Villanueva C, Colomo A, Bosch A, et al. Transfusion Strategies for Acute Upper Gastrointestinal Bleeding. N Engl J Med. 2013;368(1): 11-21. doi:10.1056/NEJMoa121180.

41. Gralnek IM, Stanley AJ, Morris AJ, et al. Endoscopic diagnosis and management of nonvariceal upper gastrointestinal hemorrhage (NVUGIH): European Society of Gastrointestinal Endoscopy (ESGE) Guideline – Update 2021. Endoscopy. 2021;53(03):300 332. doi:10.1055/a-1369-5274.

42. Roberts I, Shakur-Still H, Afolabi A, et al. Effects of a high-dose 24 h infusion of tranexamic acid on death and thromboembolic events in patients with acute gastrointestinal bleeding (HALT-IT): an international randomised, double-blind, placebo-controlled trial. The Lancet. 2020;395(10241):1927-1936. doi:10.1016/S0140 6736 (20)30848-5.

43. Krag M, Marker S, Perner A, et al. Pantoprazole in Patients at Risk for Gastrointestinal Bleeding in the ICU. N Engl J Med. 2018;379(23):2199-2208. doi:10.1056/NEJMoa1714919.

44. The PEPTIC Investigators for the Australian and New Zealand Intensive Care Society Clinical Trials Group, Alberta Health Services Critical Care Strategic Clinical Network, and the Irish Critical Care Trials Group, Young PJ, Bagshaw SM, et al. Effect of Stress Ulcer Prophylaxis With Proton Pump Inhibitors vs Histamine-2 Receptor Blockers on In-Hospital Mortality Among ICU Patients Receiving Invasive Mechanical Ventilation: The PEPTIC Randomized Clinical Trial. JAMA. 2020;323(7):616. doi:10.1001/jama.2019.22190.

45. Gunst J, Debaveye Y, Güiza F, et al. Tight Blood-Glucose Control without Early Parenteral Nutrition in the ICU. N Engl J Med. 2023;389(13):1180-1190. doi:10.1056/NEJMoa2304855.

46. Pradilla G, Ratcliff JJ, Hall AJ, et al. Trial of Early Minimally Invasive Removal of Intracerebral Hemorrhage. N Engl J Med. 2024;390(14): 1277-1289. doi:10.1056/NEJMoa2308440.

47. Smit L, Slooter AJC, Devlin JW, et al. Efficacy of haloperidol to decrease the burden of delirium in adult critically ill patients: the EuRIDICE randomized clinical trial. Crit Care. 2023;27(1):413. doi:10.1186/s13054-023-04692-3.

48. Donovan J, Bang ND, Imran D, et al. Adjunctive Dexamethasone for Tuberculous Meningitis in HIV-Positive Adults. N Engl J Med. 2023;389(15):1357-1367. doi:10.1056/NEJMoa2216218.

49. Turgeon AF, Fergusson DA, Clayton L,et al. Liberal or Restrictive Transfusion Strategy in Patients with Traumatic Brain Injury. N Engl J Med. 2024 Aug 22;391(8):722-735.

50. Xiong Y, Campbell BCV, Schwamm LH, et al. Tenecteplase for Ischemic Stroke at 4.5 to 24 Hours without Thrombectomy. N Engl J Med. 2024 Jul 18;391(3):203-212.

51. Gao Y, Chen W, Pan Y, Jing J, Wang C, Johnston SC, et al. Dual Antiplatelet Treatment up to 72 Hours after Ischemic Stroke. N Engl J Med. 2023 Dec 28;389(26):2413-2424.

52. Greenberg SM, Ziai WC, Cordonnier C, et al. 2022 Guideline for the Management of Patients With Spontaneous Intracerebral Hemorrhage: A Guideline From the American Heart Association/ American Stroke Association. Stroke. 2022;53(7). doi:10.1161/ STR.0000000000000407.

53. Steiner T, Salman RAS, Beer R, et al. European Stroke Organisation (ESO) Guidelines for the Management of Spontaneous Intracerebral Hemorrhage. International Journal of Stroke. 2014;9(7):840-855. doi:10.1111/ijs.12309.

54. Vespa P, Hanley D, Betz J, et al. ICES (Intraoperative Stereotactic Computed Tomography-Guided Endoscopic Surgery) for Brain Hemorrhage: A Multicenter Randomized Controlled Trial. Stroke. 2016;47(11):2749-2755. doi:10.1161/STROKEAHA.116.013837.

55. Hanley DF, Thompson RE, Rosenblum M, et al. Efficacy and safety of minimally invasive surgery with thrombolysis in intracerebral haemorrhage evacuation (MISTIE III): a randomised, controlled, open-label, blinded endpoint phase 3 trial. The Lancet. 2019;393 (10175):1021-1032. doi:10.1016/S0140-6736(19)30195-3.

56. Stollings JL, Kotfis K, Chanques G, Pun BT, Pandharipande PP, Ely EW. Delirium in critical illness: clinical manifestations, outcomes, and management. Intensive Care Med. 2021;47(10):1089-1103. doi:10.1007/s00134-021-06503-1.

57. Girard TD, Exline MC, Carson SS, et al. Haloperidol and Ziprasidone for Treatment of Delirium in Critical Illness. N Engl J Med. 2018;379(26):2506-2516. doi:10.1056/NEJMoa1808217.

58. Andersen-Ranberg NC, Poulsen LM, Perner A, et al. Haloperidol for the Treatment of Delirium in ICU Patients. N Engl J Med. 2022;387(26):2425-2435. doi:10.1056/NEJMoa2211868.

59. Thwaites GE, Bang ND, Dung NH, et al. Dexamethasone for the Treatment of Tuberculous Meningitis in Adolescents and Adults. N Engl J Med. 2004;351(17):1741-1751. doi:10.1056/NEJMoa040573.

60. Whitworth LJ, Troll R, Pagán AJ, et al. Elevated cerebrospinal fluid cytokine levels in tuberculous meningitis predict survival in response to dexamethasone. Proc Natl Acad Sci USA. 2021;118(10): e2024852118. doi:10.1073/pnas.2024852118.

CHAPTER 16

Medical Therapies for Lung Cancer

Authors: Dr. Tejas Menon Suri, Dr. Archana Sasi

Reviewer: Dr. Anant Mohan

INTRODUCTION

Lung cancer is the leading cause of cancer-related deaths worldwide, with over 1.8 million fatalities in 2020.[1] Lung cancer is also the most common cause of cancer among males in India.[2] There are various subtypes of lung cancer. Around 80 to 85 percent of all cases are due to non-small cell lung cancer (NSCLC), which in turn is subclassified into predominantly adenocarcinoma and squamous cell carcinoma. There has been an increase in the proportion of adenocarcinoma in recent years, particularly among younger patients, females, and non-smokers.[3] Another 10 to 15 percent of cases are due to small-cell lung cancer (SCLC). A small fraction of cases are due to rare subtypes.[1]

The majority of lung cancer patients present at an advanced stage. Hence, the outcomes of incident lung cancer have historically been dismal, with a 5-year survival rate of around 10% in the 1980s and 90s. However, over the past two decades, genotype-directed therapies and immunotherapies have rapidly developed, revolutionized the management of locally advanced and distant metastasized NSCLC. This has improved the 5-year overall survival of all NSCLC patients to approximately 28 percent in the United States. Among them, those with distant involvement have a 5-year overall survival of 9%.[4] Nonetheless, SCLC is an aggressive form of lung cancer for which no significant improvement in survival has been noted to date.[5]

The research into lung cancer therapeutics is advancing at a phenomenal pace. In this review, we will summarize the findings of the latest trials in the medical management of lung cancer and discuss them in the context of the existing guidelines.

Methodology

A search was conducted on the MEDLINE database using the MeSH term "lung cancer." Filters were applied to select English language studies conducted on human adults, with full texts available, published between 1st August 2023 and 1st August 2024. A total of 454 results were obtained. Subsequently, title and abstract screening were performed to include articles that were phase-3 randomized controlled trials of medical therapies in lung cancer management. Studies that were reporting radiotherapeutic, surgical, or supportive interventions were excluded. Subset, exploratory, and post-hoc analyses of published RCTs were also excluded. However, updated survival outcomes of previously published RCTs were included. Finally, 29 studies were included in the review.

Electronic database searched: Pubmed
Period: 1st August 2023 to 1st August 2024
Search term used : "Lung Cancer"
(n=454)

↓

Articles included
n=29

Results

1. Non-Small Cell Lung Cancer (NSCLC)

a. Adjuvant therapies for early-stage NSCLC (Stages I-IIIa)

i. Perioperative Pembrolizumab for Early-Stage Non-Small-Cell Lung Cancer. (NEJM. 2023)[6]

- *Population:* Patients with resectable early-stage NSCLC (stage II, IIIA, or IIIB N2 stage). (n=797)
- *Intervention:* Perioperative pembrolizumab (200 mg) given every 3 weeks combined with cisplatin-based chemotherapy for 4 cycles, followed by surgery and adjuvant pembrolizumab (200 mg) every 3 weeks for up to 13 cycles. (n=397)
- *Comparator:* Placebo combined with cisplatin-based chemotherapy, followed by surgery and adjuvant placebo. (n=400)
- *Outcome:* **Pembrolizumab significantly improved 24-month EFS (62.4% vs. 40.6%; HR 0.58, P<0.001).** Grade 3 or higher treatment-related adverse events occurred in 44.9% of the pembrolizumab group compared to 37.3% in the placebo group.
- *Conclusion*: Perioperative pembrolizumab combined with chemotherapy and followed by surgery significantly improved event-free survival in patients with resectable early-stage NSCLC.

ii. Perioperative Nivolumab in Resectable Lung Cancer. (NEJM. 2024)[7]

- *Population:* Adults with resectable stage IIA to IIIB NSCLC. (n=922)
- *Intervention:* Neoadjuvant nivolumab plus chemotherapy (3-weekly for four cycles) followed by surgery and adjuvant nivolumab (4-weekly) for one year. (n=461)
- *Comparator:* Neoadjuvant chemotherapy plus placebo (3-weekly for four cycles) followed by surgery and adjuvant placebo (4-weekly) for one year. (n=461)
- *Outcome:* **The 18-month event-free survival was 70.2% in the nivolumab group compared to 50.0% in the chemotherapy group**. Pathological complete response was seen in 25.3% of patients in the nivolumab group versus 4.7% in the chemotherapy group. Grade 3 or 4 treatment-related adverse events occurred in 32.5% of the nivolumab group and 25.2% of the chemotherapy group.
- *Conclusion*: Perioperative treatment with nivolumab significantly improved event-free survival and pathological responses compared to standard chemotherapy in patients with resectable NSCLC.

iii. Perioperative Durvalumab for Resectable Non-Small-Cell Lung Cancer. (NEJM. 2023)[8]

- *Population:* Patients with resectable NSCLC (stage II to IIIB). (n=802)
- *Intervention:* Platinum-based chemotherapy plus durvalumab administered intravenously every 3 weeks for 4 cycles before surgery, followed by adjuvant durvalumab administered intravenously every 4 weeks for 12 cycles. (n=400)
- *Comparator:* Platinum-based chemotherapy plus placebo administered intravenously every 3 weeks for 4 cycles before surgery, followed by adjuvant placebo administered intravenously every 4 weeks for 12 cycles. (n=402)
- *Outcome:* **Event-free survival (EFS) was significantly longer with durvalumab compared to placebo**, with a stratified hazard ratio (HR) for disease progression, recurrence, or death of 0.68 (95% CI, 0.53 to 0.88; P = 0.004). At the 12-month landmark analysis, 73.4% of patients who received durvalumab were event-free (95% CI, 67.9 to 78.1) compared to 64.5% of patients who received placebo (95% CI, 58.8 to 69.6). Grade 3 or 4 adverse events occurred in 42.4% of patients receiving durvalumab and in 43.2% receiving placebo.
- *Conclusion*: Perioperative durvalumab plus neoadjuvant chemotherapy improved event-free survival in patients with resectable NSCLC compared to neoadjuvant chemotherapy alone.

iv. Overall survival with adjuvant atezolizumab after chemotherapy in resected stage II-IIIA non-small-cell lung cancer (IMpower010): A randomised, multicentre, open-label, phase III trial. (Ann Oncol. 2023)[9]

- *Population:* Adults with completely resected stage IB (≥4 cm)-IIIA NSCLC, who received adjuvant platinum-based chemotherapy. (n=1005)
- *Intervention:* Atezolizumab 1200 mg every 3 weeks for 16 cycles. (n=507)
- *Comparator:* Best supportive care (BSC). (n=498)
- *Outcome:* At a median follow-up of 45.3 months, median overall survival (OS) was not estimable in the intention-to-treat (ITT) population. The stratified hazard ratios for OS were 0.995 for the ITT population, 0.95 for stage II-IIIA, 0.71 for PD-L1 tumor cell (TC) ≥1%, and 0.43 for PD-L1 TC ≥50%.
- *Conclusion*: The data suggest a benefit of atezolizumab, particularly in patients with high PD-L1 expression, although overall survival data for the ITT population remain immature.

v. Perioperative Toripalimab Plus Chemotherapy for Patients with Resectable Non-Small Cell Lung Cancer: The Neotorch Randomized Clinical Trial. (China). (JAMA. 2024)[10]

- *Population:* Patients with stage III resectable NSCLC (excluding EGFR or ALK alterations). (n=404)
- *Intervention:* Toripalimab 240 mg combined with platinum-based chemotherapy for 3 cycles before surgery and 1 cycle after surgery, followed by toripalimab 240 mg alone once every 3 weeks for up to 13 cycles. (n=202)
- *Comparator:* Placebo combined with platinum-based chemotherapy for the same regimen as the intervention group, followed by placebo alone once every 3 weeks for up to 13 cycles. (n=202)
- *Outcome:* The primary outcome of event-free survival was significantly longer in the toripalimab group (median not estimable; 95% CI, 24.4 months to not estimable) compared to the placebo group (median 15.1 months; 95% CI, 10.6 to 21.9 months; HR 0.40, 95% CI, 0.28 to 0.57; P < .001). The pathological complete response rate was 24.8% (95% CI, 19.0%-31.3%) in the toripalimab group versus 1.0% (95% CI, 0.1%-3.5%) in the placebo group.
- *Conclusion*: The addition of toripalimab to perioperative chemotherapy significantly improved event-free survival in patients with resectable stage III NSCLC. There were no unexpected treatment-related toxic effects.

vi. Alectinib in Resected ALK-Positive Non-Small-Cell Lung Cancer. (NEJM. 2024)[11]

- *Population:* Completely resected, ALK-positive NSCLC of stage IB (tumors $\geq$4 cm), II, or IIIA. (n=257)
- *Intervention:* Oral alectinib (600 mg twice daily) for 24 months. (n=130)
- *Comparator:* Intravenous platinum-based chemotherapy in four 21-day cycles. (n=127)
- *Outcome:* **The 2-year disease-free survival rate was 93.8% in the alectinib group versus 63.0% in the chemotherapy group for stage II or IIIA patients**. Alectinib also provided a significant benefit in CNS disease-free survival with a hazard ratio of 0.22.
- *Conclusion*: Adjuvant alectinib significantly improved disease-free survival compared to platinum-based chemotherapy, particularly in preventing CNS recurrence, with no unexpected safety concerns.

vii. Five-Year Overall Survival Analysis of the JIPANG Study: Pemetrexed or Vinorelbine Plus Cisplatin for Resected Stage II-IIIA Nonsquamous Non-Small-Cell Lung Cancer. (J Clin Oncol. 2023)[12]

- *Population:* Patients with stage II-IIIA nonsquamous NSCLC. (n=783)
- *Intervention:* Pemetrexed plus cisplatin (PemP) as adjuvant chemotherapy. (n=389)
- *Comparator:* Vinorelbine plus cisplatin (NP). (n=384)
- *Outcome:* The median recurrence-free survival (RFS) was 37.5 months for vinorelbine plus cisplatin (NP) and 43.4 months for pemetrexed plus cisplatin (PemP), with a hazard ratio of 0.95. At 5 years, overall survival (OS) was similar between the groups: 75.6% for NP and 75.0% for PemP (hazard ratio 1.04).
- *Conclusion*: This long-term follow-up analysis demonstrates that PemP has similar efficacy to NP in terms of RFS and OS in patients with stage II-IIIA nonsquamous NSCLC.

b. Genotype-directed therapies for advanced NSCLC (EGFR alterations)

i. Osimertinib with or without Chemotherapy in EGFR-Mutated Advanced NSCLC (FLAURA 2 trial). (NEJM. 2023)[13]

- *Population:* Patients with EGFR-mutated (exon 19 deletion or L858R mutation) advanced NSCLC who were treatment naive. (n=557)
- *Intervention:* Osimertinib (80 mg once daily) with chemotherapy (pemetrexed plus either cisplatin or carboplatin). (n=279)
- *Comparator:* Osimertinib monotherapy (80 mg once daily). (n=278)
- *Outcome:* **Progression-free survival (PFS) was significantly longer in the osimertinib-chemotherapy group compared to the osimertinib group (hazard ratio HR. for disease progression or death, 0.62; 95% CI, 0.49 to 0.79; P<0.001),** with median response durations of 24.0 months (95% CI, 20.9 to 27.8) and 15.3 months (95% CI, 12.7 to 19.4), respectively. At 24 months, 57% of patients in the osimertinib-chemotherapy group were alive and progression-free compared to 41% in the osimertinib group.
- *Conclusion*: First-line treatment with osimertinib plus chemotherapy significantly extended progression-free survival compared to osimertinib monotherapy in patients with EGFR-mutated advanced NSCLC.

ii. Lazertinib Versus Gefitinib as First-Line Treatment in Patients With EGFR-Mutated Advanced Non-Small-Cell Lung Cancer: Results From LASER301. (J Clin Oncol. 2023)[14]

- *Population:* Treatment-naïve patients with EGFR-mutated (exon 19 deletion/L858R mutation) locally advanced or metastatic NSCLC, including those with neurologically stable CNS metastases. (n=393)
- *Intervention:* Lazertinib 240 mg orally once daily. (n=196)
- *Comparator:* Gefitinib 250 mg orally once daily. (n=197)
- *Outcome:* **Lazertinib significantly extended median progression-free survival (PFS) to 20.6 months compared to 9.7 months with gefitinib (HR 0.45, P < .001).** Both treatments had manageable safety profiles consistent with previous reports.
- *Conclusion*: Lazertinib demonstrated superior efficacy in terms of PFS compared to gefitinib, making it a promising first-line treatment option for patients with EGFR-mutated advanced NSCLC.

iii. Amivantamab plus chemotherapy with and without lazertinib in EGFR-mutant advanced NSCLC after disease progression on osimertinib: primary results from the phase III MARIPOSA-2 study. (Ann Oncol. 2024)[15]

- *Population:* Patients with EGFR-mutated (exon 19 deletions or L858R) locally advanced or metastatic NSCLC who had progressed after osimertinib treatment. (n=657)
- *Intervention:* Amivantamab-lazertinib-chemotherapy (amivantamab plus carboplatin-pemetrexed and lazertinib started after carboplatin completion) and amivantamab-chemotherapy (amivantamab plus carboplatin-pemetrexed).
- *Comparator:* Chemotherapy alone (carboplatin-pemetrexed).
- *Outcome:* The hazard ratio (HR) for disease progression or death was 0.44 (P < 0.001; median PFS 8.3 months) for amivantamab-lazertinib-chemotherapy and 0.48 (P < 0.001; median PFS 6.3 months) for amivantamab-chemotherapy, versus 4.2 months for chemotherapy. Median intracranial PFS was also extended in the amivantamab-lazertinib-chemotherapy (12.8 months) and amivantamab-chemotherapy (12.5 months) groups compared to chemotherapy (8.3 months), with HRs for intracranial disease progression or death of 0.58 and 0.55, respectively.
- *Conclusion:* Amivantamab-chemotherapy and amivantamab-lazertinib-chemotherapy improved both PFS and intracranial PFS compared to chemotherapy alone in patients with limited treatment options after progression on osimertinib. However, high rate of hematological adverse events were encountered with amivantamab and lazertinib-containing regimens.

iv. Amivantamab plus Chemotherapy in NSCLC with EGFR Exon 20 Insertions. (NEJM. 2023)[16]

- *Population:* NSCLC with EGFR exon 20 insertions which were treatment-naive. (n=308)
- *Intervention:* Intravenous amivantamab plus carboplatin-pemetrexed (chemotherapy) (amivantamab-chemotherapy). (n=153)
- *Comparator:* Chemotherapy alone (carboplatin-pemetrexed). (n=155)
- *Outcome:* **Progression-free survival (PFS) was significantly longer in the amivantamab-chemotherapy group compared to the chemotherapy group (11.4 months vs 6.7 months; HR: 0.40; 95% CI, 0.30 to 0.53; P<0.001).** The predominant adverse events were reversible hematologic and EGFR-related toxicities, with 7% of patients discontinuing amivantamab due to adverse reactions.
- *Conclusion*: Amivantamab-chemotherapy demonstrated superior efficacy compared to chemotherapy alone as a first-line treatment for patients with advanced NSCLC with EGFR exon 20 insertions.

*v. **Osimertinib after chemoradiotherapy in stage III EGFR-mutated NSCLC. (NEJM. 2024)**[17]*

- o *Population:* Unresectable stage III NSCLC without progression following chemoradiotherapy. (n=216)
- o *Intervention:* Osimertinib till disease progression. (n=143)
- o *Comparator:* Placebo till disease progression. (n=73)
- o *Outcome:* Osimertinib prolonged the PFS compared to placebo (39.1 vs 5.6 months; HR: 0.16; 95% CI, 0.10 to 0.24; p<0.001)
- o *Conclusion*: In unresectable stage III lung cancer without progression after chemoradiotherapy, osimertinib prolongs PFS compared to placebo.

c. Genotype-directed therapies for advanced NSCLC (ALK fusions)

i. Brigatinib Versus Alectinib in ALK-Positive NSCLC After Disease Progression on Crizotinib: Results of Phase 3 ALTA-3 Trial. (J Thorac Oncol. 2023)[18]

- o *Population:* Patients with advanced ALK-positive NSCLC who progressed on crizotinib. (n=248)
- o *Intervention:* Brigatinib 180 mg once daily (with a 7-day lead-in at 90 mg). (n=125)
- o *Comparator:* Alectinib 600 mg twice daily. (n=123)
- o *Outcome:* Median progression-free survival (PFS) was 19.3 months with brigatinib and 19.2 months with alectinib (hazard ratio 0.97).
- o *Conclusion*: Brigatinib did not show superiority over alectinib in terms of PFS for crizotinib-pretreated ALK-positive NSCLC.

d. Genotype-directed therapies for advanced NSCLC (other targetable alterations)

i. Entrectinib in ROS1-positive advanced non-small cell lung cancer: the phase 2/3 BFAST trial. (Nat Med. 2024)[19]

- o *Population:* Patients aged ≥18 years with stage IIIB/IV, ROS1-positive NSCLC identified by liquid biopsies. (n=55)
- o Intervention: Entrectinib 600 mg daily.
- o *Comparator:* Comparison was made with the integrated analysis of entrectinib in patients with ROS1-positive NSCLC identified by tissue-based testing.
- o *Outcome:* The confirmed objective response rate (ORR) by the investigator was 81.5%, consistent with the ORR from the integrated analysis of entrectinib (73.4%). There were no new safety concerns.
- o *Conclusion*: These results support the clinical value of liquid biopsies as a less invasive and faster alternative to tissue-based testing for informed decision-making in advanced/metastatic NSCLC.

ii. First-Line Selpercatinib or Chemotherapy and Pembrolizumab in RET Fusion-Positive NSCLC. (NEJM. 2023)[20]

- o *Population:* Patients with advanced RET fusion-positive NSCLC. (n=212)
- o *Intervention:* First-line selpercatinib. (n=129)
- o *Comparator:* Platinum-based chemotherapy with or without pembrolizumab at the investigator's discretion. (n=83)

- *Outcome:* **Median progression-free survival (PFS) was 24.8 months with selpercatinib versus 11.2 months with control treatment (HR for progression or death, 0.46; 95% CI, 0.31 to 0.70; P<0.001)** in the intention-to-treat-pembrolizumab population. Efficacy results in the overall intention-to-treat population were consistent with those observed in the intention-to-treat-pembrolizumab population.
- *Conclusion:* Selpercatinib demonstrated significantly longer progression-free survival compared to platinum-based chemotherapy, with or without pembrolizumab, in patients with advanced RET fusion-positive NSCLC.

e. Immunotherapies for advanced NSCLC without targetable alterations (first line setting)

i. Nivolumab plus chemotherapy in first-line metastatic non-small-cell lung cancer: Results of the phase III CheckMate 227 Part 2 trial. (ESMO. 2023)[21]

- *Population:* Patients with systemic therapy-naive, stage IV/recurrent NSCLC without EGFR mutations or ALK alterations. (n=755)
- *Intervention:* Nivolumab 360 mg every 3 weeks plus chemotherapy. (n=377)
- *Comparator:* Chemotherapy alone. (n=378)
- *Outcome:* The primary endpoint, overall survival (OS) in patients with nonsquamous NSCLC, was not significantly improved with nivolumab plus chemotherapy compared to chemotherapy alone (median OS 18.8 vs. 15.6 months, HR 0.86, 95.62% CI 0.69-1.08, P = 0.1859).
- *Conclusion*: The CheckMate 227 Part 2 trial did not achieve its primary endpoint of improving OS with nivolumab plus chemotherapy in patients with metastatic nonsquamous NSCLC.

ii. Four-year clinical update and treatment switching-adjusted outcomes with first-line nivolumab plus ipilimumab with chemotherapy for metastatic non-small cell lung cancer in the CheckMate 9LA randomized trial. (J Immunother Cancer. 2024)[22]

- *Population:* Adults with stage IV/recurrent NSCLC, no sensitizing EGFR/ALK alterations, and ECOG performance status ≤1. (n=719)
- *Intervention:* Nivolumab 360 mg every 3 weeks plus ipilimumab 1 mg/kg every 6 weeks with chemotherapy (two cycles). (n=361)
- *Comparator:* Chemotherapy (four cycles, with optional maintenance pemetrexed for the nonsquamous population). (n=358)
- *Outcome:* **At a 4-year minimum follow-up, nivolumab plus ipilimumab with chemotherapy showed prolonged overall survival (OS) over chemotherapy alone (HR 0.74).** The 4-year OS rate was 21% versus 16%, regardless of tumor PD-L1 expression or histology. No new safety signals were observed.
- *Conclusion*: This 4-year update confirms the long-term efficacy of nivolumab plus ipilimumab with chemotherapy as a first-line treatment for metastatic/recurrent NSCLC.

iii. First-line nivolumab, paclitaxel, carboplatin, and bevacizumab for advanced non-squamous non-small cell lung cancer: Updated survival analysis of the ONO-4538-52/TASUKI-52 randomized controlled trial. (Japan/Korea/Taiwan). (Cancer Med. 2023)[23]

- *Population:* Patients with treatment-naïve stage IIIB/IV or recurrent non-squamous NSCLC without driver alterations in ALK, EGFR, or ROS1. (n=550)
- *Intervention:* Nivolumab plus paclitaxel, carboplatin, and bevacizumab. (n=275)
- *Comparator:* Placebo plus paclitaxel, carboplatin, and bevacizumab. (n=275)

- o *Outcome:* Median overall survival with nivolumab (30.8 months) was significantly longer compared to placebo (24.7 months; hazard ratio 0.74, 95% confidence interval 0.58-0.94).
- o *Conclusion*: **The addition of nivolumab to platinum chemotherapy and bevacizumab improved overall survival and is suggested as a viable first-line treatment for advanced non-squamous NSCLC without driver alterations.**

iv. First-line atezolizumab monotherapy versus single-agent chemotherapy in patients with non-small-cell lung cancer ineligible for treatment with a platinum-containing regimen (IPSOS): A phase 3, global, multicentre, open-label, randomised controlled study. (Lancet. 2023)[24]

- o *Population:* (i) Stage IIIB or IV NSCLC were ineligible for platinum-based chemotherapy due to an ECOG PS 2 or 3, or (ii) age 70 years or older with ECOG PS 0-1 and substantial comorbidities. (n=453)
- o *Intervention:* Atezolizumab 1200 mg intravenously every 3 weeks. (n=302)
- o *Comparator:* Single-agent chemotherapy (vinorelbine or gemcitabine). (n=151)
- o *Outcome:* **Atezolizumab improved median overall survival to 10.3 months compared to 9.2 months with chemotherapy (HR 0.78, p=0.028),** with a 2-year survival rate of 24% versus 12%. Atezolizumab also led to fewer grade 3-4 treatment-related adverse events (16% vs 33%).
- o *Conclusion*: Atezolizumab monotherapy offers improved survival, better quality of life, and a favorable safety profile, making it a viable first-line treatment option for this patient population.

v. Avelumab Versus Platinum-Based Doublet Chemotherapy as First-Line Treatment for Patients with High-Expression Programmed Death-Ligand 1-Positive Metastatic NSCLC: Primary Analysis From the Phase 3 JAVELIN Lung 100 Trial. (J Thorac Oncol. 2024)[25]

- o *Population:* Adults with PD-L1-positive ($\geq$1% of tumor cells), EGFR and ALK wild-type, previously untreated, stage IV NSCLC. (n=1214)
- o *Intervention:*

  (a) Avelumab 10 mg/kg every 2 weeks (Q2W). (n=366),

  (b) 10 mg/kg once weekly (QW) for 12 weeks, followed by Q2W. (n=322)
- o *Comparator:* Platinum-based doublet chemotherapy every 3 weeks. (n=526)
- o *Outcome:* For overall survival: (a) Avelumab Q2W vs. chemotherapy: HR 0.85 (95% CI: 0.67-1.09; one-sided p = 0.1032; median OS, 20.1 vs. 14.9 months). (b) Avelumab QW vs. chemotherapy: HR 0.79 (95% CI: 0.59-1.07; one-sided p = 0.0630; median OS, 19.3 vs. 15.3 months).
- o *Conclusion*: Avelumab showed longer median OS than platinum-based doublet chemotherapy in advanced NSCLC. However, the differences were not statistically significant, and the trial did not meet its primary objective.

vi. First-line cemiplimab monotherapy and continued cemiplimab beyond progression plus chemotherapy for advanced non-small-cell lung cancer with PD-L1 50% or more (EMPOWER-Lung 1): 35-month follow-up from a mutlicentre, open-label, randomised, phase 3 trial. (Lancet Oncol. 2023)[26]

- o *Population:* Patients with advanced NSCLC and PD-L1 tumor expression of at least 50%, without actionable biomarkers. (n=712)
- o *Intervention:* Cemiplimab administered intravenously at 350 mg every 3 weeks for up to 108 weeks. (n=357)
- o *Comparator:* Investigator's choice of chemotherapy. (n=355)

- *Outcome:* **At 35 months' follow-up, median overall survival was 26.1 months for the cemiplimab group versus 13.3 months for the chemotherapy group (hazard ratio 0.57).** Continued cemiplimab plus chemotherapy as second-line therapy resulted in a median overall survival of 15.1 months and progression-free survival of 6.6 months.
- *Conclusion*: Cemiplimab demonstrated sustained survival benefits at 35 months and may be a viable first-line treatment for advanced NSCLC. Adding chemotherapy at disease progression could offer a new second-line treatment option.

f. Immunotherapies for advanced NSCLC without targetable driver alterations (subsequent line setting)

i. *Phase III, Randomized Study of Atezolizumab Plus Bevacizumab and Chemotherapy in Patients With EGFR- or ALK-Mutated Non-Small-Cell Lung Cancer (ATTLAS, KCSG-LU19-04). (Korea). (J Clin Oncol. 2024)*[27]

- *Population:* Patients with EGFR or ALK-mutated NSCLC that progressed after tyrosine kinase inhibitor (TKI) therapy. (n=228)
- *Intervention:* Atezolizumab plus bevacizumab, paclitaxel, and carboplatin (ABCP), followed by maintenance therapy with atezolizumab plus bevacizumab. (n=154)
- *Comparator:* Pemetrexed plus carboplatin or cisplatin (PC), followed by pemetrexed maintenance. (n=74)
- *Outcome:* **Median PFS was significantly longer in the ABCP arm (8.48 months) compared to the PC arm (5.62 months) with a hazard ratio (HR) of 0.62 (95% CI, 0.45 to 0.86; P = 0.004).** The safety profile of the ABCP arm was consistent with previous reports.
- *Conclusion*: This study demonstrated the clinical benefit of atezolizumab combined with bevacizumab and chemotherapy in patients with EGFR or ALK-mutated NSCLC who have progressed on targeted therapy.

ii. *Nivolumab Plus Chemotherapy in Epidermal Growth Factor Receptor-Mutated Metastatic Non-Small-Cell Lung Cancer After Disease Progression on Epidermal Growth Factor Receptor Tyrosine Kinase Inhibitors: Final Results of CheckMate 722. (J Clin Oncol. 2024)*[28]

- *Population:* Patients with EGFR-mutated metastatic NSCLC who experienced disease progression after treatment with first- or second-generation EGFR TKIs or osimertinib. (n=294)
- *Intervention:* Nivolumab (360 mg every 3 weeks) plus platinum-doublet chemotherapy for four cycles. (n=144)
- *Comparator:* Platinum-doublet chemotherapy alone (every 3 weeks for four cycles). (n=150)
- *Outcome:* The primary outcome, PFS, was not significantly improved with nivolumab plus chemotherapy compared to chemotherapy alone (median PFS, 5.6 vs. 5.4 months; HR 0.75; P = 0.0528). Grade 3/4 treatment-related adverse events occurred in 44.7% of patients in the nivolumab plus chemotherapy group and 29.4% in the chemotherapy-alone group.
- *Conclusion*: Nivolumab plus chemotherapy did not significantly improve PFS compared to chemotherapy alone in patients with EGFR-mutated metastatic NSCLC previously treated with EGFR TKIs.

iii. *KEYNOTE-033: Randomized phase 3 study of pembrolizumab vs docetaxel in previously treated, PD-L1-positive, advanced NSCLC. (Int J Cancer. 2023)*[29]

- *Population:* Patients with previously treated, PD-L1-positive advanced NSCLC. (n=425)
- *Intervention:* Pembrolizumab 2 mg/kg every 3 weeks. (n=213)

- *Comparator:* Docetaxel 75 mg/m² every 3 weeks. (n=212)
- *Outcome:* Median OS was 12.3 months for pembrolizumab versus 10.9 months for docetaxel. The hazard ratio (HR) was 0.83 (95% CI: 0.61-1.14), with a P-value of 0.1276, not meeting the predefined significance threshold. Grade 3 to 5 treatment-related AEs were significantly lower with pembrolizumab (11.3%) than docetaxel (47.5%).
- *Conclusion*: Pembrolizumab improved OS compared to docetaxel in previously treated, PD-L1-positive NSCLC patients, though the predefined statistical significance threshold was not reached in patients with PD-L1 TPS >50%. The safety profile favored pembrolizumab, with fewer severe treatment-related adverse events.

g. Other therapies in advanced NSCLC

i. Pembrolizumab With or Without Lenvatinib for First-Line Metastatic NSCLC with Programmed Cell Death-Ligand 1 Tumor Proportion Score of at least 1% (LEAP-007): A Randomized, Double-Blind, Phase 3 Trial. (J Thorac Oncol. 2024)[30]

- *Population:* Patients with previously untreated stage IV NSCLC with a programmed cell death-ligand 1 (PD-L1) tumor proportion score of at least 1% and without targetable EGFR, ROS1, or ALK aberrations. (n=623)
- *Intervention:* Lenvatinib 20 mg once daily combined with pembrolizumab 200 mg every 3 weeks for up to 35 cycles. (n=309)
- *Comparator:* Placebo combined with pembrolizumab 200 mg every 3 weeks for up to 35 cycles. (n=314)
- *Outcome:* The median overall survival (OS) was 14.1 months (95% CI, 11.4 19.0) in the lenvatinib plus pembrolizumab group versus 16.4 months (95% CI, 12.6 20.6) in the placebo plus pembrolizumab group (HR, 1.10; 95% CI, 0.87 1.39; p = 0.79744). Grade 3 to 5 treatment-related adverse events occurred in 57.9% of patients in the lenvatinib group versus 24.4% in the placebo group.
- *Conclusion*: Lenvatinib plus pembrolizumab did not demonstrate a favorable benefit-risk profile compared to placebo plus pembrolizumab in first-line treatment of metastatic NSCLC with PD-L1 expression ≥1%.

ii. Atezolizumab and Platinum Plus Pemetrexed With or Without Bevacizumab for Metastatic Nonsquamous Non-Small Cell Lung Cancer: A Phase 3 Randomized Clinical Trial. (Japan). (JAMA. 2024)[31]

- *Population:* Patients with advanced nonsquamous NSCLC without genetic driver alterations or with genetic driver alterations who had received at least one approved tyrosine kinase inhibitor. (n=411)
- *Intervention:* Atezolizumab plus carboplatin and pemetrexed, and bevacizumab (APPB) administered for four cycles, followed by maintenance therapy with atezolizumab, pemetrexed, and bevacizumab until disease progression, unacceptable toxic effects, or two years from initiation. (n=205)
- *Comparator:* Atezolizumab plus carboplatin with pemetrexed (APP) for four cycles, followed by maintenance therapy with atezolizumab and pemetrexed. (n=206)
- *Outcome:* The median progression-free survival (PFS) as assessed by blinded independent central review (BICR) was 9.6 months with APPB versus 7.7 months with APP (HR, 0.86; 95% CI, 0.70-1.07; P = 0.92). The subgroup of patients with driver oncogenes showed improved PFS with APPB compared to APP (median, 9.7 vs 5.8 months; HR, 0.67; 95% CI, 0.46-0.98).
- *Conclusion*: The trial did not demonstrate superiority of the APPB regimen over APP in the overall population of patients with nonsquamous NSCLC. However, APPB showed improved survival and similar tolerability in patients with driver oncogenes.

2. Small Cell Lung Cancer (SCLC)

a. Initial and maintenance therapies for SCLC

☞

i. Atezolizumab Plus Carboplatin and Etoposide in Patients with Untreated Extensive-Stage Small-Cell Lung Cancer: Interim Results of the MAURIS Phase IIIb Trial. (Italy). (Oncologist. 2024)[32]

- o *Population:* Patients with newly diagnosed extensive-stage SCLC. (n=154)
- o *Intervention:* Atezolizumab combined with carboplatin/etoposide every 3 weeks for 4-6 cycles during the induction phase, followed by atezolizumab maintenance 3-weekly.
- o *Comparator:* Subgroups based on the number of induction cycles received: ≤3 cycles, 4 cycles, and 5-6 cycles.
- o *Outcome:* At a median follow-up of 10.5 months, 29.9% of patients experienced serious adverse events, with the lowest rate (19.1%) in those who received 5-6 cycles, compared with 4 cycles (34.9%) or ≤3 cycles (63.6%). The median overall survival was 10.7 months, and median progression-free survival was 5.5 months.
- o *Conclusion:* Interim results suggest that atezolizumab combined with carboplatin/etoposide is effective and has a manageable safety profile in a real-world ES-SCLC patient population.

ii. Tislelizumab Plus Platinum and Etoposide Versus Placebo Plus Platinum and Etoposide as First-Line Treatment for Extensive-Stage SCLC (RATIONALE-312): A Multicenter, Double-Blind, Placebo-Controlled, Randomized, Phase 3 Clinical Trial. (China). (J Thorac Oncol. 2024)[33]

- o *Population:* Patients with previously untreated extensive-stage SCLC. (n=457)
- o *Intervention:* Tislelizumab 200 mg plus chemotherapy (etoposide with carboplatin or cisplatin) every 3 weeks for four cycles, followed by tislelizumab maintenance. (n=227)
- o *Comparator:* Placebo plus chemotherapy (etoposide with carboplatin or cisplatin) every 3 weeks for four cycles, followed by placebo maintenance. (n=230)
- o *Outcome:* Tislelizumab plus chemotherapy showed a statistically significant improvement in overall survival (OS) with a median of 15.5 months compared to 13.5 months in the placebo group (HR = 0.75; p = 0.0040). Grade ≥3 treatment-related adverse events occurred in 86% of patients in both treatment arms.
- o *Conclusion*: Tislelizumab combined with chemotherapy offers a significant clinical benefit in OS as a first-line treatment for ES-SCLC.

b. Therapies for relapsed SCLC

i. RESILIENT Part 2: A Randomized, Open-Label Phase III Study of Liposomal Irinotecan Versus Topotecan in Adults with Relapsed Small Cell Lung Cancer. (J Clin Oncol. 2024)[34]

- o *Population:* Patients with SCLC who experienced progression after first-line platinum-based chemotherapy. (n=461)
- o *Intervention:* Intravenous (IV) liposomal irinotecan (70 mg/m² every 2 weeks in a 6-week cycle). (n=229)
- o *Comparator:* IV topotecan (1.5 mg/m² daily for 5 consecutive days, every 3 weeks in a 6-week cycle). (n=232)
- o *Outcome:* The median overall survival (OS) was 7.9 months with liposomal irinotecan versus 8.3 months with topotecan (HR, 1.11; P = .31). The ORR was 44.1% for liposomal irinotecan compared to 21.6% for topotecan. Grade ≥3 treatment-related adverse events occurred in 42.0% of the liposomal irinotecan group and 83.4% of the topotecan group.
- o *Conclusion*: Although OS was similar between the two groups, liposomal irinotecan showed a higher ORR and had a different safety profile compared to topotecan, with fewer severe adverse events.

DISCUSSION

NON-SMALL CELL LUNG CANCER (NSCLC)

(a) Adjuvant therapies for early-stage NSCLC (Stage I – IIIa)

Among patients with stage II - IIIA surgically resected NSCLC, adjuvant chemotherapy with four cycles of cisplatin-based doublet therapy has been a recommended practice because it prolongs 5-year overall survival (OS) by about 5%.[35] **Among patients with stage IB NSCLC, adjuvant chemotherapy is suggested by the National Comprehensive Cancer Network (NCCN) for patients with high-risk features, including vascular invasion, visceral pleural involvement, poorly differentiated histology, and an unknown nodal status.** However, adjuvant chemotherapy is not given to patients with stage IA NSCLC. **Available evidence shows that OS is similar between adjuvant and neoadjuvant approaches to chemotherapy among patients with surgically treated NSCLC.** However, a larger body of research is available for the adjuvant approach, which is consequently preferred.[35] Nonetheless, neoadjuvant chemotherapy is sometimes employed for resectable tumors with nodal involvement.

Over the last few years, several studies have examined targeted therapies and immunotherapies among patients with surgically treated NSCLC. **The ADAURA trial has shown that the epidermal growth factor receptor (EGFR) tyrosine kinase inhibitor (TKI), Osimertinib prolongs the disease-free survival (DFS) compared to placebo in the adjuvant setting for completely resected stage IB – IIIA NSCLC.**[36] Adjuvant chemotherapy was provided to patients before randomization according to the investigator's discretion in this trial. Hence, the **NCCN now recommends that among patients with negative margins following resection for stage IB – IIIA NSCLC with an EGFR exon 19 deletion or exon 21 L858R substitution, Osimertinib should be provided after adjuvant chemotherapy. Long-term use of osimertinib for up to three years is safe and well tolerated in this setting.**[37]

Other trials have compared EGFR TKIs directly with chemotherapy in the adjuvant setting. The **IMPACT trial** showed **gefitinib** prevented early relapse but did not prolong the DFS compared to chemotherapy.[38] In contrast, the **CTONG 1104 study** found that adjuvant gefitinib prolonged the DFS but not the OS compared to adjuvant chemotherapy.[39] The **EVIDENCE trial** conducted in China found that **icotinib** (administered for two years) prolonged the DFS compared to four cycles of chemotherapy in the adjuvant setting.[40] However, **neither gefitinib nor icotinib are approved in favor of adjuvant chemotherapy among patients with fully resected NSCLC by the NCCN. A recent study has shown that the use of alectinib for up to two years in completely resected stage Ib-IIIa, ALK-positive NSCLC substantially improved disease-free survival compared to four cycles of adjuvant chemotherapy.**[11]

The use of immunotherapy has been successfully studied in resectable NSCLC in the neoadjuvant and adjuvant settings, as well as in a combination of these two settings (i.e., perioperative immunotherapy). In the neoadjuvant setting, the combination of nivolumab with chemotherapy has been found to prolong the event-free survival (EFS) compared to chemotherapy alone among patients with NSCLC.[41] Based on this trial, the **NCCN has recommended the use of neoadjuvant nivolumab with chemotherapy for resectable NSCLC with a tumour size greater than 4 cm or positive nodal status.**

Immunotherapy agents have also been recommended by the NCCN in addition to chemotherapy in the adjuvant setting for patients with completely resected stage IIA - IIIA NSCLC without an EGFR exon 19 deletion or L858R substitution. These include pembrolizumab (irrespective of PD-L1 expression level) and atezolizumab (for PD-L1 expression ≥ 1%). The recent KEYNOTE-091 trial results support the recommendation for pembrolizumab.[42] This trial showed that up to 18 cycles of adjuvant pembrolizumab following guideline-directed adjuvant chemotherapy prolonged the DFS compared to placebo, irrespective of the PD-L1 tumor proportion score (TPS).

Over the last year, several publications have supported the benefits of perioperative immunotherapy. In these trials, four cycles of three-weekly immunotherapy agents and chemotherapy have been given in the neoadjuvant setting, followed by surgery and adjuvant immunotherapy of approximately one year). These studies have demonstrated superior disease-free survival with the combined use of chemotherapy with pembrolizumab (24-month DFS), nivolumab (12-month DFS), and durvalumab (12-month DFS) compared to placebo.[6-8]

(b) Genotype-directed therapies for advanced NSCLC (EGFR alterations)

Among patients with advanced non-squamous NSCLC, certain driver alterations allow targeted therapies to be used. EGFR was the first driver alteration against which targeted TKIs were developed. Hence, **NCCN recommended that among patients with advanced NSCLC with an EGFR exon 19 deletion or exon 21 L858R point mutation, first-line TKIs, including osimertinib, afatinib, gefitinib, erlotinib, and dacomitinib can be used as monotherapy**. These therapies have been found to prolong progression-free survival (PFS) compared to chemotherapy. **Among these agents, osimertinib may be preferable based on the results of the FLAURA trial.**[43] In this study, compared to other standard EGFR-TKIs, the use of osimertinib was associated with a superior PFS (18.9 vs 10.2 months; HR = 0.46, 95% CI = 0.37 – 0.57).

In the recently published FLAURA-2 trial 13, it has been shown that a combination of osimertinib with four cycles of platinum doublet chemotherapy may further prolong the PFS compared to osimertinib alone (24.0 vs 15.3 months; HR = 0.62, 95% CI = 0.49 – 0.79). **A combination of amivantamab and Lazertinib has also emerged as a first-line therapy for EGFR-mutated (exon 19 deletion or exon 21 L858R point mutation) lung cancer based on increased PFS compared to osimertinib alone in the MARIPOSA-1 trial.**[44] In the GAP Brain trial, the combination of chemotherapy with gefitinib among patients with intracranial metastasis resulted in superior PFS and OS compared with gefitinib alone.[45] However, combinations of chemotherapy with TKIs are associated with increased toxicity compared to TKIs alone.

The **ARCHER 1050 trial** has shown that **first-line dacomitinib is superior to gefitinib** in improving OS among patients with EGFR exon 19 deletion or exon 21 L858R substitution.[46] However, patients with brain metastasis were excluded from this trial, unlike the FLAURA trial. Furthermore, there is no head-to-head phase III RCT comparing dacomitinib with osimertinib. Hence, **the third-generation TKI, osimertinib, continues to be preferred in this setting. Lazertinib is another third-generation TKI that has recently shown remarkable benefit in PFS as a monotherapy compared to gefinitib (20.6 vs 9.7 months; HR = 0.45, p < 0.001).**[14]

Novel EGFR-TKIs including furmonertinib and aumolertinib have been compared to gefitinib in studies conducted in China.[47,48] Both furmonertinib and aumolertinib have been found to have better PFS than gefitinib in the first-line treatment of EGFR-mutated NSCLC. However, these drugs have limited availability, have not been tested in international multi-center studies, and are not recommended by the NCCN.

The addition of bevacizumab (vascular endothelial growth factor inhibitor) or placebo to erlotinib in the first-line treatment of non-squamous NSCLC with EGFR exon 19 deletion or exon 21 L858R point mutation has been studied in the Italian **BEVERLY trial and the Japanese NEJ026 trial.**[49,50] Both trials have shown that the addition of bevacizumab resulted in a superior PFS. Hence, the **NCCN has recommended the combination of erlotinib with bevacizumab as an acceptable first-line treatment in this setting. However, the comparative efficacy of this regimen against osimertinib is unknown.**

Other first-line combination regimens incorporating EGFR TKIs have been explored. The CTONG1706 study from China added apatinib (a vascular endothelial growth factor receptor-2 TKI) or placebo to gefitinib in advanced EGFR-mutated NSCLC.[51] It was found that the addition of apatinib prolonged the PFS. Results of apatinib from international trials are needed before it can be used widely.

Among patients with EGFR exon 19 deletion or exon 21 L858R point mutation who develop progressive disease on an EGFR TKI (other than osimertinib) and are found to have a T790M mutation at the time of progression, osimertinib has been found to have a benefit over chemotherapy as second-line therapy.[52] In other cases, patients should be considered for chemotherapy or immunotherapy on progression. In cases with progression on osimertinib, a recent trial has studied the addition of amivantamab with or without Lazertinib to chemotherapy for second-line therapy. They found superior PFS with amivantamab-lazertinib-chemotherapy (8.3 months, HR – 0.44, $p < 0.001$) and amivantamab-chemotherapy (6.3 months, HR – 0.48, $p < 0.001$) compared to chemotherapy alone (6.3 months).[15]

While most patients with EGFR alterations harbor the exon 19 deletion or exon 21 L858R point mutation, various rare EGFR mutations have been described (e.g., S768I mutation, L861Q mutation, and G719X mutation). **Among patients with these rare alterations, first line afatinib may have better efficacy compared to other TKIs.**[53] **Meanwhile, among patients with an EGFR exon 20 insertion, a phase III trial has found superior PFS with a combination of amivantamab and chemotherapy compared to chemotherapy alone in the first-line setting (11.4 months vs 6.7 months; HR: 0.40; 95% CI, 0.30 to 0.53; P<0.001).**[16]

The newly published LAURA trial has also validated the role of osimertinib as a maintenance therapy following chemoradiotherapy among patients with unresectable stage III EGFR-mutated NSCLC. In this trial, osimertinib prolonged PFS compared to placebo (39.1 vs 5.6 months; HR: 0.16; 95% CI, 0.10 to 0.24; p<0.001).[17]

(c) Genotype-directed therapies for advanced NSCLC (ALK fusions)

According to international data, ALK-rearranged NSCLC represents 4-5% of all metastatic NSCLC.[54] **However, in a meta-analysis of Indian literature, the pooled prevalence of ALK was 8.3% among NSCLC patients.**[55] The ALK gene rearrangement makes this subgroup of tumors highly susceptible to drugs inhibiting the ALK pathway. The FDA has approved the following TKIs for the management of ALK-rearranged metastatic NSCLC: **crizotinib** (first generation), **ceritinib** (second generation), **alectinib** (second generation), **brigatinib** (second generation), **ensartinib (second generation),** and **lorlatinib** (third generation). Crizotinib and ceritinib were found to improve overall response rates and prolong PFS in comparison to conventional chemotherapy in the first-line setting in the PROFILE-1014 and the ASCEND-4 trials, respectively.[56,57] **Alectinib, brigatinib, and lorlatinib have been found to bestow PFS benefit in the ALEX, ALTA-1L, and CROWN trials, respectively, with crizotinib being the comparator arm in each trial.**[58-60] **Ensartinib is another second-generation ALK TKI that was found to prolong PFS in comparison to crizotinib** in the eXalt3 trial conducted in China.[61] Other ALK TKIs recently found to provide superior PFS compared to crizotinib in phase III trials from China include iruplinalkib and envonalkib.[62,63] **Although crizotinib has poor efficacy for the control of CNS disease, the remaining drugs have high CNS overall response rates.**

While Phase III RCTs have shown ceritinib and alectinib to be superior to chemotherapy in later lines, lorlatinib and brigatinib have been found effective in the later-line setting in smaller single-arm trials.[64-67] Further, the recent ALTA-3 trial showed that second-line brigatinib and alectinib yield similar PFS following progression on crizotinib (19.3 vs 19.2 months).[18] The ESMO guidelines allow for flexibility in the sequencing of TKIs with allowance for first-line treatment with first, second, or third-generation drugs. However, **preference is given to second or third-generation TKIs in the NCCN guidelines. Following progression on first-line TKI, a subsequent generation TKI or chemotherapy may be administered. Repeat biopsy may be considered for testing for resistance mutations on progression.** The G1202R solvent front mutation is sensitive only to lorlatinib.

(d) Genotype-directed therapies for advanced NSCLC (other driver alterations)

Besides EGFR and ALK, there are several targetable driver mutations present among patients with NSCLC. However, besides KRAS, most of these mutations are seen infrequently. Hence, the recommendations of targeted therapies for these mutations are mainly based on phase I/II trials or case series. **A notable exception is the recently published phase III trial which showed superiority of selpercatinib against pembrolizumab-chemotherapy in prolonging PFS (24.8 vs 11.2 months,**

respectively; HR – 0.46, p < 0.001) in RET fusion-positive NSCLC.[20] A list of some of the key targeted therapies recommended for these mutations in the first line or subsequent line setting is presented in Table 1.

To date, no first-line targeted therapy has been approved for managing KRAS-mutated NSCLC. However, a recent phase III trial compared sotorasib with docetaxel in the subsequent line setting for progressive K-RAS mutated NSCLC.[68] In this study, sotorasib increased the PFS compared to docetaxel by a small but statistically significant margin (5.6 vs 4.5 months). Furthermore, sotorasib had lower toxicities compared to docetaxel. Hence, **sotorasib has been recommended in the subsequent-line setting for K-RAS mutated NSCLC by the NCCN.**

Table 1: A list of targeted therapies for driver alterations other than EGFR and ALK among patients with advanced NSCLC

Driver mutation	First line therapy	Subsequent line therapy
ROS1 rearrangement	**entrectinib, repotrectinib,** crizotinib	lorlatinib, entrectinib
NTRK gene fusion	larotrectinib, entrectinib, **repotrectinib**	larotrectinib, entrectinib, **repotrectinib**
MET exon 14 skipping mutation	Capmatinib, tepotinib, **(crizotinib - off-label)**	Capmatinib, tepotinib, **(crizotinib-off-label)**
RET rearrangement	Selpercatinib, pralsetinib	Selpercatinib, pralsetinib
MET amplification	-	**Capmatinib (off-label), crizotinib (off-label)**
KRAS G12C mutation	-	Sotorasib, adagrasib
BRAF V600E mutation	**dabrafenib plus trametinib, encorafenib plus binimetinib**	**dabrafenib plus trametinib, encorafenib plus binimetinib**
HER2 mutation	-	Fam-trastuzumab deruxtecan **(also HER2 amplification),** ado-trastuzumab emtansine

List of targeted therapies for advanced NSCLC is continuously evolving. Please check the NCCN guidelines for the latest guidance.

(e) Immunotherapies for advanced NSCLC in first-line setting

Immunotherapy is a treatment modality that leverages the body's immune system to fight against tumor cells. In the context of lung cancer, most immunotherapy agents act on either the programmed cell death protein-1 (PD-1), a cell surface protein on lymphocytes, or its ligand (PD-L1), found in cancer cells. Since the PD-1/PD-L1 interaction prevents the immune response of lymphocytes on tumor cells, the inhibition of this axis is attempted. Over the past decade, several PD-1 and PD-L1 inhibitors have been tried in both squamous and non-squamous NSCLC lacking a targetable driver alteration. The level of PD-L1 expression influences the efficacy of immunotherapy agents in NSCLC. It is described as a percentage in terms of the tumor proportion score (TPS). **Patients with a PD-L1 TPS ≥ 50% may be treated with either single-agent immunotherapy or a combination of immunotherapy and chemotherapy. The latter option is preferred among patients with a high tumor burden or rapidly progressive disease. Patients with a PD-L1 TPS < 50% are usually treated with a combination of immunotherapy and chemotherapy.** Irrespective of whether immunotherapy is given as monotherapy or in combination with chemotherapy, the immunotherapy agent is generally continued till disease progression or unmanageable toxicity or until completion of at least 2 years. The summary of the preferred and alternative agents, as suggested by NCCN, is provided in Table 2.

In the case of monotherapy among patients with PD-L1 TPS ≥ 50%, pembrolizumab was approved based on a trial that showed it had a superior median OS (26.3 vs 13.4 months) and 5-year OS (31.9% vs 16.3%) compared to chemotherapy in this setting.[69] Other single-agent immunotherapy drugs which have been found to prolong OS compared with chemotherapy include cemiplimab and atezolizumab.[26,70,71]

Among patients with a PD-L1 TPS < 50% or an unknown PD-L1 expression, a combination of pembrolizumab with chemotherapy is the preferred treatment. This recommendation is based on the results of the KEYNOTE-407 trial, which found that the combination of pembrolizumab and chemotherapy prolonged the PFS and OS compared to chemotherapy alone, regardless of the PD-L1 expression.[72] Recently, the combinations of chemotherapy with cemiplimab

(EMPOWER-Lung 3 study) and durvalumab-tremelimumab **(POSEIDON study)** have been found to prolong OS compared with chemotherapy alone in metastatic NSCLC irrespective of PD-L1 levels.[73,74] Hence, **combinations of cemiplimab and durvalumab-tremelimumab with chemotherapy have been approved by the Food & Drug Administration (FDA) and recommended by NCCN in this setting.** Furthermore, a combination of nivolumab, ipilimumab, and chemotherapy has been found to prolong the OS at 4-year follow-up compared to chemotherapy alone in the first-line setting.[22]

The choice of chemotherapy in the aforementioned regimens depends on the histology of the tumour. For non-squamous NSCLC, a combination of carboplatin and pemetrexed is used. For squamous NSCLC, a combination of carboplatin and a taxane (paclitaxel or nanoparticle albumin bound paclitaxel [nab-paclitaxel]) is given.

Among patients with metastatic non-squamous NSCLC, the combination of atezolizumab, bevacizumab and chemotherapy has been found to prolong the PFS and OS compared to bevacizumab and chemotherapy alone.[75] However, the combination of atezolizumab with carboplatin and pemetrexed has not shown to provide OS benefit in these patients.[76] **The recent Tasuki-52 trial conducted in East Asian countries has found OS benefit with the combination of nivolumab, bevacizumab and chemotherapy compared to placebo, bevacizumab, and chemotherapy in metastatic non-squamous NSCLC.**[23]

Other immunotherapy agents that have been found to have PFS benefits in combination with chemotherapy irrespective of PD-L1 expression in metastatic NSCLC include camrelizumab, tislelizumab, sugemalimab, toripalimab, sintilimab, and penpulimab.[77-85] **Most of these agents have been studied in China and have not been included in the NCCN guidelines.**

A chemotherapy-free regimen that has been tried among advanced NSCLC patients irrespective of PD-L1 expression is the combination of immunotherapy agents, nivolumab and ipilimumab. Unlike other immunotherapy drugs which act of PD-1 or PD-L1, ipilimumab acts as a cytotoxic T-lymphocyte antigen-4 (CTLA-4) inhibitor. In the CheckMate 227 trial, this combination was found to result in superior PFS and OS compared to chemotherapy, irrespective of the PD-L1 TPS.[86]

Table 2: Selected list of first-line immunotherapy agents for advanced NSCLC lacking a targetable driver mutation

Non-squamous NSCLC		Squamous NSCLC	
PD-L1 > 50%	**PD-L1 < 50%**	**PD-L1 > 50%**	**PD-L1 < 50%**
-Pembrolizumab -Atezolizumab -Cemiplimab -Pembrolizumab + chemotherapy	Pembrolizumab + chemotherapy	-Pembrolizumab -Atezolizumab -Cemiplimab -Pembrolizumab + chemotherapy	Pembrolizumab + chemotherapy

List is non-exhaustive, refer to NCCN guidelines for a comprehensive list of alternative regimens

(f) Immunotherapies for advanced NSCLC in subsequent line settings

Among patients with advanced NSCLC who progress on non-immunotherapy-containing regimens, the use of immunotherapy as a subsequent-line treatment has been found useful in various studies. In the CheckMate 078 study, nivolumab was compared to docetaxel in previously treated NSCLC and was found to significantly prolong the median OS (11.9 vs 9.5 months) irrespective of PD-L1 TPS.[87] In the phase III OAK study, atezolizumab was found to be significantly better than docetaxel in prolonging OS (13.3 vs 9.8 months) in previously treated NSCLC regardless of PD-L1 expression. In the KEYNOTE-010 study, among NSCLC patients with PD-L1 TPS $\geq$ 1%, the use of subsequent-line pembrolizumab was found to result in superior 5-year OS compared to docetaxel (15.6% vs 6.5%).[88] Based on these results, the NCCN recommends the use of nivolumab (any PD-L1 level), atezolizumab (any PD-L1 level), and pembrolizumab (PD-L1 $\geq$ 1%) in progressive NSCLC not previously treated with immunotherapy. Additional immunotherapy agents that have been found to prolong the OS compared to docetaxel in the subsequent-line setting are sintilimab (ORIENT-3 study) and tislelizumab (RATIONALE-303 study).[89,90] In **the setting of EGFR or ALK-mutated NSCLC with progression on TKI, the use of chemotherapy combined with atezolizumab-bevacizumab has**

been found to prolong the PFS compared to chemotherapy (8.5 vs 5.6 months, respectively).[27] However, the combination of chemotherapy with nivolumab was not found to prolong the PFS compared to chemotherapy alone.[28]

A special setting wherein immunotherapy has been found beneficial as a maintenance treatment is among patients with unresectable stage III NSCLC following chemoradiotherapy. In the PACIFIC trial, durvalumab (given for 1 year) was found to result in a better 5-year OS compared to placebo (42.9% vs 33.4%) following chemoradiotherapy in stage III NSCLC.[91]

(g) Other therapies in advanced NSCLC

The poly (ADP-ribose) polymerase (PARP) inhibitors act by preventing DNA repair in tumour cells and have been approved for treating ovarian and breast cancer. The PARP inhibitor, veliparib has been studied in combination with chemotherapy in advanced NSCLC but has not been found to result in OS benefit.[92,93] Further research is needed before the role of PARP inhibitors in lung cancer management is established.

SMALL CELL LUNG CANCER (SCLC)

(a) Initial and maintenance therapies for SCLC

SCLC is staged as a limited stage or extensive stage SCLC for therapeutic decision-making. Limited stage SCLC (LC-SCLC) refers to non-metastatic SCLC (any T/any N/M0) which can be encompassed within a single radiation field; a disease that is metastatic or localized but spreading beyond a single radiation field is referred to as extensive stage disease.

The NCCN and ESMO guidelines endorse surgical management for patients with early T1-2N0 SCLC. NCCN allows consideration for stereotactic body radiotherapy in place of surgery in patients who are medically unfit for surgery. Before surgery, mediastinal staging is essential. **Following surgery, adjuvant chemotherapy is to be given to all patients.[94] Four cycles of a regimen using cisplatin and etoposide is preferred.** The use of carboplatin was found to confer similar survival benefit in a meta-analysis.[95] In patients found to have N1/N2 disease or have postoperative surgical margins positive, concurrent cisplatin-etoposide-based chemoradiotherapy is preferred.[96] **Patients who are frail or unfit for concurrent chemoradiotherapy may be considered for sequential chemoradiotherapy.**

Patients with extensive-stage SCLC (EC-SCLC) are managed primarily with chemotherapy. The first-line regimen comprises four to six cycles of cisplatin or carboplatin and etoposide. The addition of atezolizumab or durvalumab along with chemotherapy followed by maintenance immunotherapy has been seen to prolong overall survival in the Impower133 and CASPIAN trials, respectively, and may be considered in patients who can access these drugs.[97,98] **The use of novel immunotherapeutic agents adebrelimab, serplulimab, and tislelizumab in combination with chemotherapy have been found to confer survival benefit in recent Chinese randomised trials; however, further confirmation of their efficacy in different populations may be required before the incorporation of these drugs into practice in ES-SCLC.[33,99,100]**

Both the NCCN and ESMO guidelines recommend that patients with LS-SCLC who have completed adjuvant systemic and local therapy and patients with ES-SCLC who have a complete or partial response to systemic therapy may be considered for prophylactic cranial irradiation (PCI). However, the role of PCI in early-stage T1-2N0 tumors is controversial. Data from a recent randomized trial suggests that there may not be a role for PCI if baseline and follow-up MRI scans are used for surveillance for CNS spread.[101] Thus, regular MRI follow-up may be an option for patients not considered for PCI. Patients with ES-SCLC with response to systemic therapy may also be considered for consolidative thoracic radiotherapy.

(b) Therapies for relapsed SCLC

Patients with relapsed SCLC may be categorised into platinum-sensitive disease (response with platinum-based therapy lasting more than three months), platinum-resistant disease (response with platinum-based therapy lasting less than three months) and platinum-refractory disease (disease progressing on platinum-based chemotherapy).

Patients with platinum sensitive disease may be considered for rechallenge with platinum-etoposide. This approach was found to improve survival in comparison with topotecan in a randomised trial. Patients with platinum-resistant or refractory disease may be treated with second line chemotherapy using topotecan or lurbinectedin based on ESMO and NCCN recommendations. Topotecan was found to improve overall survival in comparison to best supportive care and was non-inferior to a multi-drug regimen using cyclophosphamide, doxorubicin, and vincristine.[102] Meanwhile, a recent trial showed similar efficacy with liposomal irinotecan and topotecan in this setting, however with lower toxicity in the liposomal irinotecan arm.[34] Lurbinectedin was found to have impressive responsive rates of 45% and 22.2% in the platinum-sensitive and platinum-resistant settings respectively in a single-arm phase II trial in patients with relapsed ES-SCLC.[103] **Immunotherapeutic strategies have had poor response rates and have not been found superior to traditional chemotherapy in maintenance or subsequent-line settings in ES-SCLC.**[104-107]

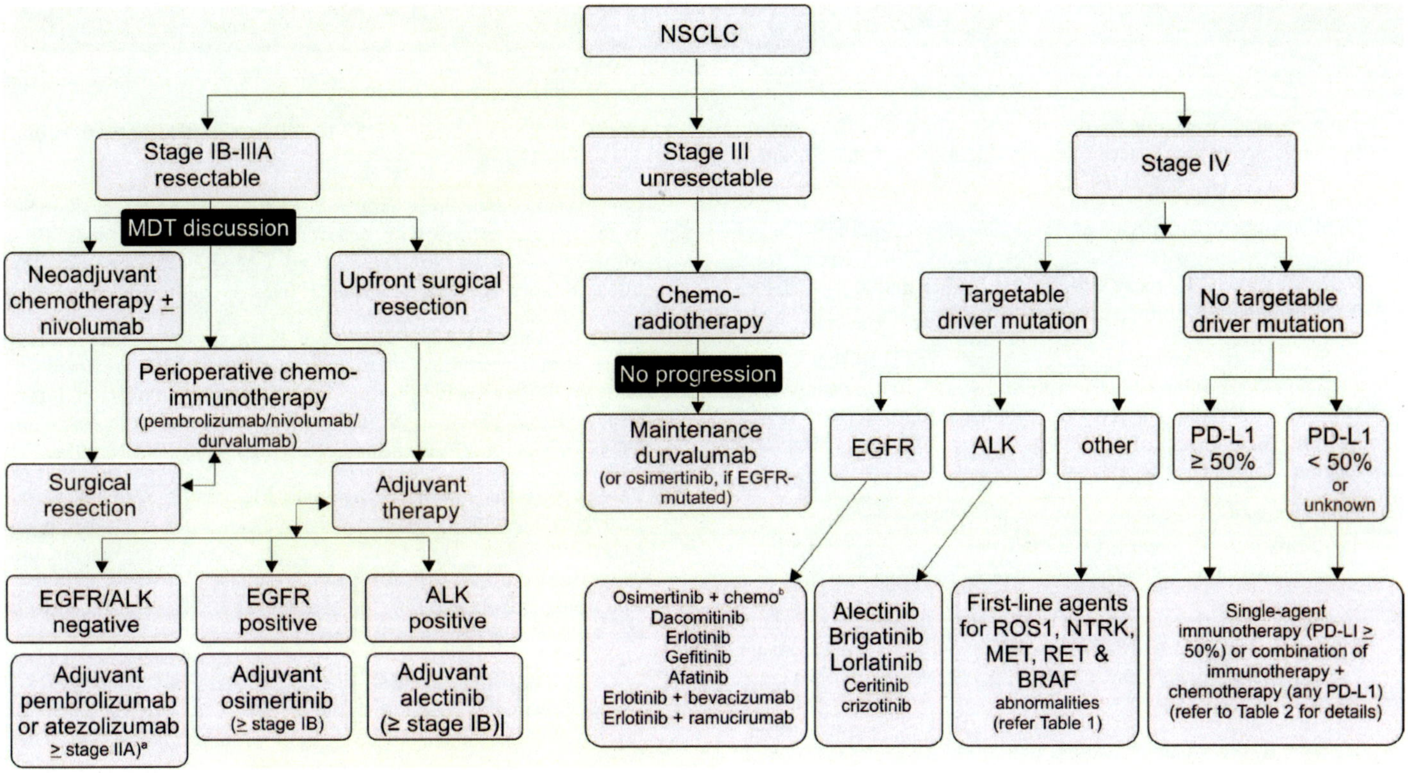

Figure 1: Simplified general algorithm for the first line management of non-small cell lung cancer (please refer to NCCN guidelines for detailed guidance for each step)

[a] Adjuvant pembrolizumab can be given irrespective of PD-L1 level and adjuvant atezolizumab can be given for PD-L1 ≥ 1%.
[b] The preferred agent

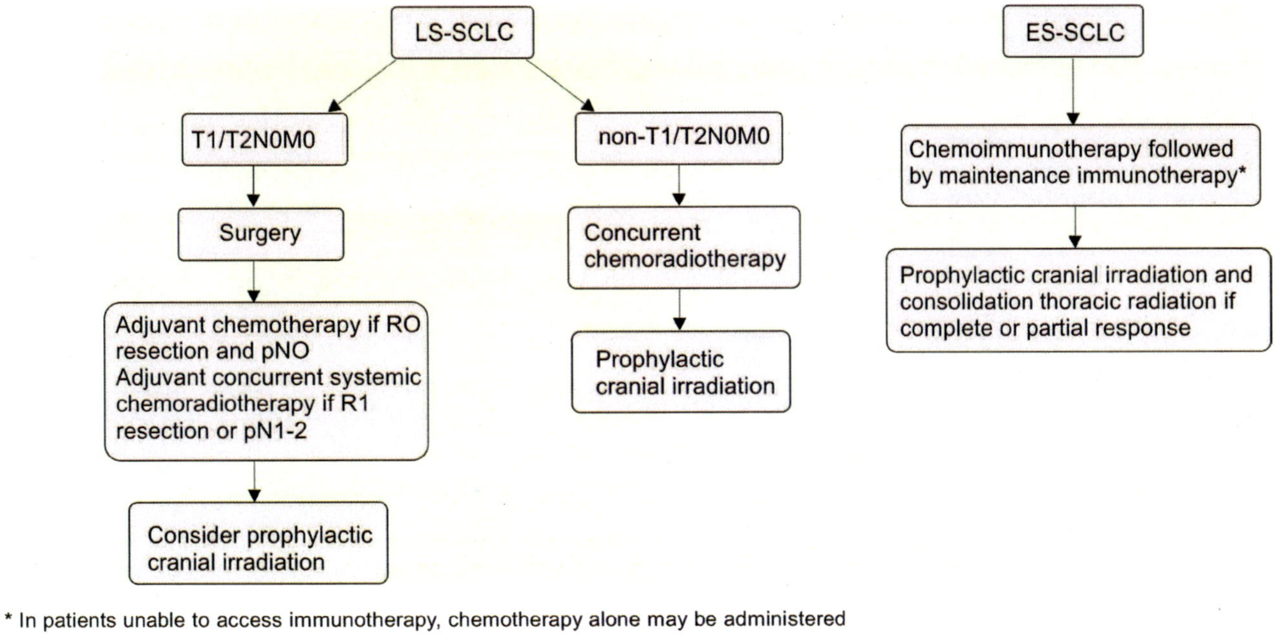

Figure 2: Simplified general algorithm for the first line management of small cell lung cancer (please refer to NCCN guidelines for detailed guidance for each step)

REFERENCES

1. Thandra KC, Barsouk A, Saginala K, Aluru JS, Barsouk A. Epidemiology of lung cancer. Contemp Oncol 2021;25:45–52. https://doi.org/10.5114/wo.2021.103829.

2. Sathishkumar K, Chaturvedi M, Das P, Stephen S, Mathur P. Cancer incidence estimates for 2022 & projection for 2025: Result from National Cancer Registry Programme, India. Indian J Med Res 2022;156:598–607. https://doi.org/10.4103/ijmr.ijmr_1821_22.

3. Mohan A, Garg A, Gupta A, Sahu S, Choudhari C, Vashistha V, et al. Clinical profile of lung cancer in North India: A 10-year analysis of 1862 patients from a tertiary care center. Lung India Off Organ Indian Chest Soc 2020;37:190–7. https://doi.org/10.4103/lungindia.lungindia_333_19.

4. Lung Cancer Survival Rates | 5-Year Survival Rates for Lung Cancer n.d. https://www.cancer.org/cancer/types/lung-cancer/detection-diagnosis-staging/survival-rates.html (accessed May 5, 2023).

5. Howlader N, Forjaz G, Mooradian MJ, Meza R, Kong CY, Cronin KA, et al. The Effect of Advances in Lung-Cancer Treatment on Population Mortality. N Engl J Med 2020;383:640–9. https://doi.org/10.1056/NEJMoa1916623.

6. Wakelee H, Liberman M, Kato T, Tsuboi M, Lee S-H, Gao S, et al. Perioperative Pembrolizumab for Early-Stage Non-Small-Cell Lung Cancer. N Engl J Med 2023;389:491–503. https://doi.org/10.1056/NEJMoa2302983.

7. Cascone T, Awad MM, Spicer JD, He J, Lu S, Sepesi B, et al. Perioperative Nivolumab in Resectable Lung Cancer. N Engl J Med 2024;390:1756–69. https://doi.org/10.1056/NEJMoa2311926.

8. Heymach JV, Harpole D, Mitsudomi T, Taube JM, Galffy G, Hochmair M, et al. Perioperative Durvalumab for Resectable Non-Small-Cell Lung Cancer. N Engl J Med 2023;389:1672–84. https://doi.org/10.1056/NEJMoa2304875.

9. Felip E, Altorki N, Zhou C, Vallières E, Martínez-Martí A, Rittmeyer A, et al. Overall survival with adjuvant atezolizumab after chemotherapy in resected stage II-IIIA non-small-cell lung cancer (IMpower010): a randomised, multicentre, open-label, phase III trial. Ann Oncol Off J Eur Soc Med Oncol 2023;34:907–19. https://doi.org/10.1016/j.annonc.2023.07.001.

10. Lu S, Zhang W, Wu L, Wang W, Zhang P, Fang W, et al. Perioperative Toripalimab Plus Chemotherapy for Patients With Resectable Non-Small Cell Lung Cancer: The Neotorch Randomized Clinical Trial. JAMA 2024;331:201–11. https://doi.org/10.1001/jama.2023.24735.

11. Wu Y-L, Dziadziuszko R, Ahn JS, Barlesi F, Nishio M, Lee DH, et al. Alectinib in Resected ALK-Positive Non-Small-Cell Lung Cancer. N Engl J Med 2024;390:1265–76. https://doi.org/10.1056/NEJMoa2310532.

12. Kenmotsu H, Yamamoto N, Misumi T, Yoh K, Saito H, Sugawara S, et al. Five-Year Overall Survival Analysis of the JIPANG Study: Pemetrexed or Vinorelbine Plus Cisplatin for Resected Stage II-IIIA Nonsquamous Non-Small-Cell Lung Cancer. J Clin Oncol Off J Am Soc Clin Oncol 2023;41:5242–6. https://doi.org/10.1200/JCO.23.00179.

13. Planchard D, Jänne PA, Cheng Y, Yang JC-H, Yanagitani N, Kim S-W, et al. Osimertinib with or without Chemotherapy in EGFR-Mutated Advanced NSCLC. N Engl J Med 2023;389:1935–48. https://doi.org/10.1056/NEJMoa2306434.

14. Cho BC, Ahn M-J, Kang JH, Soo RA, Reungwetwattana T, Yang JC-H, et al. Lazertinib Versus Gefitinib as First-Line Treatment in Patients With EGFR-Mutated Advanced Non-Small-Cell Lung Cancer: Results From LASER301. J Clin Oncol Off J Am Soc Clin Oncol 2023;41:4208–17. https://doi.org/10.1200/JCO.23.00515.

15. Passaro A, Wang J, Wang Y, Lee S-H, Melosky B, Shih J-Y, et al. Amivantamab plus chemotherapy with and without lazertinib in EGFR-mutant advanced NSCLC after disease progression on osimertinib: primary results from the phase III MARIPOSA-2 study. Ann Oncol Off J Eur Soc Med Oncol 2024;35:77–90. https://doi.org/10.1016/j.annonc.2023.10.117.

16. Zhou C, Tang K-J, Cho BC, Liu B, Paz-Ares L, Cheng S, et al. Amivantamab plus Chemotherapy in NSCLC with EGFR Exon 20 Insertions. N Engl J Med 2023;389:2039–51. https://doi.org/10.1056/NEJMoa2306441.

17. Lu S, Kato T, Dong X, Ahn M-J, Quang L-V, Soparattanapaisarn N, et al. Osimertinib after Chemoradiotherapy in Stage III EGFR-Mutated NSCLC. N Engl J Med 2024;391:585–97. https://doi.org/10.1056/NEJMoa2402614.

18. Yang JC-H, Liu G, Lu S, He J, Burotto M, Ahn M-J, et al. Brigatinib Versus Alectinib in ALK-Positive NSCLC After Disease Progression on Crizotinib: Results of Phase 3 ALTA-3 Trial. J Thorac Oncol Off Publ Int Assoc Study Lung Cancer 2023;18:1743–55. https://doi.org/10.1016/j.jtho.2023.08.010.

19. Peters S, Gadgeel SM, Mok T, Nadal E, Kilickap S, Swalduz A, et al. Entrectinib in ROS1-positive advanced non-small cell lung cancer: the phase 2/3 BFAST trial. Nat Med 2024;30:1923–32. https://doi.org/10.1038/s41591-024-03008-4.

20. Zhou C, Solomon B, Loong HH, Park K, Pérol M, Arriola E, et al. First-Line Selpercatinib or Chemotherapy and Pembrolizumab in RET Fusion-Positive NSCLC. N Engl J Med 2023;389:1839–50. https://doi.org/10.1056/NEJMoa2309457.

21. Borghaei H, O'Byrne KJ, Paz-Ares L, Ciuleanu T-E, Yu X, Pluzanski A, et al. Nivolumab plus chemotherapy in first-line metastatic non-small-cell lung cancer: results of the phase III CheckMate 227 Part 2 trial. ESMO Open 2023;8:102065. https://doi.org/10.1016/j.esmoop.2023.102065.

22. Carbone DP, Ciuleanu T-E, Schenker M, Cobo M, Bordenave S, Juan-Vidal O, et al. Four-year clinical update and treatment switching-adjusted outcomes with first-line nivolumab plus ipilimumab with chemotherapy for metastatic non-small cell lung cancer in the CheckMate 9LA randomized trial. J Immunother Cancer 2024;12. https://doi.org/10.1136/jitc-2023-008189.

23. Kim HR, Sugawara S, Lee J-S, Kang J-H, Inui N, Hida T, et al. First-line nivolumab, paclitaxel, carboplatin, and bevacizumab for advanced non-squamous non-small cell lung cancer: Updated survival analysis of the ONO-4538-52/TASUKI-52 randomized controlled trial. Cancer Med 2023;12:17061–7. https://doi.org/10.1002/cam4.6348.

24. Lee SM, Schulz C, Prabhash K, Kowalski D, Szczesna A, Han B, et al. First-line atezolizumab monotherapy versus single-agent chemotherapy in patients with non-small-cell lung cancer ineligible for treatment with a platinum-containing regimen (IPSOS): a phase 3, global, multicentre, open-label, randomised controlled study. Lancet Lond Engl 2023;402:451–63. https://doi.org/10.1016/S0140-6736(23)00774-2.

25. Reck M, Barlesi F, Yang JC-H, Westeel V, Felip E, Özgüroðlu M, et al. Avelumab Versus Platinum-Based Doublet Chemotherapy as First-Line Treatment for Patients With High-Expression Programmed Death-Ligand 1-Positive Metastatic NSCLC: Primary Analysis From the Phase 3 JAVELIN Lung 100 Trial. J Thorac Oncol Off Publ Int Assoc Study Lung Cancer 2024;19:297–313. https://doi.org/10.1016/j.jtho.2023.09.1445.

26. Özgüroðlu M, Kilickap S, Sezer A, Gümüþ M, Bondarenko I, Gogishvili M, et al. First-line cemiplimab monotherapy and continued cemiplimab beyond progression plus chemotherapy for advanced non-small-cell lung cancer with PD-L1 50% or more (EMPOWER-Lung 1): 35-month follow-up from a mutlicentre, open-label, randomised, phase 3 trial. Lancet Oncol 2023;24:989–1001. https://doi.org/10.1016/S1470-2045(23)00329-7.

27. Park S, Kim TM, Han J-Y, Lee G-W, Shim BY, Lee Y-G, et al. Phase III, Randomized Study of Atezolizumab Plus Bevacizumab and Chemotherapy in Patients With EGFR- or ALK-Mutated Non-Small-Cell Lung Cancer (ATTLAS, KCSG-LU19-04). J Clin Oncol Off J Am Soc Clin Oncol 2024;42:1241–51. https://doi.org/10.1200/JCO.23.01891.

28. Mok T, Nakagawa K, Park K, Ohe Y, Girard N, Kim HR, et al. Nivolumab Plus Chemotherapy in Epidermal Growth Factor Receptor-Mutated Metastatic Non-Small-Cell Lung Cancer After Disease Progression on Epidermal Growth Factor Receptor Tyrosine Kinase Inhibitors: Final Results of CheckMate 722. J Clin Oncol Off J Am Soc Clin Oncol 2024;42:1252–64. https://doi.org/10.1200/JCO.23.01017.

29. Ren S, Feng J, Ma S, Chen H, Ma Z, Huang C, et al. KEYNOTE-033: Randomized phase 3 study of pembrolizumab vs docetaxel in previously treated, PD-L1-positive, advanced NSCLC. Int J Cancer 2023;153:623–34. https://doi.org/10.1002/ijc.34532.

30. Yang JC-H, Han B, De La Mora Jiménez E, Lee J-S, Koralewski P, Karadurmus N, et al. Pembrolizumab With or Without Lenvatinib for First-Line Metastatic NSCLC With Programmed Cell Death-Ligand 1 Tumor Proportion Score of at least 1% (LEAP-007): A Randomized, Double-Blind, Phase 3 Trial. J Thorac Oncol Off Publ Int Assoc Study Lung Cancer 2024;19:941–53. https://doi.org/10.1016/j.jtho.2023.12.023.

31. Shiraishi Y, Kishimoto J, Sugawara S, Mizutani H, Daga H, Azuma K, et al. Atezolizumab and Platinum Plus Pemetrexed With or Without Bevacizumab for Metastatic Nonsquamous Non-Small Cell Lung Cancer: A Phase 3 Randomized Clinical Trial. JAMA Oncol 2024;10:315–24. https://doi.org/10.1001/jamaoncol.2023.5258.

32. Bria E, Morgillo F, Garassino MC, Ciardiello F, Ardizzoni A, Stefani A, et al. Atezolizumab Plus Carboplatin and Etoposide in Patients with Untreated Extensive-Stage Small-Cell Lung Cancer: Interim Results of the MAURIS Phase IIIb Trial. The Oncologist 2024;29:e690–8. https://doi.org/10.1093/oncolo/oyad342.

33. Cheng Y, Fan Y, Zhao Y, Huang D, Li X, Zhang P, et al. Tislelizumab Plus Platinum and Etoposide Versus Placebo Plus Platinum and Etoposide as First-Line Treatment for Extensive-Stage SCLC (RATIONALE-312): A Multicenter, Double-Blind, Placebo-Controlled, Randomized, Phase 3 Clinical Trial. J Thorac Oncol Off Publ Int Assoc Study Lung Cancer 2024;19:1073–85. https://doi.org/10.1016/j.jtho.2024.03.008.

34. Spigel DR, Dowlati A, Chen Y, Navarro A, Yang JC-H, Stojanovic G, et al. RESILIENT Part 2: A Randomized, Open-Label Phase III Study of Liposomal Irinotecan Versus Topotecan in Adults With Relapsed Small Cell Lung Cancer. J Clin Oncol Off J Am Soc Clin Oncol 2024;42:2317–26. https://doi.org/10.1200/JCO.23.02110.

35. Postmus PE, Kerr KM, Oudkerk M, Senan S, Waller DA, Vansteenkiste J, et al. Early and locally advanced non-small-cell lung cancer (NSCLC): ESMO Clinical Practice Guidelines for diagnosis, treatment and follow-up. Ann Oncol Off J Eur Soc Med Oncol 2017;28:iv1–21. https://doi.org/10.1093/annonc/mdx222.

36. Herbst RS, Wu Y-L, John T, Grohe C, Majem M, Wang J, et al. Adjuvant Osimertinib for Resected EGFR-Mutated Stage IB-IIIA Non-Small-Cell Lung Cancer: Updated Results From the Phase III Randomized ADAURA Trial. J Clin Oncol Off J Am Soc Clin Oncol 2023;41:1830–40. https://doi.org/10.1200/JCO.22.02186.

37. John T, Grohé C, Goldman JW, Shepherd FA, de Marinis F, Kato T, et al. Three-Year Safety, Tolerability, and Health-Related Quality of Life Outcomes of Adjuvant Osimertinib in Patients With Resected Stage IB to IIIA EGFR-Mutated NSCLC: Updated Analysis From the Phase 3 ADAURA Trial. J Thorac Oncol Off Publ Int Assoc Study Lung Cancer 2023;18:1209–21. https://doi.org/10.1016/j.jtho.2023.05.015.

38. Tada H, Mitsudomi T, Misumi T, Sugio K, Tsuboi M, Okamoto I, et al. Randomized Phase III Study of Gefitinib Versus Cisplatin Plus Vinorelbine for Patients With Resected Stage II-IIIA Non-Small-Cell Lung Cancer With EGFR Mutation (IMPACT). J Clin Oncol Off J Am Soc Clin Oncol 2022;40:231–41. https://doi.org/10.1200/JCO.21.01729.

39. Zhong W-Z, Wang Q, Mao W-M, Xu S-T, Wu L, Wei Y-C, et al. Gefitinib Versus Vinorelbine Plus Cisplatin as Adjuvant Treatment for Stage II-IIIA (N1-N2) EGFR-Mutant NSCLC: Final Overall Survival Analysis of CTONG1104 Phase III Trial. J Clin Oncol Off J Am Soc Clin Oncol 2021;39:713–22. https://doi.org/10.1200/JCO.20.01820.

40. He J, Su C, Liang W, Xu S, Wu L, Fu X, et al. Icotinib versus chemotherapy as adjuvant treatment for stage II-IIIA EGFR-mutant non-small-cell lung cancer (EVIDENCE): a randomised, open-label, phase 3 trial. Lancet Respir Med 2021;9:1021–9. https://doi.org/10.1016/S2213-2600(21)00134-X.

41. Forde PM, Spicer J, Lu S, Provencio M, Mitsudomi T, Awad MM, et al. Neoadjuvant Nivolumab plus Chemotherapy in Resectable Lung Cancer. N Engl J Med 2022;386:1973–85. https://doi.org/10.1056/NEJMoa2202170.

42. O'Brien M, Paz-Ares L, Marreaud S, Dafni U, Oselin K, Havel L, et al. Pembrolizumab versus placebo as adjuvant therapy for completely resected stage IB-IIIA non-small-cell lung cancer (PEARLS/KEYNOTE-091): an interim analysis of a randomised, triple-blind, phase 3 trial. Lancet Oncol 2022;23:1274–86. https://doi.org/10.1016/S1470-2045(22)00518-6.

43. Soria J-C, Ohe Y, Vansteenkiste J, Reungwetwattana T, Chewaskulyong B, Lee KH, et al. Osimertinib in Untreated EGFR-Mutated Advanced Non–Small-Cell Lung Cancer. N Engl J Med 2018;378:113–25. https://doi.org/10.1056/NEJMoa1713137.

44. Cho BC, Lu S, Felip E, Spira AI, Girard N, Lee J-S, et al. Amivantamab plus Lazertinib in Previously Untreated EGFR-Mutated Advanced NSCLC. N Engl J Med n.d.;0. https://doi.org/10.1056/NEJMoa2403614.

45. Hou X, Li M, Wu G, Feng W, Su J, Jiang H, et al. Gefitinib Plus Chemotherapy vs Gefitinib Alone in Untreated EGFR-Mutant Non-Small Cell Lung Cancer in Patients With Brain Metastases: The GAP BRAIN Open-Label, Randomized, Multicenter, Phase 3 Study. JAMA Netw Open 2023;6:e2255050. https://doi.org/10.1001/jamanetworkopen.2022.55050.

46. Mok TS, Cheng Y, Zhou X, Lee KH, Nakagawa K, Niho S, et al. Updated Overall Survival in a Randomized Study Comparing Dacomitinib with Gefitinib as First-Line Treatment in Patients with Advanced Non-Small-Cell Lung Cancer and EGFR-Activating Mutations. Drugs 2021;81:257–66. https://doi.org/10.1007/s40265-020-01441-6.

47. Shi Y, Chen G, Wang X, Liu Y, Wu L, Hao Y, et al. Furmonertinib (AST2818) versus gefitinib as first-line therapy for Chinese patients with locally advanced or metastatic EGFR mutation-positive non-small-cell lung cancer (FURLONG): a multicentre, double-blind, randomised phase 3 study. Lancet Respir Med 2022;10:1019–28. https://doi.org/10.1016/S2213-2600(22)00168-0.

48. Lu S, Dong X, Jian H, Chen J, Chen G, Sun Y, et al. AENEAS: A Randomized Phase III Trial of Aumolertinib Versus Gefitinib as First-Line Therapy for Locally Advanced or MetastaticNon-Small-Cell Lung Cancer With EGFR Exon 19 Deletion or L858R Mutations. J Clin Oncol Off J Am Soc Clin Oncol 2022;40:3162–71. https://doi.org/10.1200/JCO.21.02641.

49. Piccirillo MC, Bonanno L, Garassino MC, Esposito G, Dazzi C, Cavanna L, et al. Addition of Bevacizumab to Erlotinib as First-Line Treatment of Patients With EGFR-Mutated Advanced Non-squamous NSCLC: The BEVERLY Multicenter Randomized Phase 3 Trial. J Thorac Oncol Off Publ Int Assoc Study Lung Cancer 2022;17:1086–97. https://doi.org/10.1016/j.jtho.2022. 05.008.

50. Kawashima Y, Fukuhara T, Saito H, Furuya N, Watanabe K, Sugawara S, et al. Bevacizumab plus erlotinib versus erlotinib alone in Japanese patients with advanced, metastatic, EGFR-mutant non-small-cell lung cancer (NEJ026): overall survival analysis of an open-label, randomised, multicentre, phase 3 trial. Lancet Respir Med 2022;10:72–82. https://doi.org/10.1016/S2213-2600(21)00166-1.

51. Zhao H, Yao W, Min X, Gu K, Yu G, Zhang Z, et al. Apatinib Plus Gefitinib as First-Line Treatment in Advanced EGFR-Mutant NSCLC: The Phase III ACTIVE Study (CTONG1706). J Thorac Oncol Off Publ Int Assoc Study Lung Cancer 2021;16:1533–46. https://doi.org/10.1016/j.jtho.2021.05.006.

52. Mok TS, Wu Y-L, Ahn M-J, Garassino MC, Kim HR, Ramalingam SS, et al. Osimertinib or Platinum–Pemetrexed in EGFR T790M–Positive Lung Cancer. N Engl J Med 2017;376:629–40. https://doi.org/10.1056/NEJMoa1612674.

53. Yang JC-H, Sequist LV, Geater SL, Tsai C-M, Mok TSK, Schuler M, et al. Clinical activity of afatinib in patients with advanced non-small-cell lung cancer harbouring uncommon EGFR mutations: a combined post-hoc analysis of LUX-Lung 2, LUX-Lung 3, and LUX-Lung 6. Lancet Oncol 2015;16:830–8. https://doi.org/10.1016/S1470-2045(15)00026-1.

54. Soda M, Choi YL, Enomoto M, Takada S, Yamashita Y, Ishikawa S, et al. Identification of the transforming EML4-ALK fusion gene in non-small-cell lung cancer. Nature 2007;448:561–6. https://doi.org/10.1038/nature05945.

55. Raman R, Ramamohan V, Rathore A, Jain D, Mohan A, Vashistha V. Prevalence of highly actionable mutations among Indian patients with advanced non-small cell lung cancer: A systematic review and meta-analysis. Asia Pac J Clin Oncol 2023;19:158–71. https://doi.org/10.1111/ajco.13802.

56. Solomon BJ, Mok T, Kim D-W, Wu Y-L, Nakagawa K, Mekhail T, et al. First-Line Crizotinib versus Chemotherapy in ALK-Positive Lung Cancer. N Engl J Med 2014;371:2167–77. https://doi.org/10.1056/NEJMoa1408440.

57. Soria J-C, Tan DSW, Chiari R, Wu Y-L, Paz-Ares L, Wolf J, et al. First-line ceritinib versus platinum-based chemotherapy in advanced ALK-rearranged non-small-cell lung cancer (ASCEND-4): a randomised, open-label, phase 3 study. Lancet Lond Engl 2017;389:917–29. https://doi.org/10.1016/S0140-6736(17)30123-X.

58. Camidge DR, Kim HR, Ahn M-J, Yang JCH, Han J-Y, Hochmair MJ, et al. Brigatinib Versus Crizotinib in ALK Inhibitor-Naive Advanced ALK-Positive NSCLC: Final Results of Phase 3 ALTA-1L Trial. J Thorac Oncol Off Publ Int Assoc Study Lung Cancer 2021;16:2091–108. https://doi.org/10.1016/j.jtho.2021.07.035.

59. Peters S, Camidge DR, Shaw AT, Gadgeel S, Ahn JS, Kim D-W, et al. Alectinib versus Crizotinib in Untreated ALK-Positive Non–Small-Cell Lung Cancer. N Engl J Med 2017;377:829–38. https://doi.org/10.1056/NEJMoa1704795.

60. Shaw AT, Bauer TM, de Marinis F, Felip E, Goto Y, Liu G, et al. First-Line Lorlatinib or Crizotinib in Advanced ALK-Positive Lung Cancer. N Engl J Med 2020;383:2018–29. https://doi.org/10.1056/NEJMoa2027187.

61. Horn L, Wang Z, Wu G, Poddubskaya E, Mok T, Reck M, et al. Ensartinib vs Crizotinib for Patients With Anaplastic Lymphoma Kinase-Positive Non-Small Cell Lung Cancer: A Randomized Clinical Trial. JAMA Oncol 2021;7:1617–25. https://doi.org/10.1001/jamaoncol.2021.3523.

62. Shi Y, Chen J, Yang R, Wu H, Wang Z, Yang W, et al. Iruplinalkib (WX-0593) Versus Crizotinib in ALK TKI-Naive Locally Advanced or Metastatic ALK-Positive NSCLC: Interim Analysis of a Randomized, Open-Label, Phase 3 Study (INSPIRE). J Thorac Oncol Off Publ Int Assoc Study Lung Cancer 2024;19:912–27. https://doi.org/10.1016/j.jtho.2024.01.013.

63. Yang Y, Min J, Yang N, Yu Q, Cheng Y, Zhao Y, et al. Envonalkib versus crizotinib for treatment-naive ALK-positive non-small cell lung cancer: a randomized, multicenter, open-label, phase III trial. Signal Transduct Target Ther 2023;8:301. https://doi.org/10.1038/s41392-023-01538-w.

64. Novello S, Mazières J, Oh I-J, de Castro J, Migliorino MR, Helland Å, et al. Alectinib versus chemotherapy in crizotinib-pretreated anaplastic lymphoma kinase (ALK)-positive non-small-cell lung cancer: results from the phase III ALUR study. Ann Oncol Off J Eur Soc Med Oncol 2018;29:1409–16. https://doi.org/10.1093/annonc/mdy121.

65. Huber RM, Hansen KH, Rodríguez LP-A, West HL, Reckamp KL, Leighl NB, et al. Brigatinib in Crizotinib-Refractory ALK+ NSCLC: 2-Year Follow-up on Systemic and Intracranial Outcomes in the Phase 2 ALTA Trial. J Thorac Oncol 2020;15:404–15. https://doi.org/10.1016/j.jtho.2019.11.004.

66. Shaw AT, Felip E, Bauer TM, Besse B, Navarro A, Postel-Vinay S, et al. Lorlatinib in non-small-cell lung cancer with ALK or ROS1 rearrangement: an international, multicentre, open-label, single-arm first-in-man phase 1 trial. Lancet Oncol 2017;18:1590–9. https://doi.org/10.1016/S1470-2045(17)30680-0.

67. Solomon BJ, Besse B, Bauer TM, Felip E, Soo RA, Camidge DR, et al. Lorlatinib in patients with ALK-positive non-small-cell lung cancer: results from a global phase 2 study. Lancet Oncol 2018;19:1654–67. https://doi.org/10.1016/S1470-2045(18)30649-1.

68. de Langen AJ, Johnson ML, Mazieres J, Dingemans A-MC, Mountzios G, Pless M, et al. Sotorasib versus docetaxel for previously treated non-small-cell lung cancer with KRAS(G12C) mutation: a randomised, open-label, phase 3 trial. Lancet Lond Engl 2023;401:733–46. https://doi.org/10.1016/S0140-6736(23)00221-0.

69. Reck M, Rodríguez-Abreu D, Robinson AG, Hui R, Csõszi T, Fülöp A, et al. Five-Year Outcomes With Pembrolizumab Versus Chemotherapy for Metastatic Non-Small-Cell Lung Cancer With PD-L1 Tumor Proportion Score ≥ 50. J Clin Oncol Off J Am Soc Clin Oncol 2021;39:2339–49. https://doi.org/10.1200/JCO.21.00174.

70. Sezer A, Kilickap S, Gümüþ M, Bondarenko I, Özgüroðlu M, Gogishvili M, et al. Cemiplimab monotherapy for first-line treatment of advanced non-small-cell lung cancer with PD-L1 of at least 50%: a multicentre, open-label, global, phase 3, randomised, controlled trial. Lancet Lond Engl 2021;397:592–604. https://doi.org/10.1016/S0140-6736(21)00228-2.

71. Herbst RS, Giaccone G, de Marinis F, Reinmuth N, Vergnenegre A, Barrios CH, et al. Atezolizumab for First-Line Treatment of PD-L1-Selected Patients with NSCLC. N Engl J Med 2020;383:1328–39. https://doi.org/10.1056/NEJMoa1917346.

72. Novello S, Kowalski DM, Luft A, Gümüþ M, Vicente D, Mazières J, et al. Pembrolizumab Plus Chemotherapy in Squamous Non-Small-Cell Lung Cancer: 5-Year Update of the Phase III KEYNOTE-407 Study. J Clin Oncol Off J Am Soc Clin Oncol 2023;41:1999–2006. https://doi.org/10.1200/JCO.22.01990.

73. Johnson ML, Cho BC, Luft A, Alatorre-Alexander J, Geater SL, Laktionov K, et al. Durvalumab With or Without Tremelimumab in Combination With Chemotherapy as First-Line Therapy for Metastatic Non-Small-Cell Lung Cancer: The Phase III POSEIDON Study. J Clin Oncol Off J Am Soc Clin Oncol 2023;41:1213–27. https://doi.org/10.1200/JCO.22.00975.

74. Gogishvili M, Melkadze T, Makharadze T, Giorgadze D, Dvorkin M, Penkov K, et al. Cemiplimab plus chemotherapy versus chemotherapy alone in non-small cell lung cancer: a randomized, controlled, double-blind phase 3 trial. Nat Med 2022;28:2374–80. https://doi.org/10.1038/s41591-022-01977-y.

75. Socinski MA, Jotte RM, Cappuzzo F, Orlandi F, Stroyakovskiy D, Nogami N, et al. Atezolizumab for First-Line Treatment of Metastatic Nonsquamous NSCLC. N Engl J Med 2018;378:2288–301. https://doi.org/10.1056/NEJMoa1716948.

76. Nishio M, Saito H, Goto K, Watanabe S, Sueoka-Aragane N, Okuma Y, et al. IMpower132: Atezolizumab plus platinum-based chemotherapy vs chemotherapy for advanced NSCLC in Japanese patients. Cancer Sci 2021;112:1534–44. https://doi.org/10.1111/cas.14817.

77. Zhong H, Sun S, Chen J, Wang Z, Zhao Y, Zhang G, et al. First-line penpulimab combined with paclitaxel and carboplatin for metastatic squamous non-small-cell lung cancer in China (AK105-302): a multicentre, randomised, double-blind, placebo-controlled phase 3 clinical trial. Lancet Respir Med 2024;12:355–65. https://doi.org/10.1016/S2213-2600(23)00431-9.

78. Zhou C, Chen G, Huang Y, Zhou J, Lin L, Feng J, et al. Camrelizumab plus carboplatin and pemetrexed versus chemotherapy alone in chemotherapy-naive patients with advanced non-squamous non-small-cell lung cancer (CameL): a randomised, open-label, multicentre, phase 3 trial. Lancet Respir Med 2021;9:305–14. https://doi.org/10.1016/S2213-2600(20)30365-9.

79. Ren S, Chen J, Xu X, Jiang T, Cheng Y, Chen G, et al. Camrelizumab Plus Carboplatin and Paclitaxel as First-Line Treatment for Advanced Squamous NSCLC (CameL-Sq): A Phase 3 Trial. J Thorac Oncol Off Publ Int Assoc Study Lung Cancer 2022;17:544–57. https://doi.org/10.1016/j.jtho.2021.11.018.

80. Wang J, Lu S, Yu X, Hu Y, Sun Y, Wang Z, et al. Tislelizumab Plus Chemotherapy vs Chemotherapy Alone as First-line Treatment for Advanced Squamous Non-Small-Cell Lung Cancer: A Phase 3 Randomized Clinical Trial. JAMA Oncol 2021;7:709–17. https://doi.org/10.1001/jamaoncol.2021.0366.

81. Lu S, Wang J, Yu Y, Yu X, Hu Y, Ai X, et al. Tislelizumab Plus Chemotherapy as First-Line Treatment for Locally Advanced or Metastatic Nonsquamous NSCLC (RATIONALE 304): A Randomized Phase 3 Trial. J Thorac Oncol Off Publ Int Assoc Study Lung Cancer 2021;16:1512–22. https://doi.org/10.1016/j.jtho.2021.05.005.

82. Zhou C, Wang Z, Sun Y, Cao L, Ma Z, Wu R, et al. Sugemalimab versus placebo, in combination with platinum-based chemotherapy,

as first-line treatment of metastatic non-small-cell lung cancer (GEMSTONE-302): interim and final analyses of a double-blind, randomised, phase 3 clinical trial. Lancet Oncol 2022;23:220–33. https://doi.org/10.1016/S1470-2045(21)00650-1.

83. Wang Z, Wu L, Li B, Cheng Y, Li X, Wang X, et al. Toripalimab Plus Chemotherapy for Patients With Treatment-Naive Advanced Non-Small-Cell Lung Cancer: A Multicenter Randomized Phase III Trial (CHOICE-01). J Clin Oncol Off J Am Soc Clin Oncol 2023;41:651–63. https://doi.org/10.1200/JCO.22.00727.

84. Zhou C, Wu L, Fan Y, Wang Z, Liu L, Chen G, et al. Sintilimab Plus Platinum and Gemcitabine as First-Line Treatment for Advanced or Metastatic Squamous NSCLC: Results From a Randomized, Double-Blind, Phase 3 Trial (ORIENT-12). J Thorac Oncol Off Publ Int Assoc Study Lung Cancer 2021;16:1501–11. https://doi.org/10.1016/j.jtho.2021.04.011.

85. Zhang L, Wang Z, Fang J, Yu Q, Han B, Cang S, et al. Final overall survival data of sintilimab plus pemetrexed and platinum as First-Line treatment for locally advanced or metastatic nonsquamous NSCLC in the Phase 3 ORIENT-11 study. Lung Cancer Amst Neth 2022;171:56–60. https://doi.org/10.1016/j.lungcan.2022.07.013.

86. Brahmer JR, Lee J-S, Ciuleanu T-E, Bernabe Caro R, Nishio M, Urban L, et al. Five-Year Survival Outcomes With Nivolumab Plus Ipilimumab Versus Chemotherapy as First-Line Treatment for Metastatic Non-Small-Cell Lung Cancer in CheckMate 227. J Clin Oncol Off J Am Soc Clin Oncol 2023;41:1200–12. https://doi.org/10.1200/JCO.22.01503.

87. Lu S, Wang J, Cheng Y, Mok T, Chang J, Zhang L, et al. Nivolumab versus docetaxel in a predominantly Chinese patient population with previously treated advanced non-small cell lung cancer: 2-year follow-up from a randomized, open-label, phase 3 study (CheckMate 078). Lung Cancer Amst Neth 2021;152:7–14. https://doi.org/10.1016/j.lungcan.2020.11.013.

88. Herbst RS, Garon EB, Kim D-W, Cho BC, Gervais R, Perez-Gracia JL, et al. Five Year Survival Update From KEYNOTE-010: Pembrolizumab Versus Docetaxel for Previously Treated, Programmed Death-Ligand 1-Positive Advanced NSCLC. J Thorac Oncol Off Publ Int Assoc Study Lung Cancer 2021;16:1718–32. https://doi.org/10.1016/j.jtho.2021.05.001.

89. Shi Y, Wu L, Yu X, Xing P, Wang Y, Zhou J, et al. Sintilimab versus docetaxel as second-line treatment in advanced or metastatic squamous non-small-cell lung cancer: an open-label, randomized controlled phase 3 trial (ORIENT-3). Cancer Commun Lond Engl 2022;42:1314–30. https://doi.org/10.1002/cac2.12385.

90. Zhou C, Huang D, Fan Y, Yu X, Liu Y, Shu Y, et al. Tislelizumab Versus Docetaxel in Patients With Previously Treated Advanced NSCLC (RATIONALE-303): A Phase 3, Open-Label, Randomized Controlled Trial. J Thorac Oncol Off Publ Int Assoc Study Lung Cancer 2023;18:93–105. https://doi.org/10.1016/j.jtho.2022.09.217.

91. Spigel DR, Faivre-Finn C, Gray JE, Vicente D, Planchard D, Paz-Ares L, et al. Five-Year Survival Outcomes From the PACIFIC Trial: Durvalumab After Chemoradiotherapy in Stage III Non-Small-Cell Lung Cancer. J Clin Oncol Off J Am Soc Clin Oncol 2022;40:1301–11. https://doi.org/10.1200/JCO.21.01308.

92. Ramalingam SS, Novello S, Guclu SZ, Bentsion D, Zvirbule Z, Szilasi M, et al. Veliparib in Combination With Platinum-Based Chemotherapy for First-Line Treatment of Advanced Squamous Cell Lung Cancer: A Randomized, Multicenter Phase III Study. J Clin Oncol Off J Am Soc Clin Oncol 2021;39:3633–44. https://doi.org/10.1200/JCO.20.03318.

93. Govindan R, Lind M, Insa A, Khan SA, Uskov D, Tafreshi A, et al. Veliparib Plus Carboplatin and Paclitaxel Versus Investigator's Choice of Standard Chemotherapy in Patients With Advanced Non-Squamous Non-Small Cell Lung Cancer. Clin Lung Cancer 2022;23:214–25. https://doi.org/10.1016/j.cllc.2022.01.005.

94. Yang C-FJ, Chan DY, Speicher PJ, Gulack BC, Wang X, Hartwig MG, et al. Role of Adjuvant Therapy in a Population-Based Cohort of Patients With Early-Stage Small-Cell Lung Cancer. J Clin Oncol Off J Am Soc Clin Oncol 2016;34:1057–64. https://doi.org/10.1200/JCO.2015.63.8171.

95. Rossi A, Di Maio M, Chiodini P, Rudd RM, Okamoto H, Skarlos DV, et al. Carboplatin- or cisplatin-based chemotherapy in first-line treatment of small-cell lung cancer: the COCIS meta-analysis of individual patient data. J Clin Oncol Off J Am Soc Clin Oncol 2012;30:1692–8. https://doi.org/10.1200/JCO.2011.40.4905.

96. Ernani V, Ganti AK. Surgery for limited-stage small cell lung cancer: ready for prime-time? J Thorac Dis 2017;9:3576–8. https://doi.org/10.21037/jtd.2017.09.43.

97. Liu SV, Reck M, Mansfield AS, Mok T, Scherpereel A, Reinmuth N, et al. Updated Overall Survival and PD-L1 Subgroup Analysis of Patients With Extensive-Stage Small-Cell Lung Cancer Treated With Atezolizumab, Carboplatin, and Etoposide (IMpower133). J Clin Oncol Off J Am Soc Clin Oncol 2021;39:619–30. https://doi.org/10.1200/JCO.20.01055.

98. Goldman JW, Dvorkin M, Chen Y, Reinmuth N, Hotta K, Trukhin D, et al. Durvalumab, with or without tremelimumab, plus platinum-etoposide versus platinum-etoposide alone in first-line treatment of extensive-stage small-cell lung cancer (CASPIAN): updated results from a randomised, controlled, open-label, phase 3 trial. Lancet Oncol 2021;22:51–65. https://doi.org/10.1016/S1470-2045(20)30539-8.

99. Wang J, Zhou C, Yao W, Wang Q, Min X, Chen G, et al. Adebrelimab or placebo plus carboplatin and etoposide as first-line treatment for extensive-stage small-cell lung cancer (CAPSTONE-1): a multicentre, randomised, double-blind, placebo-controlled, phase 3 trial. Lancet Oncol 2022;23:739–47. https://doi.org/10.1016/S1470-2045(22)00224-8.

100. Cheng Y, Han L, Wu L, Chen J, Sun H, Wen G, et al. Effect of First-Line Serplulimab vs Placebo Added to Chemotherapy on Survival in Patients With Extensive-Stage Small Cell Lung Cancer: The ASTRUM-005 Randomized Clinical Trial. JAMA 2022;328:1223–32. https://doi.org/10.1001/jama.2022.16464.

101. Takahashi T, Yamanaka T, Seto T, Harada H, Nokihara H, Saka H, et al. Prophylactic cranial irradiation versus observation in patients with extensive-disease small-cell lung cancer: a multicentre, randomised, open-label, phase 3 trial. Lancet Oncol 2017;18:663–71. https://doi.org/10.1016/S1470-2045(17)30230-9.

102. von Pawel J, Schiller JH, Shepherd FA, Fields SZ, Kleisbauer JP, Chrysson NG, et al. Topotecan versus cyclophosphamide, doxorubicin, and vincristine for the treatment of recurrent small-cell lung cancer. J Clin Oncol Off J Am Soc Clin Oncol 1999;17:658–67. https://doi.org/10.1200/JCO.1999.17.2.658.

103. Trigo J, Subbiah V, Besse B, Moreno V, López R, Sala MA, et al. Lurbinectedin as second-line treatment for patients with small-cell lung cancer: a single-arm, open-label, phase 2 basket trial. Lancet Oncol 2020;21:645–54. https://doi.org/10.1016/S1470-2045(20)30068-1.

104. Owonikoko TK, Park K, Govindan R, Ready N, Reck M, Peters S, et al. Nivolumab and Ipilimumab as Maintenance Therapy in Extensive-Disease Small-Cell Lung Cancer: CheckMate 451. J Clin Oncol Off J Am Soc Clin Oncol 2021;39:1349–59. https://doi.org/10.1200/JCO.20.02212.

105. Spigel DR, Vicente D, Ciuleanu TE, Gettinger S, Peters S, Horn L, et al. Second-line nivolumab in relapsed small-cell lung cancer: CheckMate 331(&). Ann Oncol Off J Eur Soc Med Oncol 2021;32:631–41. https://doi.org/10.1016/j.annonc.2021.01.071.

106. Pujol J-L, Greillier L, Audigier-Valette C, Moro-Sibilot D, Uwer L, Hureaux J, et al. A Randomized Non-Comparative Phase II Study of Anti-Programmed Cell Death-Ligand 1 Atezolizumab or Chemotherapy as Second-Line Therapy in Patients With Small Cell Lung Cancer: Results From the IFCT-1603 Trial. J Thorac Oncol 2019;14:903–13. https://doi.org/10.1016/j.jtho.2019.01.008.

107. Gadgeel SM, Pennell NA, Fidler MJ, Halmos B, Bonomi P, Stevenson J, et al. Phase II Study of Maintenance Pembrolizumab in Patients with Extensive-Stage Small Cell Lung Cancer (SCLC). J Thorac Oncol 2018;13:1393–9. https://doi.org/10.1016/j.jtho.2018.05.002.

CHAPTER 17

Lung Transplantation

Systematic Review of Recent Literature

Author: Dr. Srinivas Rajagopala

Reviewer: Dr. Shweta Bansal

INTRODUCTION

Lung transplantation (LT) is the only definitive treatment for end-stage lung diseases with chronic respiratory failure and an estimated 6000 lung transplants occur annually across the globe. Significant improvements have occurred in surgical techniques, post-transplant care, donor lung management and expanding the donor pool with ex-situ perfusion techniques, utilisation of HCV-infected lungs and older donors. These concerted efforts are improving outcomes after lung transplantation with sicker recipients at transplant, with experienced centers reporting a median survival of 10 years. With better outcomes and increasing numbers, research is now focussed on further expanding the donor pool safely, reducing wait-list mortality and reducing chronic lung allograft dysfunction in recipients. CLAD, however, remains the main determinant of long-term survival post-lung transplantation. Translational research is now focussing on improving donor lung utilisation by proteomics and genomics approach, followed by transplantation. This update pertains to important research published in the field of lung transplantation within the last year relevant to practicing pulmonologists. This is not meant to be an exhaustive or comprehensive review of lung transplantation for which the reader may refer to the International Society for heart and lung transplantation (ISHLT) documents.

Methodology

A PubMed search was carried out with search term (lung OR Pulmonary) AND Transplant. Articles between the time span of August 1, 2023 to August 1, 2024 were reviewed. This yielded 6153 results. After including only articles published in English, humans as subjects, and including Clinical Trial, Meta-Analysis, Randomized Controlled Trial, guidelines and reviews, this resulted in 1106 citations whose titles were individually scanned for inclusion. This was further supplemented by direct search of the references of retrieved relevant articles and our personal databases. Both the abstracts and full text articles, where available, were reviewed. Only studies directly relevant to clinical practice of Pulmonologists were accepted for inclusion. We excluded studies on surgical techniques, pharmacokinetics studies, coronary artery disease interventions, interventions involving consent, attitudes and adherence to medications post-transplant. The below review summarizes the important studies that were identified to be of importance to clinical practice. A detailed list of articles of interest retrieved and those of practice relevance reviewed in the manuscript is provided in the Appendix.

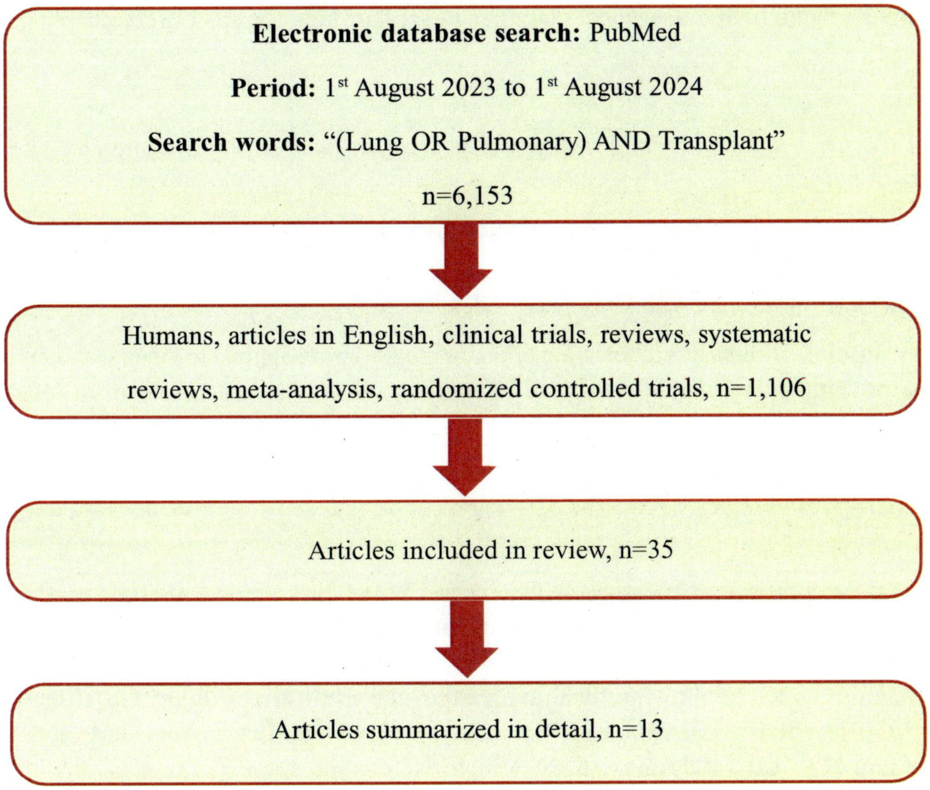

Analysis of literature

Recipient selection for lung transplantation

Interstitial lung diseases are the most common indication for referral to lung transplant in North America and in India, for differing reasons. In the U.S., the CAS (combined allocation score) system favors allocation for ILDs whereas in India, it is due to referral bias. There are no robust evidence-based data to support the timing of referral and subsequently, listing for lung transplant. This is guided by cohort-level data of patients with IPF. This is further complicated by the fact that our mortality prediction models for Idiopathic pulmonary fibrosis (IPF) and Progressive fibrosing ILDs (PF-ILDs) are poor, antifibrotics attenuate progression and mortality, and real-world data on current survival is lacking. **Currently, consensus-based evidence in the ISHLT document[1] recommends *referral* to lung transplant at any of the below time points; for usual interstitial pneumonia (UIP), irrespective of lung function at the time of diagnosis; lung function decline (relative forced vital capacity [FVC] decline of ≥10% over six months or FVC decline >5% with radiographic worsening, relative diffusion capacity for carbon monoxide [DLco] decline ≥15%); FVC<80%, DLco <40% at diagnosis; desaturation to ≤88% or walking <250 m at a six minutes-walk test or decline in walk distance ≥50 meters over six months; any oxygen requirement, even if only on exertion and pulmonary hypertension on right heart catheterization.** For inflammatory ILDs, failure to improve on appropriate anti-inflammatory therapy is an indication for referral while maximizing therapy.

Indications for listing for lung transplantation include absolute FVC decline of >10% or FVC decline >5% with radiographic worsening, absolute DLco decline >15%; and hospitalization because of respiratory decline, pneumothorax, or acute exacerbation of ILD.[2] Unfortunately, all of these clinical variables are evidence of established worsening lung disease and frailty in a given patient. Frailty impacts post-transplant survival and hence better predictors are needed, especially in IPF and

PF-ILD.[3,4] It is in this context that a multidimensional classifier to support lung transplant referral in patients with pulmonary fibrosis has been evaluated.

- ***A multidimensional classifier to support lung transplant referral in patients with pulmonary fibrosis. (J Heart Lung Transplant. 2024)***[5]

  - o *Population:* Patients were recruited from a prospective cohort study of interstitial lung disease (ILD). The IPF derivation, IPF validation, and non-IPF ILD validation cohorts consisted of 314, 105, and 295 patients, respectively. Cohorts were restricted to patients aged ≤72 years with body mass index 18 to 32.
  - o *Intervention:* Least absolute shrinkage and selection operator method were applied to clinical and proteomic data generated to derive clinical, proteomic, and multidimensional logistical models of near-term death or lung transplant within 18 months of blood draw.

    Model-fitted values were dichotomized at the point of maximal sensitivity and specificity, and decision curve analysis was used to select the best-performing classifier. The derivation cohort was separate from the validation cohorts (IPF & non-IPF).
  - o *Outcomes:* 93% of this cohort were Caucasians with a mean FVC of 66.1 (16.1) and DLco of 41.3 (16.4). 83% were on anti-fibrotics. Over 18 months, 25.5% had met the study endpoint; 13.1% had died and another 12.4% had undergone lung transplantation. A multidimensional model comprising 2 clinical variables and 20 proteins outperformed stand-alone clinical and proteomic models. Following dichotomization, the **multidimensional classifier predicted near-term outcomes with 70% sensitivity and 92% specificity in the IPF validation cohort and 70% sensitivity and 80% specificity in the non-IPF ILD validation cohort.** A high-risk classification was associated with a >7-fold increase in outcome risk; in the high-risk classification, nearly 80% died or needed a transplant within 18 months whereas <10% in the low-risk classification met this outcome over the same period.
  - o *Conclusion:* **The individual proteomic variables in the 20 proteins are unclear and the model did not perform well in non-IPF PF-ILDs, where it is most needed.** About 50% of the baseline cohort met referral criteria for lung transplant according to current criteria at study entry; the addition of a predictive model in these seems superfluous. Finally, the model needs to be validated in a non-Caucasian independent cohort of newly diagnosed IPF and PF-ILDs with follow-up to see the predictive power for progression, which remains the main criteria for referral to transplant as per ISHLT criteria.

Antifibrotics are now the standard of therapy for IPF and other fibrotic PF-ILDs.[6] The use of nintedanib pre-operatively in IPF patients was initially viewed with concern given the potential for increased bleeding complications intra-operatively and airway dehiscence/wound healing problems postoperatively.[7] Subsequently, publications showed the safety of continuing nintedanib till transplant.[8] With increasing experience with this approach, a recent publication has shown an interesting effect of nintedanib on post-transplant outcomes.

- ***Effect of antifibrotic agents on postoperative complications after lung transplantation for idiopathic pulmonary fibrosis. (Respirology. 2024)***[9]

  - o *Population:* Multi-centre, nationwide, retrospective, observational study of French IPF patients undergoing LT between 2011 and 2018. (n=205)
  - o *Intervention:* Antifibrotics.
  - o *Comparator:* IPF patients undergoing LT who were not on antifibrotics at the time of transplant.
  - o *Outcomes:* 205 patients were included. 58 (28%) had received antifibrotics within 4 weeks before LT: pirfenidone in 37 (18.0%) and nintedanib in 21 (10.2%). The median duration of treatment before LT was 13.8 (5.6–24) months. The

treatment and control groups did not significantly differ in airway, bleeding or skin healing complications (p = 0.91, p = 0.12 and p = 0.70, respectively). Primary graft dysfunction was less frequent in the antifibrotics group than in controls (26% vs. 43%, p = 0.02), and the 90-day mortality was lower (7% vs. 18%, p = 0.046).

- o *Conclusion:* **21.8% of the control group were on antifibrotics at transplant and the control group had lower total lung capacity, DLco*%pred,* and walk distance than the antifibrotics group.** This large real-world experience surprisingly revealed that continuing antifibrotics was associated with lower PGD and mortality. These effects could be modulated by better stability while on the waitlist, lower bridging, and lower intra-operative bleeding. However, the pre-operative bridging rates were similar (9.3-11.6%), and intraoperative bleeding rates and the need for postoperative ECMO (as a surrogate for PGD) were again similar. Intra-operative ECMO was numerically actually lower in the control arm (53.6% vs 47.6%, p=0.12). Interestingly, any PGD (26% vs. 43%, p = 0.02), PGD grade 3 at 72 hours (25.2% vs 12.1%, p=0.04) and its consequence, mechanical ventilation hours (96 vs 48 hours) and tracheostomy (27.7% vs 19%) were higher in the control group, suggesting that this was the main driver of the observed effects. This paper shows evidence of the superiority of continuing antifibrotics while waiting for a transplant in terms of better stability, lower PGD, and lower 90-day mortality. This is now the standard of care.

The ISHLT document remains the main consensus for the timing of referral for various causes of chronic lung diseases.[2] Notably, while the 2019 iteration includes more etiologic categories, several newer indications and their outcomes need clarification. Cohort-level data of several rarer aetiologies of chronic respiratory failure are clarifying their natural history and timing of lung transplantation. An important paper on Lymphangioleiomyomatosis was reviewed in the last update.[10] Pleuro-parenchymal fibroelastosis (PPFE) is one such entity that has no currently available specific treatment.[11] A French multicentric retrospective study recently looked at the outcomes of lung transplantation for PPFE.

- ***Outcomes of lung transplantation for pleuroparenchymal fibroelastosis: A French multicentric retrospective study. (J Heart Lung Transplant. 2024)***[12]
  - o *Population:* Nation-wide multicentric retrospective study in patients who underwent lung or heart-lung transplantation for chronic end-stage lung disease secondary to PPFE between 2012 and 2022 in France. (n=31)
  - o *Outcomes:* 31 patients were included. Median age was 48 years [IQR 35–55]; 64.5% were women. 21(67.7%) had idiopathic PFFE. 16 (52%) had bilateral LT, 10 (32%) had single LT, 4 (13%) had lobar transplantation and one (3%) had heart-lung transplantation. Operative mortality was 3.2% and early mortality (< 90 days or during the first hospitalization) was 32%. 11(35.5%) underwent re-exploration. Length of stay in intensive care unit and hospital were 34 [IQR 18–73] and 64 [IQR 36–103] days, respectively. Bronchial complications were seen in 10 (30.8%). Median survival was 21 months. Post-transplant survival rates after 1, 2, and 5 years were 57.9%, 42.6% and 38.3% respectively. **Low albuminemia (p = 0.046), FVC (p = 0.021), FEV1 (p = 0.009), and high emergency lung transplantation (p = 0.04) were associated with increased early mortality.**
  - o *Conclusion:* This is a sobering first large series for PPFE which shows a dismally high rate of re-exploration, early mortality, airway complications, longer ICU and hospital stays, and poor overall survival. These correlate with the low BMI, and frailty that is seen in these patients. **Extensive pleural adhesions intra-operative bleeding, and transfusion requirements are higher in these patients and correlate with PGD and poor survival; however, this was not captured in this study.** Also, this study had a small number over a decade; data on whether survival improved over this time frame is unclear. This data is similar to a single-center experience and literature review (Faccioli, E Lung Transplantation for Pleuro-parenchymal Fibroelastosis: A Single-Center Experience with Revision of Literature).[13] Careful case selection, attention to pre-transplant nutrition, and rehabilitation are needed for patients with PPFE with avoidance of pre-operative bridging to improve outcomes.

The COVID-19 pandemic brought the feasibility of lung transplantation for persistent non-resolving ARDS to the limelight.[14] Carefully selected multi-centric studies showed feasibility[15] and good short-term outcomes.[16] The long-term outcomes were unclear but a large number of transplants had already been performed across the U.S. for COVID-19-related ARDS and fibrosis. The 1-year outcomes have now been reported.

- ***Lung transplantation for COVID-2019 respiratory failure in the United States: Outcomes 1-year posttransplant and the impact of preoperative extracorporeal membrane oxygenation support. (J Thorac Cardiovasc Surg. 2024)***[17]
  - o *Population:* Nation-wide (U.S) multicentric retrospective study in patients who underwent lung or heart-lung transplantation for COVID-19 related respiratory failure from August 2020 through March 2022 using UNOS database. (n=305)
  - o *Outcomes:* 305 patients with COVID-19-related respiratory failure underwent LT in the study period; this included 188 patients with COVID-19-related acute respiratory distress syndrome and 117 patients with post-COVID-19 pulmonary fibrosis. Pre-transplant ECMO support (median 66 days) was required in 191 patients (63%), and veno-venous ECMO was used in 91.2% of patients. 1-, 6-, and 12-month survival was not significantly different between patients requiring ECMO and patients without ECMO (95.8% vs 99.1%, 93.1% vs 96.4%, 84.8% vs 90.9%, P=0.2). 10% needed postoperative dialysis. 1-year survival was similar in recipients requiring ECMO for COVID-19 lung failure and recipients requiring ECMO for non-COVID-19 restrictive lung failure (84.8% vs 78.0%, P=0.1).
  - o *Conclusion:* **This paper showed that LT is a viable option with comparable survival in carefully selected patients with COVID-19-related ARDS and fibrosis despite the complex postoperative course and prolonged ECMO support.** The mean LAS was 88.0 pre-transplant and 75.4% needed prolonged ventilation post-operatively. While the rates of PGD were not evaluated, 26% of the cohort needed postoperative ECMO, including new postoperative initiation in 10.5% indicating at least a third of the cohort had significant PGD. 1-year survival, however, was similar in these highly experienced centers. More data on CLAD and long-term survival is needed. **A literature review of LT for non-COVID-19 persistent ARDS also showed that LT is an effective therapy in carefully selected patients with single-organ failure in experienced centers with multi-disciplinary teams, attention to minimizing sedation, and awake ECMO.**[18]

Coronary artery disease is common among LT candidates increasingly as more aged recipients are being listed for transplant. The optimal method of management of CAD before LT remains unclear, ranging from delisting to combined LT plus CABG. The Temple group recently published their experience over 10 years to clarify this conundrum.

- ***Lung transplant survival with past and concomitant cardiac revascularization. (J Heart Lung Transplant. 2023)***[19]
  - o *Population:* All single and double lung transplant patients from Feb, 2012 to Aug, 2021 at Temple, Philadelphia, U.S (n=880)
  - o *Intervention:* Re-vascularisation; this was grouped into 1) pre-operative PCI; 2) pre-operative CABG; 3) LT plus CABG.
  - o *Comparator:* LT without revascularization.
  - o *Outcomes:* There were 880 LTs in this period; 724 did not need revascularisation; 57 underwent preoperative PCI, 43 underwent preoperative CABG, and 56 underwent concurrent LT plus CABG. The no-revascularisation group was younger, had more women and non-Caucasians, and had higher LAS scores at LT. More patients in the concurrent CABG+LT group underwent Single LT (69.6% vs 63.5%, p = 0.014). Survival rates were similar between the groups (p = 0.471).
  - o *Conclusion:* This paper showed that LT can be safely performed with revascularisation in patients with stable CAD before or during LT. The choice of technique and timing of revascularisation generally depends on the number of lesions and their morphology, the disease severity of the patient, and the time available before transplant with a decision generally taken after a team discussion.

Donor selection and management for lung transplantation

Static ice storage has long been the standard of care for lung preservation. However, **freezing injury limits cold ischemic time (CIT). Data from the Toronto group showed that suggests that controlled hypothermic storage (CHS) at an increased temperature (6-10°C) protects organ quality and mitochondrial health better without compromising the outcome.**[20] Several centers have now started to implement this approach and noted that this approach introduces time flexibility and increases CIT safety. Data on this was published recently from a multicenter experience (Prague, Leuven and Boston), showing that a CIT of >15 hours was feasible and safe.

- ***Extended ischemic time (>15 hours) using controlled hypothermic storage in lung transplantation: A multicenter experience. (J Heart Lung Transplant. 2024)***[21]
  - *Population:* Adult patients who underwent bilateral LT at Leuven (Belgium), Prague (Czech Republic) and Boston (US) between April and October 2023 with an ischemic time >15 hours were included. (n=13)
  - *Intervention:* Donor's lungs were stored in the LUNGguard (Paragonix, Boston, USA) system at 7 (5-9.3)°C.
  - *Outcomes:* 13 patients underwent LT in this period with a CIT>15 hours (12%, 13/113). 4/13 had PGD grade 3 within 72 hours and 0/13 at 72 hours. Post-LT mechanical ventilation was 29 (7-442) hours. ICU stay was 9 (5-28) and hospital stay 30 (16-90) days. Four patients needed postoperative ECMO. One patient died (day 7) following mal-positioning of the ECMO cannula.
  - *Conclusion:* **This paper showed that LT with CIT>15 hours can be achieved and is a viable option with comparable survival in carefully selected recipient-donor combinations using a proprietary system.**

Peri-transplant management of lung transplantation-matching, cardiorespiratory support and primary graft dysfunction

Primary Graft Dysfunction is a multifactorial cause of early delayed graft dysfunction occurring within 72 hours of transplantation and affects up to 25% of recipients. Beyond hypoxemia and the need for additional therapies, including ECMO, PGD is associated with excess of short-term mortality, delayed weaning, and prolonged hospital stay. It also reduces long-term survival through its interaction with baseline lung allograft function and chronic lung allograft dysfunction.[22] With sicker recipients being prioritized, the incidence of PGD has been increasing.[23] Better predictive models are needed to predict, and if possible, subsequently ameliorate PGD incidence by modulating modifiable risk factors. Recently, a predictor has been developed to predict PGD incidence at the time of transplant but needs independent validation.

- ***Development and validation of primary graft dysfunction predictive algorithm for lung transplant candidates. (J Heart Lung Transplant. 2024)***[24]
  - *Population:* The Lung transplant Outcomes Group (LTOG) is a prospective multicenter, National Institutes of Health–sponsored cohort study. Patients aged 18 to 80 years transplanted at LTOG centers between 2012 and 2018 were included. Donor data was retrieved using data from the Organ Procurement and Transplantation Network (OPTN). The derived score was validated in a contemporaneous external cohort of patients from the Washington University School of Medicine. (n=1,167)
  - *Outcomes:* During the study period, there were 3,831 transplants performed at participating centers, 1,527 subjects enrolled in the cohort, and 1,167 with complete data. The overall PGD incidence overall was 26.3% (307/1,167) and varied more than 5-fold across the centers (8.6% [6/70] to 44.7% [46/108]). The developed model included center volume, donor smoking, death mechanism of death, donor gender, recipient age, gender, diagnosis, BMI, LAS, pulmonary hypertension, and distance of donor offers from recipient hospital, and recipient TLC. Using a standard donor and a matched recipient pTLC, the score predicts a PGD of 29.3% for most lung transplants.

- *Conclusion:* This paper shows that risk factors tend to cluster for sicker patients awaiting LT. The model offers decision-making net benefit in the PGD risk range of 10-75% in the derivation centers but only between 2-10% in the validation cohort. The score does not capture size-matching directly and ignores intraoperative bleeding and transfusion, which are also major predictors of PGD.

The association of intraoperative bleeding and PGD has been evaluated by a paper recently.

- ***Intraoperative Red Blood Cell Transfusion and Primary Graft Dysfunction After Lung Transplantation. (Transplantation. 2023)***[25]
  - *Population:* The Extracorporeal Life Support in LT Registry includes data on LT recipients from 9 high-volume (>40 transplants/year) transplant centers (2 from Europe, 7 from the United States). Adult patients who underwent bilateral orthotopic lung transplant from January 2016 to January 2020 were included retrospectively. (n=729)
  - *Intervention:* Retrospective, tertiles of transfusion; intraoperative PRBC transfusion (0, 1-4, and >4 units)
  - *Outcomes:* 729 patients underwent LT between January 2016 and November 2020 in these centers. LT recipient population tertiles based on the amount of intraoperative PRBC transfusion (0, 1-4, and >4 units) were significantly different in terms of diagnosis, age, gender, body mass index, mean pulmonary artery pressure, lung allocation score, hemoglobin, prior chest surgery, preoperative hospitalization, and extracorporeal membrane oxygenation requirement as expected. Inverse probability treatment weighting logistic regression showed that intraoperative PRBC transfusion of >4 units was significantly ($P < 0.001$) associated with grade 3 PGD within 72 h (odds ratio [95% confidence interval], 2.2 [1.6-3.1]). Excluding patients with ECMO produced similar findings (O.R, 95% CI, 2.4 [1.7-3.4], $P < 0.001$).
  - *Conclusion:* **This paper shows that risk factors tend to cluster for sicker patients awaiting LT.** As the disease worsens, pulmonary hypertension develops, frailty worsens, the need for bridging increases, and intraoperative transfusion requirement increases; all these increase the incidence of PGD and impact post-transplant outcomes. **This once again reiterates the need for appropriate early referral and listing for lung transplant as most of these are modifiable recipient risk factors.**

Pleural adhesions, prior thoracic surgery, PPFE as the etiology for chronic lung disease, and prior pleurodesis all increase the difficulty of surgical dissection, bleeding, and intraoperative transfusion requirements. Unfortunately, none of them are modifiable. One potentially modifiable risk factor is the use of intraoperative plasmapheresis (PLEX) for the presence of pre-formed donor-specific antibody (DSA) at the time of transplant. This is a controversial area of therapeutics, with decision-making ranging from "do not cross DSA" to full intraoperative PLEX, followed by a postoperative protocol.[26-29] There has been concern about the impact of intraoperative PLEX on surgical bleeding, given the potential removal of clotting factors. This has hindered the adoption of this approach beyond a few centers, including the Toronto group which has pioneered this approach. They recently looked at the impact of intraoperative PLEX on intraoperative bleeding in lung transplantation and its outcomes.

- ***Impact of intraoperative therapeutic plasma exchange on bleeding in lung transplantation. (J Heart Lung Transplant. 2024)***[30]
  - *Population:* All first-time LT recipients at Toronto between 2014 and 2019 retrospectively. (n=897)
  - *Intervention:* Patients undergoing intra-operative PLEX.
  - *Comparison:* No PLEX.
  - *Outcomes:* 897 Patients were included; this had 142 (16%) with PLEX and 755 (84%) without PLEX. The number of perioperative pRBC transfusions was higher among patients who received PLEX (4.2 vs 2.9) than those who did not. PLEX was associated with increased odds of requiring large-volume perioperative transfusion (O.R 1.9; 95% C.I: 1.2-2.9, p-value = 0.007) but was not associated with an increased incidence of hemothorax (5% in both groups, $p = 0.99$) or 30-day posttransplant mortality (3.5% vs 2.1%, $p = 0.31$).

- o *Conclusion:* Bleeding is a real concern while using intraoperative PLEX to cross DSA at transplant. In experience centers, this is not associated with higher mortality or complications, but this may not hold in small-volume centers. An alternate approach is the use of postoperative PLEX protocol championed by the Edmonton group.[31]

Complications after lung transplantation-acute rejection, infections and airway complications

Acute rejection affects up to 30% of LT recipients in the first year. Recurrent acute rejection is associated with the development of CLAD. The implication of grade 1 acute cellular rejection (A1ACR) is less certain and asymptomatic A1ACR is not treated.[32] However, a small proportion of patients with minimal ACR develop early CLAD within 2-4 years. It has been unclear what drives CLAD in this setting; recurrent minimal A1ACR is certainly one of them along with unrecognized higher-grade ACR.

Recently, the Toronto group looked at deep immunological profiling of patients with asymptomatic A1 ACR to see if there was a spectrum and distribution of intra-graft T-cell phenotype at A1ACR on subsequent CLAD onset.

- ***The CD8(+) T cell content of transbronchial biopsies from patients with a first episode of clinically stable grade A1 cellular rejection is associated with future chronic lung allograft dysfunction. (J Heart Lung Transplant 2024)***[33]
  - o *Population:* Patients who received a primary, bilateral lung transplant in the Toronto Lung Transplant Program between January 1, 2010 and December 18, 2016. (n=82)
  - o *Comparison:* Patients experiencing a first episode of Asymptomatic A1R (lack of a ≥10% decline from a prior reference FEV1) in the first 13 months post-transplant that was not preceded by ACR grade ≥1. Transbronchial biopsies (TBB) were compared to those without A1ACR. FEV1.Exclusion criteria included significant pathogens in BAL or lung tissue, concurrent antimicrobial treatment, or evidence of concurrent B grade ≥1. From this cohort, patients were selected if they remained CLAD-free for 5 or more years (no early CLAD) or if they developed CLAD within 2 years (early CLAD).
  - o *Outcomes:* 82 patients met the criteria outlined above. PhenoGraph unsupervised clustering on Imaging mass cytometry revealed 50 unique immune cell subpopulations.

    Methylation and immunofluorescence analyses demonstrated no significant differences in Tregs between early-CLAD and no early-CLAD groups. Immunofluorescence revealed that patients who developed CLAD within 2 years of lung transplantation showed greater CD8+ T cell infiltration compared to those who remained CLAD-free for 5 or more years.
  - o *Conclusion:* This paper showed that graft-infiltrating CD8 T-cells have a role in the development of CLAD. Whether subsets of Tregs and their paucity are as important is unclear as subgrouping was not done.

There is considerable controversy over the utility of surveillance TBBs for post-lung transplant allograft surveillance given its risks, costs, and yield. Donor-specific antibody (DSA) testing of blood is another cornerstone of graft assessment. However, it is also subject to major variations in the interpretation of results and has poor predictive value. Alternatives are needed. One approach is microarrays in endobronchial biopsies; these are performed as well as TBBs.[34] Unfortunately, this has not been validated externally yet or refined for clinical practice. There is immense interest in alternate non-invasive platforms for allograft surveillance. This includes donor-derived cell-free DNA, miRNA expression, exosomes, and Torque teno virus load.[35]

Donor cfDNA is the most advanced in this regard. cfDNA consists of short fragments of DNA released by necrotic or apoptotic cells, making them a direct marker of tissue injury. They can also, in some cases, be secreted by healthy cells. They circulate, bound to histones, with a half-life between 15 and 120 minutes. cfDNA is degraded by DNase I and then eliminated by macrophages in the liver and spleen and by glomerular filtration. cfDNA is normally rapidly cleared, but if excessive production outstrips clearance, it leads to accumulation. In healthy individuals, cfDNA level correlates with age and sex. Levels of donor-derived cfDNA (dd-cfDNA), expressed as a fraction of total cfDNA, correlate with damage to the allograft due to any cause. **In LT recipients without rejection or infection, dd-cfDNA levels are highly elevated during the first 2 weeks post-transplant, due to organ injury after reperfusion. dd-cfDNA levels then subsequently decrease over time, reaching a steady-state level 2-4 months after LT. Compared to other SOTs, LT recipients have an elevated dd-cfDNA (range 2-5%) throughout their post-transplant course** comparable to liver SOTs; this is likely related to the mass of the organ. At a threshold of ≥1% dd-cfDNA fraction, it has a sensitivity of 89.1% (95% CI 76.2–100.0%), a specificity of 82.9% (95% CI 73.3–92.4%), a positive predictive value of 51.9% (95% CI 37.5–66.3%) and a negative predictive value of 97.3% (95% CI 94.3–100%) for ACR. Dd-cfDNA has limited utility in AMR. Currently, the negative predictive value of the dd-cfDNA fraction may have utility but it has very limited specificity. Also, a normal value of dd-cfDNA fraction might therefore be insufficient to rule out the diagnosis of low-grade ACR, especially in cases of high clinical suspicion. A recent study has added another piece to the puzzle, moving dd-cfDNA towards routine clinical practice.

- ***Extreme elevations of donor-derived cell-free DNA increases the risk of chronic lung allograft dysfunction and death, even without clinical manifestations of disease. (J Heart Lung Transplant. 2024)***[36]
  - *Population:* Multicentric prospective cohort study from the US. (n=238)
  - *Intervention:* Serial plasma samples were collected for dd-cfDNA measurement by shotgun sequencing. Extreme molecular Injury (EMI) was defined as a dd-cfDNA above the third quartile of levels observed for acute rejection which was defined by a dd-cfDNA level of ≥5% occurring after 45 days post-transplant. EMI was categorized as Secondary if associated with coexisting acute rejection, infection, or PFT decline; or Primary if unassociated with any of the above.
  - *Outcomes:* 238 LT recipients were included. EMI developed in 16% of patients at a median 343.5 (IQR: 177.3–535.5) days post-transplant. Over 50% of EMI episodes were classified as Primary. EMI was associated with an increased risk of severe CLAD or death (HR: 2.78, 95% CI: 1.26–6.22, $p = 0.012$). The risk remained consistent for the Primary EMI subgroup (HR: 2.34, 95% CI 1.18–4.85, $p = 0.015$). Time to first EMI episode was a significant predictor of the likelihood of developing CLAD or death (AUC=0.856, 95% CI=0.805–0.908, $p < 0.001$).
  - *Conclusion:* At least 50% of EMI is unassociated with infection or rejection. EMI is associated with an increased risk of severe CLAD or death, independent of concomitant transplant complications. This finding, if replicated, signifies an independent role of cfDNA in allograft monitoring beyond infection or ACR.

Late complications after lung transplantation-chronic lung allograft dysfunction, cancer, infections and renal failure

Chronic lung allograft dysfunction affects 50% of recipients by 5 years and is the main determinant of intermediate and long-term survival post-LT. There has been considerable controversy regarding the optimal immunosuppression regimen in reducing CLAD incidence. Studies cleared demonstrated the advantage of tacrolimus over cyclosporine about ACR but had inconsistent effects on CLAD and survival. A recent large trial has clarified this question.

- ***Effect of once-per-day tacrolimus versus twice-per-day ciclosporin on 3-year incidence of chronic lung allograft dysfunction after lung transplantation in Scandinavia (ScanCLAD): A multicentre randomised controlled trial. (Lancet Respir Med. 2024)***[37]
  - *Population:* Open-label, multicentre, randomized, controlled trial in Scandinavia enrolling patients 18–70 years undergoing BLT between Oct 21, 2016, and July 10, 2019. Surveillance biopsies were done at 1, 3, and 12 months. (n=383)
  - *Intervention:* Anti-thymocyte globulin induction followed by sustained-release tacrolimus (once per day 0.1-0.2 mg/kg/day), mycophenolate mofetil, and corticosteroids targeted to 10–14 ng/mL at 0–3 months, 8–12 ng/mL at 3–6 months, 8–10 ng/mL at 6–12 months, and 6–8 ng/mL beyond 12 months.

- *Comparator:* Cyclosporin (twice per day) 2-3 mg/kg, mycophenolate mofetil, and Corticosteroids targeted to 250–300 ng/mL at 0–3 months, 200–250 ng/mL at 3–6 months, 150–200 ng/mL at 6–12 months, and 100–150 ng/mL beyond 12 months
- *Outcomes:* CLAD was assessed at 36 months post-transplantation, determined by repeated lung function tests and adjudicated by an independent committee, and was assessed with a competing-risks analysis with death and re-transplantation as competing events in the mITT population (at least 1 dose of Tacrolimus). 383 patients were assessed for eligibility and 249 of these were included in the mITT population. 125 (50%) in the cyclosporin group and 124 (50%) in the tacrolimus group. The mean age of 55·2 (10·2) years; COPD and ILD accounted for 62% of all transplants. About 15 early deaths occurred and had no PFT values (6 in the cyclosporin arm and 9 in the tacrolimus arm) and 21 in the cyclosporin arm crossed over to tacrolimus (13 before CLAD, 8 after CLAD) and 2 in the tacrolimus crossed over to cyclosporine. ACR occurred in 57% of the cyclosporin arm vs 40% in the tacrolimus group (p=0.011). CLAD occurred in 48 (cumulative 39% [95% CI 31–48]) in the cyclosporin group and in 16 (13% [8–21]) in the tacrolimus group at 36 months post-transplantation (HR 0·28 [95% CI 0·15–0·52], p<0·0001). Overall survival did not differ between groups at 3 years (74% [65–81] for cyclosporin vs 79% [70–85] for tacrolimus; HR 0·72 [95% CI 0·41–1·27], p=0·25). In those with at least lung function post-transplant, allograft survival was significantly better in the tacrolimus group (HR 0·49 [95% CI 0·26–0·91], p=0·021). Adverse events, mostly infections, were similar and frequent in either arm (90%). Fungal infections occurred in 34% of the cyclosporin arm and 45% of the tacrolimus arm.
- *Conclusion:*This large study showed a usually large number of ACR in either arm. Events were fragile; the addition of a few patients who did not take the drug as per protocol nullified the effects on survival. The tacrolimus arm showed a very low rate of CLAD that needs to be re-examined in real-world scenarios. Once-a-day tacrolimus (Advagraf) is proprietary and has not been used widely in the lung transplantation population outside a few centers. Finally, the rates of infections seem excessive and is likely related to the ATG induction that was used.

Esophageal motility abnormalities, microaspiration, and reflux have long been suspected of being related to early CLAD. Studies, however, have not been conclusive and may be related to the airway biomarker (pepsin and pepsinogen) related to aspiration not being evaluated. The Toronto group evaluated airway pepsinogen A4 (PGA4) as it is not expressed in the airway to identify microaspiration in lung transplant recipients and found that it predicts chronic lung allograft dysfunction.

- ***Airway pepsinogen A4 identifies lung transplant recipients with microaspiration and predicts chronic lung allograft dysfunction. (J Heart Lung Transplant. 2024)***[38]
  - *Population:* LT recipients (LTRs) in the Toronto Lung Transplant Program from 2010 to 2015 with post-transplant 24-hour pH/impedance testing and available post-transplant Large Airway Bronchial Wash/bronchoalveolar lavage (BAL) samples collected 60 to 120 days post-transplant were included in this study.
  - *Outcomes:* PGA4 was expressed in a healthy human stomach but not lungs. Airway PGA4, but not total pepsin, was associated with aspiration. Airway PGA4 was associated with an increased risk of CLAD in two independent cohorts of LTRs on multivariable analysis (time to CLAD H.R 2.28, 95% C.I 1.17-4.47, p=0.02) but not to time to death and retransplant (H.R 1.44, 95% C.I 0.76-2.73, p=0.26). Anti-reflux surgery was associated with reduced airway PGA4 (N=5). The use of proton pump inhibitors was not associated with reduced PGA4.
  - *Conclusion:* Airway PGA4 is a marker of aspiration that predicts CLAD in LTRs. However, there are immense number of biases in the inclusion design of this cohort and it needs to be replicated in a prospective cohort. **Measuring PGA4 at surveillance bronchoscopies can help triage high-risk LTRs for anti-reflux surgery.** The lack of availability of a biomarker can explain the negative results of anti-reflux surgery post-LT due to confounding.[39] More clarification with trials enriched with patients having biomarker-high microaspiration is needed to elucidate the role of anti-reflux surgery post-LT.[40,41]

DISCUSSION

Indications for transplantation

The most common indications for lung transplant remain interstitial lung diseases (IPF and Progressive pulmonary fibrosis), advanced COPD, worsening cystic fibrosis, and pulmonary arterial hypertension associated with intermediate-high or high-risk scores (ESC/ERS) on appropriate therapy during follow-up (Figure 1 and Tables 1 and 2). Such patients should be referred to a transplant center for assessment of the risks and benefits of transplantation, optimization, and listing in the absence of contraindications (Table 3). In the Indian context, challenges arise from 1) absence of cohort-level data on survival for the above indications associated with a clinician's overestimation of survival from chronic lung disease (immortal time bias, with only those surviving coming for follow-up) and 2) number of lung transplant centers and robust follow-up data. The latter is likely to change with lung transplants now being offered routinely. At least five centers in Chennai have an in-house program in 2024 with another two programs each in Hyderabad and New Delhi; more are associating with these programs to establish new ones (Bengaluru, Mumbai, Pune, Ahmedabad, and New Delhi). As numbers and experience accumulate, outcomes will mature and this will further strengthen the pulmonologist's perception of better outcomes post-lung transplantation. Certainly, there are several lung transplant recipients (LTRs) doing well years after their index lung transplantation in India.

The ISHLT document guideline on recipient selection is a comprehensive one. In the Indian context, particular challenges include our high rates of ILDs referred for transplant (65% of all cases, often with advanced pulmonary hypertension and frailty). This cohort frequently needs bridging (BTT) and this leads to additional costs and poorer outcomes (typically 15% lower 1-year and 3-year survival). As pulmonologists' acceptance of lung transplantation as an option increase, early referral will lead to better outcomes (>90% survival at 1 year and >70% at 5 years). These outcomes will remain far superior with the additional outcomes of better quality of life and lower medical costs after lung transplantation. **Additional differences in our context include bronchiectasis (not associated with cystic fibrosis) and post-tuberculous lung disease as an indication for transplantation.** While these patients may often have a prolonged stable disease course, those referred for transplantation are those with severe pulmonary hypertension and on domiciliary oxygen and BiPAP. Low BMI, poor documentation of tuberculosis treatment regimen, and colonization with Aspergillus and resistant bacteria are additional challenges in this cohort. Cohort-level data of patients with advanced bronchiectasis and advanced post-tuberculous lung disease will help better case selection for lung transplantation.

Induction immunosuppression

Induction immunosuppression refers to the use of Anti-thymocyte globulin, basiliximab (anti-IL-2R), or alemtuzumab (anti-CD52, now discontinued) in the intra- or early postoperative period for reducing the chances of immune-mediated acute allograft rejection and dysfunction. This also enables a lower maintenance immunosuppression to be used subsequently. **High-dose glucocorticoids are routinely used just before re-perfusion of either side of lung allografts (methylprednisolone 1000mg in total) and this is not considered part of induction immunosuppression.** Cohort studies indicate a possible reduction in mortality and acute rejection with the use of induction therapy while a systematic review of small RCTs indicates no benefit and a high risk of bias in published studies. There is insufficient data to recommend induction over none or one agent over the other. Certainly, large programs with >200 transplants annually have good outcomes without induction immunosuppression. **In India, any additional immunosuppression must be balanced against the risk of postoperative infections, which remain the most common cause of early mortality.** It is however, common practice to use Basiliximab intra-operatively to delay tacrolimus initiation post-operatively when there is an anticipated risk of acute kidney injury (severe PH, bleeding).

Maintenance immunosuppression

Maintenance immunosuppression regimen is life-long and it is easier to prevent rejection rather than to treat it.

A combination of immunosuppressive agents is used and this varies with the transplant center. **Available evidence and consensus guidelines prefer a combination of three drugs; steroids, a Calcineurin Inhibitor (Cyclosporine, CYC or Tacrolimus, TAC) and a cell cycle inhibitor (Mycophenolate, MMF or Azathioprine, AZA).** Steroids are initially dosed at 0.75 mg per kg per day prednisone or equivalent. **Among CNI, TAC is preferred due to better pharmacokinetics and lower acute rejection rates**; data on clinically relevant outcomes like Bronchiolitis obliterans rates and mortality is variable. **Among anti-metabolites, there is no data to choose one over another**; MMF is often used. MMF has no advantage in efficacy over AZA in a TAC-containing regimen. Anti-proliferative agents, primarily mammalian targets of rapamycin inhibitors (mTORi)have been studied in lung transplant recipients to reduce side effects, BOS, and for their anti-cancer properties. There are several caveats; their labeling lists that they are not to be used for liver/lung recipients; mTORi should not be started within 90 days of transplant due to high rate of anastomotic dehiscence; sirolimus and everolimus have a 1-4% incidence of interstitial lung disease that might be progressive despite discontinuation; both carry a 16% risk of venous thromboembolism and the dose of CNI has to be reduced while on mTORi. They have a different list of metabolic complications compared to CNIs. **Both CNI and mTORi interact with many commonly used drugs via CYP3A4 and p-glycoprotein efflux pump mechanisms. At present, mTORi are reserved for patients beyond 3 months intolerant of both AZA and MMF, patients with CNI-related kidney injury (to lower TAC trough), and occasionally in recipients with post-transplant lymphoproliferative disease.**

Post-transplant infections

Infection is an important cause of morbidity, re-admission, and mortality during the post-transplant course. The rate of infections depends on the "net state of immunosuppression" of the patient; prior exposures (tuberculosis, farming, travel, pets); vaccination status, and planned prophylaxis and its duration. "The net state of immunosuppression" depends on

(a) Immunosuppression: Type, temporal sequence, intensity, Induction

(b) Prior Rx: Chemotherapy, anti-microbials

(c) Mucocutaneous integrity: Lines, catheters

(d) Neutropenia, lymphopenia, hypogammaglobulinemia

(e) Technical complications: graft injury, collections, wound

(f) Immune defects: autoimmune dis, polymorphisms

(g) Metabolic: uremia, diabetes, malnutrition, age, alcoholism

(h) Viral infection: Herpes, RSV, influenza, HIV/HBV/HCV

A discussion on "safe living post-lung transplantation" is crucial before discharge in lung recipients. There is an anticipated timeline of infections post-lung transplant (Table 4); the initial approach to a recipient with suspected infection utilizes this table and the radiologic findings to narrow the differential diagnosis. It is crucial to review the intensity of immunosuppression when unanticipated infections happen in the recipient.

Viral Infections: Influenza is the most common respiratory viral infection (CARV) and annual vaccination of both the recipient and their household is an important part of post-transplant optimization. Infection is treated with oseltamivir and a brief steroid surge/taper. Similar concerns currently exist on vaccination, prevention of COVID-19 (and its variants-related surges), and its treatment with nirmatrelvir-ritonavir. The drug interactions between nirmatrelvir-ritonavir and CNIs and the possibility of relapse with a 5-day course must be addressed. The challenges in managing RSV CARV were discussed above. CARVs may be followed by fungal infections and these events may increase the risk of subsequent chronic lung allograft dysfunction (CLAD).

CMV is an important middle-period infection in LTRs. The rates of anticipated CMV infection without prophylaxis is 20-25% in CMV R+ recipients and approaches 70% in the case of CMV mismatch (Donor CMV IgG+/Recipient CMV IgG-); CMV disease occurs in 10% and 25% respectively. Prophylaxis is administered for 12 months for mismatch and six months for CMV IgG+ recipients, with subsequent CMV DNA PCR monitoring till the end of the first year. CMV prophylaxis is also administered to cover periods of intensification of immunosuppression (Pulse steroids, ATG). **Treatment of CMV disease is based on the severity of the clinical syndrome; CMV pneumonitis is typically treated with ganciclovir parenterally, with subsequent conversion to Valganciclovir after 2-3 weeks of clinical response**. In non-severe disease or CMV syndrome, oral valganciclovir is as efficacious as ganciclovir. With the use of prophylaxis, late-onset CMV disease after cessation of prophylaxis is common and needs monitoring. Epstein-Barr virus infection related to a mismatch is linked to early post-transplant lymphoproliferative disease.

Bacterial Infections: **Early period bacterial infections are nosocomial derived and related to ventilation and catheters (bloodstream related, urinary tract)**. Clostridiodes difficile can also occur in this period. Donor-derived bacterial pneumonia and bacteremia is common, especially with the use of extended donors. **Perioperative antibiotic prophylaxis is recommended as per local nosocomial infection antibiogram for at least 72 hours in uncomplicated cases. Positive donor cultures are treated with appropriate antibiotics for at least 2 weeks.** Bacterial infections again occur in the late period and reflect pathogens in the community.

Fungal infection: Among fungal infections, **Candida predominates in the first 30 days, and molds especially Aspergillus predominate after 30 days.** Candida prophylaxis is also not universal, except for central ECMO during surgery, post-operative ECMO utilization, and Candida isolation from the airways. **International society guidelines recommend either universal prophylaxis (administration of antifungals to all recipients) or pre-emptive therapy (antifungals on detection of colonization on routine surveillance investigations including BAL Galactomannan); there is considerable controversy over which is the best approach.** All patients with pre-transplant mold isolation should receive antifungal prophylaxis. **Echinocandins are the choice to cover Candida or instead of azoles for molds in the presence of hepatitis. Nebulized liposomal amphotericin B with or without voriconazole is used as mold active universal prophylaxis or pre-emptive therapy for three months. Indefinite prophylaxis against *Pneumocystis jirovecii* pneumonia is recommended.**

Parasitic infections: Pre-transplant screening for Strongyloidiasis by ELISA and eradication therapy in those positive is the standard of care in Western countries. **In tropical countries, pre-transplant Universal eradication with ivermectin and albendazole (for Ascariasis) is utilized in all potential recipients.** Another potential parasitic infection of concern is Toxoplasma gondii, especially in heart-lung transplants. **Those with positive IgG ELISA for T. gondii are treated with daily Cotrimoxazole (double strength) prophylaxis life-long post-heart Lung Transplantation.**

Airway complications (Table 5): The lungs contain a dual blood supply from the pulmonary artery and the bronchial circulation. Post-lung transplantation, bronchial circulation is not typically restored, and the allograft is dependent on (deoxygenated) pulmonary artery blood for its viability till those connections are spontaneously restored (typically in 4 weeks). Post-transplant airway complications are common, occurring in up to 1 in 5 patients; interventions may be needed in 2-5% of patients. Airway complications can be ischemia, dehiscence, stenosis, or malacia. **Ischemia and dehiscence are early complications and are related to surgical techniques, donor lung preservation and post-operative recipient complications, including prolonged ventilation, need for ECMO and airway fungal infections. A short donor bronchus length is crucial to reduce anastomotic complications. Stenosis and/or malacia are late (>3 months) complications and may need balloon dilatation and/or stenting.**

Acute rejection: Acute cellular rejection (ACR) is the most common type of acute lung rejection and is due to a T-lymphocyte mediated response against donor Human leukocyte antigens (HLA) in the allograft. Patients may be asymptomatic or can have fever, dyspnea, cough or sputum production along with a decline in lung function. Evaluation includes spirometry and bronchoscopy with bronchoalveolar lavage (BAL) to rule out infection; **diagnosis is typically made on transbronchial lung biopsies with at least four adequate pieces needed.** ACR is common, occurring in 20-25% of recipients in the first year. The diagnosis is made on transbronchial lung biopsies and is graded from A0 to A4 for perivascular infiltrates and B0 to B2 for peri-bronchial lymphoid aggregates with immunological damage. **Unrecognized ACR is a risk factor for chronic lung allograft dysfunction (CLAD). Several centers utilize surveillance BAL and biopsies at around 1, 3-, 6-, 9- and 12-months post-transplant as an acceptable schedule to identify asymptomatic infection or rejection but this is controversial.**

Acute cellular rejection is treated with a methylprednisolone pulse of 10 mg/kg IV for 3 days followed by a tapering steroid regimen. Refractory ACR is treated with ATG. Switching maintenance immunosuppression to tacrolimus from cyclosporine and MMF for azathioprine is also frequently practiced.

Antibody-mediated rejection (AMR) is mediated by antibodies directed against HLA or other antigens in the allograft. **Hyperacute rejection occurs in the first few minutes to hours of reperfusion mediated by pre-existing donor-specific antibodies and is virtually unknown in the current era as recipients are routinely screened for pre-transplant anti-HLA antibodies.** The diagnosis of AMR is made with variable confidence (definite, probable, possible) depending on the presence of needed components of the diagnosis. The diagnosis is based on ISHLT guidelines which mandate all four of acute allograft dysfunction, presence of donor-specific antibodies, lung injury (capillaritis, diffuse alveolar damage or acute fibrinous organizing pneumonia) on histopathology, subendothelial C4d deposition in alveolar capillaries, and exclusion of other causes for allograft dysfunction. Categories of AMR include subclinical AMR and clinical AMR. **Treatment of AMR is often unsatisfactory and is directed at the removal of the offending antibodies, prevention of complement-mediated damage, and prevention of subsequent IgG formation; available options include IVIG, plasmapheresis, ATG, Rituximab, bortezomib, and eculizumab.**

Chronic lung allograft dysfunction (CLAD)

CLAD is defined as a substantial and persistent decline in measured FEV1 ≥20% from the reference (baseline) value persisting for beyond 3 months. The reference baseline value is computed as the mean of the best two postoperative FEV1 measurements taken >3 weeks apart. CLAD does not equate to chronic rejection and represents the end-stage response to a variety of insults which may be infectious, alloimmune, autoimmune, and dysfunctional injury-repair mechanisms (PGD, GERD) in the lung. The inferior outcome of lung transplantation compared to other solid organ transplants is primarily because of the frequency of chronic lung allograft dysfunction (CLAD). **While short-term outcomes have significantly improved, late morbidity and mortality, which is driven by CLAD, have remained the same over the last decade, affecting 50% by 5 years. CLAD remains the most common cause of death in 1-year survivors of lung transplantation, causing 45% of all deaths after 1 year of transplant.**

The diagnosis of CLAD involves ruling out reversible causes of allograft dysfunction and confounders (Tables 6 and 7).

Phenotypically, CLAD can be classified into

1. **Bronchiolitis obliterans syndrome (BOS): is the predominant form of CLAD, occurring in 65-70% and is manifest clinically as obstructive lung disease, defined by a FEV1/FVC<0.7.** BOS is characterized by an obstructive pulmonary function, air trapping on CT and obliterative bronchiolitis (OB) on histopathology. It is the clinical counterpart of predominant histologic dense fibrous scar tissue affecting the small airways (bronchiolitis obliterans, BO).
2. **Restrictive allograft syndrome (RAS): ISHLT has defined RAS in 2019 as a persistent ≥20% decline in FEV1 (± FVC) compared with the reference or baseline value; (2) a decrease in total lung capacity (TLC) to ≤90% compared with baseline, defined as the average of the 2 measurements obtained at the same time as or very near to the best 2 post-operative FEV1 measurements (since TLC subsequently may be higher with BOS); and (3) the presence of persistent opacities on chest imaging (chest X-ray [CXR] and/or computed tomography [CT]).** A CT is recommended but not obligated and should show parenchymal and/or pleural opacities. RAS is characterized by upper lobe-predominant fibrotic changes and restrictive pulmonary function tests all of which persist for more than 3 months. Predominant RAS occurs in 15-30% of CLAD but biopsies often show areas of BO simultaneously. RAS, especially lower-lobe predominant and associated with diffuse CT abnormalities and/or peripheral or BAL eosinophilia is associated with poor outcomes (when compared to BOS). **ISHLT statement recommends obtaining Body Plethysmography at 3, 6 months, and then at annual intervals** given the difficulty of using the FEV1/FVC & FVC surrogate in hyperinflation & pseudo-restriction due to raised IRC. Also, FEV1/FVC may be <0.7 in the presence of a true restriction in single allografts for COPD, anastomotic strictures, and when a BOS phenotype changes to RAS. RAS is now referred to as a restrictive type of CLAD (rCLAD).

3. **Mixed CLAD:** Where RAS develops after BOS has been established (mixed phenotype CLAD), the baseline for TLC should be taken as the last TLC measured in BOS to minimize the effect that gas trapping may have on the calculation of the FVC. If a restrictive defect is implied by changes in spirometry, as discussed in what follows, then an appellation of "probable" RAS can be applied, if facilities to measure TLC are not available.
4. Unclassified CLAD (Tables 6 and 7).

Management of CLAD

There are no proven therapies for CLAD except re-transplantation in carefully selected patients. Current options include:

1. **Avoiding high-dose steroids** (defined as >30 mg/day) except in those patients where ACR is a component.
2. **Azithromycin for patients with proven CLAD; typically, this is 250 mg weekly thrice.** The duration of therapy in those with a response is unknown but possibly life-long. If there is no response (typically defined as >10% increase in FEV1 by 3 months), it is again unknown whether it can be safely stopped. The role of azithromycin in RAS-type CLAD is also unknown.
3. **Montelukast has been used for the treatment of BOS-type CLAD,** but the database is not robust.
4. **Change in immunosuppression:** Tacrolimus over cyclosporine and Mycophenolate over azathioprine. The exact benefit of CLAD uncomplicated by ACR is unclear.
5. **ECP (Extracorporeal photopheresis)** for the management of progressive BOS (NCT02181257) is currently active.
6. **Mesenchymal stromal cell therapy** is of unclear benefit.
7. **Supplemental oxygen** improves breathlessness in those who are hypoxic.
8. **Supervised pulmonary rehabilitation** improves breathlessness.

CLAD is the main driver of re-transplants, accounting for 5% of all transplants in large centers. A four-center 10-year retrospective study of re-transplantation for CLAD included 143 patients [94 BOS (66%) and 49 rCLAD (34%)].[42] 88% of these were re-do double lung transplants. More patients were bridged toward re-LTx using ECMO in the rCLAD group compared to BOS ($p<0.011$) (23% in rCLAD vs. 7% in BOS) and there was more transfusion in the RAS arm (pleural fibrosis). Adjusted survival after re-LTx for RAS was worse compared to BOS (HR=2.61, 1.51–4.51; $p<0.0006$, respectively), which itself has poor survival compared to first transplants. Careful patient selection is crucial and most centers do not bridge RAS-type CLAD to re-transplantation.

Algorithmic approach has been described in Figure 1.

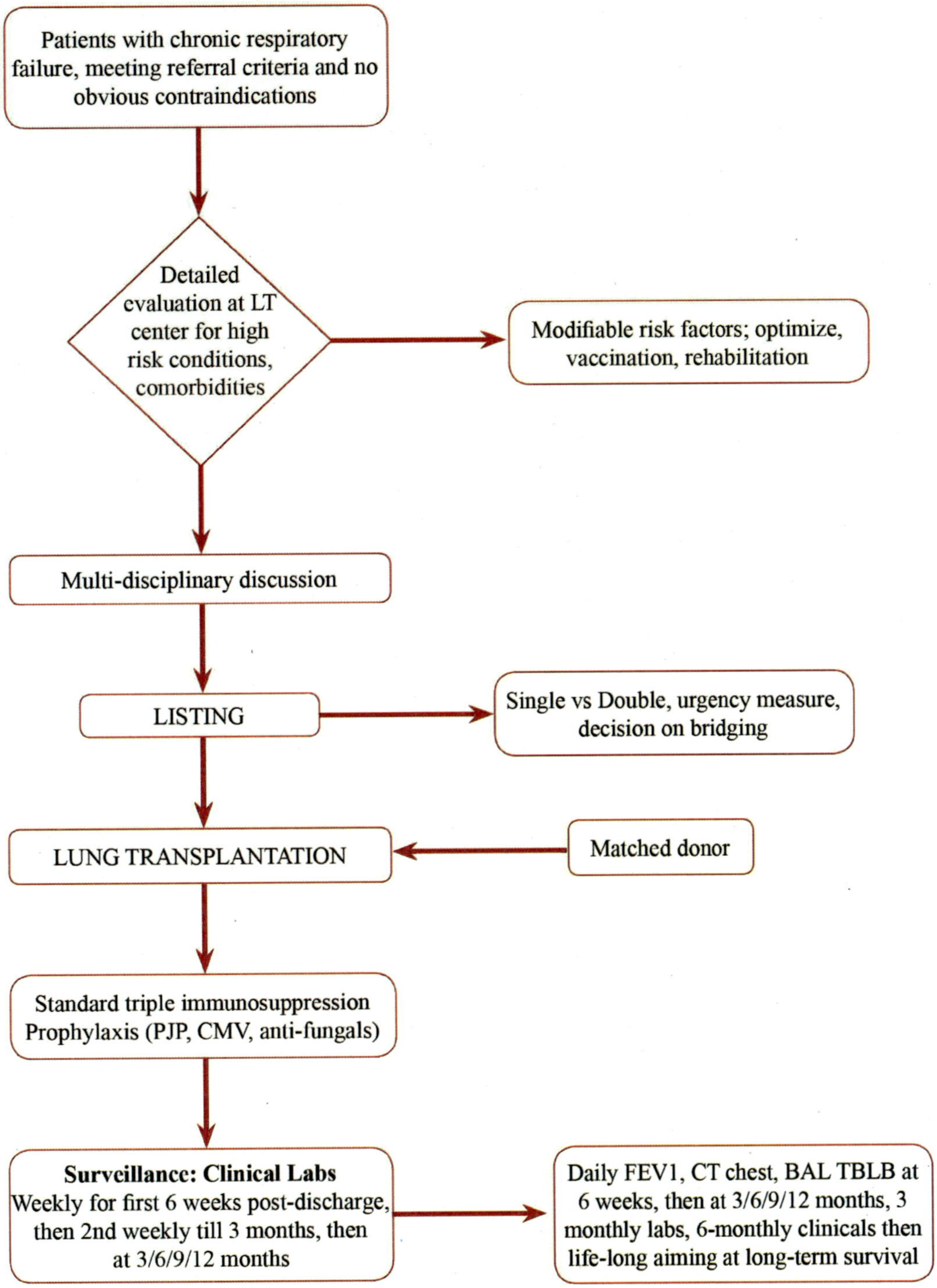

Figure 1: Algorithmic Approach: Abridged Algorithmic Pathway in Lung Transplant

Table 1: Disease-specific indications for lung transplantation (Modified from)[1]

Disease	Referral	Listing
Interstitial lung disease^	For UIP, irrespective of lung function, at the time of diagnosis**	FVC decline of ≥ 10% over 6 months or FVC decline > 5% with radiographic worsening
	FVC < 80%, DLco < 40%	DLco decline of ≥ 10% over 6 months
	Relative decline in: FVC decline ≥ 10%, DLco decline ≥ 15%, FVC decline ≥ 5% with clinical or CT progression over previous 2 years^	Desaturation to ≤ 88% or walking < 250 m at 6 minutes or decline in ≥ 50 meters over 6 months
	Any oxygen requirement, even if only on exertion	Pulmonary hypertension on RHC
	For inflammatory ILD, failure to improve on appropriate anti-inflammatory therapy	Hospitalization because of respiratory decline, pneumothorax, or acute exacerbation
Cystic fibrosis[@]	FEV1< 30% or falling rapidly on optimal therapy, especially in female gender	Chronic respiratory failure (PaO_2 < 60 mm Hg, $PaCO_2$ > 50)
	FEV1< 40% in adults and 6MWD < 400 m, $PaCO_2$ > 50 mm Hg, hypoxemia at rest/exertion, PAH, worsening nutritional status, ≥ 2 exacerbations needing IV therapy, massive hemoptysis, pneumothorax	FEV1 < 25%, Rapid decline in FEV1 or progressive symptoms (> 30% relative decline in FEV1 over 12 months)
		Any exacerbation requiring mechanical ventilation
	FEV1 < 50% and rapidly declining	Frequent hospitalization (> 28 days hospitalized preceding year)
	Any exacerbation needing non-invasive ventilation	PAH > 50 mm Hg, RV dysfunction, BMI < 18 kg/m^2, massive hemoptysis needing bronchial artery embolization, WHO IV
		Chronic respiratory failure associated with increasing oxygen requirements or needing long-term NIPPV
COPD	Disease is progressive, despite maximal treatment including medications, pulmonary rehabilitation and oxygen	BODE 7-10 with one additional factor prompting listing include any one: FEV1 < 20%, moderate-severe pulmonary hypertension, chronic hypercapnia
	BODE 5-6 with additional risk factor for mortality: frequent exacerbations, increase in BODE>1 in 24 months, PA/Ao >1 on CT, FEV1 20-25% Pred	
	Poor quality of life unacceptable to the patient	≥ 1 Severe exacerbation with acute hypercapnic respiratory failure
	Simultaneous referral for LVRS is acceptable	
Pulmonary vascular disease^	ESC/ERS intermediate or high risk or REVEAL score > 8 despite appropriate therapy	ESC/ERS high risk or REVEAL risk score > 10 on appropriate PAH therapy, including IV or SC prostacyclin analogues
	Significant right ventricular dysfunction despite appropriate therapy	Progressive hypoxemia, especially in patients with PVOD or PCH
	Need for IV or SC prostacyclin therapy	Progressive, but not end-stage, liver or kidney dysfunction due to pulmonary hypertension
	Consideration or proven PVOD/PCH	
	Progressive disease despite appropriate therapy or recent hospitalization for PAH worsening	
	Secondary liver or kidney dysfunction, recurrent hemoptysis	Life-threatening hemoptysis

Contd.

Contd.

Comments:

**In India, this is unlikely to be feasible given the disparity between disease incidence and number of transplant centers; referral on progression (while on anti-fibrotics) may be reasonable.

^ Early referral is recommended given poor outcomes for IPF and PPF. Patients with expected poor outcomes on the basis of clinical findings must be prioritized for referral. Patients with CTD-ILD, Chronic hypersensitivity pneumonitis, fNSIP, Familial ILD and unclassifiable ILD are managed using the same criteria.

@ FEV1 <30% of predicted was associated with a 2-year mortality of approximately 40% in men and 55% in women.

Liou *et al.* developed a model using the CF Foundation database and identified female sex, diabetes mellitus, B cepacia infection, and the number of exacerbations negatively correlated better than FEV1 alone. These are to be fulfilled after a trial of medical management of elexacaftor / tezacaftor / ivacaftor if eligible and available. For non-CF bronchiectasis, similar criteria may be applied as for CF, though these patients have slower decline in lung function and prolonged survival without transplantation.

Patients with CF colonized by cenocepacia have a higher rate of progression and poorer outcomes post-transplantation; centers managing these patients must evolve options for them.

BODE index 5-6 [BMI, airflow limitation (forced expiratory volume in one second), dyspnea and 6-minute walk distance], was the basis for listing in earlier guidelines. Comparative studies of expected mortality by BODE index and observed mortality in the lung transplant candidate cohort found that original BODE index-overestimated mortality. Referral criteria has been updated to BODE index 5-6 along with an additional factor for increased mortality (frequent exacerbations, increase in BODE index > 1 over last 2 years, pulmonary artery to aorta diameter >1, FEV1 20-25% predicted).

COPD presenting with acute hypercapnic respiratory failure has an in-hospital mortality of 10%, and patients who survive the hospital admission have a mortality rate of 43% at 1 year and 49% at 2 years post-admission.

LVRS and Tx can be assessed at the same meeting; in some patients with FEV1 > 20% < 25%, DLco > 20% and heterogeneous upper lobe predominant emphysema, LVRS can be offered first and may help the patients become more suitable for transplant.

^ Most of the patients being bridged using ECLS are in this cohort; typical strategies include an Avalon VV-ECMO to improve oxygenation. However, this may not offload the right ventricle. In patients with severe right ventricular failure, V-AV ECMO, Protek duo or Novalung may be needed to offload the right ventricle. Patients can then ambulate after extubation and be bridged to transplant.

Table 2: LAS grouping for lung transplantation

LAS Group A	LAS Group B	LAS Group C	LAS Group D*
COPD	iPAH	CF	IPF
α1-AT deficiency Bronchopulmonary dysplasia, Ehlers-Danlos Granulomatous LD	Eisenmenger's syndrome Congenital malformation	CVID Fibrocavitory disease Schwachmann-Diamond	Wegener's/CREST/HHTN-restrictive/SSc-ILD/PAP/Amyloidosis/BOOP/LIP/IPH/Fibrosing mediastinitis
Bronchiectasis ABPA Constrictive bronchiolitis	Specific pulmonary vascular diseases (CTEPH, PVOD/PCH, Porto-pulmonary, secondary PH) CREST-PH HHTN SSc-PH PS/Hypoplastic lung	Hypogammaglobinemia	HP/GVHD/Hermansky-Pudlack
LAM			ARDS/Pneumonia
Sarcoidosis mPAP ≤ 30 mm Hg Inhalation/burns PCD/Kartagener's Tuberous sclerosis Wegener's granulomatosis-bronchiectasis			Bronchoalveolar carcinoma/ Carcinoid
			Lung re-transplant/graft failure
			RA-ILD/MCTD-ILD/PSS-ILD/Polymyositis/Lupus/ Paraneoplastic pemphigus Castleman's/silicosis
			Sarcoidosis with mPAP > 30 mm Hg, surfactant B deficiency

Table 3: Contraindications for lung transplantation (Modified from)[1]		
Absolute contraindications	**High or substantially high risk**	**Risk factors**
Lack of patient acceptance of transplant	Age > 70 years*	Age 65-70 years
Malignancy with high risk of recurrence or death	Severe CAD requiring CABG at transplant, LVEF < 40%	GFR 40-60 mL/min/1.73 m^2
GFR< 40 mL/min/1.73 m^2 (unless multi-organ transplant)	Significant cerebrovascular disease	Mild to moderate coronary artery disease
Acute coronary syndrome or myocardial infarction within 30 days	Severe esophageal dysmotility	Severe CAD requiring PCI prior to LTx
Stroke within 30 days	Untreatable hematologic disorders including bleeding diathesis, thrombophilia, or severe bone marrow dysfunction	Prior coronary artery bypass grafting, LVEF 50-60%, Peripheral vascular disease
Liver cirrhosis with portal hypertension or synthetic dysfunction	BMI >35 kg/m^2 or < 16 kg/m^2	Connective tissue diseases (scleroderma, lupus, myopathies)
Acute liver failure	Limited functional status with potential for rehabilitation	Severe GER, esophageal dysmotility
Acute renal failure or on dialysis with low chance of recovery	Psychiatric, psychological or cognitive conditions affecting adherence	Persistent Thrombocytopenia, leukopenia, or anemia
Septic shock	Unreliable support system or caregiving plan	Osteoporosis
Active extrapulmonary or disseminated infection	Lack of understanding of disease and/or transplant	BMI 30-34.9 kg/m^2 or 16-17 kg/m^2
Active tuberculosis infection	Mycobacterium abscessus infection	Frailty, Hypoalbuminemia
HIV infection with detectable viral load	Lomentosporaprolificans infection	Diabetes that is poorly controlled
Limited functional status with poor potential for rehabilitation	Burkholderia cenocepacia or gladioli infection	Scedosporium apiospermum infection
Progressive cognitive impairment	Hepatitis B or C infection with detectable viral load and liver fibrosis	HIV with undetectable viral load
Repeated episodes of non-adherence	Chest wall or spinal deformity expected to cause restriction	Previous thoracic surgery, pleurodesis
Active substance use or dependence including current tobacco use, vaping, marijuana smoking, or IV drug use	Extracorporeal life support	Mechanical ventilation
Other severe uncontrolled medical condition expected to limit survival after transplant	Retransplant < 1 year, reTx for RAS and reTx for AMR	Retransplant for obstructive CLAD > 1 year

Comments: Carefully selected patients between 65 and 70 years have similar survival post-lung transplantation.

Abbreviations: GFR: Glomerular filtration rate, LVEF: Left ventricular ejection fraction, BMI: Body mass index, reTx: retransplantation, CAD: Coronary artery disease, PCI: Percutaneous coronary intervention, LTx: Lung transplantation, GER: Gastro-esophageal reflux disease. HIV: Human immunodeficiency virus, CLAD: Chronic lung allograft dysfunction.

Table 4: A timeline of infections post-lung transplantation relevant to the Indian context

<1 month	**1-12 months**	**>12 months**
Prophylaxis (Septra/ Valganciclovir/ voriconazole)	**Prophylaxis (Septran/ Valganciclovir)**	**Prophylaxis (Septran)**
Recipient/nosocomial derived	Viral: HCV, adenovirus, influenza, BK virus	CARVs, bacterial pneumonia
CRE Gram-negatives, espcarbapenemases (prolonged ventilation in donor)	Bacterial: Clostridium difficile	Infection with Aspergillus, other molds
MRSA, VRE, Candida	Mycobacterial reactivation	Tuberculosis, Late NTM disease
Aspiration	Early NTM disease	Late Viral infections
Catheter-related infection	Stronglyloides infection	CMV
Anastomotic site infection	Cryptococcus infection	Hepatitis (HBV, HCV)
Clostridium difficile	Rare: leishmaniasis, mucor	JC polyoma virus encephalitis
PreTx colonization-derived	All the Herpes virus infections are prevented by Valganciclovir for 6-9 months; Septran prevents PJP, toxoplasmosis, listeria, susceptible nocardiosis, Isospora belli, Cyclospora cayetanensis, UTI, GI, sinus and respiratory infections	EBV: PTLD
Pseudomonas, Aspergillus		
Donor-derived (bacteria, viruses, fungi)		
CMV, EBV		
Uncommon: HSV, Rabies, HIV		

Table 5: Summary of various classification systems of airway complications post-lung transplantation

Classification system	Year	Includes	Comments
Couraud *et al.*	1992	Macroscopic appearance on D15; system describes anastomotic ischemia and necrosis	No distal airway findings or other manifestations (stenosis, granulation, dehiscence)
Shennib and Massard	1994	Comprehensive assessment of ischemia and necrosis	Limited in description of stenosis simultaneous pathologies not defined
Chhajed *et al.*	2004	TEGLA system T-Mucosal injury thickness E-Circumferential extent G-Granulation extent L-Loose sutures A-Anastomoses and airway (distal)	No standardization of extent Dehiscence and stenosis are dichotomous Severity and extent have to be entered separately
Thistlethwaite *et al.*	2008	Extent of stenosis; various sites and severity	Did not include measures of severity Other features not included
Santa Cruz and Mehta	2009	Described 6 manifestations	dehiscence not separate from necrosis; not a grading system per se (descriptive)
Dutau *et al.*	2013	Macroscopic, Diameter, Suture system (MDS)	Ischemia and necrosis not graded
ISHLT, 2018	Ischemia	Perianastomotic (<1 cm from anastomoses)	< 50% circumferential ischemia
		Extending >1 cm from anastomosis to major airways (bronchus intermedius and distal left mainstem)	> 50-100% circumferential ischemia
		Extending >1 cm from anastomosis into lobar or segmental airways	< 50% circumferential necrosis
			> 50-100% circumferential necrosis
	Dehiscence	Cartilaginous	0-25% circumference
		Membranous	> 25-50% circumference
		Both	> 50-75% circumference
			> 75% circumference
	Stenosis	Anastomotic	0-25% reduction in cross-sectional area
		Anastomotic plus lobar/segmental	> 25-50% reduction in CSA
		Both	> 50% but < 100% reduction in CSA
			100% Obstruction
	Malacia	Perianastomotic <1 cm of anastomosis	
		Diffuse (involving anastomosis and > 1 cm)	

Table 6: Factors that have to be ruled out during evaluation of allograft dysfunction
Factors where recalculation/resetting of the FEV1 reference value may be valid (if FEV1 remains stable for at least 6 months)
1. Decreasing lung function due to the normal aging process
2. Surgical factors
Transplant lung resection, chest-wall surgery, phrenic nerve damage
3. Mechanical factors
Airway: Airway stenosis
Parenchyma: Persistent lung edema due to significant kidney/heart/liver failure
Parenchyma: Localized infection with chronic scarring: Abscess/empyema/mycetoma
Pleural: Persistent pleural effusion
Neuromuscular: Myopathy, neuropathy and Parkinson disease
SLT: Native lung hyperinflation after single lung
General: Weight gain
Failing to reach normal predicted lung function (i.e., low FEV1 reference value such that FEV1 is ≤ 80% of the recipient predicted value
Age difference between donor and recipient where older donor lungs are implanted or when an intra-operative allograft reduction surgery/lobectomy is performed
Factors that cannot be differentiated easily from CLAD and do not ever allow recalculation/resetting of the FEV1 reference value
1. Any from (A) above where there is not a period of at least 6 months of stability
2. Acute/subacute generalized infection
3. Acute/subacute cellular or antibody-mediated rejection
4. Acute/subacute effects of aspiration
5. Drug or other induced pulmonary toxicity (e.g., sirolimus, methotrexate, amiodarone, radiotherapy)
6. Pulmonary arterial strictures or emboli
7. Infiltration of the allograft with proven disease recurrence from the underlying transplant indication (e.g., LAM, sarcoidosis, etc.)
8. Infiltration with tumor

Table 7: Current ISHLT requirements to classify CLAD Phenotypes			
	Obstruction (FEV1/FVC < 0.7)	**Restriction (TLC decline ≥ 10% from baseline)**	**[c]CT opacities**
[a]BOS	Yes	No	No
[b]RAS	No	Yes	Yes
[d]Mixed	Yes	No	Yes
[e]Unclassified	Yes	Yes	No
	No	No	Yes

[a] Obstruction is defined by a fall in FEV1 ≥ 20% and associated with other indices of airflow limitation (FEV1/FVC ratio < 0.70).

[b] Restriction is properly defined as a ≥10% reduction in baseline TLC.

[c] Refers to parenchymal opacities and/or increasing pleural thickening consistent with a diagnosis of pulmonary and/or pleural fibrosis and likely to cause a restrictive physiology, rather than the airway-based changes consistent with bronchiectasis. Although the 2 (opacities and bronchiectasis) may coexist, in some cases, the presence of bronchiectasis may reflect traction changes on airways due to fibrotic parenchymal opacities.

[d] By definition, all cases that transition from a BOS phenotype to an RAS phenotype and vice-versa, will meet these criteria, which is in accord with histopathologic findings at explant/post mortem.

[e] Undefined means definite CLAD, but with 2 possible combinations of variables, making it difficult to categorize in the upper panels (BOS, RAS, or mixed phenotype).

REFERENCES

1. Leard LE, Holm AM, Valapour M, Glanville AR, Attawar S, Aversa M, et al. Consensus document for the selection of lung transplant candidates: An update from the International Society for Heart and Lung Transplantation. J Heart Lung Transplant. 2021; 40(11):1349-1379.

2. Holm AM. Candidate selection for lung transplantation - considerations beyond the medical evidence. Curr Opin Pulm Med. 2024; 30(4): 405-409.

3. Agarwal A, Neujahr DC. Frailty in Lung Transplantation: Candidate Assessment and Optimization. Transplantation. 2021 Oct 1;105(10):2201–12.

4. Singer JP, Diamond JM, Gries CJ, McDonnough J, Blanc PD, Shah R, et al. Frailty Phenotypes, Disability, and Outcomes in Adult Candidates for Lung Transplantation. Am J Respir Crit Care Med. 2015 Dec 1;192(11):1325–34.

5. Pugashetti JV, Kim JS, Combs MP, Ma SF, Adegunsoye A, Linderholm AL, et al. A multidimensional classifier to support lung transplant referral in patients with pulmonary fibrosis. J Heart Lung Transplant. 2024 Jul;43(7):1174–82.

6. Raghu G, Remy-Jardin M, Richeldi L, Thomson CC, Inoue Y, Johkoh T, et al. Idiopathic Pulmonary Fibrosis (an Update) and Progressive Pulmonary Fibrosis in Adults: An Official ATS/ERS/JRS/ALAT Clinical Practice Guideline. Am J Respir Crit Care Med. 2022 May 1;205(9):e18–47.

7. Mora Cuesta VM, Iturbe Fernández D, Aguado Ibáñez S, Anguera de Francisco G, Margallo Iribarnegaray J, Carrillo Hernández-Rubio J, et al. Antifibrotics and lung transplantation: A Spanish multicentre case-controlled study. Respirology. 2022 Dec;27(12):1054–63.

8. Zhu MZL, Huang JY, Liu DH, Snell GI. Does continuation of antifibrotics before lung transplantation influence post-transplant outcomes in patients with idiopathic pulmonary fibrosis? Interact Cardiovasc Thorac Surg. 2022 Jan 18;34(2):250–4.

9. Moncomble E, Weisenburger G, Picard C, Dégot T, Reynaud-Gaubert M, Nieves A, et al. Effect of antifibrotic agents on postoperative complications after lung transplantation for idiopathic pulmonary fibrosis. Respirology. 2024 Jan;29(1):71–9.

10. Palipana AK, Gecili E, Song S, Johnson SR, Szczesniak RD, Gupta N. Predicting Individualized Lung Disease Progression in Treatment-Naive Patients With Lymphangioleiomyomatosis. Chest. 2023 Jun;163(6):1458–70.

11. Cottin V, Si-Mohamed S, Diesler R, Bonniaud P, Valenzuela C. Pleuroparenchymal fibroelastosis. Curr Opin Pulm Med. 2022 Sep 1;28(5):432–40.

12. Clermidy H, Mercier O, Brioude G, Mordant P, Fadel G, Picard C, et al. Outcomes of lung transplantation for pleuroparenchymal fibroelastosis: A French multicentric retrospective study. J Heart Lung Transplant. 2024 Oct;43(10):1727–36.

13. Faccioli E, Verzeletti V, Giraudo C, Schiavon M, Calabrese F, Loy M, et al. Lung Transplantation for Pleuroparenchymal Fibroelastosis: A Single-Center Experience with Revision of Literature. Biomedicines. 2023 May 23;11(6).

14. Cypel M, Keshavjee S. When to consider lung transplantation for COVID-19. Lancet Respir Med. 2020 Oct;8(10):944–6.

15. Bharat A, Querrey M, Markov NS, Kim S, Kurihara C, Garza-Castillon R, et al. Lung transplantation for patients with severe COVID-19. Sci Transl Med. 2020 Dec 16;12(574).

16. Early outcomes after lung transplantation for severe COVID-19: a series of the first consecutive cases from four countries. Vol. 9. England; 2021.

17. Bermudez C, Bermudez F, Courtwright A, Richards T, Diamond J, Cevasco M, et al. Lung transplantation for COVID-2019 respiratory failure in the United States: Outcomes 1-year posttransplant and the impact of preoperative extracorporeal membrane oxygenation support. J Thorac Cardiovasc Surg. 2024 Jan;167(1):384-395.e3.

18. Hoetzenecker K, Schwarz S, Keshavjee S, Cypel M. Lung transplantation for acute respiratory distress syndrome. J Thorac Cardiovasc Surg. 2023 Apr;165(4):1596–601.

19. Tran T, Kashem MA, Firoz A, Yanagida R, Shigemura N, Toyoda Y. Lung transplant survival with past and concomitant cardiac revascularization. J Heart Lung Transplant. 2023 Oct;42(10):1334–40.

20. Abdelnour-Berchtold E, Ali A, Baciu C, Beroncal EL, Wang A, Hough O, et al. Evaluation of 10°C as the optimal storage temperature for aspiration-injured donor lungs in a large animal transplant model. J Heart Lung Transplant. 2022 Dec;41(12):1679–88.

21. Novysedlak R, Provoost AL, Langer NB, Van Slambrouck J, Barbarossa A, Cenik I, et al. Extended ischemic time (>15 hours) using controlled hypothermic storage in lung transplantation: A multicenter experience. J Heart Lung Transplant. 2024 Jun;43(6): 999–1004.

22. Snell GI, Yusen RD, Weill D, Strueber M, Garrity E, Reed A, et al. Report of the ISHLT Working Group on Primary Lung Graft Dysfunction, part I: Definition and grading-A 2016 Consensus Group statement of the International Society for Heart and Lung Transplantation. J Heart Lung Transplant. 2017 Oct;36(10):1097–103.

23. Cantu E, Diamond JM, Cevasco M, Suzuki Y, Crespo M, Clausen E, et al. Contemporary trends in PGD incidence, outcomes, and therapies. J Heart Lung Transplant. 2022 Dec;41(12):1839–49.

24. Diamond JM, Anderson MR, Cantu E, Clausen ES, Shashaty MGS, Kalman L, et al. Development and validation of primary graft dysfunction predictive algorithm for lung transplant candidates. J Heart Lung Transplant. 2024 Apr;43(4):633–41.

25. Subramaniam K, Loor G, Chan EG, Bottiger BA, Ius F, Hartwig MG, et al. Intraoperative Red Blood Cell Transfusion and Primary Graft Dysfunction After Lung Transplantation. Transplantation. 2023 Jul 1;107(7):1573–9.

26. Courtwright AM, Kamoun M, Diamond JM, Kearns J, Ahya VN, Christie JD, et al. Lung transplantation outcomes after crossing low-level donor specific antibodies without planned augmented immunosuppression. Clin Transplant. 2021 Nov;35(11):e14447.

27. Wang M, Campbell P, Lien DC, Varughese R, Weinkauf J, Nagendran J, et al. Safety of Crossing Donor-specific Antibodies in Lung Transplantation. Transplantation. 2023 May 1;107(5):1172–9.

28. Aversa M, Martinu T, Patriquin C, Cypel M, Barth D, Ghany R, et al. Long-term outcomes of sensitized lung transplant recipients after peri-operative desensitization. Am J Transplant. 2021 Oct;21(10): 3444–8.

29. Roux A, Hachem RR. Point-Counterpoint: Desensitization to improve the likelihood of lung transplantation. Hum Immunol. 2023 Jan;84(1):43–5.

30. Saddoughi SA, Martinu T, Patriquin C, Barth D, Huszti E, Ghany R, et al. Impact of intraoperative therapeutic plasma exchange on bleeding in lung transplantation. J Heart Lung Transplant. 2024 Mar;43(3):414–9.

31. Halloran K, Hirji A, Weinkauf J, Nagendran J, Campbell P. Exploring a postoperative alternative to intraoperative therapeutic plasma exchange for sensitized lung transplant recipients. J Heart Lung Transplant. 2024 May;43(5):859–60.

32. Levy L, Huszti E, Tikkanen J, Ghany R, Klement W, Ahmed M, et al. The impact of first untreated subclinical minimal acute rejection on risk for chronic lung allograft dysfunction or death after lung transplantation. Am J Transplant. 2020 Jan;20(1):241–9.

33. Beber SA, Moshkelgosha S, White M, Zehong G, Cheung M, Hedley D, et al. The CD8(+) T cell content of transbronchial biopsies from patients with a first episode of clinically stable grade A1 cellular rejection is associated with future chronic lung allograft dysfunction. J Heart Lung Transplant. 2024 Oct;43(10):1654–64.

34. Halloran K, Mackova M, Parkes MD, Hirji A, Weinkauf J, Timofte IL, et al. The molecular features of chronic lung allograft dysfunction in lung transplant airway mucosa. J Heart Lung Transplant. 2022 Dec;41(12):1689–99.

35. Pradère P, Zajacova A, Bos S, Le Pavec J, Fisher A. Molecular monitoring of lung allograft health: is it ready for routine clinical use? Eur Respir Rev. 2023 Dec 31;32(170).

36. Keller MB, Newman D, Alnababteh M, Ponor L, Shah P, Mathew J, et al. Extreme elevations of donor-derived cell-free DNA increases the risk of chronic lung allograft dysfunction and death, even without clinical manifestations of disease. J Heart Lung Transplant. 2024 Sep;43(9):1374–82.

37. Dellgren G, Lund TK, Raivio P, Leuckfeld I, Svahn J, Holmberg EC, et al. Effect of once-per-day tacrolimus versus twice-per-day ciclosporin on 3-year incidence of chronic lung allograft dysfunction after lung transplantation in Scandinavia (ScanCLAD): a multicentre randomised controlled trial. Lancet Respir Med. 2024 Jan;12(1): 34–44.

38. Ramendra R, Duong A, Zhang CYK, Huszti E, Zhou X, Havlin J, et al. Airway pepsinogen A4 identifies lung transplant recipients with microaspiration and predicts chronic lung allograft dysfunction. J Heart Lung Transplant. 2024 Jun;43(6):973–82.

39. Frankel A, Kellar T, Zahir F, Chambers D, Hopkins P, Gotley D. Laparoscopic fundoplication after lung transplantation does not appear to alter lung function trajectory. J Heart Lung Transplant. 2023 May;42(5):603–9.

40. Latorre-Rodríguez AR, Razia D, Omar A, Bremner RM, Mittal SK. Pulmonary and esophageal function in lung transplantation: Fundamental principles and clinical application. Transplant Rev (Orlando). 2024 Jan;38(1):100796.

41. Ahmad U. Commentary: Esophageal aperistalsis should not preclude lung transplant candidacy in well-selected patients. J Thorac Cardiovasc Surg. 2020 Dec;160(6):1629–30.

42. Halloran K, Aversa M, Tinckam K, Martinu T, Binnie M, Chaparro C, Chow CW, Waddell T, McRae K, Pierre A, de Perrot M, Yasufuku K, Cypel M, Keshavjee S, Singer LG. Comprehensive outcomes after lung retransplantation: A single-center review. Clin Transplant. 2018 Jun;32(6):e13281.

CHAPTER 18

Interventional Pulmonology

Authors: Dr. Manu Madan, Dr. Yash Kedia

Reviewer: Dr. Karan Madan

INTRODUCTION

Interventional pulmonology is associated with both diagnostics and therapeutics, thus proving to be an integral part of pulmonary medicine. Field of Interventional pulmonology is a dynamic field with novelties coming in very frequently, thus it is important to keep pace with newer advancements.

Methodology

We systematically searched pubmed using the search term "Peripheral pulmonary nodule" OR "central airway obstruction" OR "EBUS FNA" OR "endobronchial ultrasound" OR "EBUS" OR "Cone beam CT" OR "Bronchoscopy" OR "Tracheal stent" OR "Bronchial stent" OR "Argon plasma coagulation" OR "cryotherapy" OR "endobronchial valve" OR "bronchial thermoplasty" OR "Interventional pulmonology" OR "Thoracoscopy", for a period between 01/08/2023 to 01/08/2024. We got 3302 results from the term and finally selected 47 articles for the review.

Electronic database search: PubMed

Period: 1st August 2023 to 1st August 2024

Search words: "Peripheral pulmonary nodule" OR "central airway obstruction" OR "EBUS FNA" OR "endobronchial ultrasound" OR "EBUS" OR "Cone beam CT" OR "Bronchoscopy" OR "Tracheal stent" OR "Bronchial stent" OR "Argon plasma coagulation" OR "cryotherapy" OR "endobronchial valve" OR "bronchial thermoplasty" OR "Interventional pulmonology" OR "Thoracoscopy"
(n=3,302)

↓

Articles included in the review
(n=47)

Analysis of literature

1. BRONCHOSCOPY

a. *Sedation and Anaesthesia*

☞

- ***Five Versus 10 Pharyngeal Sprays of 10% Lignocaine for Topical Anesthesia During Flexible Bronchoscopy: A Multicenter, Randomized Controlled Trial (J Bronchology Interv Pulmonol. 2023)***[1]
  - o *Population:* Patients undergoing flexible bronchoscopy (n=284). This study was conducted in India (AIIMS, New Delhi).
  - o *Intervention:* 5 sprays of 10% lidocaine. (n=143)
  - o *Comparator:* 10 sprays of 10% lidocaine. (n=141)
  - o *Outcome:* The operator-rated overall procedure satisfaction, the VAS scores of patient-rated cough, and operator-rated cough, the time to reach vocal cords, overall procedure duration, mean doses of sedatives, and complications were similar between the two groups.
  - o *Conclusion:* During bronchoscopy, there was no difference in operator-rated overall procedure satisfaction between topical anesthesia with 5 sprays of 10% lidocaine vs 10 sprays, and so, 5 sprays can be preferred due to the lower cumulative lidocaine dose compared with 10 sprays.

- ***Comparison of remifentanil and esketamine in combination with propofol for patient sedation during fiberoptic bronchoscopy (BMC Pulm Med. 2023)***[2]
  - o *Population:* Patients undergoing fiberoptic bronchoscopy. (n=84)
  - o *Intervention:* Propofol/ remifentanil. (PR group; n=42)
  - o *Comparator:* Propofol/esketamine. (PK group; n=42)
  - o *Outcome:* The dosage of propofol in the PR group was significantly higher than that in the PK group (144 ± 38 mg vs. 125 ± 35 mg, P = 0.012). Patients in the PR group showed more transient hypoxia (SpO_2 < 95%), more intraoperative choking, postoperative vomiting and vertigo. Bronchoscopists in the PK group showed more satisfaction.
  - o *Conclusion:* Compared with remifentanil, the combination of esketamine with propofol in fiberoptic bronchoscopy leads to more stable hemodynamics, lower dosage of propofol, lower and greater bronchoscopists satisfaction.

- ***Safety and efficacy of remimazolam compared with midazolam during bronchoscopy: A single-center, randomized controlled study (Scientific reports. 2023)***[3]
  - o *Population:* Patients undergoing flexible bronchoscopy. (n=100)
  - o *Intervention:* Remimazolam as sedative. (n=49)
  - o *Comparator:* Midazolam as sedative. (n=51)
  - o *Outcome:* The time taken to reach peak sedation and the time from the end of the procedure to full alertness was significantly shorter in the remimazolam group than in the midazolam group. Hypotension, hypoxemia, tachycardia, the degree of patient and physician satisfaction were similar between the two groups.

- *Conclusion:* Remimazolam is effective and safe for achieving adequate sedation, with a shorter onset time and faster neuropsychiatric recovery than midazolam.

- ***Bolus administration of remimazolam was superior to midazolam for deep sedation in elderly patients undergoing diagnostic bronchoscopy: A randomized, double-blind, controlled trial. (Medicine (Baltimore. 2024)*** [4]
  - *Population:* Elderly patients (age range 65–80 yr; American Society of Anesthesiologists Physical Status I–III) undergoing bronchoscopy. (n=94)
  - *Intervention:* Remimazolam (0.135 mg/kg) for sedation induction. (n=46)
  - *Comparator:* Midazolam (0.045 mg/kg) for sedation induction. (n=48)
  - *Outcome:* The success rate of sedation at a single induced dose to achieve target depth (Ramsay sedation score = 4) was higher with remimazolam and the incidence of extra sleep within 6 hours after procedure was lower in the remimazolam group. No statistically significant differences were observed between the 2 groups regarding hemodynamic fluctuations, incidence of hypoxemia, and cough response during the procedure, as well as postoperative recall, willingness to undergo re-examination, and other post-bronchoscopy adverse events.
  - *Conclusion:* Bolus administration of remimazolam offers advantages over midazolam for deep sedation in elderly patients undergoing bronchoscopy, in terms of a higher success rate of sedation and a lower incidence of sleepiness post procedure.

- ***The Safety and Efficacy of Remimazolam Compared to Dexmedetomidine for Awake Tracheal Intubation by Flexible Bronchoscopy: A Randomized, Double-Blind, Controlled Trial. (Drug Des Devel Ther. 2024)*** [5]
  - *Population:* Patients undergoing Awake Tracheal Intubation by Flexible Bronchoscopy. (n=90)
  - *Intervention:* Dexmedetomidine 0.6 μg/kg + sufentanil (group DS) (n=30) vs remimazolam 0.073 mg/kg + sufentanil (group R_1S). (n=30)
  - *Comparator:* Remimazolam 0.093 mg/kg + sufentanil (group R_2S). (n=30)
  - *Outcome:* The success rates of sedation in groups R_2S and DS were higher than that in group R_1S. Group R_2S had shorter intubation times than groups R_1S and DS ($P = 0.003$), and a higher incidence of tracheal intubation amnesia than group DS.
  - *Conclusion:* Both dexmedetomidine and high dose remimazolam were effective in successful sedation and better intubation conditions, with minor respiratory depression. However, as compared to dexmedetomidine, remimazolam was associated with shorter intubation time and more anterograde amnesia.

- ***Clinical usefulness of nebulized dexmedetomidine for conscious sedation in daycare flexible bronchoscopy in Southern India. (Indian J Pharmacol. 2024)*** [6]
  - *Population:* Patients undergoing diagnostic bronchoscopy. (n=60)
  - *Intervention:* Nebulized dexmedetomidine. (n=30)
  - *Comparator:* Nebulized 0.9% normal saline. (n=30)
  - *Outcome:* The intensity of pain and mean cough score were lower in the dexmedetomidine group compared to the placebo.
  - *Conclusion:* Dexmedetomidine in the nebulized form improves the comfort of patients during the procedure.

- ***The different doses of sufentanil combined with nalmefene in bronchoscopy: A systematic review and meta-analysis. (J Thorac Dis. 2024)***[7]
    - *Population:* Different doses of sufentanil combined with nalmefene in bronchoscopies as evaluated in 6 studies. (n=774)
    - *Intervention:* Sufentanil plus Nalmefene
    - *Comparator:* Conventional therapy
    - *Outcome:* Compared to conventional therapy, combined use of sufentanil and nalmefene was associated with better hemodynamic outcomes, including stable blood pressure, heart rate and oxygen saturation, with better sedative effects. Subgroup analysis of different doses shows that sufentanil at 0.4 μg/kg was the most effective, with fewer side effects.
    - *Conclusion:* Use of sufentanil plus nalmefene may improve patient hemodynamics and better sedation in patients undergoing bronchoscopy.

- ***Dexmedetomidine-ketamine combination versus fentanyl-midazolam for patient sedation during flexible bronchoscopy: A prospective, single-blind, randomized controlled trial. (BMC Pulm Med. 2024)***[8]
    - *Population:* Patients undergoing diagnostic bronchoscopy. (n=50)
    - *Intervention:* Dexmedetomidine-ketamine (DK) for sedation. (n=25)
    - *Comparator:* Midazolam-fentanyl (MF) for sedation. (n=25)
    - *Outcome:* There was no significant difference in critical desaturation events and hemodynamic between the two groups. DK achieved deeper maximum sedation levels (higher Ramsay - lower Riker scale) and was associated with longer recovery times. Patient satisfaction was similar between the two groups, but bronchoscopist satisfaction was higher with the DK combination.
    - *Conclusion:* Use of dexmedetomidine-ketamine as compared to midazolam-fentanyl was associated with better bronchoscopist satisfaction during bronchoscopy, but there was no difference in patient hemodynamics and oxygenation.

- ***The Influence of Piriform Recess Instillation with Lidocaine Before Bronchoscopy on Post-General Anesthesia Cough: A Randomized Controlled Trial. (Drug Des Devel Ther. 2024)***[9]
    - *Population:* Patients undergoing bronchoscopy under general anaesthesia with laryngeal mask ventilation. (n=88)
    - *Intervention:* Piriform recess instillation with 2 mL 2% lidocaine. (n=44)
    - *Comparator:* 2 ml normal saline instillation. (n=44)
    - *Outcome:* The severity of cough and sore throat score at 10 min after extubation in lidocaine group was significantly lower as compared to the saline group. The subject-rated overall anesthesia satisfaction score was significantly higher in lignocaine group.
    - *Conclusion:* Piriform recess instillation with lidocaine before bronchoscopy can reduce cough intensity.

b. Oxygenation and Ventilation during Bronchoscopy

- ***Efficacy of different respiratory supports to prevent hypoxia during flexible bronchoscopy in patients of COPD: A triple-arm, randomised controlled trial. (BMJ Open Respiratory Research. 2023)***[10]
  - *Population:* COPD patients undergoing flexible bronchoscopy (n=90). This study was conducted in India (PGIMS, Rohtak)
  - *Intervention:*

    a. Bronchoscopy on NIV. (n=30)

    b. Bronchoscopy on HFOT. (n=30)
  - *Comparator:* Bronchoscopy on conventional oxygen therapy (COT). (n=30)
  - *Outcome:* SpO_2 and respiratory rate during flexible bronchoscopy were worst in COT group. Post bronchoscopy PaO_2 was highest in NIV arm, while post bronchoscopy $PaCO_2$ was similar in all three arms. Operator's ease-of-performing-procedure was least in the NIV group and a higher number of NIV group participants reported nasal pain as compared with the other two arms.
  - *Conclusion:* NIV and HFOT are superior to conventional oxygen therapy in preventing hypoxia during bronchoscopy, but NIV is associated with poor patient-tolerance and inferior operator's ease of doing procedure.

- ***Supraglottic Jet Oxygenation and Ventilation to Minimize Hypoxia in Patients Receiving Flexible Bronchoscopy Under Deep Sedation: A 3-Arm Randomized Controlled Trial. (Anesth Analg. 2024)***[11]
  - *Population:* Adult patients scheduled to undergo flexible bronchoscopy. (n=132)
  - *Intervention:* Supraglottic jet oxygenation and ventilation (SJOV) via Wei nasal jet tube (WNJ). (n=44)
  - *Comparator:* Oxygen supplementation via WNJ alone (n=44) or nasal catheter (NC). (n=44)
  - *Outcome:* Number of hypoxic events were significantly higher among patients receiving oxygen supplementation via WNJ alone and nasal catheter as compared to SJOV group. The percentage of subclinical respiratory depression was also significantly diminished in patients with SJOV (39%) compared with patients with NC (100%) or patients with LPLF (96%).
  - *Conclusion:* Supraglottic jet oxygenation and ventilation via Wei nasal jet tube effectively reduces the incidence of hypoxia during FB under deep sedation.

- ***Optimal flow of high-flow nasal cannula oxygenation to prevent desaturation during sedation for bronchoscopy: A randomized controlled study. (Ther Adv Respir Dis. 2024)***[12]
  - *Population:* Patients undergoing diagnostic bronchoscopy. (n=240)
  - *Intervention:* HFNC with propofol sedation (fraction of inspired oxygen, 100%) at flow of 10 (n=40), 20 (n=40) and 30 (n=40) L/min.
  - *Comparator:* HFNC with propofol sedation (fraction of inspired oxygen, 100%) at flow of 40 (n=40), 50 (n=40), and 60 (n=40) L/min.
  - *Outcome:* The incidence of desaturation significantly decreased by increasing the oxygen flow rate. The optimal oxygen flow rate for HFNC determined by probit regression to effectively prevent desaturation in 95% of patients was 43.20 (95% confidence interval, 36.43–55.96) L/min.
  - *Conclusion:* An HFNC flow rate of 40-50 L/min could prevent desaturation during sedation for bronchoscopy.

- ***The effectiveness of transnasal high flow nasal cannula in bronchoscopy under sedation: A systematic review and meta-analysis. (Front Med (Lausanne). 2024)***[13]
  - o *Population:* Application of high flow nasal cannula in patients undergoing bronchoscopy as evaluated in 12 studies. (n=1631)
  - o *Intervention:* Use of HFNC during flexible bronchoscopy.
  - o *Comparator:* Other oxygen therapy (Nasal cannula (n=8), NIV (n=2), HFNC with lower flow rate (n=1), not mentioned. (n=1))
  - o *Outcome:* HFNC significantly reduced the incidence of hypoxemia and improved the minimum oxygen saturation, reduced procedure time and improved PaO_2 at the end of the procedure compared to conventional oxygen therapy.
  - o *Conclusion:* HFNC in comparison to conventional oxygen therapy during flexible bronchoscopy is associated with significantly better oxygenation and fewer episodes of hypoxemia.

c. Sampling in Flexible Bronchoscopy

- ***Prophylactic epinephrine attenuates severe bleeding in lung transplantation patients undergoing transbronchial lung biopsy: Results of the PROPHET randomized trial. (J Heart Lung Transplant. 2023)***[14]
  - o *Population:* Lung transplant recipients undergoing transbronchial lung biopsy. (n=66)
  - o *Intervention:* 1:10,000-diluted topical epinephrine administered prophylactically into the target segmental airway. (n=46)
  - o *Comparator:* Saline placebo administered prophylactically into the target segmental airway. (n=54)
  - o *Outcome:* Severe or very severe hemorrhage occurred in 4 cases (8%) in the prophylactic epinephrine group and in 13 cases (24%) in the control group (p = 0.04).
  - o *Conclusion:* Prophylactic administration of 1:10,000-diluted topical epinephrine into the target segmental airway before trans bronchial lung biopsy attenuates the incidence of significant endobronchial hemorrhage without conveying a significant cardiovascular risk.

☞

- ***Bronchoscopic Electrocautery Versus Adrenaline and Cold Saline Instillation for Prophylactic Haemostasis Prior to Biopsy of Endobronchial Lesions (BEVACS): A Randomized Controlled Trial. (J Bronchology Interv Pulmonol. 2024)***[15]
  - o *Population:* Patients undergoing bronchoscopy with endobronchial biopsy for endobronchial lesion (n=60). This study was conducted in India (AIIMS, Jodhpur).
  - o *Intervention:* Prophylactic electrocautery using 15 watts.
  - o *Comparator:* Prophylactic adrenaline and cold saline.
  - o *Outcome:* Even though there was significantly lesser bleed in the electrocautery arm, there was no significant difference in the proportion of grade 2 or higher bleeding between the two arms.
  - o *Conclusion:* There was no difference in post biopsy bleed between the application of electrocautery or instillation of cold saline plus adrenaline before biopsy of those endobronchial lesions which were likely to bleed more after biopsy.

☞

- **Assessment of a randomized controlled trial on the safety of pre-placing bronchial balloons in transbronchial lung cryobiopsy for diagnosing interstitial lung disease.** ***(Eur J Med Res, 2024)***[16]
  - o *Population:* Patients with suspected ILD undergoing transbronchial lung cryobiopsy. (n=250)
  - o *Intervention:* Pre-placed balloon group. (n=125)
  - o *Comparator:* Non-pre-placed balloon group. (n=125)
  - o *Outcome:* There were no significant differences in severe bleeding between the none-pre-placed balloon group and pre-placed balloon group, while more moderate bleeding occurred in the non-pre-placed balloon group (26.4% vs. 6.4%, adjusted $p = 0.001$), as well as more use of haemostatic drug.
  - o *Conclusion:* A pre-placed bronchial balloon can reduce the incidence of moderate bleeding and increase the confidence of the bronchoscopists.

☞

- **A Randomized Control Trial Comparing the Yield of Bronchoalveolar Lavage Using Three Different Techniques in Patients Undergoing Flexible Bronchoscopy (BAL-3T).** ***(J Bronchology Interv Pulmonol, 2024)***[17]
  - o *Population:* Patients undergoing flexible bronchoscopy and bronchoalveolar lavage (n=942). This study was conducted in India (PGIMER, Chandigarh).
  - o *Intervention:* BAL using wall mount suction (WMS) (n=314), BAL using manual suction (MS) (n=314).
  - o *Comparator:* BAL using manual suction with tubing (MST). (n=314)
  - o *Outcome:* The optimal yield (defined as at least 30% return of volume instilled and <5% bronchial cells) was similar in all the groups. The proportion of patients with BALF return >30% was significantly higher in the WMS and MS than in the MST arm. There was no difference in the complication rate across the groups.
  - o *Conclusion:* There is no difference in optimal yield of BAL obtained by using wall mount suction vs manual suction.

d. Simulation for Flexible Bronchoscopy Training

- ***Effectiveness of Flexible Bronchoscopy Simulation-Based Training: A Systematic Review. (Chest. 2023)***[18]
  - o *Population:* Simulation-based training (SBT) to teach flexible bronchoscopy (FB) skills to novice trainees as evaluated in 14 studies. (n=367)
  - o *Intervention:*
    - a. Virtual reality simulator. (n=12 studies)
    - b. Part task trainer. (n=1 study)
    - c. Simulation equipment not mentioned. (n=1)
  - o *Comparator:* Conventional training.
  - o *Outcome:* 11 out of the 14 studies reported positive effects of simulation training programs on their outcome measures (procedure time, percentage of segments entered, wall contact, time in redout etc., there was no consensus among investigators on outcome measures).
  - o *Conclusion:* Flexible bronchoscopy simulation-based training is effective in improving skills when evaluated in a simulation setting.

- ***Simulation-based bronchoscopy training: Randomized trial comparing worked example to video introduction. (Pediatr Pulmonol. 2023)***[19]
    - o *Population:* Medical students participating in a simulator-based bronchoscopy training program using AccuTouch Flexible Bronchoscopy Simulator. (n=60)
    - o *Intervention:* Participants who received modeling example. (n=30)
    - o *Comparator:* Participants who received a video lesson. (n=30)
    - o *Outcome:* Simulation-based training was effective for both groups, based on simulator metrics. The modeling example group outperformed the control group in all measures, i.e, bronchoscopy execution time, number of collisions on the bronchial wall, red out time, percentage of bronchi examined and percentage of bronchi examined/minute.
    - o *Conclusion:* The modeling example group showed substantial benefits over the control group, both in reducing the cognitive load in learning and in retaining knowledge and skill after 15 days and 12 months.

- ***Artificial Intelligence Improves Novices' Bronchoscopy Performance: A Randomized Controlled Trial in a Simulated Setting. (Chest.2024)***[20]
    - o *Population:* Novices without former bronchoscopy experience practiced on a mannequin. (n=20)
    - o *Intervention:* Practiced on AI-based automatic bronchial segment identification feedback (Feedback group). (n=10)
    - o *Comparator:* Conventional training. (n=10)
    - o *Outcome:* The feedback group performed significantly better on all three outcome measures: diagnostic completeness, structured progress, and procedure time.
    - o *Conclusion:* Training guided by AI makes novices perform more complete, more systematic, and faster bronchoscopies.

d. Miscellaneous

- ***Bronchoscopy-guided antimicrobial therapy for cystic fibrosis. (Cochrane Database Syst Rev. 2024)***[21]
    - o *Population:* Patients with cystic fibrosis from two RCTs. (n=185)
    - o *Intervention:* Antimicrobial therapies guided by the results of bronchoscopy.
    - o *Comparator:* Antimicrobial therapies guided by any other type of sampling.
    - o *Outcome:* Antimicrobial therapy directed by the use of BAL or standard of care did not make significant difference in lung functions after two years as measured by the change from baseline in lung clearance index and FEV1, chest scores assessed by computed tomography (CT) scan at either two or five years and nutritional parameters or in the number of positive isolates of P aeruginosa per participant per year.
    - o *Conclusion:* There is no evidence to support the routine use of BAL for the diagnosis and management of pulmonary infection in patients with CF compared to the standard practice of providing treatment based on results of oropharyngeal culture and clinical symptoms.

☞

- ***World Association for Bronchology and Interventional Pulmonology (WABIP) guidelines on airway stenting for malignant central airway obstruction (MCAO). (Respirology. 2024)***[22]

Recommendations:

- o In patients with MCAO, airway stenting should be done to improve quality of life (Grade 2B).
- o In patients with MCAO, airway stenting can lead to improvement in survival (Grade 2C).
- o In patients with respiratory failure requiring invasive mechanical ventilation due to MCAO, airway stenting should be considered, as it may lead to early liberation from ventilatory support (Grade 1C).
- o In patients with MCAO requiring airway stenting, pulmonary hygiene measures should be implemented to reduce the incidence of stent-related complications (Expert Consensus).
- o In patients with MCAO requiring airway stenting, surveillance bronchoscopies after stenting should be performed to detect stent-related complications in asymptomatic patients (Grade 2C).
- o In patients with MCAO requiring airway stenting, either silicone or hybrid metallic stents should be used (Grade 2B).

2. ENDOBRONCHIAL ULTRASOUND (EBUS)

a. *Sedation and Analgesia*

- ***Esketamine Combined with Propofol TCI versus Propofol TCI for Deep Sedation during Endobronchial Ultrasound-Guided Transbronchial Needle Aspiration: A Prospective, Randomized, and Controlled Trial. (Int J Clin Pract. 2023)***[23]
  - o *Population:* Patients undergoing EBUS TBNA. (n=135)
  - o *Intervention:* 0.3 mg/kg esketamine, propofol Target controlled infusion (TCI), and 0.2 mg/kg/h esketamine with midazolam (0.01–0.03 mg/kg) and oxycodone (0.07–0.08 mg/kg) – Group E. (n=68)
  - o *Comparator:* Propofol TCI with midazolam (0.01–0.03 mg/kg) and oxycodone (0.07–0.08 mg/kg) – Group P. (n=67)
  - o *Outcome:* Patients in group E required significantly less lidocaine spraying frequency than group P. The cough score and mean arterial pressure were significantly better in group E. There were no significant differences between the two groups in terms of sedation-related adverse events and side effects, recovery time, endoscopist satisfaction, and patient satisfaction.
  - o *Conclusion:* Esketamine in combination with propofol TCI for deep sedation for EBUS-TBNA can improve the sedation effect, reduce coughing reaction during the procedure, and obtain more stable blood pressure.

b. *EUS vs EUS-B*

☞

- ***Performance of EUS-FNA and EUS-B-FNA for the diagnosis of left adrenal glands metastases in patients with lung cancer: A systematic review and meta-analysis. (Lung Cancer. 2023)***[24]
  - o *Population:* Patients undergoing EUS and/or EUS-B to diagnose left adrenal gland metastases in adults with (suspected) lung cancer from 19 studies. (n=1712)

- *Intervention:* EUS-B to visualized and sample left adrenal gland.
- *Comparator:* EUS to visualize and sample left adrenal gland
- *Outcome:* Both EUS and EUS-B had good ability to visualize and to sample with the left adrenal gland with good adequacy. Average malignancy detection rate was 0.42 (95 % CI 0.34–0.49). Ability to visualize was slightly higher for EUS than EUS-B.
- *Conclusion:* Both EUS and EUS-B have good performance and are safe for left adrenal gland analysis in patients with lung cancer.

c. Route: Oral vs Nasal

☞

- ***Comparison of Patient's Procedural Tolerance of EBUS-TBNA Performed Through Nasal Versus Oral Route: The NO-EBUS Randomized Clinical Trial. (J Bronchology Interv Pulmonol. 2024)***[25]
  - *Population:* Adults posted for a linear EBUS-TBNA examination under conscious sedation were randomized (n=180). This study was conducted in India (AIIMS, Rishikesh).
  - *Intervention:* EBUS via nasal route. (n=98)
  - *Comparator:* EBUS via oral route. (n=82)
  - *Outcome:* Subject-rated procedural tolerance, overall satisfaction, operator's ease of performing the procedure and subject's willingness to undergo a repeat procedure were found to be equivalent in the 2 groups.
  - *Conclusion:* Nasal route for EBUS-TBNA could be considered where it is feasible for the patient as well as the operator.

d. Needle

☞

- ***Diagnostic Yield and Safety of the 19-Gauge versus 22-Gauge Endobronchial Ultrasound-Guided Transbronchial Needle Aspiration Needle in Subjects with Sarcoidosis (GUESS). (Respiration. 2024)***[26]
  - *Population:* Consecutive subjects with suspected sarcoidosis and enlarged thoracic lymph nodes undergoing EBUS-TBNA (n=150). This study was conducted in India (PGIMER, Chandigarh).
  - *Intervention:* EBUS TBNA using 19G needle. (n=75)
  - *Comparator:* EBUS TBNA using 22G needle. (n=75)
  - *Outcome:* The diagnostic sensitivity, adequacy of aspirates and operator assessed cough intensity was similar in the 19-G and the 22-G needle groups. However, the operators had significantly greater difficulty puncturing lymph nodes with the 19-G needle. (p = 0.03)
  - *Conclusion:* 19G needle is not superior to 22G needle in obtaining adequate and diagnostic samples in patients with suspected sarcoidosis undergoing EBUS TBNA.

e. Cryobiopsy and Forceps biopsy

- ***Is the diagnostic yield of mediastinal lymph node cryobiopsy (cryoEBUS) better for diagnosing mediastinal node involvement compared to endobronchial ultrasound-guided transbronchial needle aspiration (EBUS-TBNA)? A systematic review. (Respir Med. 2023)[27]***
  - o *Population:* Patients undergoing mediastinal lymph node sampling from 7 studies. (n=555)
  - o *Intervention:* CryoEBUS of mediastinal LN.
  - o *Comparator:* EBUS TBNA of mediastinal LN.
  - o *Outcome:* The overall diagnostic usefulness of cryoEBUS was higher compared to EBUS-TBNA (92% vs. 80%). CryoEBUS was especially useful in cases of lymphomas or non-pulmonary carcinomas and in benign cases, with no significant differences being found in specific cases of lung cancer. Genetic studies and immunohistochemical determination of PD-L1 was possible better with cryoEBUS.
  - o *Conclusion:* CryoEBUS improves the diagnostic yield of mediastinal lymph nodes over EBUS TBNA, especially in benign diseases and lymphomas.

- ***Comparison of cryobiopsy and forceps biopsy for the diagnosis of mediastinal lesions: A randomised clinical trial. (Pulmonology. 2024)[28]***
  - o *Population:* Patients undergoing EBUS in diagnosing mediastinal disease. (n=155)
  - o *Intervention:* EBUS cryobiopsy followed by forceps biopsy. (n=78)
  - o *Comparator:* EBUS forceps biopsy followed by cryobiopsy. (n=77)
  - o *Outcome:* Overall diagnosis was made in 92.9% of patients. TBNA plus cryobiopsy achieved diagnosis in more patients than TBNA plus forceps, but the difference was insignificant. All samples collected by TBNA plus cryobiopsy were suitable for lung cancer genomic and PD-L1 immunohistochemical testing, while this fraction was lower for TBNA plus forceps biopsy ($P = 0.036$). Cryobiopsy provided a higher diagnostic yield in lung cancer cases, rare tumours, and benign disorders than forceps biopsy.
  - o *Conclusion:* Transbronchial mediastinal cryobiopsy might be a promising complementary tool to supplement traditional needle biopsy for increased diagnostic yield and tissue harvesting.

- ***Comparative yield of transbronchial cryo-nodal biopsy, transbronchial intra-nodal forceps biopsy, and transbronchial needle aspiration for mediastinal lesions at a tertiary care center in India (COLD-FORCEPS study). (Monaldi Arch Chest Dis. 2024)[29]***
  - o *Population:* Patients undergoing EBUS for mediastinal lesions after an inconclusive EBUS TBNA or TBNA P-ROSE negative (n=34). This study was conducted in India (Safdarjung hospital, New Delhi).
  - o *Intervention:* EBUS TBNA followed by transbronchial cryo-nodal biopsy followed by transbronchial intra-nodal forceps biopsy. (n=34)
  - o *Comparator:* None.
  - o *Outcome:* The addition of cryobiopsy and forceps biopsy did not improve the diagnostic yield of EBUS TBNA significantly.
  - o *Conclusion:* EBUS guided mediastinal cryobiopsy and intra-nodal forceps biopsy may not be superior to an adequately performed EBUS-TBNA and should not be done routinely as an upfront procedure.

- ***Endobronchial Ultrasound-Guided Transbronchial Mediastinal Cryobiopsy versus Endobronchial Ultrasound-Guided Transbronchial Needle Aspiration for Mediastinal Disorders: A Meta-Analysis. (Respiration. 2024)*** [30]
  - o *Population:* EBUS transbronchial mediastinal cryo-nodal biopsy to diagnose mediastinal disease as evaluated in 10 studies. (n=538)
  - o *Intervention:* EBUS Transbronchial mediastinal cryobiopsy.
  - o *Comparator:* EBUS transbronchial needle aspiration.
  - o *Outcome:* The overall diagnostic yield of EBUS TMC was significantly higher (89.59%) than EBUS TBNA (77.13%), especially in the diagnosis of lymphoma and benign disorders.
  - o *Conclusion:* EBUS-TMC enhanced overall diagnostic yield compared to EBUS-TBNA, particularly for diagnosing benign disease and lymphoma.

☞

- ***Utility and safety of endobronchial ultrasound-guided transbronchial mediastinal cryobiopsy (EBUS-TMC): A systematic review and meta-analysis. (Lung India. 2024)*** [31]
  - o *Population:* EBUS transbronchial mediastinal cryo-nodal biopsy to diagnose mediastinal disease as evaluated in 14 studies (n=869). This study was conducted in India (AIIMS, New Delhi).
  - o *Intervention:* EBUS Transbronchial mediastinal cryobiopsy.
  - o *Comparator:* EBUS transbronchial needle aspiration.
  - o *Outcome:* The overall diagnostic yield of EBUS TMC was 92%, as compared to 81% of EBUS TBNA. (Risk difference in yield 11%), favouring EBUS TMC over EBUS TBNA. There was no significant difference in reported complications between the two methods.
  - o *Conclusion:* EBUS-TMC have better overall diagnostic yields compared to EBUS-TBNA, with good safety profile.

☞

- ***Additional yield of transbronchial cryo-node biopsy over endobronchial ultrasound-guided transbronchial needle aspiration for mediastinal lesions at a tertiary care center in India (COLD-FORCEPS-2 study). (Monaldi Arch Chest Dis. 2024)*** [32]
  - o *Population:* Consecutive patients undergoing EBUS for mediastinal lesions (n=101). This study was conducted in India (Safdarjung hospital, New Delhi).
  - o *Intervention:* EBUS transbronchial needle aspiration followed by transbronchial cryo-nodal biopsy for mediastinal lesions. (n=101)
  - o *Comparator:* None.
  - o *Outcome:* Diagnostic yields achieved in EBUS-TBNA and EBUS-TBNA with mediastinal cryobiopsy were 67.32% and 86.13%, respectively (p=0.001). No significant complications were observed with the addition of cryobiopsy.
  - o *Conclusion:* EBUS guided mediastinal cryobiopsy when added to EBUS-TBNA improved the diagnostic yield significantly, without significant risk of any severe complications.

3. PERIPHERAL PULMONARY NODULE

a. Radial EBUS

☞

- ***Cryobiopsy with radial-endobronchial ultrasound (Cryo-Radial) has comparable diagnostic yield with higher safety in comparison to computed tomography-guided transthoracic biopsy for peripheral pulmonary lesions: An exploratory randomised study. (Intern Med J. 2023)***[33]
  - o *Population:* Patients with nodules >1 cm on CT thorax. (n=48)
  - o *Intervention:* Cryobiopsy via radial EBUS guidance - conventional R-EBUS sample with either brush, forceps or needle aspiration through the guide sheath f/b cryobiopsy (minimum 3 samples) using 1.9mm cryoprobe, with 4 seconds freezing time (Intention to treat n=26, Per protocol n = 20).
  - o *Comparator:* Computed tomography-guided transthoracic biopsy (minimum 2 samples) using 17-19G needle (CT-TTB) (Intention to treat n = 22, Per protocol n = 16).
  - o *Outcome:* There was no significant difference between the diagnostic yield and sample adequacy for EGFR testing of CT-TTB and Cryo-Radial EBUS. Incidence of pneumothorax occurrence was significantly lower with Cryo-Radial (p=0.004).
  - o *Conclusion:* Cryo-Radial is comparable in diagnostic yield and ability to perform EGFR testing with a significantly lower risk of pneumothorax, compared with CT-TTB. Cryo-Radial has the additional advantage of mediastinal staging during the same procedure using Linear-EBUS.

- ***Radial Endobronchial Ultrasound-guided Transbronchial Cryobiopsy versus Forceps Biopsy for the Diagnosis of Solitary Pulmonary Nodules: A Prospective Randomised Trial. (Open Respir Med J. 2023)***[34]
  - o *Population:* Patients with pulmonary nodules requiring radial EBUS with guide sheath under fluoroscopy guidance. (n=28)
  - o *Intervention:* Transbronchial cryobiopsy. (n=12)
  - o *Comparator:* Conventional radial EBUS with forceps biopsy. (n=16)
  - o *Outcome:* The diagnostic yield in the cryobiopsy arm and the forceps arm was not significantly different, however, the median biopsy sizes were consistently larger for the cryobiopsy arm at 7.0mm compared to 2.5mm(p<0.0001).
  - o *Conclusion:* Transbronchial cryobiopsy under the guidance of fluoroscopy and radial EBUS facilitates larger biopsy specimens without a significant increase in major complications.

☞

- ***Clinical outcomes of transbronchial cryobiopsy using a 1.1-mm diameter cryoprobe for peripheral lung lesions: A prospective pilot study. (Respir Med. 2023)***[35]
  - o *Population:* Patients with peripheral pulmonary lesion <30mm. (n=50)
  - o *Intervention:* 1.1-mm diameter cryoprobe with radial endobronchial ultrasound (RP-EBUS), virtual bronchoscopic navigation and fluoroscopy. (n=49)

- *Comparator:* None.
- *Outcome:* The overall diagnostic yield of TBCB was 90%. There was no difference in the diagnostic yield between size (20 mm vs. 20-30 mm), RP-EBUS findings (concentric vs. others), and acute angle location (apical segment of both upper lobes vs. others).
- *Conclusion:* TBCB using a 1.1-mm diameter cryoprobe is an effective, reasonable method for the diagnosis of PLLs regardless of its size, RP-EBUS finding, and anatomical location without serious complication.

- ***Radial endobronchial ultrasound - guided bronchoscopy for the diagnosis of peripheral pulmonary lesions: A systematic review and meta-analysis of prospective trials. (Heliyon. 2024)***[36]
  - *Population:* Patients undergoing r-EBUS for diagnosing peripheral pulmonary lesions as evaluated in 46 studies. (n=7252)
  - *Intervention:* r-EBUS for diagnosing peripheral pulmonary lesions.
  - *Comparator:* None.
  - *Outcome:* The pooled diagnostic yield of r-EBUS was 73.4 %. PPLs located in the middle or lower lobe, >2 cm in size, malignant in type, solid in appearance on computerized tomography (CT), present in bronchus sign, the within probe location, and the addition of rapid on-site evaluation (ROSE) were associated with increased diagnostic yield.
  - *Conclusion:* r-EBUS is a good diagnostic modality for diagnosis of peripheral pulmonary lesions, with acceptable risks.

b. Robotic assisted bronchoscopy

☞

- ***Diagnostic Performance and Safety Profile of Robotic-assisted Bronchoscopy: A Systematic Review and Meta-Analysis. (Ann Am Thorac Soc. 2023)***[37]
  - *Population:* Peripheral pulmonary lesions sampled using one of the robotic assisted bronchoscopy (RAB) systems as evaluated in 25 studies. (n=1779)
  - *Intervention:* Use of robotic assisted bronchoscopy systems for diagnostic interventions.
  - *Comparator:* None.
  - *Outcome:* The pooled diagnostic yield of RAB was 84.3%. Lesion size > 2 cm, the presence of a computed tomography bronchus sign, and concentric radial endobronchial ultrasound view were associated with a statistically significant increase in the odds of diagnosis with RAB.
  - *Conclusion:* RAB systems could potentially increase the diagnostic yield of bronchoscopic procedures, but well-designed RCTs are needed to better understand their role in diagnostic bronchoscopy.

- ***Robotic-assisted bronchoscopy for the diagnosis of peripheral pulmonary lesions: A systematic review and meta-analysis. (Thorac Cancer. 2024)***[38]
  - *Population:* Peripheral pulmonary lesions sampled using one of the robotic assisted bronchoscopy (RAB) systems as evaluated in 10 studies. (n=725)
  - *Intervention:* Robotic assisted bronchoscopy for peripheral pulmonary lesions.
  - *Comparator:* None.

- *Outcome:* RAB had a pooled diagnostic yield of 80.4%. Lesion size of >30 mm, presence of a bronchus sign, and a concentric radial endobronchial ultrasound view were associated with a statistically significantly higher diagnostic yield. Studies using cryoprobes reported better yields than those without cryoprobes.
- *Conclusion:* RAB is an effective and safe technique for PPLs diagnosis. Head-to-head studies with conventional bronchoscopies are required to prove its superiority.

c. CT guided biopsy

- ***Computed tomography-guided biopsy for sub-centimetre pulmonary nodules: A meta-analysis. (Kardiochir Torakochirurgia Pol. 2023)***[39]
  - *Population:* Studies enrolling patients with sub-centimetre peripheral nodules undergoing CT-guided biopsy procedures. (n=10)
  - *Intervention:* CT guided biopsy for peripheral pulmonary lesions <1cm.
  - *Comparator:* None.
  - *Outcome:* The pooled diagnostic yield and diagnostic accuracy were 60% and 91% respectively, with the incidence of pulmonary haemorrhage and pneumothorax being 11% and 24% respectively. A substantial difference in diagnostic accuracy was observed when comparing biopsy procedures performed using fine- and core-needle biopsy approaches (85% vs. 95%), whereas the use of the co-axial method or the selected guidance approach (conventional vs. cone-beam CT) had no impact on diagnostic accuracy.
  - *Conclusion:* CT-guided biopsy represents an effective means of accurately diagnosing sub-centimetre PN, with some risk of complications like pneumothorax and pulmonary haemorrhage.

d. Electromagnetic navigational bronchoscopy

- ***A Multicenter, Single-Arm, Prospective Trial Assessing the Diagnostic Yield of Electromagnetic Bronchoscopic and Transthoracic Navigation for Peripheral Pulmonary Nodules. (Am J Respir Crit Care Med. 2023)***[40]
  - *Population:* Participants with pulmonary nodules (<3 cm). (n=160)
  - *Intervention:* Staged procedure with same-day CT, EBUS, Electromagnetic navigational bronchoscopy (ENB), and electromagnetic navigational transthoracic biopsy (EMN-TTNA).
  - *Comparator:* The procedures were staged such that, when a diagnosis had been achieved via rapid on-site pathologic evaluation, the procedure was ended and subsequent biopsy modalities were not attempted.
  - *Outcome:* The diagnostic yield of the combined procedure was 59%. The yield of ENB alone was 49%, that of EMN-TTNA alone was 27% and that of ENB plus EMN-TTNA was 53%. When EMN-TTNA was performed, the pneumothorax rate was 30%.
  - *Conclusion:* The high complication rate and low diagnostic yield of EMN-TTNA do not support the routine use of electromagnetic navigational bronchoscopy and electromagnetic navigational transthoracic biopsy.

- ***Diagnostic Yield of Cone-beam-Derived Augmented Fluoroscopy and Ultrathin Bronchoscopy Versus Conventional Navigational Bronchoscopy Techniques. (J Bronchology Interv Pulmonol. 2023)***[41]
  - o *Population:* Patients with peripheral pulmonary nodule. (n=116)
  - o *Intervention:* Cone-beam computed tomography (CBCT)+ radial endobronchial ultrasound (r-EBUS) guided biopsy. (n=27)
  - o *Comparator:*

    a. CBCT+ ultrathin bronchoscope (UTB)+r-EBUS guided biopsy. (n=30)

    b. r-EBUS without CBCT or fluoroscopy guidance. (n=59)
  - o *Outcome:* The diagnostic yield of r-EBUS group (44.5%) was significantly lower than CBCT + UTB + r-EBUS group (85.0%). There was no statistically significant difference in the incidence of pneumothorax in the three groups. However, the median dose of radiation was very high in the CBCT group as compared to r-EBUS group.
  - o *Conclusion:* Compared with the r-EBUS group, CBCT + UTB + r-EBUS was associated with higher navigational success, and a higher diagnostic yield.

e. *Ultrathin Bronchoscope*

- ***Diagnostic yield and the number of tumor cells of ultrathin bronchoscopy for peripheral lung lesions: A comparison with thin bronchoscopy. (PLoS One. 2023)***[42]
  - o *Population:* Retrospective study - Patients with NSCLC in peripheral lung lesions obtained using an ultrathin bronchoscope (3mm OD, working channel 1.7mm) and a thin bronchoscope (4.2mm OD, working channel 2mm) with EBUS.
  - o *Intervention:* Biopsy proven NSCLC via ultrathin bronchoscopy. (n=38)
  - o *Comparator:* Biopsy proven NSCLC via thin bronchoscopy. (n=64)
  - o *Outcome:* In histologically NSCLC cases (n = 102), the maximum number of tumor cells per slide as the primary endpoint was similar.
  - o *Conclusion:* The yield of NSCLC tumor cells was not different between the samples obtained by the ultrathin bronchoscope and those obtained by the thin bronchoscope.

4. PERSISTENT AIR LEAK

- ***Bronchial Valves for Persistent Air Leak: A Systematic Review and Meta-analysis. (J Bronchology Interv Pulmonol. 2024)***[43]
  - o *Population:* Studies evaluating the efficacy and safety of bronchial valve for persistent air leak. (n=28)
  - o *Intervention:* Bronchial valve for persistent air leak.
  - o *Comparator:* None.
  - o *Outcome:* The pooled success rate of bronchial valves in PAL was 82% (95% confidence intervals, 75 to 88). A higher success rate was seen in studies using intrabronchial valves versus endobronchial valves (84% vs. 72%).
  - o *Conclusion:* Bronchial valves are an effective and safe option for treating persistent air leak.

- ***Embolization coils in treating postoperative bronchopleural fistula: A systematic review. (Front Med (Lausanne). 2024)***[44]
    - o *Population:* Studies evaluating efficacy of embolization coils to treat postoperative BPF (n=9, 20 patients)
    - o *Intervention:* Embolization coils to treat postoperative BPF
    - o *Comparator:* None
    - o *Outcome:* The median number of embolization coils inserted per patient was 3 (range: 1–10). The embolization coils resulted in complete closure rate in 80% patients with postoperative BPF, with sizes ranging from 2 to 3.1 mm. During a median follow-up period of 12 months, no fistula recurrence was reported.
    - o *Conclusion:* Embolization coils might offer a minimally invasive and cost effective method, with few complications and recurrences, in patients with post operative BPF.

5. INTERVENTIONS IN COPD

- ***Research on the effectiveness and safety of bronchial thermoplasty in patients with chronic obstructive pulmonary disease. (Eur J Med Res. 2023)***[45]
    - o *Population:* Moderate-to-severe COPD patients who received high doses of ICS in the past year and were using LABAs and LAMAs. (n=57)
    - o *Intervention:* Conventional medical treatment combined with BT ablation. (n=28)
    - o *Comparator:* Conventional medical treatment. (n=29)
    - o *Outcome:* The Intervention group showed greater improvement in FEV_1, FEV_1(%, predicted), mMRC, 6MWT and CAT scores and the total number of COPD acute exacerbations and hospitalizations due to COPD in intervention group significantly decreased relative to those in the control group at 1 year after treatment.
    - o *Conclusion:* Combined BT therapy is superior to conventional medical treatment in improving lung function and quality of life of COPD patients, and it also significantly reduces the COPD exacerbation risk without causing serious adverse events.

☞

- ***Impact of bronchoscopic thermal vapor ablation on lung volume reduction in patients with emphysema: A meta-analysis. (BMC Pulmonary Medicine. 2023)***[46]
    - o *Population:* Patients undergoing bronchoscopic thermal vapor ablation in upper lobe emphysema as evaluated in 4 studies. (n=112 patients)
    - o *Intervention:* Bronchoscopic thermal vapor ablation.
    - o *Comparator:* Standard medical management.
    - o *Outcome:* FEV1, residual volume (RV), total lung capacity (TLC), 6-min walk distance (6MWD) and St George's Respiratory Questionnaire (SGRQ) were significantly improved in patients with emphysema following BTVA treatment between 6 months vs. baseline. The magnitude of benefit was higher at 3 months compared to 6 months. The most common complications at 6 months were treatment-related COPD exacerbations and pneumonia.
    - o *Conclusion:* BTVA can result in short term improvement in lung functions in patients with upper lobe predominant emphysema.

- ***Sustained Clinical Benefits of Spiration Valve System in Patients with Severe Emphysema: 24-Month Follow-Up of EMPROVE. (Annals of American Thoracic Society. 2024)***[47]
    - o *Population:* Patients who had undergone spiration valve placement for severe emphysema in EMPROVE trial. (n=142)
    - o *Intervention:* Spiration valve placement with medical management. (n=98)
    - o *Comparator:* Medical management alone. (n=44)
    - o *Outcome:* A significant improvement in FEV1, mMRC grade of dyspnea, the St. George's Respiratory Questionnaire and the COPD Assessment Test was maintained at 24 months in the SVS treatment group. There was no significant difference in COPD exacerbations between the two groups.
    - o *Conclusion:* SVS treatment resulted in statistically significant improvements in lung function, respiratory symptoms, and QOL for at least 24 months while maintaining an acceptable safety profile.

DISCUSSION

Bronchoscopy

Sedation and anaesthesia

The 2019 Indian guidelines suggest that although there is an option to perform flexible bronchoscopy without sedation, the administration of sedation/anaesthesia can make the procedure more comfortable and tolerable.[48] **The current evidence suggests that the combination of an opioid with a non-opioid agent for sedation has good efficacy, patient tolerance, and low reuse dose requirement.**[49] Few recent studies have supported the use of remimazolam over midazolam as the sedative, given faster patient recovery from sedation, but at present there is insufficient evidence to support the use of one agent over another.[3-5]

As for topical anaesthesia, "the spray as you go" and "cricothyroid injection of lignocaine" techniques are the popular choices for the application of lignocaine to the vocal cords and the trachea during bronchoscopy and are recommended by the Indian bronchoscopy guidelines. Dose of lignocaine needs to be titrated to keep it below 8mg/kg body weight to avoid toxicity. **The Indian bronchoscopy guidelines recommend 3-5 sprays of 10% lignocaine for pharyngeal anaesthesia. A recent study found that 5 sprays of 10% lignocaine were effective to reduce cough and improve patient comfort, which is also found to be non-inferior to 10 sprays of 10% lignocaine.**[1,48] Therefore, 5 sprays of 10% lignocaine may be considered for pharyngeal anaesthesia during bronchoscopy.

Oxygenation and Ventilation

Bronchoscopy can be associated with significant hypoxemia, especially in patients with chronic obstructive pulmonary disease (COPD) and interstitial lung disease (ILD). Non-invasive ventilation (NIV), high-frequency nasal cannula (HFNC) and supraglottic jet ventilation improve oxygenation in patients undergoing bronchoscopy, although use of NIV might be uncomfortable for some patients.[10–12] In the latest meta-analysis by Wei et al,[13] HFNC was shown to be superior to conventional oxygen therapy in reducing episodes of hypoxemia and maintaining better oxygenation during bronchoscopy. As per the Indian Bronchoscopy guidelines, NIV should be used in patients with mild to moderate ARDS undergoing bronchoscopy, and an experienced bronchoscopist should perform the procedure, with the backup of invasive ventilatory support at their disposal.[48] While using HFNC, a flow rate of 40-50L/min is shown to be optimal to prevent desaturations. **We also do not recommend routine use of NIV or HFNC in bronchoscopy and may be restricted to high-risk bronchoscopies like patients with hypoxemia wherein a bronchoscopic examination is deemed necessary.**

Sampling in flexible bronchoscopy

Bleeding during bronchoscopy procedures is a potential threat and requires proper management to maintain adequate ventilation during the procedure. **The Indian bronchoscopy guidelines recommend the use of intrabronchial adrenaline and cold saline for moderate bleeding, and the placement of catheters, bronchial blockers and fibrin in case of severe bleeding.**[14,48] **Prophylactic placement of balloons or prophylactic administration of adrenaline is not recommended.** Bronchoscopic electrocautery can be used but has no added advantage over cold saline and adrenaline.[15]

Obtaining lower respiratory tract samples via bronchoalveolar lavage (BAL) is the most common indication of flexible bronchoscopy. There are three methods described in literature to obtain BAL – using wall mount suction, using manual suction and using manual suction with tubing. In a one of its kind study, comparing the three methods to obtain BAL, it was shown that the yield obtained was similar using any of the three methods.[17]

Simulation for flexible bronchoscopy training

Performing flexible bronchoscopies require good anatomical knowledge and technical skills. Simulators can help to improve these skills. Various studies have shown that simulation based training before performing bronchoscopies on actual patients can help improve the skills and the time to completion among new medical trainees.[18-20]

Miscellaneous

Patients with cystic fibrosis (CF) are at a high risk of recurrent bacterial infections and adequate treatment with suitable antibiotics is essential. Best method to obtain a lower respiratory sample is a bronchoscopy and BAL. However, a **Cochrane review showed that there is no evidence to support the routine use of BAL for the diagnosis and management of pulmonary infection in patients with CF compared to the standard practice of providing treatment based on results of oropharyngeal culture and clinical symptoms, thus routine use of BAL in cystic fibrosis patients cannot be recommended.**[21]

Endobronchial Ultrasound

Sedation and Analgesia

EBUS TBNA can be done under moderate sedation or general anaesthesia. General anaesthesia requires additional procedure time and cost but is associated with better patient comfort. **The Indian guidelines recommend that EBUS TBNA can be done under either moderate sedation or general anaesthesia, based on operator comfort and experience. A combination of sedative agents is preferred over single agent alone.**[50] Even for deep sedation, combination of agents improves patient comfort and hemodynamics.[23]

EUS vs EUS-B

EUS-B uses the EBUS scope via the esophagus to approach the mediastinal lymph nodes and can also help to sample the left adrenal gland. **A recent study showed that both EUS and EUS-B have good performance and are safe to sample the left adrenal gland.**[24]

Route: Oral vs Nasal

The Indian EBUS guidelines prefer the oral route over the nasal route for insertion of the EBUS scope.[50] **The NO EBUS trial showed that both routes had similar patient tolerance and operator comfort for performing EBUS.**[25] For EBUS-TBNA performed under sedation, either oral or nasal route for scope insertion may be chosen based on operator comfort. In case of any difficulty with nasal introduction, the approach should be promptly changed to oral.

Needle size

The Indian EBUS guidelines recommend that either 21G or 22G needles may be used, however, they did not make any recommendation for or against the use of other needles. Recent studies have also shown similar results, that needle size had no significant impact on obtaining adequate and diagnostic samples.[26]

Cryobiopsy and Forceps Biopsy

The diagnostic yield of EBUS TBNA in various studies have been shown to be around 70-80%. So various new modalities are being studied to improve the diagnostic yield of EBUS, among which cryobiopsy and forceps biopsy are being extensively used now. **Various studies have shown that transbronchial mediastinal cryobiopsy has a superior yield in the diagnosis of mediastinal lesions, especially in benign diseases and lymphoma.**[27-32] **The Indian EBUS guidelines recommend to use transbronchial mediastinal cryobiopsy in patients with negative rapid-on-site evaluation (ROSE), or prior non-diagnostic EBUS-TBNA.**[50] Decision to perform mediastinal cryobiopsy should be on a case to case basis.

Peripheral Pulmonary Nodule

Peripheral lesions are difficult to biopsy and those approachable percutaneously are best sampled under ultrasound or CT guidance. However, the problem lies in sampling those lesions which cannot be approached percutaneously. Thus, research into newer modalities is ongoing to improve the diagnostic yield of peripheral pulmonary nodules. Table 1 compares the diagnostic yield of various modalities for sampling peripheral lesions.

Table 1: Diagnostic yield for various modalities for sampling peripheral lesions		
Sr no	**Modality**	**Diagnostic yield**
1.	Radial EBUS	Overall yield: 73.4% [36] Using ultrathin bronchoscope: 70.8% [36] Addition of ROSE: 80.7% [36] Using fluoroscopy: 75.5% [36] Using VBN/EBN: 75.6% [36] Using ultrathin bronchoscope + CBCT: 85% [41] Using cryo-biopsy: 91.7% [34]
2.	Robotic assisted bronchoscopy	80.4% [38] With radial EBUS: 89.4% [38] With cryoprobe: 90% [38] With CBCT: 80.6% [38]
3.	CT guided biopsy	93.8% [33] In sub-centimetric nodule: 60% [39]
4.	Electromagnetic navigational biopsy	49% [40]

CBCT: Cone Beam CT, ENB: Electromagnetic Navigation Bronchoscopy, ROSE: Rapid Onsite Evaluation, VBN: Virtual Bronchoscopic Navigation

Radial EBUS

Radial EBUS has been in use for a considerable amount of time now. However, the diagnostic yield is still poor. The diagnostic yield of radial EBUS is around 73% as per a recent meta-analysis, and the addition of rapid onsite evaluation (ROSE) improves the diagnostic yield significantly from 72.9% to 80.7%.[36] Cone beam CT (CBCT) is a type of computed tomography (CT) that uses a cone-shaped X-ray beam to create 3D images of the lungs. It provides high-resolution images of the lung tissue and can even detect small lesions. however, cone beam CT exposes the patient to a higher amount of radiation as compared to other modalities, which can be a cause for concern. However, studies have shown that adding CBCT to radial EBUS significantly increases the diagnostic yield to 85%.[36] Cryobiopsy has revolutionized the field of interventional pulmonology and has found significant success with transbronchial lung biopsy and transbronchial mediastinal biopsy. **A recent RCT showed that radial EBUS-guided cryobiopsy had a comparable diagnostic yield to CT-guided biopsy, with a significantly lesser risk of pneumothorax.**[33] Two separate RCTs demonstrated the diagnostic yield using radial EBUS guided cryobiopsy to be more than 90%.[34,35] Thus, cryobiopsy appears to be a promising tool to sample peripheral pulmonary lesions via radial EBUS.

Robotic-assisted bronchoscopy

Robotic-assisted bronchoscopy (RAB) is a minimally invasive medical procedure that uses a robotic system to assist in the examination of the airways and lungs. The robotic system helps to control the movement of the bronchoscope and provides high-definition 3D views of the airways, making it easier for the bronchoscopist to obtain adequate samples with reduced chances of complications. Recent meta-analyses have shown the diagnostic yield of RAB is more than 80%.[37,38] Addition of radial EBUS improves the diagnostic yield significantly. Other factors associated with improved yield were the presence of a bronchus sign on the CT scan and lesion size >2cm. Thus, **combining RAB with r-EBUS could be the next step in improving the diagnostic yield of peripheral pulmonary nodules, the only limitation being the cost of the two instruments.**

Electromagnetic navigational bronchoscopy

Electromagnetic navigational bronchoscopy (ENB) is a form of guided bronchoscopy that consists of a conventional bronchoscope, coupled with an electromagnetic sensor and computer software with the patient's CT Thorax images. Using this CT, before the procedure, the software creates a virtual path through the bronchial trees to reach the target lesion. The electromagnetic probe is part of an extended working channel that can be passed via the bronchoscope, and this probe allows the computer to track the location of the probe in the patient's lungs. Thus, it accurately allows us to reach the target lesion and obtain adequate samples.

A recent prospective study showed that ENB did not improve the diagnostic yield significantly and there was no significant reduction in the risk of pneumothorax.[40]

Ultrathin bronchoscopes

Ultrathin bronchoscopes have the advantage of reaching up to the subsegmental levels, however, the smaller sizes of working channels could pose a challenge in obtaining adequate samples. **A recent study concluded that the number of tumor cells per slide was similar using either a conventional bronchoscope or an ultrathin bronchoscope. Thus, ultrathin bronchoscopes can be used as a tool to access peripheral lesions.**[42]

CT guided biopsy

CT Guided biopsy has been the 'go-to' procedure for sampling a peripheral pulmonary lesion and has shown to have a good diagnostic yield, especially if the lesion is subpleural. However, deeper lesions are associated with higher risks of complications, particularly pneumothorax. A recent study has shown that for sub-centimetric lesions, CT-guided biopsy has a diagnostic yield of 60%.[39]

Persistent air leak

Air leaks in cases of pneumothorax, which last for more than 5-7 days are defined as persistent air leaks. **The 2023 British Thoracic Guidelines (BTS) guidelines recommend thoracic surgical consultation in case of persistent air leak, and if a patient is not considered fit for surgery, autologous blood pleurodesis or endobronchial therapies should be considered for the treatment of pneumothorax with a persistent air leak in adults.**[51]

In a first-of-its-kind case series, an air leak was identified using thoracoscopy and an autologous blood patch was instilled under thoracoscopic guidance at the exact site of the leak. This led to the successful resolution of the air leak in both cases in the series. This could be a novel treatment option for treating persistent air leaks, which is associated with significant morbidity. However, the authors also reported potential challenges during the intervention, such as the inability to localize the site of the leak or the inability to make the leak in a dependent position, to put the autologous blood over it.[52]

Bronchial valves are one-way valves, that prevent air from going towards the distal airways and thus reduce the air leak. Endobronchial valves have shown to have a success rate of 82% in resolving persistent air leaks and are considered as one of the therapies.[43]

Embolization coils originally designed to occlude bleeding blood vessels, have shown good efficacy in the treatment of persistent air leaks as well. These coils have shown to be a cost-effective, easy-to-perform, minimally invasive bronchoscopy intervention in the treatment of persistent air leak, showing a success rate of around 80%.[44]

Interventions in COPD

Bronchial thermoplasty

Bronchial thermoplasty has found good utility in treating uncontrolled bronchial asthma. It uses radiofrequency, which is converted into heat energy and ablates the bronchial smooth muscles. It is done over three sessions, ablating the right lower lobe, the left lower lobe, and bilateral upper lobes sequentially. A study was recently conducted to evaluate the utility of bronchial thermoplasty in moderate to severe COPD patients. As compared to conventional medical management, patients treated with bronchial thermoplasty showed greater improvements in lung functions and functional capacity.[45] However, the severity of emphysema on CT Thorax, as scored using the Goddard et al method, was lower in the BT arm as compared to the conventional therapy arm, and thus, the results should be interpreted with caution. Moreover, the discontinuation of bronchial thermoplasty sales by the company itself has put the future of bronchial thermoplasty in uncertainty.

Bronchial thermal vapour ablation

Bronchoscopic lung volume reduction can be achieved using bronchial valves, coils, and thermal vapor ablation. BTVA is the only bronchoscopy method that can be used even in the presence of collateral ventilation. It leads to parenchymal thermal damage and fibrosis, causing lung volume reduction in the targeted regions. **A recent meta-analysis concluded that BTVA as compared to standard medical management is associated with improved lung functions, clinical symptoms, and functional capacity. However, the effects seemed to reduce over the long term, indicating that potential re-intervention might be required. However, further studies are required to conclude the same.**

Endobronchial valves

In a 24 month follow up of the EMPROVE study.[53] evaluating the utility of endobronchial valves in patients with COPD and heterogenous emphysema, it was shown that lung functions, functional lung capacity and symptom scores were significantly better in the arm treated with endobronchial valve as compared to the medical management arm.[47] However, there was no significant difference in number of COPD exacerbations between the two groups, thus raising a query on it's utility, considering the expenses.

REFERENCES

1. Iyer H, Mishra M, Sindhwani G, Mittal S, Tiwari P, Hadda V, et al. Five Versus 10 Pharyngeal Sprays of 10% Lignocaine for Topical Anesthesia During Flexible Bronchoscopy: A Multicenter, Randomized Controlled Trial. J Bronchology Interv Pulmonol. 2023 Jul 1;30(3):232–7.
2. Nie J, Chen W, Jia Y, Zhang Y, Wang H. Comparison of remifentanil and esketamine in combination with propofol for patient sedation during fiberoptic bronchoscopy. BMC Pulm Med. 2023 Jul 11;23(1):254.
3. Kim SH, Cho JY, Kim M, Chung JM, Yang J, Seong C, et al. Safety and efficacy of remimazolam compared with midazolam during bronchoscopy: a single-center, randomized controlled study. Sci Rep. 2023 Nov 22;13(1):20498.
4. Wu Q, Xu R, Zhou X, Wang L, Sheng C, Ding M, et al. Bolus administration of remimazolam was superior to midazolam for deep sedation in elderly patients undergoing diagnostic bronchoscopy: A randomized, double-blind, controlled trial. Medicine (Baltimore). 2024 Mar 22;103(12):e37215.
5. Chen Q, Qin B, Zhang M, Zhou Y, Shi X, Xie Y. The Safety and Efficacy of Remimazolam Compared to Dexmedetomidine for Awake Tracheal Intubation by Flexible Bronchoscopy: A Randomized, Double-Blind, Controlled Trial. Drug Des Devel Ther. 2024;18:967–78.
6. Antony T, Acharya KV, Acharya PR, Kotian H, Kamath S. Clinical usefulness of nebulized dexmedetomidine for conscious sedation in daycare flexible bronchoscopy in Southern India. Indian J Pharmacol. 2024 Mar 1;56(2):105–11.
7. Zhao Z, Zhang J, Wang Z, Petrella F. The different doses of sufentanil combined with nalmefene in bronchoscopy: a systematic review and meta-analysis. J Thorac Dis. 2024 Jun 30;16(6):3956–66.
8. Apostolos F, Nikolaos Z, Charalampos M, Kyriakos K, Sotirios F, Gregorios V. Dexmedetomidine-ketamine combination versus fentanyl-midazolam for patient sedation during flexible bronchoscopy: a prospective, single-blind, randomized controlled trial. BMC Pulm Med. 2024 Jun 26;24:301.
9. Min K, Wang Y, Feng D, Jin T, Zhu W, Duan R, et al. The Influence of Piriform Recess Instillation with Lidocaine Before Bronchoscopy on Post-General Anesthesia Cough: A Randomized Controlled Trial. Drug Des Devel Ther. 2024;18:2883–90.
10. Sharma VK, Singh PK, Govindagoudar MB, Thulasi A, Chaudhry D, Shriram CP, et al. Efficacy of different respiratory supports to prevent hypoxia during flexible bronchoscopy in patients of COPD: a triple-arm, randomised controlled trial. BMJ Open Respir Res. 2023 Nov;10(1):e001524.
11. Wei J, Zhang X, Min K, Zhou H, Shi X, Deng H, et al. Supraglottic Jet Oxygenation and Ventilation to Minimize Hypoxia in Patients Receiving Flexible Bronchoscopy Under Deep Sedation: A 3-Arm Randomized Controlled Trial. Anesth Analg. 2024 Feb 1;138(2):456–64.
12. Zhang W, Yuan X, Shen Y, Wang J, Xie K, Chen X. Optimal flow of high-flow nasal cannula oxygenation to prevent desaturation during sedation for bronchoscopy: a randomized controlled study. Ther Adv Respir Dis. 2024;18:17534666241246637.
13. Wei C, Ma S, Wang J, Yang N, Wang D, Yuan L, et al. The effectiveness of transnasal high flow nasal cannula in bronchoscopy under sedation: a systematic review and meta-analysis. Front Med (Lausanne). 2024;11:1428431.
14. Kalchiem-Dekel O, Tran BC, Glick DR, Ha NT, Iacono A, Pickering EM, et al. Prophylactic epinephrine attenuates severe bleeding in lung transplantation patients undergoing transbronchial lung biopsy: Results of the PROPHET randomized trial. J Heart Lung Transplant. 2023 Sep;42(9):1205–13.
15. Shahul S A, Chauhan NK, Dutt N, Chakraborti A, Elhence P, Jalandra R. Bronchoscopic Electrocautery Versus Adrenaline and Cold Saline Instillation for Prophylactic Haemostasis Prior to Biopsy of Endobronchial Lesions (BEVACS): A Randomized Controlled Trial. J Bronchology Interv Pulmonol. 2024 Apr 1;31(2):199–204.
16. Bian Y, Zhou G, Gao Q, Deng M, Tong R, Xia Y, et al. Assessment of a randomized controlled trial on the safety of pre-placing bronchial balloons in transbronchial lung cryobiopsy for diagnosing interstitial lung disease. Eur J Med Res. 2024 May 3;29(1):268.
17. Sehgal IS, Kaur G, Gupta N, Dhooria S, Prasad KT, Bal A, et al. A Randomized Control Trial Comparing the Yield of Bronchoalveolar Lavage Using Three Different Techniques in Patients Undergoing Flexible Bronchoscopy (BAL-3T). J Bronchology Interv Pulmonol. 2024 Oct 1;31(4):e0979.
18. Gerretsen ECF, Chen A, Annema JT, Groenier M, van der Heijden EHFM, van Mook WNKA, et al. Effectiveness of Flexible Bronchoscopy Simulation-Based Training: A Systematic Review. Chest. 2023 Oct;164(4):952–62.
19. Vieira LMN, Ibiapina C da C, Camargos PAM, Brand PLP. Simulation-based bronchoscopy training: Randomized trial comparing worked example to video introduction. Pediatr Pulmonol. 2023 Nov;58(11):3227–34.
20. Cold KM, Xie S, Nielsen AO, Clementsen PF, Konge L. Artificial Intelligence Improves Novices' Bronchoscopy Performance: A Randomized Controlled Trial in a Simulated Setting. Chest. 2024 Feb;165(2):405–13.
21. Jain K, Wainwright CE, Smyth AR. Bronchoscopy-guided antimicrobial therapy for cystic fibrosis. Cochrane Database Syst Rev. 2024 May 3;5(5):CD009530.
22. Chaddha U, Agrawal A, Kurman J, Ortiz-Comino R, Dutau H, Freitag L, et al. World Association for Bronchology and Interventional Pulmonology (WABIP) guidelines on airway stenting for malignant central airway obstruction. Respirology. 2024 Jul;29(7):563–73.
23. Cui S, Huang P, Wei Z, Guo T, Zhang A, Huang L. Esketamine Combined with Propofol TCI versus Propofol TCI for Deep Sedation

during Endobronchial Ultrasound-Guided Transbronchial Needle Aspiration: A Prospective, Randomized, and Controlled Trial. Int J Clin Pract. 2023;2023:1155126.

24. Moretti A, Kovacevic B, Vilmann P, Annema JT, Korevaar DA. Performance of EUS-FNA and EUS-B-FNA for the diagnosis of left adrenal glands metastases in patients with lung cancer: A systematic review and meta-analysis. Lung Cancer. 2023 Dec;186:107391.

25. Mishra M, Chowdhury N, Krishnadas Padmanabhan A, Banerjee S, Kumar Saini L, Sharma P, et al. Comparison of Patient's Procedural Tolerance of EBUS-TBNA Performed Through Nasal Versus Oral Route: The NO-EBUS Randomized Clinical Trial. J Bronchology Interv Pulmonol. 2024 Apr 1;31(2):215–23.

26. Dhooria S, Sehgal IS, Prasad KT, Muthu V, Dogra P, Saini M, et al. Diagnostic Yield and Safety of the 19-Gauge versus 22-Gauge Endobronchial Ultrasound-Guided Transbronchial Needle Aspiration Needle in Subjects with Sarcoidosis (GUESS). Respiration. 2024;103(6):336–43.

27. Botana-Rial M, Lojo-Rodríguez I, Leiro-Fernández V, Ramos-Hernández C, González-Montaos A, Pazos-Area L, et al. Is the diagnostic yield of mediastinal lymph node cryobiopsy (cryoEBUS) better for diagnosing mediastinal node involvement compared to endobronchial ultrasound-guided transbronchial needle aspiration (EBUS-TBNA)? A systematic review. Respir Med. 2023 Nov;218:107389.

28. Cheng TL, Huang ZS, Zhang J, Wang J, Zhao J, Kontogianni K, et al. Comparison of cryobiopsy and forceps biopsy for the diagnosis of mediastinal lesions: A randomised clinical trial. Pulmonology. 2024 Jan 4;S2531-0437(23)00240-4.

29. Madan M, Mahendran AJ, Kumar R, Kedia Y, Kaushik R, Ish P, et al. Comparative yield of transbronchial cryo-nodal biopsy, transbronchial intra-nodal forceps biopsy, and transbronchial needle aspiration for mediastinal lesions at a tertiary care center in India (COLD-FORCEPS study). Monaldi Arch Chest Dis. 2024 Jan 15;

30. Zhang Z, Li S, Bao Y. Endobronchial Ultrasound-Guided Transbronchial Mediastinal Cryobiopsy versus Endobronchial Ultrasound-Guided Transbronchial Needle Aspiration for Mediastinal Disorders: A Meta-Analysis. Respiration. 2024 Apr 8;

31. Chandragiri PS, Tayal A, Mittal S, Madan NK, Tiwari P, Hadda V, et al. Utility and safety of endobronchial ultrasound-guided transbronchial mediastinal cryobiopsy (EBUS-TMC): A systematic review and meta-analysis. Lung India. 2024 Jul 1;41(4):288–98.

32. Madan M, Kumar R, Ish P, Kedia Y, Mahendran AJ, Kaushik R, et al. Additional yield of transbronchial cryo-node biopsy over endobronchial ultrasound-guided transbronchial needle aspiration for mediastinal lesions at a tertiary care center in India (COLD-FORCEPS-2 study). Monaldi Archives for Chest Disease [Internet]. 2024 Jul 24 [cited 2024 Jul 26]; Available from: https://www.monaldi-archives.org/macd/article/view/3054

33. Herath S, Wong C, Dawkins P, Veale A, Yap E, Williamson J, et al. Cryobiopsy with radial-endobronchial ultrasound (Cryo-Radial) has comparable diagnostic yield with higher safety in comparison to computed tomography-guided transthoracic biopsy for peripheral pulmonary lesions: An exploratory randomised study. Intern Med J. 2023 Aug;53(8):1390–9.

34. Brown M, Nguyen P, Jersmann H, Holmes M, Wong M. Radial Endobronchial Ultrasound-guided Transbronchial Cryobiopsy versus Forceps Biopsy for the Diagnosis of Solitary Pulmonary Nodules: A Prospective Randomised Trial. Open Respir Med J. 2023;17: e187430642309190.

35. Kim SH, Mok J, Kim S, Yoo WH, Jo EJ, Kim MH, et al. Clinical outcomes of transbronchial cryobiopsy using a 1.1-mm diameter cryoprobe for peripheral lung lesions - A prospective pilot study. Respir Med. 2023 Oct;217:107338.

36. Tian S, Li X, Liu J, Wang X, Chen H, Dai Z, et al. Radial endobronchial ultrasound - guided bronchoscopy for the diagnosis of peripheral pulmonary lesions: A systematic review and meta-analysis of prospective trials. Heliyon. 2024 Apr 30;10(8):e29446.

37. Ali MS, Ghori UK, Wayne MT, Shostak E, De Cardenas J. Diagnostic Performance and Safety Profile of Robotic-assisted Bronchoscopy: A Systematic Review and Meta-Analysis. Ann Am Thorac Soc. 2023 Dec;20(12):1801–12.

38. Zhang C, Xie F, Li R, Cui N, Herth FJF, Sun J. Robotic-assisted bronchoscopy for the diagnosis of peripheral pulmonary lesions: A systematic review and meta-analysis. Thorac Cancer. 2024 Mar;15(7):505–12.

39. Feng JL, Fu YF, Li Y. Computed tomography-guided biopsy for sub-centimetre pulmonary nodules: a meta-analysis. Kardiochir Torakochirurgia Pol. 2023 Sep;20(3):139–45.

40. Thiboutot J, Pastis NJ, Akulian J, Silvestri GA, Chen A, Wahidi MM, et al. A Multicenter, Single-Arm, Prospective Trial Assessing the Diagnostic Yield of Electromagnetic Bronchoscopic and Transthoracic Navigation for Peripheral Pulmonary Nodules. Am J Respir Crit Care Med. 2023 Oct 15;208(8):837–45.

41. DiBardino DM, Kim RY, Cao Y, Andronov M, Lanfranco AR, Haas AR, et al. Diagnostic Yield of Cone-beam-Derived Augmented Fluoroscopy and Ultrathin Bronchoscopy Versus Conventional Navigational Bronchoscopy Techniques. J Bronchology Interv Pulmonol. 2023 Oct 1;30(4):335–45.

42. Yatani A, Katsurada N, Fukui T, Yamada J, Satoh H, Mimura C, et al. Diagnostic yield and the number of tumor cells of ultrathin bronchoscopy for peripheral lung lesions: A comparison with thin bronchoscopy. PLoS One. 2023 Aug 24;18(8):e0290609.

43. Damaraju V, Sehgal IS, Muthu V, Prasad KT, Dhooria S, Aggarwal AN, et al. Bronchial Valves for Persistent Air Leak: A Systematic Review and Meta-analysis. J Bronchology Interv Pulmonol. 2024 Jul 1;31(3):e0964.

44. Luo X, Zhan K, Bai Y. Embolization coils in treating postoperative bronchopleural fistula: a systematic review. Front Med (Lausanne). 2024 Jun 20;11:1364994.

45. Wang T, Fu P, Long F, Liu S, Hu S, Wang Q, et al. Research on the effectiveness and safety of bronchial thermoplasty in patients with chronic obstructive pulmonary disease. Eur J Med Res. 2023 Sep 9;28(1):331.

46. Zhi L, Liao L, Wu Z, Wang T, Ye Y, Li H, et al. Impact of bronchoscopic thermal vapor ablation on lung volume reduction in patients with emphysema: a meta-analysis. BMC Pulm Med. 2023 Oct 26;23(1):405.

47. Criner GJ, Mallea JM, Abu-Hijleh M, Sachdeva A, Kalhan R, Hergott CA, et al. Sustained Clinical Benefits of Spiration Valve System in Patients with Severe Emphysema: 24-Month Follow-Up of EMPROVE. Ann Am Thorac Soc. 2024 Feb;21(2):251–60.

48. Mohan A, Madan K, Hadda V, Tiwari P, Mittal S, Guleria R, et al. Guidelines for diagnostic flexible bronchoscopy in adults: Joint Indian Chest Society/National College of chest physicians (I)/Indian association for bronchology recommendations. Lung India. 2019 Jul;36(Supplement):S37–89.

49. Yan Q, Sheng B, Huang X, Lin K, Lin J, Ye X. Effect of different doses of midazolam combined with fentanyl during painless bronchoscopy in adults. Am J Transl Res. 2023 Jan 15;15(1): 563–72.

50. Mohan A, Madan K, Hadda V, Mittal S, Suri T, Shekh I, et al. Guidelines for endobronchial ultrasound-transbronchial needle aspiration (EBUS-TBNA): Joint Indian Chest Society (ICS)/Indian Association for Bronchology (IAB) recommendations. Lung India. 2023;40(4):368–400.

51. Roberts ME, Rahman NM, Maskell NA, Bibby AC, Blyth KG, Corcoran JP, et al. British Thoracic Society Guideline for pleural disease. Thorax. 2023 Jul;78(Suppl 3):s1–42.

52. Kedia Y, Madan M, Kaushik R, Kumar R, Mahendran AJ, Ish P, et al. Thoracoscopic blood patch instillation for persistent air leak in pneumothorax: a case series and systematic review. Monaldi Arch Chest Dis. 2024 Apr 5.

53. Criner GJ, Delage A, Voelker K, Hogarth DK, Majid A, Zgoda M, et al. Improving Lung Function in Severe Heterogenous Emphysema with the Spiration Valve System (EMPROVE). A Multicenter, Open-Label Randomized Controlled Clinical Trial. Am J Respir Crit Care Med. 2019 Dec 1;200(11):1354–62.

CHAPTER

19 Pulmonary Physiological Tests

Author: Dr. Shweta Bansal

Reviewer: Dr. Rahul Roshan

INTRODUCTION

Pulmonary function tests are the physiological tests that help to evaluate dyspnoea, diagnose various lung diseases, and monitor progression of disease and response to particular treatment e.g., inhaled corticosteroids in asthma and antifibrotics in various progressive fibrosing interstitial lung disease (PFILDs). These, however, do not provide specific diagnosis and should be interpreted in the background of relevant clinical history, physical examination, and chest radiology.

Methodology and Discussion

In the PubMed search using the terms: "pulmonary function test" OR "spirometry" OR "lung function test", 4164 articles were found. However, there has been no relevant randomized controlled trial (RCT) or meta-analysis in the last 3 years pertaining particularly to PFT. Recent ERS/ATS guidelines were updated in 2022 which focussed on strategies for how to interpret PFTs for routine lung functions and relevant changes have been made.[1] The guideline mainly focussed on:

- Reference equations and limits of normal of the healthy population to identify those with unexpectedly low or high values.
- Interpretation strategies or bronchodilator responsiveness testing.
- Interpretation of measurements made by spirometry, lung volumes, and gas transfer and providing updated classification and protocols for common patterns of lung impairments.

Few important changes have been made and few differences between the American Thoracic Society (ATS) and European Respiratory Society (ERS) 2005 and 2021 interpretation standards are as follows.[2,3]

1. Selection of reference values for pulmonary function tests

Predicted values of pulmonary function depend upon the patient's age, sex, height, and ethnicity. The latest ERS/ATS guidelines recommend **the use of Global Lung Function Initiative (GLI) reference equations for spirometry, lung volumes, and diffusing capacity**. These reference values should be used to define healthy individuals' expected range of values.

Previously, 2005 ATS/ERS guidelines for lung functions recommended the use of the National Health and Nutrition Examination Survey (NHANES) III spirometry reference equations. They derived separate equations for Mexican Americans and Caucasians, and no specific equations were recommended for the European population.[2]

In 2021, ERS released official technical standards on Global Lung Function Initiative reference values for static lung volumes [total lung capacity (TLC), functional residual capacity (FRC), residual volume (RV), inspiratory capacity, vital capacity, expiratory reserve volume, and RV/TLC] in individuals of European ancestry between the age of 5 and 80 years.[3]

For the diffusion capacity of lungs for carbon monoxide (DLCO) also, GLI Reference equations have been recommended which are derived from the Caucasian population.[4]

A further modification was done in the latest ATS/ERS 2023 official statement on race and ethnicity in pulmonary function test interpretation in which GLI Global, is the recommended race-neutral average reference equation. It is an alternative equation derived as a weighted average of available GLI data from European, African American, North East

Asian, and South East Asian racial/ethnic groups. It can be applied universally and has wider limits of normal than the previous ones.[5]

So, the emphasis is on following the reference equations provided by the Global Lung Function Initiative (GLI) which is one of the most important advancements of the recent document. The main aim was to avoid uncertainties in reference values due to older subjects, the transition from adolescence to adult age, and ethnic differences especially for spirometry.[6]

2. *Upper and Lower Limits of Normality*

The 5th and 95th percentile limits of the healthy population, i.e. lower limit of normality (LLN) and upper limit of normality (ULN) should be used to identify individuals with unusually low or high results respectively. The 5th percentile means only 5% of the healthy population will have a result below the lower limits of normality (LLN).

Global Initiative for Chronic Obstructive Lung Disease (GOLD) and the ATS/ERS guidelines on COPD recommended a fixed FEV1/FVC value of 0.7 to define an obstructive ventilatory impairment.[7] However, the latest guidelines strongly discourage its use as it tends to under-diagnose younger individuals and over-diagnose older individuals with airflow obstruction. The use of LLN reduces this misclassification. For LLN, the 5th percentile and for ULN, the 95th percentile is used.

Another important change has been the introduction of the 'Z-score'. Z-scores provide an estimate of the uncertainty in ruling disease in or out disease and express how much an observed lung function value deviates from the predicted value after taking into account age, sex, height, and genetics.[6] It is expressed in standard deviations. **Z-score is used to grade the severity of lung function impairment for all the measures. As the 5th percentile occurs at 1.65 standard deviations below the mean, it corresponds to a 'Z-score' of -1.65. It is considered abnormal if the Z-score is lower than -1.65.**

3. *Changes in FEV1 and FVC following Bronchodilator Responsiveness (BDR) Testing*

This parameter should be expressed as the percent change relative to the individual's predicted value as it helps to minimize sex and height differences in the assessment of bronchodilator response. **In the recent update, a change $\geq$10% of the predicted value of FEV_1 or FVC indicates a positive response. The previous guidelines recommended a positive response as an increase in the FEV_1 or FVC of more than 12 percent and greater than 0.2 L.**[1] However, GINA 2024 continues to use the older cut-offs for BDR.

4. *Interpretation of PFT Reproducibility*

Two approaches have been recommended: Conditional change scores for children and FEV1Q for adults. FEV1Q is defined as FEV1 divided by the sex-specific 1st percentile values of the absolute FEV1 values found in adults with lung disease (0.4 L for women and 0.5 L for men).

5. To recognize the different patterns and physiology found in lung diseases, the recommendation is to focus on values of airflow, lung volumes, and gas transfer measurements which help in the proper interpretation of PFT values.

Interpretation of normal values

Few common patterns are as:

1. **Obstructive impairment:** FEV1/FVC (or VC) below the LLN (defined as the 5th percentile of a normal population).

   It contrasts with the widely used definitions suggested by the Global Initiative for Chronic Obstructive Lung Disease and the ATS/ERS guidelines on COPD, which use a fixed FEV1/FVC value of 0.7 to define an obstructive ventilator impairment.[8,9]

   - Thus, a Fixed FEV1/FVC value of 0.7 is not recommended.
   - Use of LLN reduces this misclassification.
   - Cut-offs of 80% of predicted for FEV1 (% predicted=observed×100/predicted) to define normal is also not recommended

Guading of obstruction severity

	ATS 2005[2]	GOLD Guidelines[7]	ATS/ERS 2022[1]
Normal			Z-scores > -1.65
Mild	> 70 %	≥ 80%	Between -1.65 and -2.5
Moderate	60%-69%	≥ 50% and < 80%	Between -2.51 and -4
Moderately severe	50%-59%	NA	
Severe	35%-49%	≥ 30% and < 50%	<-4.1
Very severe	< 35%	< 30%	
FEV1/FVC cutoff	Below the LLN	< 70%	Not recommended

2. **Restrictive impairment:** Reduction in TLC below the LLN. When FVC is reduced, FEV1/FVC is normal or increased, restrictive impairment may be suspected, however, confirmation is by reduced TLC below LLN. New terminologies suggested are:
   - **Simple restriction:** FEV1, FVC, and TLC are typically reduced in roughly the same proportion.
   - **Complex restriction:** It refers to a reduction in FVC that is out of proportion to the reduction in TLC, with normal FEV1/FVC e.g., obesity, neuromuscular disease, chest wall restriction, or small airway disease with gas trapping.

     The three-level system used for obstructive impairment is used to assess the severity of lung function impairment (Z-scores > -1.645 are normal, Z-scores between -1.65 and -2.5 are mild, Z-scores between -2.51 and -4 are moderate, and Z-scores < -4.1 are severe).
   - When Z-scores are not available, the percentage of predicted normal values may be an alternative.

3. **Low FEV1/FVC ratio with normal range FEV1:** Such a pattern can be explained by "dysanaptic" or unequal growth of the airways and lung parenchyma and may be a normal physiological variant. This pattern may have the propensity to develop obstructive lung disease.

4. **Non-specific pattern (NSP):** Defined as reduced FVC and/or FEV1, normal FEV1/FVC and normal TLC.
   - If the patient fails to inhale or exhale completely, it may falsely lead to reduced FEV1 and FVC. Flow–volume curve may appear concave downward towards the end of the maneuver in this scenario and may be helpful to differentiate poor effort and glottis closure.
   - **It has been found that about a third of patients with NSP tend to develop restrictive or obstructive patterns later, during a 3-year follow-up.**
   - NSP may indicate an early restrictive pattern which may be confirmed by performing TLC.
   - In an individual who has sustained maximal effort, and has NSP, it is recommended to repeat spirometry after treatment with an inhaled bronchodilator. Significant improvement in FEV1, FVC, or both suggests the presence of some degree of bronchial responsiveness.
   - **Preserved ratio impaired spirometry (PRISM):** Individuals with FEV1/FVC ≥ 0.7 after bronchodilation but FEV1 < 80% of reference, after bronchodilation.[7] **This phenotype may be associated with a normal or obstructive pattern of spirometry on follow-up and needs careful monitoring.**

5. **Mixed ventilatory impairment:** Presence of both obstruction and restriction and is defined when both FEV1/FVC and TLC are below the LLN.
   - This pattern can be due to poor effort, a restrictive ventilatory impairment or early small airway disease with air trapping and/or emphysema. Measurement of a low TLC is necessary to confirm restriction.
   - Compare FVC to slow vital capacity (SVC). If SVC is significantly larger than FVC (>100 mL), it may suggest airway collapse occurring due to the forced exhalation.
   - Air trapping is indicated when the RV or RV/TLC is increased (>ULN); hyperinflation is indicated when the FRC and/or TLC are increased (>ULN). Thus, in the setting of COPD with obstruction on spirometry and a low vital capacity, measurement of lung volumes can help determine if there is a superimposed restrictive disorder or if VC is decreased due to air trapping or hyperinflation.

6. Gas transfer impairments defined by DLco

- All interpretations must have reference values adjusted for hemoglobin content.
- DLco=KCO × VA.
  KCO (the measured carbon monoxide concentration changes over time).
  VA (the volume of gas containing carbon monoxide measured by the dilution of an inert tracer gas in the inspired volume)
- Grading of severity done as follows.

	Preferred (latest) grading[1]	**ATS/ERS 2005 grading**[2]
Abnormally high	Z-score > -1.645	
Normal	Z-scores between -1.645 and 1.645	
Mild	Z-scores between -1.65 and -2.5	DLco % pred > 60% and < LLN
Moderate	Z-scores between -2.51 and -4.0	DLco % pred 40-60%
Severe	Z-scores <-4.0	DLco % pred < 40%

Summary of differences between the American Thoracic Society (ATS) and European Respiratory Society (ERS) 2005 and 2021 interpretation standards[1,3]

	2005 recommended strategy	**2021/2022 recommended strategy**
Aim of PFT	Assist in making clinical diagnosis	Classify physiology rather making a clinical diagnosis
Reference equations	Use of race/ethnic-specific equations preferred overusing adjustment factors	Global Lung Function Initiative (GLI) average equation is a recommended race neutral average reference equation–biological sex, not gender be used to interpret lung function
Normal range	General use of LLN=5th percentile	• Use of fixed ratio FEV1/FVC < 0.7 not recommended as in GOLD • General use of LLN=5th percentile and ULN=95th percentile recommended
Bronchodilator response	Increase of ⩾12% and 200 mL in FEV1 and/or FVC from baseline • 4 doses of 100 μg salbutamol and to wait 15 min	> 10% of predicted value in FEV1 or FVC • Choice of protocol for administering broncho-dilator not specified
	• **Using FEV1 (includes obstruction or restriction):** *Mild:* FEV1 > 70% predicted *Moderate:* 60–69% predicted *Moderate-to-severe:* 50–59% predicted *Severe:* 35–49% predicted *Very severe:* <35% predicted • **DLCO:** *Mild:* > 60% predicted and < LLN *Moderate:* 40–60% predicted *Severe:* < 40% predicted	• **Use of Z-score for all the measures:** *Mild:* −1.65 to −2.5 *Moderate:* −2.51 to −4.0 *Severe:* <−4.1
Categories of pattern	Airflow Obstruction, Restrictive pattern and mixed	Airflow Obstruction, and newer terms – dysanapsis; non-specific pattern and PRISm, Simple versus complex restriction, Mixed pattern

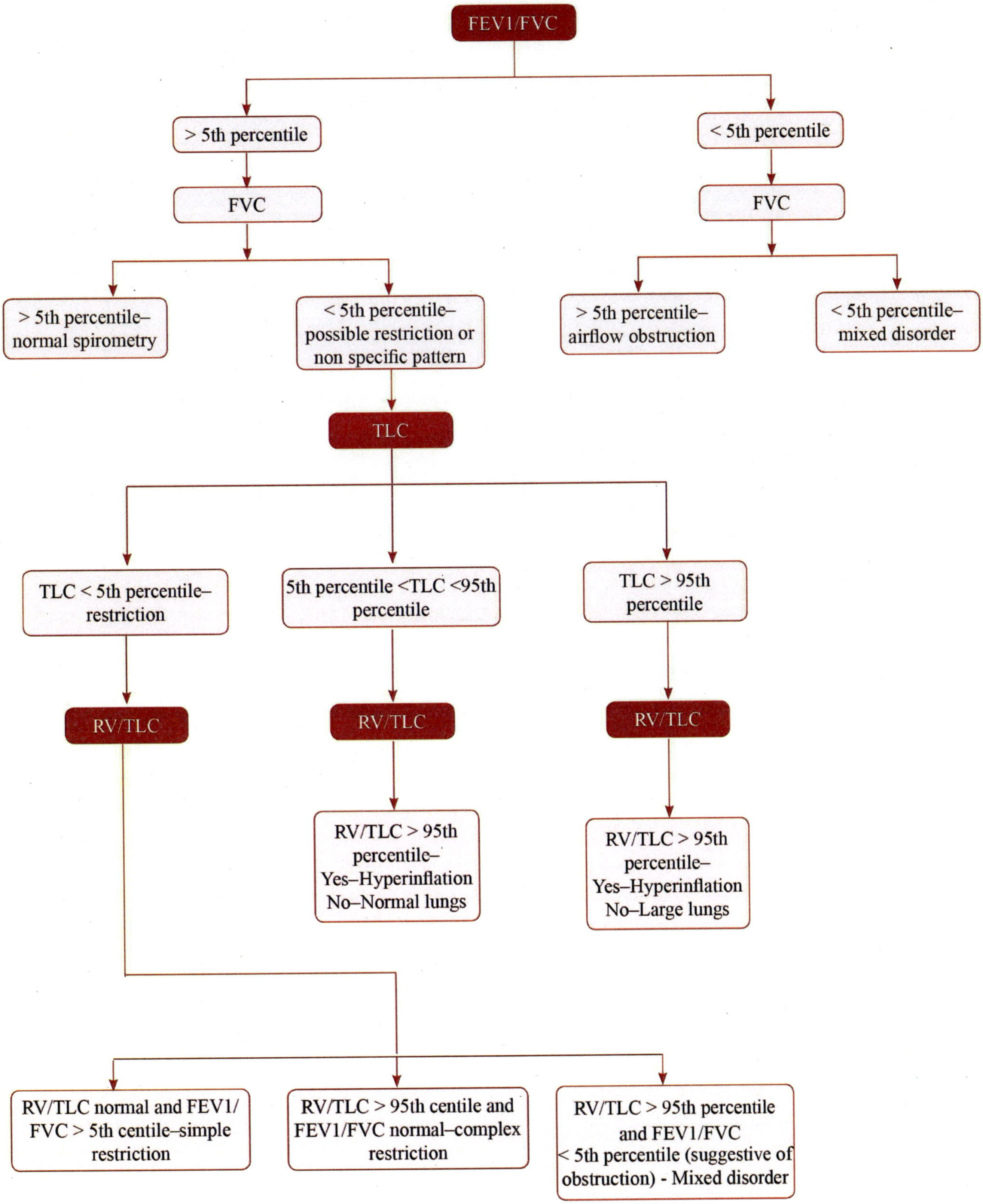

Flowchart 1: Interpretation of Pulmonary Function Tests[1]

- ***FEV1/FVC Severity Stages for Chronic Obstructive Pulmonary Disease. (AJRCCM. 2023)***[10]
  - o *Population:* Current and former smokers aged 45–80 years. (n=12,149)
  - o *Intervention:* Patients underwent pre and post-bronchodilator spirometry. The new severity classification (STAR) was derived using approximately the 25th, 50th, and 75th percentiles of FEV1/FVC ratios of the participants with FEV1/FVC ratio less than 0.70. FEV1/FVC values of >0.60 to 0.70, >0.50 to 0.60, >0.40 to 0.50, and less than 0.40 respectively were divided into 4 stages respectively.
  - o *Outcome:* Between GOLD and the new FEV1/FVC ratio severity stages, the agreement was found to be 0.89. The new STAR classification provided significant discrimination between the absence of airflow obstruction and stage 1 for all-cause mortality, respiratory quality of life, dyspnea, airway wall thickness, exacerbations, and lung function decline. There were no major differences for emphysema, small airway disease, and 6-minute walk distance, and identified more patients with stage 3/4 disease.
  - o *Conclusion:* The Staging of Airflow obstruction using the Ratio (STAR) classification scheme may help to differentiate patients' symptoms, burden of the disease, and prognosis better than the present classification which is based on the percent predicted FEV1. Moreover, the new classification is less sensitive to race/ethnicity and other demographic characteristics. Further studies may be needed for the validation.

IMPULSE OSCILLOMETERY (IOS)

INTRODUCTION

Though spirometry is the gold standard for demonstrating various physiological parameters of different lung diseases, it has its limitations. Younger patients, especially pediatric age groups less than 5 years of age, elderly patients, and patients with neuromuscular diseases are not able to generate adequate forced expiration. Thus, spirometry may not be useful in such patients. In about 28% of patients who are able to do the test properly, the diagnosis is either missed or over diagnosed. It may not reliably diagnose peripheral airway and parenchymal diseases.[11] In such cases, IOS may be a useful tool. Also called the Forced Oscillation Technique, it is a much simpler technique, is non-invasive, easy to perform, requires only tidal breathing, and thus is an effort-independent technique to assess lung functions. It can help to differentiate between the degree of central and peripheral airway obstruction.[12]

Differences[11,12]

	Spirometry	**IOS**
Principle	Measure flow rates and lung volumes	Sound waves (IOS) are pushed into the lungs as pressure waves to measure respiratory resistance and reactance[12]
Breathing maneuver	**Forced expiration and maneuver required**	**Normal tidal breathing**
Age	Children > 7 years	> 2 years
Patient cooperation	**Needed**	**Very less**
Peripheral airway obstruction	Less sensitive	More sensitive
Aerosol generation	More	Very minimal
Main parameters measured	FVC, FEV1, FEV1/FVC	R5, R20, X5
Reference values	Present	Need more studies

Terminology

Impedance (Z): Impedance measured at any frequency is the ratio of the difference in pressure and changes in the flow at that frequency. Pressure difference at the mouth and in the alveoli gives information about the impedance of the airways while the difference at the mouth and pleural pressures give the total impedance of the lung.[13] So in IOS, the pressure is first measured at the mouth which is compared to the pressure outside the chest wall, that is, atmospheric pressure. This is called respiratory system impedance (Zrs). It includes the real in-phase component which is known as the resistive component and an imaginary out-of-phase component which is called the reactive component.

Resistance (R) includes resistance due to central airways, peripheral airways, lung tissue, and chest wall. **In adults, central airways contribute to 80% of the airway resistance, and the rest 20% is by small airways (defined as <2 mm in diameter). Resistance (R) values are considered normal within the range of 150% of predicted values.** Resistance is independent of the frequency in healthy subjects. In central airway obstruction, the resistance at all frequencies increases, while, in small airway obstruction, the resistance at lower frequencies increases but is unchanged at higher frequencies that do not reach the small airways. R5 and R20 are resistance values at 5 Hz and 20 Hz frequencies.

Reactance (X): Reactance includes two components, the inertia of the air column to move (inertance) and the capacitance of the lung. Capacitance can be interpreted as a property that reflects the elasticity of the lung. The capacitance component of the reactance is defined to be negative in sign and inertance is defined as positive.

Reactance is frequency dependent. Xf, for example, is measured at 5 Hz, X5 is reactance at 5 Hz.

In either fibrosis or emphysema or small airway disease, the reaction at lower frequencies would change in the same direction, i.e., become even more negative. Hence, the direction of change of reactance does not differentiate between obstructive or restrictive diseases.[13]

Resonant frequency (Fres): It is the arbitrary frequency number at which capacitive and inertial forces equalize and reactance becomes zero.[11]

Reactance area (Ax): It is the triangular area limited by Fres (on the right side) and reactance at 5 Hz (on the left side).[11]

Coherence: To determine the quality of the test and validate the results. It reflects the reproducibility of the impedance measurements. **It is a value between 0 and 1 and, ideally, should be >0.8 at 5 Hz and >0.9 at 20 Hz for the measurement to be considered valid.**

Interpretation.[11]

- Total, central, and small airway resistances are represented as R5, R20, and R5–R20.
- *In peripheral airway obstruction, R5 will increase with normal R 20.*
- *In larger airway obstruction, both R5 and R 20 will rise with normal R5–R20.*
- *There will not be any change in any of these in restrictive lung diseases.*
- *Reactance (X) is more negative in both peripheral airway obstruction and lung parenchymal disease and is not affected by large airway obstruction.*
- Resonant frequency (Fres): It increases in both restrictive and peripheral airway obstructive diseases, and is not affected by central airway obstruction.
- Reactance area (Ax): It increases in both small airway obstruction and restrictive diseases and is not affected by central airway disorders.
- **Decrease in R5 by 40% is considered as a positive bronchodilator response.**

RECENT UPDATE

Methodology

PubMed search of key words "impulse oscillometry" OR "forced oscillatory impedance". 191 results were found – one metanalysis and one technical standard guideline update has been published in last 3 years.

Analysis of literature and Discussion

Meta analysis in children in 2021 by Ling et al was published to determine the usefulness of IOS in predicting acute asthma attacks in children.[14]

- ***The predictive value of impulse oscillometry for asthma exacerbations in childhood: A systematic review and meta analyses. (Pediatric Pulmonology. 2021)***[14]
  - o *Population*: Participants were children (≤14 years old) with asthma exacerbations or poorly controlled asthma, which was diagnosed according to the Global Initiative for Asthma or relevant guidelines from 6 trials. (n=615)
  - o *Intervention*: Common IOS parameters were measured and analyzed.
  - o *Outcome*:
    - – Elevated R5 levels may indicate the risk of asthma exacerbations (weighted mean difference [WMD] = -1.21, 95% CI: -1.55 to –0.87, p < .001).
    - – R20 (WMD = -0.81, 95% CI: -1.95 to 0.32, p = .161) and R5 20 (WMD = -0.68, 95% CI: -1.61 to 0.25, p = .151) did not show a good correlation with the acute attack of asthma.
    - – X5 (WMD = 0.81, 95% CI: 0.56 to 1.01, p < .001), Fres (WMD = -1.34, 95% CI: -2.03 to -0.65, p = .018) and AX (WMD = -7.35, 95% CI: -9.94 to -4.76, p < .001) were also significantly related to the loss of asthma control.
  - o *Conclusion:* R5, AX, Fres, and X5 had significant correlation with asthma exacerbations while R20 and R5-R20 could not. However, the data is heterogenous. The severity of asthma exacerbations, baseline patient characteristics (race, age, sex, and height) and treatments given varied considerably among the studies, so more RCTs needed to confirm the potential relationship between the two.

An update of the 2003 European Respiratory Society (ERS) technical standards document on IOS was published in 2020.[15]

Main differences between current and previous European Respiratory Society technical standards for oscillometry.

- The ideal forcing frequency when applied to spontaneous breathing is ≥4 Hz (changed from ≥2 Hz).
- *Coherence* :
  - o New guidelines recommend not using the coherence function for quality control, rather using Coefficient of variation (CoV%) – CoV ≤10% in adults and ≤15% in children for 2 sets of R5
- 2003 guidelines did not define bronchodilator responsiveness by oscillometry. The recent recommended thresholds for both children and adults are –40% in Rrs5, +50% in Xrs5 and –80% in AX. For future definition of a significant response, Z-scores are recommended.
- Apart from these, there have been a few changes in manufacturer instructions, which have been modified to report device accuracy for measuring test loads.

- It has been recommended to perform oscillometry before tests which require a deep breath, e.g., spirometry, exhaled nitric oxide. Whenever IOS report is prepared, the order of tests and period of withholding deep breaths should be mentioned.
- Changes have been made in the modern analysis tools to allow the removal of entire breaths that are affected by artifacts to obtain a technically acceptable acquisition.

LITERATURE FROM 2023-24

- ***Impulse Oscillometry as an Alternative Lung Function Test for Hospitalized Adults. (Respiratory Care. 2024)***[16]
  - o *Population*: Sixty-one subjects hospitalized either with unexplained dyspnea or for pre-surgery evaluation.
  - o *Intervention*: All subjects underwent PFTs and IOS test.
  - o *Outcome:* The study found a good correlation between IOS results and PFT values. The resonant frequency was an independent predictor and had the best predictive ability for abnormal FEV1/FVC (area under the ROC curve 0.732 [95% CI 0.57–0.90], optimal cutoff 17 Hz, 87% sensitivity, 62% a good predictive ability for abnormal FEV1/FVC (area under the ROC curve 0.716 and 0.730, respectively).
  - o *Conclusion:* In hospitalized patients, who are quite dysneic to perform PFT or in non-cooperative patients, IOS might serve as an alternative to standard PFTs.

- ***Impulse oscillometry and its independent role in the diagnosis of chronic obstructive pulmonary disease. (Heliyon. 2024)***[17]
  - o *Population:* Retrospective study of 115 patients.
  - o *Intervention*: All subjects underwent PFTs and IOS test.
  - o *Outcome*: A capital of area under reactance (AX) and airway resistance (predicted R5% × resonant frequency) in relation to body mass index (BMI) were found to be the best parameters assessed for diagnosis of COPD based on spirometry. BMI-adjusted airway resistance had an area under the curve (0.782; 95 % confidence interval: 0.620–0.945) value that was larger than the corresponding AX when the post-BD FEV1/FVC ratio was <0.6.
  - o *Conclusion:* BMI-adjusted airway resistance value of >160 moderately predicted spirometry-based COPD diagnosis.

Integrating oscillometry with spirometry in guidelines can improve the detection of uncontrolled asthma, anticipate future exacerbations, and aid in identifying potential targeted treatments. Peripheral airway impairment has been shown to correlate significantly with poor asthma control. It is a strong predictor of asthma exacerbation, even more so than spirometry. Notably, this impairment can also occur in a substantial number of patients who are deemed well-controlled according to guidelines.

Thus, IOS is a useful tool for the diagnosis and evaluation of pediatric and adult patients with asthma and other obstructive lung diseases. It is also useful in uncooperative patients, and may also help to predict exacerbations in young children. It should be interpreted carefully considering clinical features and the existing guidelines.

UPDATE IN FRACTIONAL EXHALED NITRIC OXIDE (FENO)

Introduction

Diagnosis of asthma can be a real challenge in day-to-day practice. It is essentially a clinical diagnosis; however, sometimes clinical symptoms are not sufficient to make the diagnosis and spirometry is often normal. As bronchial asthma is pathophysiologically characterized by both Th1 and Th2 inflammation due to exposure to different allergens, tobacco smoke or pollution, infections, exercise, exposure to cold air, etc., direct measurement of inflammation may be useful for the diagnosis.[18]

There has been a paradigm shift in the management of asthma in recent years with more emphasis being given to identifying the different phenotypes driven by different endotypes. The early recognition of the phenotypes is mainly based on the family history, atopy, presence of nasal polyps, lung functions, sputum, and blood eosinophils levels. Identifying these phenotypes, including type 2 and non–type 2 asthma allows a better understanding of disease mechanisms and the personalization of treatment and prescribing the targeted therapy like biologicals. [19] Biomarkers including FENO, blood and sputum eosinophils, and serum IgE are now widely used tests to identify type 2 inflammation.

Fractional exhaled nitric oxide (FENO) is a point-of-care test for measuring nitric oxide in an exhaled sample of a patient's breath. In atopic asthma, eosinophilic inflammation leads to upregulation of inducible nitric oxide synthase (iNOS) expression due to an increase in Th2 mediated cytokines (IL- 4 and IL- 13) increasing nitric oxide (NO) production.[20] **Measuring the fraction of NO during a steady-state exhalation is a standardized and quantitative method and helps in identifying type 2 asthma.** The sample is collected by having the patient breathe slowly and steadily into a mouthpiece that is attached to a machine. Even children as young as 5 years of age can perform this test adequately.[21]

FENO is a noninvasive, easy-to-perform tool and it may be useful for both asthma diagnosis and management.[18] FENO can help to predict and monitor the patient's response to inhaled steroids as well as to optimize their dose for asthma control. Recently, ample data has emerged regarding its role in predicting and monitoring the treatment with biological drugs as well. [22]

FENO levels increase with acute exacerbations and decrease with treatment not only in asthma, but there have been a few case reports and evidence of its utility in COPD, cystic fibrosis, Sjögren's syndrome, and a few other lung diseases. [23]

The last full guidelines regarding the interpretation of FENO for clinical applications were published in 2011.[24] The cut-off values for FENO in the guidelines is as follows and also summarized in Flowchart 2.

- *Low FENO of less than 25 ppb in adults and 20 ppb in children indicate that eosinophilic inflammation and response to corticosteroids is less likely (Strong recommendation, moderate quality of evidence).*
- *FENO greater than 50 ppb in adults and >35 ppb in children indicates eosinophilic inflammation and, suggests likely responsiveness to corticosteroids in symptomatic patients (Strong recommendation, moderate quality of evidence).*
- *FENO values between 25 ppb and 50 ppb in adults and between 20–35 ppb in children should be interpreted cautiously in the context of clinical background. (Strong recommendation, low quality of evidence).*
- *Significant increase in FENO is defined as greater than 20% for values over 50 ppb or more than 10 ppb for values lower than 50 ppb from one visit to the next (weak recommendation, low quality of evidence).*
- *Reduction of at least 20% in FENO for values over 50 ppb or more than 10 ppb for values lower than 50 ppb as the cut point to indicate a significant response to anti-inflammatory therapy (weak recommendation, low quality of evidence).*

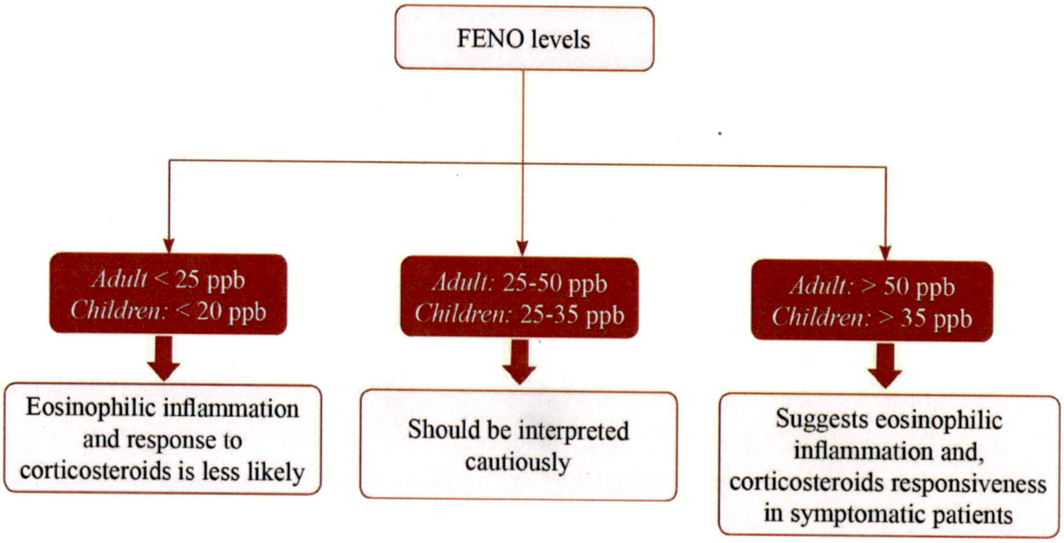

Flowchart 2: Interpretation of FENO Levels

Analysis of Literature and Discussion

There has been a recent update to the previous guidelines on FENO by ATS in 2021.[21]

- *Question:* Patients with asthma in whom treatment is being considered, whether they should undergo FENO testing or not
- *Comparator*: FENO-based care compared with usual care.
- *Outcomes assessed:* Asthma control as assessed by using any validated questionnaire, the use of oral corticosteroids, the acute asthma exacerbation rate, the frequency of emergency room/urgent care visits, and the frequency of asthma-related hospitalizations
- *Conclusion*: FENO can be used in addition to usual care rather than usual care alone (conditional recommendation).
- *Critical appraisal:* The guideline did not recommend any speciûc cut points for initiating or escalating the dose of an ICS.

Thus, the role of FENO in the diagnosis of asthma and predicting its response to ICS is well established, however, a recent systematic analysis was published by Pianigiani et al in 2023 which looked into the published data in the following areas regarding the utility of FENO with respect to various biologicals.[25]

- ***Exploring the Interaction between Fractional Exhaled Nitric Oxide and Biologic Treatment in Severe Asthma: A Systematic Review. (Antioxidants. 2023)***[25]
  - *Population:* Severe Asthma patients from 58 studies were included in the metanalysis.
  - *Intervention:* Use of FENO as a biomarker.
  - *Outcomes Assessed:*

    1. Use of FENO as a predictive biomarker of response to biological treatment.
    2. Influence of biologic treatment in FENO values.
    3. FENO as a Predictor of Exacerbations and/or Biomarker of Asthma Control in Patients Treated with Biologic Drugs.
  - *Outcome 1*: Use of FENO as a predictive biomarker of response to biological treatment.
  - *Conclusions:*

    (i) The evidence concluded that the FENO measurement is a predictor of response to omalizumab treatment and can be used to predict its response before initiating the therapy. Though there are no specific cut-off confounding factors such as the use of systemic or inhaled steroids may contribute to alter the FENO results.

    (ii) FENO levels do not provide an added benefit in predicting response to anti-IL5 drugs as FENO values are strictly related to the IL-4 and -13 pathways and much less to IL-5 expression.

    (iii) It has a role in predicting a good response to dupilumab in severe asthmatic patients as dupilumab inhibits both IL-4 and -13 pathways, Therefore, FENO can be used to identify patients with severe type 2-asthma who will benefit from dupilumab treatment.

This evidence is supported by the study published in NEJM – the phase 3 LIBERTY ASTHMA QUEST study, in which the maximum benefits from dupilumab treatment in terms of annual rate of severe asthma exacerbations were observed in patients with higher FENO ($\geq$25 to <50 parts per billion [ppb] or $\geq$50 ppb) than among those with a lower value (<25 ppb).[26]

- *Outcome 2:* Influence of biological treatment in FENO values.

- *Conclusions:*
  - (i) Conflicting data in omalizumab and overall influence on FENO remains unclear
  - (ii) Data showed a reduction trend of FENO levels after mepolizumab or benralizumab treatment.

    Real-world data from a recent metanalysis of 21 studies has been published in 2022.[27] It included 7 studies that examined the effect of mepolizumab on FENO and concluded moderate-quality evidence for a reduction in FENO after treatment with mepolizumab. 3 trials examined the effect of benralizumab on FENO indicating no significant change in FENO after treatment with benralizumab (low-quality evidence).
  - (iii) Dupilumab reduces FENO levels in patients with severe asthma, and this effect appeared to be quick and sustained throughout the treatment period. A recent systematic review and meta-analysis published by Zaazouee et al in 2022 included 13 trials and 4482 patients showed the drug significantly reduced the FENO levels at 12th and 24th week which was sustained up to 52 weeks as compared to the placebo.[28]
- *Outcome 3:* FENO as a predictor of exacerbations and/or biomarker of asthma control in patients treated with biologic drugs
- *Conclusions:* Higher baseline values of FENO are associated with a greater benefit in terms of reduction of exacerbation rate and improvement of clinical control, especially for omalizumab and dupilumab.
  - (i) In a multicentric study that investigated the long-term effectiveness of omalizumab by Ledford et al[29] reported that in subjects in whom omalizumab was withdrawn, a rise in FENO at week 12 was still predictive of an increased risk of exacerbation. However, in patients who continued to be treated with anti-IgE treatment, FENO levels remained relatively stable and, in case of any exacerbation, the rise of FENO levels was negligible or smaller than the patients in whom omalizumab was withheld. According to this study, measurement of FENO levels may be helpful in the management of severe asthmatic patients and in predicting exacerbations who are on omalizumab.
  - (ii) FENO is not useful for predicting exacerbations in patients who are being treated with mepolizumab and benralizumab
  - (iii) No studies are available for this topic in dupilumab.

- ***Effectiveness of FENO-guided treatment in adult asthma patients: A systematic review and meta-analysis. (Clinical & Experimental Allergy. 2023)*** [30]
  - *Population:* Adult asthma patients from 12 RCTs (n=2,116 patients).
  - *Intervention:* Comparing FENO-guided treatment and usual (symptom-guided) treatment in adult asthma patients.
  - *Outcome:* FENO-guided treatment of bronchial asthma reduced the number of patients having $\geq$1 exacerbation and the rate of exacerbation (moderate certainty), however the difference is not clinically significant. No effect was found on severe exacerbations, quality of life, FEV1 and treatment dosage.
  - *Conclusion:* The treatment of asthma guided by FENO measurement may lead to a decrease in the number of exacerbations but has no effects on other outcomes.

The role of FENO in COVID-19 patients

Till 2022, the COVID-19 pandemic caused by severe acute respiratory syndrome coronavirus 2 (SARS and CoV-2) has been the most important health problem in the world.[22] Since infection with this virus has been postulated to be associated with the dysregulated immune response of the inflammatory system, the role of NO as a potential marker for predicting the severity of the infection and post-COVID sequel was proposed. In the PubMed search for keywords: FENO, COVID-19, exhaled nitric oxide and COVID, coronavirus, and FENO- 24 studies were found. There has been no meta-analysis, systematic review, or RCT. Important observational studies have been tabulated below. However, the results of the studies are mixed and still, it is inconclusive regarding the potential role of NO in COVID patients, and larger studies are required to conclude.

Summary of studies published on FENO and COVID

Author/year	Type of study	Study subjects	Results and conclusions
Betancor D *et al.*[31]	Retrospective observational	82 COVID patients (25 mild, 26 mod, 31 severe)	No significant differences in FENO values according to disease severity or atopy history, 29 hospitalized had significant decrease in FENO, however all received systemic steroids
Kerget Burga *et al.* 2022[23]	Observational study	106 COVID and 40 control Moderate COVID-19 (group 1) Severe COVID-19 without macrophage activation syndrome (MAS) (group 2) Severe COVID-19 with MAS (group 3)	FENO levels were higher in Groups 2 and 3 than in the control group ($p = 0.001$) during the admission FENO level at discharge were higher in group 3 than in group 2 *Conclusion:* FENO may be useful for evaluating for parenchymal infiltration in the diagnosis and follow-up of COVID-19 patients
Cameli P *et al.* 2021[32]	Prospective observational study	20 patients hospitalized for COVID-19 22 healthy controls	Post-COVID-19 patients showed significantly higher FENO 350 mL/s, no difference after stratification according to age > 65 years, COVID-19 severity, need for oxygen supplementation or mechanical ventilation, ICU, use of steroids and/or remdesivir and/or interleukin-6 inhibitors
Lior *et al.* 2022[33]	Single-center prospective cohort study	56 COVID patients–Severe outcome patients n = 14 (group 1), Discharge patients = 42 (group 2)	FENO lower in group 1 ($P = .008$) Time to severe outcome among patients with FENO measurements ≤ 11.8 PPB was significantly shorter compared with patients whose FENO measured >11.8 PPB An admission FENO ≤ 11.8 PPB was a significant risk factor for severe outcomes
Maniscalcom *et al.* 2022[34]	Prospective study	68 post-COVID patients	FENO value in post-COVID-19 patients was not statistically significant as compared to healthy control-concluded FENO not useful as a biomarker in post-COVID-19 patient
Balci A *et al.* 2021[35]	Retrospective study	102 COVID patients	FENO value was significantly higher in COVID-19 patients as compared to control, 31.73 ± 14.80 mmol/lt and 15.48 ± 6.64 mmol/lt respectively

REFERENCES

1. Stanojevic S, Kaminsky DA, Miller MR, Thompson B, Aliverti A, Barjaktarevic I, et al. ERS/ATS technical standard on interpretive strategies for routine lung function tests. Eur Respir J 2022; 60(1): 2101499.
2. Pellegrino R. Interpretative strategies for lung function tests. Eur Respir J. 2005; 26(5): 948–68.
3. Hall GL, Filipow N, Ruppel G, Okitika T, Thompson B, Kirkby J, et al. Official ERS technical standard: Global Lung Function Initiative reference values for static lung volumes in individuals of European ancestry. Eur Respir J. 2021; 57(3): 2000289.
4. Stanojevic S, Graham BL, Cooper BG, Thompson BR, Carter KW, Francis RW, et al. Official ERS technical standards: Global Lung Function Initiative reference values for the carbon monoxide transfer factor for Caucasians. Eur Respir J. 2017; 50(3): 1700010.
5. Bhakta NR, Bime C, Kaminsky DA, McCormack MC, Thakur N, Stanojevic S, et al. Race and Ethnicity in Pulmonary Function Test Interpretation: An Official American Thoracic Society Statement. Am J Respir Crit Care Med. 2023; 207(8): 978-995.
6. Brusasco V, Pellegrino R. Pulmonary function interpretative strategies: from statistics to clinical practice. Eur Respir J. 2022; 60(1): 2200317.
7. Agustí A, Celli BR, Criner GJ, Halpin D, Anzueto A, Barnes P, et al. Global Initiative for Chronic Obstructive Lung Disease 2023 Report: GOLD Executive Summary. Eur Respir J. 2023; 61(4): 2300239.
8. Singh D, Agusti A, Anzueto A, Barnes PJ, Bourbeau J, Celli BR, et al. Global Strategy for the Diagnosis, Management, and Prevention of Chronic Obstructive Lung Disease: the GOLD science committee report 2019. Eur Respir J. 2019; 53(5): 1900164.
9. Qaseem A, Wilt TJ, Weinberger SE, Hanania NA, Criner G, van der Molen T, Marciniuk DD, Denberg T, Schünemann H, Wedzicha W, MacDonald R, Shekelle P; American College of Physicians; American College of Chest Physicians; American Thoracic Society; European Respiratory Society. Diagnosis and management of stable chronic obstructive pulmonary disease: a clinical practice guideline update from the American College of Physicians, American College of Chest Physicians, American Thoracic Society, and European Respiratory Society. Ann Intern Med. 2011; 155(3): 179-9.
10. Bhatt SP, Nakhmani A, Fortis S, Strand MJ, Silverman EK, Sciurba FC, et al. FEV1/FVC Severity Stages for Chronic Obstructive Pulmonary Disease. Am J Respir Crit Care Med. 2023; 208(6): 676–84.
11. Gupta N, Sachdev A, Gupta D, Gupta S. Oscillometry – The future of estimating pulmonary functions. Karnataka Paediatr J. 2021; 35(2): 79–87.
12. Brashier B, Salvi S. Measuring lung function using sound waves: Role of the forced oscillation technique and impulse oscillometry system. Breathe 2015; 11: 57–65.
13. Desiraju K, Agrawal A. Impulse oscillometry: The state-of-art for lung function testing. Lung India Off Organ Indian Chest Soc. 2016; 33(4): 410–6.
14. Ling Y, Si M, Niu Y, Han Y, Xu Y. The predictive value of impulse oscillometry for asthma exacerbations in childhood: A systematic review and meta analyses. Pediatr Pulmonol. 2021; 56(7): 1850–6.
15. King GG, Bates J, Berger KI, Calverley P, de Melo PL, Dellacà RL, et al. Technical standards for respiratory oscillometry. Eur Respir J. 2020; 55(2): 1900753.
16. Kleinhendler E, Rosman M, Fireman E, Freund O, Gershman I, Pumin I, et al. Impulse Oscillometry as an Alternative Lung Function Test for Hospitalized Adults. Respir Care. 2024; 69(4): 415-421.
17. Chen KY, Hung MH, Kao KC. Impulse oscillometry and its independent role in the diagnosis of chronic obstructive pulmonary disease. Heliyon. 2024; 10(1): e23627.
18. Heffler E, Carpagnano GE, Favero E, Guida G, Maniscalco M, Motta A, et al. Fractional Exhaled Nitric Oxide (FENO) in the management of asthma: a position paper of the Italian Respiratory Society (SIP/IRS) and Italian Society of Allergy, Asthma and Clinical Immunology (SIAAIC). Multidiscip Respir Med. 2020; 15(1): 36.
19. Loewenthal L, Menzies-Gow A. FENO in Asthma. Semin Respir Crit Care Med. 2022; 43(5): 635–45.
20. Hoggins R, Velpula M, Woodward S, Tighe MP. How to use the fractional exhaled nitric oxide test. Arch Dis Child Educ Pract Ed. 2022; 107(2): 133-140.
21. Khatri SB, Iaccarino JM, Barochia A, Soghier I, Akuthota P, Brady A, et al. Use of Fractional Exhaled Nitric Oxide to Guide the Treatment of Asthma: An Official American Thoracic Society Clinical Practice Guideline. Am J Respir Crit Care Med. 2021; 204(10): e97–109.
22. Escamilla-Gil JM, Fernandez-Nieto M, Acevedo N. Understanding the Cellular Sources of the Fractional Exhaled Nitric Oxide (FENO) and Its Role as a Biomarker of Type 2 Inflammation in Asthma. BioMed Res Int. 2022; 2022: 5753524.
23. Kerget B, Araz Ö, Akgün M. The role of exhaled nitric oxide (FENO) in the evaluation of lung parenchymal involvement in COVID-19 patients. Intern Emerg Med. 2022; 17(7): 1951–8.
24. Dweik RA, Boggs PB, Erzurum SC, Irvin CG, Leigh MW, Lundberg JO, et al. An official ATS clinical practice guideline: interpretation of exhaled nitric oxide levels (FENO) for clinical applications. Am J Respir Crit Care Med. 2011; 184(5): 602–15.
25. Pianigiani T, Alderighi L, Meocci M, Messina M, Perea B, Luzzi S, et al. Exploring the Interaction between Fractional Exhaled Nitric Oxide and Biologic Treatment in Severe Asthma: A Systematic Review. Antioxidants. 2023; 12(2): 400.

26. Castro M, Corren J, Pavord ID, Maspero J, Wenzel S, Rabe KF, et al. Dupilumab Efficacy and Safety in Moderate-to-Severe Uncontrolled Asthma. N Engl J Med. 2018; 378(26): 2486–96.

27. Charles D, Shanley J, Temple SN, Rattu A, Khaleva E, Roberts G. Real-world efficacy of treatment with benralizumab, dupilumab, mepolizumab and reslizumab for severe asthma: A systematic review and meta-analysis. Clin Exp Allergy. 2022; 52(5): 616–27.

28. Zaazouee MS, Alwarraqi AG, Mohammed YA, Badheeb MA, Farhat AM, Eleyan M, et al. Dupilumab efficacy and safety in patients with moderate to severe asthma: A systematic review and meta-analysis. Front Pharmacol. 2022;13: 992731.

29. Ledford D, Busse W, Trzaskoma B, Omachi TA, Rosén K, Chipps BE, et al. A randomized multicenter study evaluating Xolair persistence of response after long-term therapy. J Allergy Clin Immunol. 2017; 140(1): 162-169.e2.

30. Korevaar DA, Damen JA, Heus P, Moen MJ, Spijker R, van Veen IH, et al. Effectiveness of FENO-guided treatment in adult asthma patients: A systematic review and meta-analysis. Clin Exp Allergy. 2023; 53(8): 798–808.

31. Betancor D, Olaguibel J, Sastre J. The Discrepant Role of Fractional Exhaled Nitric Oxide in SARS-CoV-2 Infection. J Investig Allergol Clin Immunol. 2022; 32(5): 417–8.

32. Cameli P, Bargagli E, Bergantini L, d'Alessandro M, Giugno B, Gentili F, et al. Alveolar Nitric Oxide as a Biomarker of COVID-19 Lung Sequelae: A Pivotal Study. Antioxidants. 2021 25; 10(9): 1350.

33. Lior Y, Yatzkan N, Brami I, Yogev Y, Riff R, Hekselman I, et al. Fractional exhaled Nitric Oxide (FENO) level as a predictor of COVID-19 disease severity. Nitric Oxide. 2022; 124: 68–73.

34. Maniscalco M, Ambrosino P, Poto R, Fuschillo S, Poto S, Matera MG, et al. Can FENO be a biomarker in the post-COVID-19 patients monitoring? Respir Med. 2022; 193: 106745.

35. Balcý A, Yýldýz E, Selendýlý O, Günay E. A predictive and prognostic marker in COVID-19 patients: Exhaled nitric oxide (FENO). Acta Medica Mediterr. 2021; 841–6.

CHAPTER

20 Drugs and Machines

Authors: Dr. Sreyas Sharma, Dr. Nitesh Gupta, Dr. Sumita Agrawal

INTRODUCTION

The rapid advances in medical research are instrumental in helping to better understand and unravel the complex pathogenesis of diseases, develop new diagnostic modalities, and explore newer prospective treatment pathways, helping provide better patient care and improving medical outcomes. Each year, new drugs and medical devices are approved because of continuous ongoing research efforts. This chapter will focus on the latest medicines and medical devices approved by the US-FDA/ European Medicines Agency (EMA) in 2023-2024.

NEW DRUGS APPROVED FROM MARCH 2023 TO AUGUST 2024 [In Chronological Order]

1. **REZAFUNGIN:** It is a **semi-synthetic echinocandin** indicated in patients 18 years of age or older for **treating candidemia and invasive candidiasis.** It acts by **inhibiting the 1,3-β-D-glucan synthase enzyme complex, which is present in fungal cell walls but not in mammalian cells.** This results in concentration-dependent in vitro fungicidal activity against Candida spp. It received US-FDA approval in March 2023 based on the results of the **ReSTORE trial.**[1] This trial was a multicentre, double-blind, double-dummy, randomized phase 3 trial done at 66 tertiary care centres in 15 countries. Adults (≥18 years) with systemic signs and mycological confirmation of candidemia or invasive candidiasis were randomly assigned (1:1) to receive intravenous rezafungin once a week (400 mg in week 1, followed by 200 mg weekly for a total of two to four doses) or intravenous caspofungin (70 mg loading dose on day 1, followed by 50 mg daily) for no more than 4 weeks. **Rezafungin was found to be non-inferior to caspofungin** for the primary endpoints of global cure (consisting of clinical cure, radiological cure, and mycological eradication) at day 14 and 30-day all-cause mortality. There were no concerning trends in treatment-emergent or serious adverse events. The most common adverse reactions (incidence ≥5%) are hypokalemia, pyrexia, diarrhea, anemia, vomiting, nausea, hypomagnesemia, abdominal pain, constipation, and hypophosphatemia. **It has not yet received DCGI approval in India.**

2. **SULBACTAM-DURLOBACTAM:** It is a **novel β-lactam-β-lactamase inhibitor indicated** in patients 18 years of age and older for the **treatment of hospital-acquired bacterial pneumonia and ventilator-associated bacterial pneumonia (HABP/VABP), caused by susceptible isolates of Acinetobacter baumannii-calcoaceticus complex.** It received US-FDA approval in May 2023 based on the results of phase 3, a pathogen-specific, multicentre randomized controlled **ATTACK trial.**[2] This trial compared the efficacy and safety of sulbactam–durlobactam versus colistin, both in combination with imipenem–cilastatin as background therapy. The primary efficacy endpoint was 28-day all-cause mortality. The primary safety endpoint was the incidence of nephrotoxicity. Results showed that **sulbactam–durlobactam was non-**

inferior to colistin, both agents given in combination with imipenem–cilastatin, for the primary endpoint of 28-day all-cause mortality. Hence, the authors concluded that sulbactam–durlobactam was well tolerated and could effectively reduce mortality from serious infections caused by carbapenem-resistant ABC, including multidrug-resistant strains. The most common adverse reactions (incidence > 10%) were liver test abnormalities, diarrhea, anemia, and hypokalemia. **It has not yet received DCGI approval in India.**

3. **PAXLOVID: It includes nirmatrelvir, a severe acute respiratory syndrome coronavirus 2 (SARS-CoV-2) main protease (Mpro: also referred to as 3CLpro or nsp5 protease) inhibitor, and ritonavir, an HIV-1 protease inhibitor and CYP3A inhibitor, is indicated for the treatment of mild-to-moderate coronavirus disease 2019 (COVID-19)** in adults who are at high risk for progression to severe COVID-19, including hospitalization or death. It received US FDA approval in May 2023 based on the results of Phase 2/3, a randomized, double-blind, placebo-controlled **EPIC-HR trial.**[3] This trial assessed the efficacy and safety of paxlovid. 2246 adults were randomly assigned to receive paxlovid or placebo every 12 hours for 5 days. The primary outcome was the incidence of COVID-19-related hospitalization or death from any cause by day 28 in patients. **Treatment of symptomatic COVID-19 with nirmatrelvir plus ritonavir resulted in a risk of progression to severe COVID-19 that was 89% lower than the risk with placebo, without evident safety concerns.** It is not approved as pre-exposure or post-exposure prophylaxis to prevent COVID-19. Dysgeusia and diarrhea were the most frequent adverse effects. **It has not yet received DCGI approval in India.**

4. **GEFAPIXANT:** It is an **oral P2X3 receptor antagonist indicated for the management of refractory chronic cough and unexplained chronic cough.** It received EMA approval in September 2023 based on the results of double-blind, randomized, parallel-group, placebo-controlled, phase 3 trials [COUGH-1 (N=732) and COUGH-2 (N=1317)].[4] These trials enrolled participants who were 18 years or older with a diagnosis of refractory chronic cough or unexplained chronic cough of 1-year duration or more along with cough severity visual analog scale score of 40 mm or more at screening and baseline. Participants were randomly allocated (1:1:1) to one of three treatment groups: placebo, gefapixant 15 mg twice daily, or gefapixant 45 mg twice daily. Participants were treated over a 12 weeks main study period in COUGH-1 and a 24 weeks main study period in COUGH-2, followed by extension periods for up to 52 weeks of treatment in both trials. The primary outcome was a placebo-adjusted mean change in 24-hour cough frequency at 12 weeks in COUGH-1 and 24 weeks in COUGH-2. Gefapixant 45 mg twice daily showed significant reductions in 24-hour cough frequency compared with placebo at week 12 in COUGH-1 (p=0·041) and at week 24 in COUGH-2 (p=0·031). **Gefapixant 15 mg twice daily did not significantly reduce cough frequency compared to placebo in both studies. The most commonly reported adverse events were taste disturbances. It has not yet received US-FDA and DCGI approval.**

☞

5. **REPOTRECTINIB:** It is a tyrosine kinase inhibitor indicated for treating adult patients with **locally advanced or metastatic ROS1-positive non-small cell lung cancer (NSCLC)**. It received US FDA approval in November 2023 based on the results of a multicentre, single-arm, open-label, multi-cohort clinical trial **(TRIDENT-1 trial).**[5] This trial was conducted at 152 sites in the United States and outside. There were 154 patients treated in the United States and 290 treated outside the United States. TRIDENT-1 trial evaluated the efficacy and safety of repotrectinib. Patients with symptomatic brain metastases were excluded from this trial. The major efficacy outcome measures were overall response rate (ORR) and duration of response (DOR) according to Response Evaluation Criteria in Solid Tumors, version 1.1. (RECIST v1.1). Response occurred in 56 of the 71 patients (79%) with *ROS1* fusion-positive NSCLC who had not previously received a ROS1 TKI; the median duration of response was 34.1 months, and the median progression-free survival was 35.7 months. Response occurred in 21 of the 56 patients (38%) with *ROS1* fusion-positive NSCLC who had previously received one ROS1 TKI and had never received chemotherapy; the median duration of response was

14.8 months, and median progression-free survival was 9.0 months. Ten of the 17 patients (59%) with the *ROS1* G2032R mutation had a response. The recommended dosage is 160 mg orally once daily for 14 days, then increase to 160 mg twice daily, with or without food. The most common treatment-related adverse events were dizziness (in 58% of the patients), dysgeusia (in 50%), paresthesia (in 30%), and 3% discontinued repotrectinib owing to treatment-related adverse events. **It has not yet received DCGI approval in India.**

6. **SOTATERCEPT-CSRK:** It is an **activin signaling inhibitor indicated for treating adults with pulmonary arterial hypertension (PAH, WHO Group 1) to increase exercise capacity, improve WHO functional class (FC), and reduce the risk of clinical worsening events.** It received US- FDA approval in March 2024 based on the results of a multicentre, double-blind, phase 3 trial (**STELLAR Trial**).[6] This trial enrolled adults with pulmonary arterial hypertension (World Health Organization [WHO] functional class II or III) who were receiving stable background therapy were randomly assigned in a 1:1 ratio to receive subcutaneous sotatercept (starting dose, 0.3 mg per kilogram of body weight; target dose, 0.7 mg per kilogram) or placebo every 3 weeks. The primary endpoint was the change from baseline at week 24 in the 6-minute walk distance. Nine secondary endpoints, tested hierarchically in the following order, were multi-component improvement, change in pulmonary vascular resistance, change in N-terminal pro-B-type natriuretic peptide level, improvement in WHO functional class, time to death or clinical worsening, French risk score, and changes in the Pulmonary Arterial Hypertension-Symptoms and Impact (PAH-SYMPACT) Physical Impacts, Cardiopulmonary Symptoms, and Cognitive/Emotional Impacts domain scores; all were assessed at week 24 except time to death or clinical worsening, which was assessed when the last patient completed the week 24 visit. 163 patients were assigned to receive sotatercept and 160 to receive placebo. The median change from baseline at week 24 in the 6-minute walk distance was 34.4 m in the sotatercept group and 1.0 m in the placebo group. The Hodges-Lehmann estimate of the difference between the sotatercept and placebo groups in the change from baseline at week 24 in the 6-minute walk distance was 40.8 m ($P<0.001$). The first eight secondary endpoints significantly improved with sotatercept compared with placebo, whereas the PAH-SYMPACT Cognitive/Emotional Impacts domain score was not. **The recommended starting dose is 0.3 mg/kg by subcutaneous injection, and the target dose is 0.7 mg/kg every 3 weeks. The most common adverse reactions were headache, epistaxis, rash, telangiectasia, diarrhea, dizziness, and erythema. It has not yet received DCGI approval in India.**

7. **CEFTOBIPROLE MEDOCARIL SODIUM:** It is a **cephalosporin antibacterial, indicated in adult and pediatric patients (3 months and above) with community-acquired bacterial pneumonia (CABP).** It received US-FDA approval in April 2024 based on the results of the randomized, controlled, double-blind, multinational, multicentre study (NCT00326287).[7,8] Seven hundred and six patients with CAP severe enough to require hospitalization were randomized to ceftobiprole or an expert-recommended course of ceftriaxone ± linezolid (comparator group). Clinical and microbiological outcomes were determined 7-14 days after completion of therapy. For the 469 clinically evaluable patients, cure rates were 86.6% vs. 87.4% for ceftobiprole and comparator, respectively [95% confidence interval (CI) of the difference, -6.9% to 5.3%]; in the intention-to-treat (ITT) analysis of 638 CAP patients, these cure rates were 76.4% vs. 79.3%, respectively (95% CI of the difference, -9.3% to 3.6%). A typical bacterial pathogen was identified in 29% of the ITT population. Microbiological eradication rates in the 144 microbiologically evaluable patients were 88.2% and 90.8% for the respective treatment groups (95% CI of the difference, -12.6% to 7.5%). Both study drugs were well tolerated, with a minority of patients requiring premature discontinuation due to an adverse event (6% in the ceftobiprole group and 4% in the comparator group). The overall incidence of treatment-related adverse events was higher in the ceftobiprole group, primarily owing to differences in rates of self-limited nausea (7% vs. 2%) and vomiting (5% vs. 2%). In summary, **ceftobiprole was non-inferior to the comparator (ceftriaxone ± linezolid) in all clinical and microbiological analyses conducted, suggesting that ceftobiprole has a potential role in treating hospitalized**

patients with CAP. The 30-day all-cause mortality rates in the ITT population were 5/314 (1.6%) for patients treated with ZEVTERA and 8/324 (2.5%) for patients treated with ceftriaxone ± linezolid group. The most common adverse reactions were nausea, hepatic enzyme derangement, vomiting, diarrhea, headache, rash, insomnia, abdominal pain, phlebitis, hypertension, and dizziness. **It has not yet received DCGI approval in India.**

8. **TARLATAMAB-DLLE:** It is a **bispecific T-cell engager that binds to DLL3 expressed on the surface of cells,** including tumor cells, and CD3 expressed on the surface of T-cells. It causes T-cell activation, release of inflammatory cytokines, and lysis of DLL3-expressing cells. It is indicated for the **treatment of adult patients with extensive stage small cell lung cancer (ES-SCLC) with disease progression on or after platinum-based chemotherapy.** It received US-FDA approval in May 2024 based on the results of an open-label, multicentre, multi-cohort clinical trial [NCT05060016].[9] This phase 2 trial evaluated the antitumor activity and safety of tarlatamab, administered intravenously every 2 weeks at a dose of 10 mg or 100 mg, in patients with previously treated small-cell lung cancer. The primary endpoint was objective response (complete or partial response), as assessed by a blinded independent central review according to the RECIST v1.1. Tarlatamab, administered at a 10-mg dose every 2 weeks, showed antitumor activity with durable objective responses and promising survival outcomes in patients with previously treated small-cell lung cancer. The most common adverse events were cytokine-release syndrome (in 51% of the patients in the 10-mg group and in 61% of those in the 100-mg group), decreased appetite (in 29% and 44%, respectively), and pyrexia (in 35% and 33%). **It has not yet received DCGI approval in India.**

9. **ENSIFENTRINE:** It is a **phosphodiesterase 3 (PDE3) inhibitor and phosphodiesterase 4 (PDE4) inhibitor indicated for the maintenance treatment of chronic obstructive pulmonary disease (COPD) in adult patients.** It received US-FDA approval in June 2024 based on the results of phase III, multicentre, randomized, double-blind, parallel-group, placebo-controlled trials of nebulized ensifentrine, **ENHANCE-1 Trial** [NCT04535986] and **ENHANCE-2 Trial** [NCT04542057].[10] These trials evaluated the efficacy of ensifentrine compared with placebo for lung function, symptoms, quality of life, and exacerbations in patients with COPD. Patients aged 40-80 years with moderate to severe symptomatic COPD were enrolled. **Ensifentrine treatment significantly improved average FEV1 area under the curve at 0-12 hours versus placebo** (ENHANCE-1, 87 ml [95% confidence interval, 55, 119]; ENHANCE-2, 94 ml [65, 124]; both $P < 0.001$) and also **ensifentrine treatment significantly improved symptoms (Evaluating Respiratory Symptoms) and quality of life (St. George's Respiratory Questionnaire) versus placebo** at Week 24 in ENHANCE-1 but not in ENHANCE-2. **Ensifentrine treatment reduced the rate of moderate or severe exacerbations** versus placebo over 24 weeks (ENHANCE-1, rate ratio, 0.64 [0.40, 1.00]; $P = 0.050$; ENHANCE-2, rate ratio, 0.57 [0.38, 0.87]; $P = 0.009$) and **increased time to first exacerbation** (ENHANCE-1, hazard ratio, 0.62 [0.39, 0.97]; $P = 0.038$; ENHANCE-2, hazard ratio, 0.58 [0.38, 0.87]; $P = 0.009$). Adverse event rates were similar to those for placebo. The authors concluded that ensifentrine significantly improved lung function in both trials, with results supporting exacerbation rate and risk reduction in a broad COPD population and in addition to other classes of maintenance therapies. The recommended dosage is 3 mg (one ampule) twice daily, administered by oral inhalation using a standard jet nebulizer with a mouthpiece. **It has not yet received DCGI approval in India.**

10. **LAZERTINIB:** It is a **third-generation tyrosine kinase inhibitor with good central nervous system penetration activity. It is indicated in combination with amivantamab for the first-line treatment of adult patients with locally advanced or metastatic non-small cell lung cancer (NSCLC) with epidermal growth factor receptor (EGFR) exon 19 deletions or exon 21 L858R substitution mutations.** It received US-FDA approval in August 2024 based on the results of a randomized, multicentre, MARIPOSA trial [NCT04487080].[11] This trial enrolled patients with untreated locally advanced or metastatic NSCLC with either exon 19 deletions or exon 21 L858R substitution EGFR

mutations as well as asymptomatic or previously treated patients with stable intracranial metastases. 858 patients were randomized between the two study arms, lazertinib in combination with amivantamab arm (N=429) and osimertinib monotherapy arm (N=429). Randomization was stratified by EGFR mutation type (exon 19 deletion or exon 21 L858R substitution mutation), Asian race (yes or no), and history of brain metastasis (yes or no). The major efficacy outcome measure was progression-free survival (PFS), assessed by a blinded independent central review (BICR). Additional efficacy outcome measures included overall survival (OS), overall response rate (ORR), and duration of response (DOR). **This trial demonstrated a statistically significant improvement in PFS for lazertinib in combination with amivantamab compared to osimertinib. It has not yet received DCGI approval in India.**

NEW MACHINES/ MEDICAL DEVICES AS APPROVED BY US-FDA TILL AUGUST 2024

1. **Inspire Upper Airway Stimulation:** P130008/S089

   Inspire Upper Airway Stimulation (UAS)[12] is used to treat a subset of patients with **moderate to severe obstructive sleep apnea (OSA)** (apnea-hypopnea index [AHI] of $\geq$ 15 and $\leq$ 100). **Inspire UAS is used in adult patients 22 years of age and older who have been confirmed to fail or cannot tolerate positive airway pressure (PAP) treatments (such as continuous positive airway pressure [CPAP] or bi-level positive airway pressure [BPAP] machines) and who do not have a complete concentric collapse at the soft palate level.** Inspire UAS is also indicated for use in patients between the ages of 18 to 21 years with moderate to severe OSA ($15 \leq AHI \leq 100$) and pediatric patients ages 13 to 18 years with Down syndrome and AHI >10 and < 50 who do not have complete concentric collapse at the soft palate level, contraindicated for or not effectively treated by adenotonsillectomy, have been confirmed to fail, or cannot tolerate PAP therapy despite attempts to improve compliance and have followed standard of care in considering all other alternative/adjunct therapies. It received US-FDA approval in March 2023 based on the effectiveness results from the ADHERE registry in patients with 65 <AHI<100 and $32 < BMI \leq 40$, showing consistent results with those of the STAR trial subjects. Patients with $AHI \leq 100$ and $BMI \leq 40$ demonstrated significant reductions in the severity of OSA and improved quality of life. Contraindications for use are (1) Central + mixed apneas > 25% of the total apnea–hypopnea index (AHI), (2) Any anatomical finding that would compromise the performance of upper airway stimulation, such as the presence of complete concentric collapse of the soft palate, (3) Any condition or procedure that has compromised neurological control of the upper airway (4) Patients who are unable or do not have the necessary assistance to operate the sleep remote (5) Patients who are pregnant or plan to become pregnant due lack of safety data, (6) Patients with an implantable device (7) Patients who require magnetic resonance imaging (MRI) other than what is specified in the MR Conditional labeling. The Inspire UAS system consists of implanted components, including the implantable pulse generator (IPG), stimulation lead, and sensing lead, as well as external components such as the physician programmer and the patient remote. Figure 1 depicts the implantable components and their relative positioning. The IPG detects the patient's respiratory effort and maintains airway patency with mild hypoglossal nerve stimulation during inspiration. The physician can configure the stimulation settings using the external physician programmer. The patient sleep remote allows the patient to turn therapy on before they go to sleep and turn it off when they wake up. It also provides the ability to pause therapy and adjust stimulation amplitude within physician-defined limits within the therapeutic range of treatment.

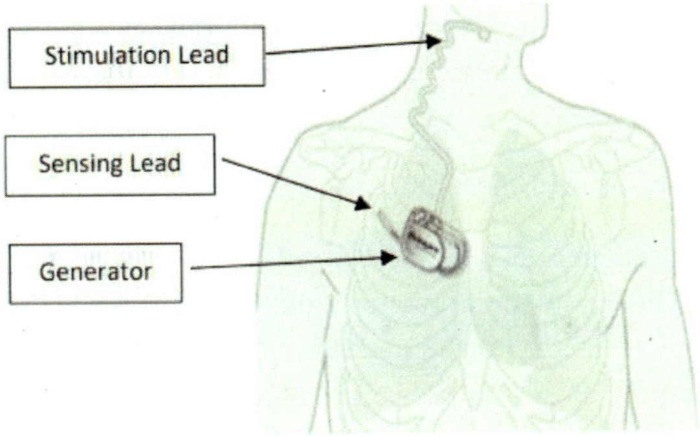

Figure 1: Inspire Upper Airway Stimulation apparatus

2. **NeuRx Diaphragm Pacing System:** P200018

The NeuRx Diaphragm Pacing System (NeuRx DPS)[13, 14] (Figure 2) is an **intramuscular, percutaneous, motor point diaphragm stimulation system. It is intended for use in patients with stable, high spinal cord injuries with resultant loss of diaphragmatic control.** It received US FDA approval in March 2023 for use in patients 18 years or older. The device is indicated to allow the patients to breathe without the assistance of a mechanical ventilator for at least 4 continuous hours a day. The Pivotal Study of the NeuRx DPS system was conducted at 5 investigational sites as a prospective, non-randomized, multicentre study to demonstrate the safety and effectiveness of the NeuRx device utilizing a patient as their control. Patients were implanted between March 2000 and March 2008. The primary effectiveness endpoint was defined as the use of the NeuRx DPS to breathe without the assistance of a mechanical ventilator for at least 4 continuous hours a day. It was reported that 96.2% (51/53) of patients achieved at least 4 continuous hours of daily use compared to the performance goal (PG) of 45% (p value<0.01). In addition, it was found that 58% of subjects achieved at least 24 hours of daily use. The device's intramuscular electrodes are implanted using standard laparoscopic surgical techniques and are connected to a four-channel external pulse generator at a percutaneous exit site. The pulse generator (Figure 3) provides a charge-balanced, biphasic stimulation to each electrode with a common indifferent electrode placed subcutaneously. The pulse generator controls the charge delivered through clinician-programmed parameters of pulse amplitude, pulse duration, pulse frequency, pulse ramp, inspiration time, and respiratory rate. The user connects the device and turns it on for use.

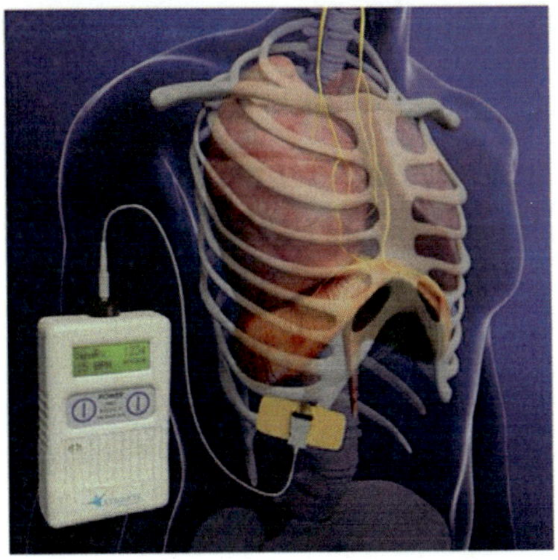

Figure 2: NeuRx Diaphragm Pacing System

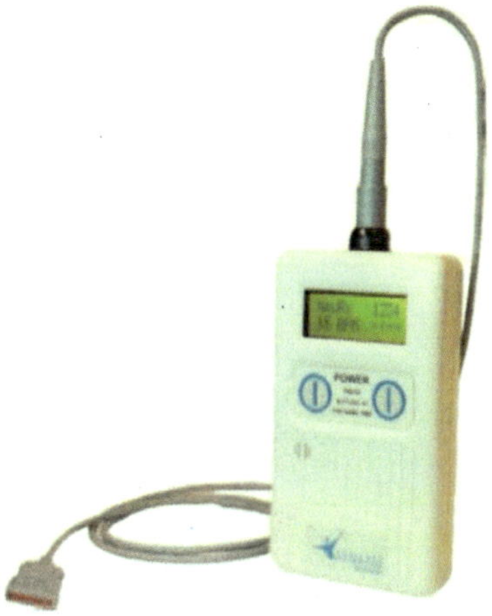

Figure 3: External pulse generator

3. **EVIS-X1 Endoscopy System compatible bronchoscopes**: The EVIS X1 Endoscopy System represents the latest in diagnostic and therapeutic bronchoscopy from Olympus. Designed with high-definition imaging, the two bronchoscopes

offer physicians a slim outer diameter when compared to predecessors, allowing access to more distal airways. Improved suction and flexibility during procedures, combined with the ability to pass a wide array of diagnostic and therapeutic devices through large working channels, provides physicians with options to successfully address the tracheal bronchial tree.

Both the diagnostic and therapeutic versions of the bronchoscopes feature a compact outer diameter and large working channel, as well as redesigned imaging and handling.

- **Large working channel:** The BF-H1100 diagnostic bronchoscope offers a large 2.2mm working channel, which provides an 11% increase in suction capability. The BF-1TH1100 therapeutic bronchoscope offers a 3.0mm working channel that provides a 29% increase in suction and the ability to pass a broad array of endotherapy devices.
- **Slim bronchoscopes:** The BF-H1100 diagnostic bronchoscope (Figure 4) and the BF-1TH1100 therapeutic bronchoscopes have a thin outer diameter compared to their predecessors.
- **Scope handling:** The insertion tube rotation ring on the control section is connected to the insertion tube, allowing the insertion tube to turn without turning the control section. This mechanism reduces hand rotation and may reduce physical stress, providing a comfortable body position during the procedure.
- **Redesigned image sensor:** Both bronchoscopes feature a redesigned image sensor that allows for a small outer diameter while maintaining the HDTV resolution of its predecessors.

The EVIS X1 endoscopy system is Olympus' most advanced endoscopy system, offering a series of imaging technologies, including the CV-1500 video system center, which combines the video processor and an LED light source in one box. The imaging technologies, available with both bronchoscopes, include:

- **Brightness Adjustment Imaging with Maintenance of Contrast (BAI-MAC) technology** is designed to correct the brightness levels in dark areas of the endoscopic image, while maintaining the brightness of lighter areas, to increase the total distance view. BAI-MAC increases the visibility of distal areas.
- **Texture and Color Enhancement Imaging (TXI) technology** is designed to increase the visibility of potentially suspicious lesions and mucosal abnormalities by enhancing image color and texture during endoscopic screening.
- **Red Dichromatic Imaging (RDI) technology** is designed to enhance the visibility of deep blood vessels and bleeding points.
- **Narrow Band Imaging (NBI) technology** continues to be featured in the EVIS X1 endoscopy system. NBI technology enhances visual observation of mucosal and vascular patterns by utilizing specific blue and green wavelengths absorbed by hemoglobin, enhancing visualization of the capillary network and mucosal morphology.

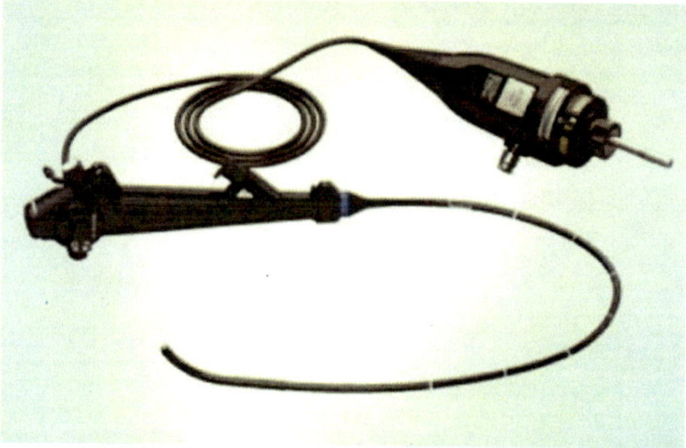

Figure 4: BF-1TH1100-EVIS X1 Video Bronchoscope

Table 1: New Approved Drugs By US-FDA 2023-2024						
S. no.	**Name of Drug and Date of US-FDA Approval**	**Indication**	**Mechanism of Action**	**Dose**	**Evidence for Approval**	**Adverse Effects**
1.	**REZAFUNGIN; 22/03/2023**	**Candidemia and invasive candidiasis**	**Inhibition of 1,3-β-D-glucan synthase enzyme complex**	Intravenous rezafungin once a week (400 mg in week 1, followed by 200 mg weekly, for a total of two to four doses)	**ReSTORE Trial[1]**	Most common adverse reactions are hypokalemia, pyrexia, diarrhea, anemia, vomiting, nausea, hypomagnesemia, abdominal pain, constipation, and hypophosphatemia.
2.	**SULBACTAM, DURLOBACTAM; 23/05/2023**	**Treatment of HAP and VAP due to susceptible isolates of *Acinetobacter baumannii-calcoaceticus complex***	**Novel β-lactam-β-lactamase inhibitor**	(1 gm of sulbactam, 1 gm of durlobactam) every 6 hours by intravenous infusion over 3 hours in patients with creatinine clearance of 45 to 129 mL/min.	**ATTACK Trial[2]**	Most common adverse reactions are liver test abnormalities, diarrhea, anemia, and hypokalemia.
3.	**PAXLOVID; 25/05/2023**	**Treatment of mild-to-moderate COVID-19 in adults at high risk for progression to severe COVID-19**	**Nirmatrelvir, (SARS-CoV-2 nsp5 protease inhibitor) and Ritonavir, (HIV-1 protease inhibitor and CYP3A inhibitor)**	300 mg nirmatrelvir with 100 mg ritonavir taken together twice daily for 5 days.	**EPIC-HR Trial[3]**	Most common adverse effects are dysgeusia and diarrhea
4.	**GEFAPIXANT; 15/09/2023**	**Management of refractory chronic cough or unexplained chronic cough**	**P2X3 receptor antagonist**	45 mg twice per day	**COUGH-1 and COUGH-2 Trials[4]**	Most common adverse effect are dysgeusia, ageusia and hypogeusia
5.	**REPOTRECTINIB; 15/11/2023**	**Adult patients with locally advanced or metastatic ROS1-positive NSCLC**	**Tyrosine kinase inhibitor**	160 mg orally once daily for 14 days, then increase to 160 mg twice daily, with or without food.	**TRIDENT-1 Trial[5]**	Most common adverse reactions are dizziness, dysgeusia, peripheral neuropathy, constipation, dyspnea, ataxia, fatigue, cognitive disorders, and muscular weakness.
6.	**SOTATERCEPT-CSRK; 26/03/2024**	**Pulmonary arterial hypertension (WHO Group-1)**	**Activin signaling inhibitor**	Recommended starting dose is 0.3 mg/kg by subcutaneous injection and recommended target dose is 0.7 mg/kg every 3 weeks by subcutaneous injection.	**STELLAR Trial[6]**	Most common adverse effects were headache, epistaxis, rash, telangiectasia, diarrhea, dizziness, and erythema

Contd.

7.	**CEFTOBIPROLE MEDOCARIL SODIUM; 03/04/2024**	**Community-acquired bacterial pneumonia**	**Inhibition of bacterial cell wall synthesis**	667mg 8 hourly for 5 to 14 days	**NCT00326287**[7,8]	Most common adverse reactions were nausea, hepatic enzyme derangement, vomiting, diarrhea, headache, rash, insomnia, abdominal pain, phlebitis, hypertension, and dizziness.
8.	**TARLATAMAB-DLLE; 16/05/2024**	**Extensive stage small cell lung cancer**	**Bispecific delta-like ligand 3 (DLL3)-directed CD3 T cell engager**	Administer as an intravenous infusion over 1-hour. Step-up dosing schedule is followed starting from 1mg dose and going to 10 mg dose)	**Study DeLLphi-301 [NCT05060016]**[9]	Most common adverse reactions are cytokine release syndrome, fatigue, pyrexia, dysgeusia, decreased appetite, musculoskeletal pain, constipation, anemia and nausea.
9.	**ENSIFENTRINE; 26/06/2024**	**Chronic obstructive pulmonary disease**	**PDE3 and PDE4 inhibitor**	Recommended Dose: 3 mg (one ampule) twice daily administered by oral inhalation using a standard jet nebulizer with a mouthpiece	**(ENHANCE-1 trial [NCT04535986] and ENHANCE-2 Trial [NCT04542057])**[10]	Most common adverse reactions include back pain, hypertension, urinary tract infection, and diarrhea
10.	**LAZERTINIB; ` 19/08/2024**	**Non-small cell lung cancer**	**Tyrosine kinase inhibitor**	Recommended dose is 240 mg orally once daily	**MARIPOSA trial [NCT04487080]**[11]	Most common adverse reactions include rash, nail toxicity, musculoskeletal pain, edema, stomatitis, venous thromboembolism, paresthesia, fatigue, diarrhea, constipation, nausea and ocular toxicity.

CONCLUSION

Several new advances in pharmacotherapy and medical equipment are expected to transform the standard paradigm of the treatment of many diseases and also give the hope of providing better care to patients and achieving desired medical outcomes.

REFERENCES

1. Thompson GR 3rd, Soriano A, Cornely OA, Kullberg BJ, Kollef M, Vazquez J, et al; ReSTORE trial investigators. Rezafungin versus caspofungin for treatment of candidaemia and invasive candidiasis (ReSTORE): a multicentre, double-blind, double-dummy, randomised phase 3 trial. Lancet. 2023 Jan 7;401(10370):49-59.

2. Kaye KS, Shorr AF, Wunderink RG, Du B, Poirier GE, Rana K, et al. Efficacy and safety of sulbactam-durlobactam versus colistin for the treatment of patients with serious infections caused by Acinetobacter baumannii-calcoaceticus complex: a multicentre, randomised, active-controlled, phase 3, non-inferiority clinical trial (ATTACK). Lancet Infect Dis. 2023 Sep; 23(9):1072-1084.

3. Hammond J, Leister-Tebbe H, Gardner A, Abreu P, Bao W, Wisemandle W, et al. EPIC-HR Investigators. Oral Nirmatrelvir for High-Risk, Nonhospitalized Adults with COVID-19. N Engl J Med. 2022 Apr 14;386(15):1397-1408.

4. McGarvey LP, Birring SS, Morice AH, Dicpinigaitis PV, Pavord ID, Schelfhout J et al. Efficacy and safety of gefapixant, a P2X3 receptor antagonist, in refractory chronic cough and unexplained chronic cough (COUGH-1 and COUGH-2): results from two double-blind, randomised, parallel-group, placebo-controlled, phase 3 trials. Lancet. 2022 Mar 5;399(10328):909-923.

5. Drilon A, Camidge DR, Lin JJ, Kim SW, Solomon BJ, Dziadziuszko R, et al. Repotrectinib in *ROS1* Fusion-Positive Non-Small-Cell Lung Cancer. N Engl J Med. 2024 Jan 11;390(2):118-131.

6. Hoeper MM, Badesch DB, Ghofrani HA, Gibbs JSR, Gomberg-Maitland M, McLaughlin VV, et al. Phase 3 Trial of Sotatercept for Treatment of Pulmonary Arterial Hypertension. N Engl J Med. 2023 Apr 20;388(16):1478-1490.

7. Nicholson SC, Welte T, File TM Jr, Strauss RS, Michiels B, Kaul P, et al. A randomised, double-blind trial comparing ceftobiprole medocaril with ceftriaxone with or without linezolid for the treatment of patients with community-acquired pneumonia requiring hospitalisation. Int J Antimicrob Agents. 2012 Mar;39(3):240-6.

8. Welte T, Scheeren TW, Overcash JS, Saulay M, Engelhardt M, Hamed K. Efficacy and safety of ceftobiprole in patients aged 65 years or older: a *post hoc* analysis of three Phase III studies. Future Microbiol. 2021 May;16:543-555. doi: 10.2217/fmb-2021-0042. Epub 2021 May 7.7.

9. Ahn MJ, Cho BC, Felip E, Korantzis I, Ohashi K, Majem M, et al. Tarlatamab for Patients with Previously Treated Small-Cell Lung Cancer. N Engl J Med. 2023 Nov 30;389(22):2063-2075.

10. Anzueto A, Barjaktarevic IZ, Siler TM, Rheault T, Bengtsson T, Rickard K, et al. Ensifentrine, a Novel Phosphodiesterase 3 and 4 Inhibitor for the Treatment of Chronic Obstructive Pulmonary Disease: Randomized, Double-Blind, Placebo-controlled, Multicenter Phase III Trials (the ENHANCE Trials). Am J Respir Crit Care Med. 2023 Aug 15;208(4):406-416.

11. Cho BC, Felip E, Hayashi H, Thomas M, Lu S, Besse B, et al. MARIPOSA: phase 3 study of first-line amivantamab + lazertinib versus osimertinib in EGFR-mutant non-small-cell lung cancer. Future Oncol. 2022 Feb;18(6):639-647.

12. Strollo PJ Jr, Gillespie MB, Soose RJ, Maurer JT, de Vries N, Cornelius J, et al. Upper Airway Stimulation for Obstructive Sleep Apnea: Durability of the Treatment Effect at 18 Months. Sleep. 2015 Oct 1;38(10):1593-8.

13. Kerwin AJ, Yorkgitis BK, Ebler DJ, Madbak FG, Hsu AT and Crandall ML. Use of diaphragm pacing in the management of acute cervical spinal cord injury. J Trauma Acute Care Surg. 2018; 85:928-31.

14. Lammertse D, Charlifue S and Berliner J. Longitudinal follow-up of individuals with implanted diaphragm pacing systems - a multi-center study. Paper presented at: American Spinal Injury Association: 2016 Annual Scientific Meeting; 2016; Philadelphia, PA.